Neville J. Bryant, A.R.T., F.A.C.B.S.

Serological Services Ltd.
Toronto, Ontario, Canada

LABORATORY IMMUNOLOGY & SEROLOGY

Third Edition

W. B. SAUNDERS COMPANY
Harcourt Brace Jovanovich, Inc.
Philadelphia London Toronto Montreal Sydney Tokyo

W. B. SAUNDERS COMPANY
Harcourt Brace Jovanovich, Inc.

The Curtis Center
Independence Square West
Philadelphia, PA 19106

Library of Congress Cataloging in Publication Data

Bryant, Neville J.
    Laboratory immunology and serology / Neville J. Bryant. — 3rd ed.
        p.   cm.
    Includes bibliographical references and index.
    ISBN 0-7216-4212-8
    1. Serology—Technique.   2. Immunodiagnosis.   I. Title.
    [DNLM: 1. Allergy and Immunology—laboratory manuals.
    2. Serology—laboratory manuals.   QW 525 B915L]
    RB46.5.B79   1992
    616.07'95—dc20
    DNLM/DLC   91-46873

Editor: Selma Ozmat

Designer: Nina McDaid Ikeda

Cover Designer: Megan Costello Connell

Production Manager: Peter Faber

Manuscript Editors: Tina Rebane and Cynthia Fairbanks

Illustration Specialist: Cecelia Roberts

Indexer: Mark Coyle

Listed here is the latest translated edition of this book together with the language of the translation and the publisher. 4/25/88, 2nd edition, Japanese, Igaku-Shoin/Saunders Tokyo, Japan.

Laboratory Immunology and Serology   ISBN 0-7216-4212-8

Printed in the United States of America.

Last digit is the print number: 9   8   7   6   5   4   3   2   1

Preface

In preparing the third edition of *Laboratory Immunology and Serology* I have tried to keep in mind that, as a student text, it should be short and to the point, present the student with necessary information to provide a solid foundation in these two sciences, and yet remain unencumbered by the research information that is of little use to the beginner. Of necessity, however, the book has grown, mainly because the discoveries that have been made during the past four or five years called for additional chapters. Realizing that a book of this size may seem like an insurmountable task for the student, I have included a section at the end of each chapter entitled "Just the Facts," which attempts to place important information in point form, allowing rapid review of the chapter when examination time rolls around. This section is not intended as a substitute for the reading of the text itself, and the student is cautioned against this, since important back-up information may be lost in this way.

The format of the text is basically the same as it was in the earlier editions, including learning objectives, review questions, and general references. These should assist the students in knowing what is expected of them, in testing their understanding of the text, and in referring them to additional material that may be required for more advanced study.

It is my hope that this book will prove a useful addition to the student's library, and I would appreciate knowing of any shortcomings or difficulties experienced in using this text. In this way, I can ensure that future editions will be even more useful.

I am grateful for the encouragement and contributions of friends and colleagues during the lengthy preparation of this third edition. Thanks are due especially to Nancy Harrison, my secretary, who is always at my right hand and always willing to do whatever I ask of her. Without her, my life would be considerably more complicated.

Thanks are also due to the people at W. B. Saunders, who are always supportive. Special thanks to Selma Ozmat, my editor, who prodded me gently, yet was always kind and encouraging.

The book now falls into the hands of students and instructors. I can only hope that you will find it useful and that it will fulfill the purpose for which it is intended.

Neville J. Bryant

Contents

1

Introduction: Nonspecific (Natural, Innate) Immunity

OBJECTIVES

The student shall know, understand, and be prepared to explain:

1. A brief history of immunology
2. Types of nonspecific immunity
3. The concepts of susceptibility and nonsusceptibility
4. The role of the epithelial barriers in nonspecific immunity
5. Inflammation, with special emphasis on the vascular and cellular responses
6. Phagocytosis, including the cells involved and encompassing the contributing mechanisms of initiation, chemotaxis, engulfment (opsonization), and digestion (degranulation)
7. The other purposes of phagocytosis
8. The screening test for phagocytic engulfment
9. The concepts of nonspecific immunity with respect to body fluids, including:
   a. "Natural antibody"
   b. Lysozyme
   c. Properdin
   d. Betalysin
   e. The cytokines, interferon, tumor necrosis factor, Interleukin-1, Interleukin-6, the Interleukin-8 family
   f. Complement
   g. Other nonspecific factors
10. The role of the acute phase plasma proteins in nonspecific immunity
11. Other aspects of nonspecific immunity, in particular the effects of age, nutrition, and allergy
12. The general principles of psychoneuroimmunology

Introduction

The science of immunology represents that area of biology that is concerned with the processes by which all living organisms (including human beings) defend themselves against infection (i.e., the study of immunity).

The term *immunity* can be used to imply "resistance" in its broadest sense, including resistance to infectious agents, foreign particles, toxins (poisonous substances), living cells, and cancer.

The principles of immunology stem from almost the earliest written observation of humankind, in which it was noted that individuals who recovered from a certain disease rarely contracted that same disease again. This observation prompted deliberate attempts to induce immunity: In A.D. 1500, the Chinese developed a custom of inhaling crusts from smallpox lesions to prevent the development of smallpox in later life. The procedure was, at best, hazardous. In 1718, the practice of injecting material from crusts or fluids from smallpox blisters (known as "variolation") was used extensively throughout the Eastern world and was introduced into Western medicine by Lady Montagu, the wife of the British ambassador to Turkey, who had her children so treated. By the time the American colonies developed into an independent nation, variolation was a reasonably common practice, and clear evidence had been obtained that it was effective in most cases. The problem that could not be overcome, however, was that the virus used could be transmitted; therefore, protection by variolation was hazardous to the community at large.

In 1798, an English physician, Jenner, published his monumental work on vaccination, describing a related, yet safe, procedure. Realizing that individuals who had had cowpox were spared in smallpox epidemics, he inoculated a boy with pus from an individual who had cowpox and subsequently reinoculated the same boy with infectious pus from a patient in the active state of smallpox. No disease state followed these inoculations, and the experiment was repeated several times with great success. The term *vaccination* (L. *vacca* = cow) was applied to the procedure and referred specifically to the injection of smallpox "vaccine." The term has now come to mean any immunizing procedure in which vaccine is injected.

Jenner's discovery provided the first clear evidence that active immunization could be used safely to prevent an infectious disease, that attenuated (thinned, weakened) viruses could be used for effective active immunization, and that resistance to infection might be related to the speed and intensity of inflammatory reactions. The concept of interference of one virus infection by another was also suggested in Jenner's work.

Almost 70 years later, these discoveries were extended by Pasteur, who showed that heat could kill bacteria, and, from this observation, the term *pasteurization* came into use. In addition, Pasteur recognized and exploited the general principles underlying vaccination through the observation that the inoculation of the causative agents of chicken cholera and anthrax in animals induced immunity against these diseases. Later, he also made the outstanding contribution of vaccination against rabies.

In the two decades before 1900, Elie Metchnikoff, a Russian biologist who was one of the major pioneers of immunology, elucidated the roles of phagocytosis and cellular immunity. Within the same period of time, killed vaccines were introduced, complement (alexin) was described, and the comparative roles of complement and cell lysis were elucidated.

Discoveries in the field of immunology during the twentieth century have been numerous and have profoundly influenced the development of every branch of medicine and surgery. In 1903, White and Douglas demonstrated that acquired immunity resulted from both humoral and cellular elements and described opsonization. As a result of these observations and discoveries, the term *antigen* (antibody + Gr. *gennan* = to produce) came into regular use to describe the agent that conferred immunity on the host by the production of specific antibody.

In 1902, Richet and Portier provided evidence that the immune reaction could be damaging as well as beneficial by showing anaphylaxis to be an immunologic reaction. The following year, the Arthus reaction was described, and, at about the same time, von Pirquet and Schick showed as part of their studies of serum sickness that diseases of the skin, heart, joints, blood vessels, and kidneys, as well as fever, could be caused by the body's immunologic reaction to foreign protein. By 1920 the immunologic basis of certain kinds of allergy had also been reported by Prausnitz and Küstner.

In another direction of inquiry, Paul Ehrlich was the first to use quantitative measurements of immune reactions. Then, in 1928, Alexander Fleming discovered penicillin, and, in 1932, Gerhard Domagk developed Prontosil, which was found to be an effective antibacterial agent against *Streptococcus*. Later, the active ingredient was found to be sulfanilamide, which proved to be active against a wide variety of organisms.

The understanding of immune reactions has been enhanced by the techniques for analysis of these processes, including the precise chemical methods for measurement of antigens and antibodies through precipitin analysis (introduced by Heidelberger, 1924–1926), immunoelectrophoresis (Grabar and Williams, 1953), and so forth.

Studies of immunodeficiency and structure-function relationships in the lymphoid system were initiated as a result of the discovery of hypogammaglobulinemia (Burton, 1952), which eventually led to the dissection of the immune system into two separate areas, known as T- and B-cell systems.

In addition, the studies of Medawar *et al.* (1944, 1945) initiated interest in transplantation and showed that the immunologic processes were clearly involved in allograft rejection of normal organs.

The field of immunology has exploded with new challenges and information over the past ten years, mainly as a result of acquired immunodeficiency syndrome (AIDS) and, to a lesser extent, the discovery of the condition known as Lyme disease. In addition, it has been discovered that the major histocompatibility complex (MHC) is important in the regulation of the immune response during antigen presentation (Schwartz, 1987).

At the present time, in fact, it is safe to say that immunology has an impact on all medical disciplines. Many patients are recognized who have immunologic deficiencies or abnormal immune responses as the sole basis for their disease. Factors such as age, nutrition, and allergy and their effects on the immunologic response have been closely studied in recent times, and it has been recognized that factors such as stress and other emotional events can play a significant role in the overall efficiency of the immune system. It is therefore clear that no other body of knowledge is as important for medical personnel to study and understand as are the fundamentals of the immune process.

NONSPECIFIC IMMUNITY

The primary function of the immune system is to protect the body against invasion by so-called nonself substances (i.e., any and all substances that are considered "foreign"). Such foreign substances include *all* things not recognized by the living organism as belonging to or being part of that organism (i.e., "self"). In a positive sense, immunity serves the organism by providing natural resistance, recovery, and acquired resistance to infectious diseases. On the negative side, immunity may result in the rejection of a life-saving organ transplant.

Two types of immunity are recognized: (1) that which is present at the time of birth or that develops during maturation ("natural") and (2) that which is acquired as a result of prior experience with a foreign substance ("acquired").

Nonspecific (natural or "innate") immunity, therefore, is the process by which all animals (including humans) resist the invasion of foreign or potentially harmful microorganisms by natural means (i.e., without the production of protective antibodies). This type of immunity is present at birth and is activated in the same manner each time the individual is subject to challenge. The mechanisms are nonspecific and include the physical barrier of the skin and mucous membranes, susceptibility and nonsusceptibility, the provision of an unfavorable environment for the infecting organism (e.g., stomach acid, which destroys most ingested organisms), and the flushing away (or capture) of particulate matter that may enter from the air (e.g., tears, urine flow, and the cilia and mucus of the respiratory tract). Innate immunity is also influenced by factors such as age and nutrition and by chemicals that are secreted by the cells (e.g., lysozyme, lactic acid, and saturated fatty acids in skin secretions and mucoprotein and interferon, which acts to prevent viral replication). Other factors that form the overall action of innate immunity include inflammation, complement, phagocytosis, and so forth. Each of these factors will now be discussed in turn.

Susceptibility and Nonsusceptibility

Certain animal species (and certain races of humans) are resistant to particular diseases, whereas other species are highly susceptible to them. This phenomenon is not clearly understood, although there is growing evidence that it is controlled to some extent by hereditary or genetic influences. An example of this would be the Fy^a and Fy^b (Duffy) receptors on the erythrocyte membrane, which are believed to be associated with susceptibility to malaria. Studies by Miller *et al.* (1975, 1976) showed that the red cells of individuals who had not inherited the Fy^a or Fy^b receptors (i.e., individuals of Duffy phenotype Fy(a−b−)) were resistant to invasion *in vitro* with *Plasmodium knowlesi*. Of 17 volunteers exposed to the bites of *Plasmodium vivax*–infected mosquitoes, only those with the red cell phenotype Fy (a−b−) were resistant to erythrocyte infection.

The concepts of susceptibility and nonsusceptibility are not confined to species differences; they are evident among different races of humans and can be affected by age and the influence of hormones.

The Epithelial Barriers

The skin and mucous membranes provide the body with a physical barrier against invasion and, in addition, possess certain active mechanisms for the killing of bacteria and other organisms. This protection is in many ways remarkable, because many epithelial surfaces consist of only a single layer and are exposed to large numbers of bacteria. Complete sterilization of these surfaces by artificial means is impossible except, perhaps, for brief periods of time.

The self-sterilizing power of the skin is achieved by desiccation (drying), epithelial desquamation (shedding), pH, and, most important, the secretion of fatty acids that have antibacterial properties. In addition, the constant renewal of the skin's epithelial cells (which serves to repair breaks) assists this protective function (as does the normal flora [microorganisms] that inhabit the skin [and mucous membranes]) by hindering the penetration of the skin by microorganisms and by assisting in the elimination of those that gain entry into the body.

Body secretions also play an important role in the defense against invading microorganisms. For example, the oil (known as sebum) produced by the sebaceous glands of the skin possesses antimicrobial properties, as does the lactic acid contained in sweat. Mucus in the nose serves to trap microorganisms, which are subsequently expelled by coughing or sneezing. Microorganisms are also prevented from entering the body by ear wax, which protects the auditory canals of the ear, and are expelled from the body by the secretions produced in the process of eliminating waste products (urine and feces). Further protection is afforded by the acidity and alkalinity of fluids in the stomach and intestinal tract as well as by acidity in the vagina. The respiratory tract is protected by the constant motion of the cilia of the tubules.

Mucosal surfaces are protected by a so-called slime layer, which has been shown to possess antibodies to the IgA class (see discussion in Chapter 2) and other antimicrobial and antiviral substances. The bacterial enzyme *lysozyme* is present in abundance in such secretions (e.g., saliva, tears), as well as in the granules of polymorphs and macrophages, and is widely distributed throughout the body fluids. This enzyme is especially effective in lysing certain bacteria (e.g., *Micrococcus lysodeikticus*).

In addition to this, a nonspecific antiviral agent known as *interferon*, which inhibits intracellular viral replication, is itself synthesized by cells in response to viral infection. It is evident that interferon is a major factor in the recovery from (as distinct from the prevention of) viral infections.

Inflammation

Inflammation is the term used to describe the condition into which tissues enter as a reaction to injury—the classic signs of which are pain, heat, redness and swelling, and sometimes a loss of function. The inflammatory process involves the *cellular defenses* of the body, which are among the most efficient and adaptive of all mechanisms available for the resistance to invasion by parasitic microorganisms. In addition, the *vascular response* aids in preventing the invasion of bacterial agents beyond the periphery of the body.

In brief, the inflammatory process is characterized by the vascular response, the cellular responses (including the emigration of neutrophils, followed by the emigration of mononuclear cells), and, finally, cellular proliferation and repair.

The Vascular Response

The primary response in acute inflammation is the localized dilation of the capillaries and venules so that more blood passes to the area of injury. This increased content of blood is termed *hyperemia* and is the reason why the inflamed area appears red. As a result of this, plasma leaks from the vessels, making the blood more viscoid; the lubricating action of the plasmatic zone is impaired and the stream of blood slows down or, in the case of severe injury, may cease completely (referred to as *stasis*). At the same time, the endothelial cells become swollen, and the spaces between adjacent cells become widened, thereby permitting plasma and cells to pass between them.

The most characteristic feature of acute inflammation is the formation of an exudate that has both a fluid and a cellular component. The fluid exudate is formed as a result of increased vascular permeability, which allows the plasma proteins to leak through the vessel wall, causing the osmotic pressure effect of the plasma proteins to be lost. In addition, there is an alteration in the "ground substance," which becomes more fluid, thus allowing the exudate to diffuse into the surrounding tissues more readily, preventing an immediate rise in tissue tension. Although it is normal for the tissues to drive fluid back into the venules, tissue tension does eventually increase, thus limiting the amount of exudate formed and causing pain.

The fluid exudate has almost the same composition as plasma, and it contains antibacterial substances (e.g., complement) as well as specific antibodies. Drugs and antibiotics, if present in the plasma, also appear in the exudate.

In addition to these effects, the fluid exudate serves to dilute any irritating chemicals and bacterial toxins that might be present. The fibrinogen that is in the exudate is converted to fibrin by the action of tissue thromboplastins, and a fibrin clot is formed. This fibrin forms a fine network of fibers, which provides a union between severed tissues, acts as a barrier against bacterial invasion, and aids phagocytosis (discussed later in this chapter).

The Cellular Response

The defense of the body against disease states is the basic function of the leukocytic (white cell) system. Many *types* of white cells exist, and each type is known to have a special function in this defense mechanism, acting both independently and in cooperation with each other.

The leukocytes, all of which play a minor or major role in the inflammatory response, can be conveniently divided into three general categories, as follows:

1. Granulocytes. These cells have a role in phagocytosis and in hypersensitivity reactions (see further discussion, below). On the basis of morphology, they can be further divided into neutrophils (which are actively phagocytic for microorganisms and other foreign material, and whose active aerobic glycolysis is responsible for the formation of lactic acid, which causes pain), eosinophils (considered to be the a homeostatic regulator of inflammation: this means that they attempt to suppress the inflammatory reaction so as to suppress the spread of the infection), and basophils (see further discussion, below).
2. Monocytes-macrophages. These are the primary phagocytic cells (see *Phagocytosis*, below).
3. Lymphocytes-plasma cells. These cells are responsible for the recognition of foreign antigen and the production of antibody (see Chapter 2). Lymphocytes are particularly found during the healing process, although in certain instances (e.g., viral infections, acute dermatitis), they are the predominant cells in the early stages of inflammation.

The cellular response in inflammation begins when the white cells move into the plasmatic zone at the site of injury and stick to the altered vessel wall. At first, this adhesion is brief, after which the cells either roll gently along the endothelial lining or get swept back into the blood stream. Later, however, the cells adhere more firmly and line the endothelium, forming masses that may even block the lumen (known as *pavementation of the endothelium*). These adhering white cells will eventually push pseudopodia between adjacent endothelial cells, penetrate the basement membrane, and emerge on the external surface of the vessel (known as *emigration of the white cells*). The gap that is left by the emigrating white cells soon closes behind them, although sometimes a few red cells escape at the same time. These red cells that appear in the tissues apparently have been passively forced through the gaps in damaged epithelium. It is the hemoglobin breakdown products that result in the purple, then green, and finally yellow color of the bruise.

A characteristic feature of the cellular exudate is that in the initial stages of development, neutrophil polymorphonuclear leukocytes (commonly called PMNs, polys, or polymorphs) predominate, but as time goes by, these are replaced by monocytes (probably due to the faster migration and limited life span of polymorphs, which die off, leaving the long-lived mononuclear cells to replace them). The emigration of significant numbers of neutrophils into the inflamed area is dependent upon chemotactic factors. In the case of immune complexes being involved in initiating the inflammation, PMNs are attracted by the chemotactic factors released during complement activation (C5a). The neutrophil granules, when released from the PMNs arriving first on the scene, are chemotactic for other PMNs. Certain bacterial products are also chemotactic for neutrophils. The amount of chemotactic factor present in the inflamed area determines the intensity and duration of the neutrophil emigration, which may last 24 to 48 hours.

Neutrophils participate in the inflammatory process in many ways:

1. They are actively phagocytic for microorganisms and other foreign material.
2. Their lysosomes contain a number of biologically active macromolecules.
3. The active aerobic glycolysis of PMNs is responsible for the formation of large amounts of lactic acid found in the inflamed tissues (which causes pain).

When a large number of neutrophils are attracted to the site of injury, this also stimulates the accumulation of fibroblasts and the proliferation and synthesis of collagen. This may result in the formation of a "walled-off" abscess, which may require drainage before healing can occur (Bach and Good, 1980).

The emigration of mononuclear cells begins about 4 hours after the initial stimulus and may reach a peak (after a *single* injury) at 16 to 24 hours. The few monocytes that are found in the early stages of inflammation are stimulated either directly by phagocytosis of debris or indirectly by products of polymorphonuclear leukocyte phagocytosis and degranulation to produce monokines

(e.g., interleukin-1 [IL-1]) (Oppenheim *et al.*, 1987). IL-1 was first known as lymphocyte-activating factor. It is also released from neutrophils, epithelial cells, fibroblasts, and other cell types. It is associated with many of the manifestations of inflammatory reactions (e.g., fever, elevation of acute phase proteins, and infiltration of inflammatory sites by leukocytes). It therefore attracts and activates other monocytes-microphages into the inflamed area. IL-1 can also stimulate T lymphocytes to produce interleukin-2 (IL-2), which, in turn, enhances the proliferation of T lymphocytes.

The final stages of the inflammatory process include resolution and repair (Bach and Good, 1980). Within 18 hours (and with a peak at 48 to 72 hours), fibroblast proliferation begins. These fibroblasts produce acidic mucopolysaccharides during proliferation, which may neutralize the effects of some of the chemical mediators that are still being released by damaged mast cells and basophils. At the end of the inflammatory process, there may be three possible effects:

1. The affected area may be completely repaired with total restoration of function.
2. The injury may lead to the formation of an abscess with at least some loss of function.
3. A granuloma (a tightly packed pocket of inflammatory cells that die and degenerate from the center out) may be formed. This is a typical end result of delayed hypersensitivity of cell-mediated immunity.

The function of the cellular exudate is to enact the process known as *phagocytosis.*

PHAGOCYTOSIS

The action of the phagocytes is one of the most remarkable and fascinating of all body defense mechanisms. Early descriptions of the phenomenon are attributed to Elie Metchnikoff (1907), a Russian-born biologist, who recognized that specialized phagocytic (eating) cells provide a defense mechanism against invasion by engulfing foreign particulate matter, which they then attempt to destroy enzymatically. Metchnikoff observed that the process is a very general one and can be observed in animals of all stages of evolution.

Cells of the Phagocytic System

The main function of polymorphonuclear leukocytes (PMNs) is phagocytosis. This is achieved by the external wall of the PMN, which adheres to and completely surrounds the offending bacterium or other particle (see further discussion, below). In addition, monocytes, which accumulate in the area of acute inflammation, are highly phagocytic.

The mononuclear-phagocyte system (originally known as the "reticuloendothelial system") is made up of the macrophage and its precursors, including promonocytes and their precursors in the bone marrow, monocytes in the circulating blood, and macrophages in tissues. All of these cells have a common origin, common functions, and similar morphology. The cells originate in the bone marrow from the multipotential stem cell, which can differentiate into either the granulocyte or monocyte-macrophage pathway, depending on the chemical reactors involved and on the microenvironment. There are various directions in which these cells mature and differentiate. Circulating monocytes may continue to have a multipotential and give rise to different types of macrophages. The most important step in the maturation of macrophages is their lymphokine-drive conversion from normal renting macrophages to activated macrophages (discussed further below). The terminal stage of development is the multinucleated giant cell (seen in granulomatous inflammatory infections such as tuberculosis).

Macrophages are known to be either "fixed" or "wandering" cells. They may be specialized like, for example, the pulmonary alveolar macrophages, which are the first line of defense against inhaled foreign particles and bacteria (the dust macrophages). Fixed macrophages line the endothelium of capillaries and the sinuses of organs such as the bone marrow, spleen, and lymph nodes.

During infection, macrophages can be converted from a normal, resting state to an activated state by the release of macrophage-activating lymphokines (e.g., interferon, gamma and granulocyte-colony–stimulating factor) from T lymphocytes specifically sensitized to antigens from the infecting microorganisms. Macrophages exposed to an endotoxin release a hormone (tumor necrosis factor, alpha-cachectin) that can itself activate macrophages under certain conditions *in vitro*.

Activated macrophages play several roles in body defense in addition to phagocytosis. These include antigen presentation and induction of the immune response and the secretion of biologically active molecules.

The Process of Phagocytosis

The mechanisms contributing to the process of phagocytosis include *initiation, chemotaxis, engulfment,* and *digestion.*

Initiation. Phagocytosis is initiated as the result of tissue damage, either through trauma or as a result of microbial multiplication. The activated phagocyte has increased surface receptors (CR3, formyl-methionyl-leucyl-phenylalanine receptors, and laminin receptors) that allow for the adherence of the bacterium to the phagocyte.

Chemotaxis. Chemotaxis is a process by which cells tend to move in a certain direction under the stimulation of chemical substances. This stimulation can cause two effects: (1) the cells may move *toward* the stimulating substance (known as *positive* chemotaxis) or (2) the cells may move *away* from the stimulating substance (known as *negative* chemotaxis). Without the influence of these chemotactic substances, cell motion is random.

Leukocytes have never been shown to display negative chemotaxis; they are always drawn *toward* the substance and therefore to the site of injury. This is a critical early step in phagocytosis.

A considerable amount of research has been devoted to the identification of the chemicals responsible for chemotaxis in acute inflammation in humans. Agents such as starch and certain bacteria have been shown to attract both polymorphs and monocytes *in vitro*. Other chemotactic agents are antigen-antibody complexes and dead tissue, although these only function if complement is present and activated (C567 and the anaphylatoxins C3a and C5a being the chemotactic agents). In addition, it has been found that formyl-methionyl-leucyl-phenylalanine and LTB_4, which activate phagocytes, also promote diapedesis (the ameboid movement of neutrophils through the vessel wall to the interstitial tissues) and chemotaxis.

The chemotactic agents therefore guide the various phagocytic cells to the site of injury.

Engulfment. Once the phagocyte has recognized that a particle is foreign, engulfment occurs by active ameboid motion (i.e., resembling an ameba in movement). The phagocyte extends its cytoplasmic membrane around the invading organism, which is eventually surrounded and completely enclosed. This final structure, containing the phagocytosed particle, is known as the phagocytic "vacuole" or "phagosome" (Fig. 1–1).

It is important to understand that certain conditions apply in determining whether or not phagocytosis can occur. These include the physical nature of both the bacteria and the phagocytic cell. The bacteria must be more hydrophobic than the phagocyte (e.g., most nonpathogenic bacteria). Bacteria with a hydrophilic capsule (e.g., *Diplococcus pneumoniae*) are not normally phagocytosed.

Of great importance in the phagocytic process is a group of antibodies known as serum opsonins (i.e., antibodies and complement components). These antibodies interact with the surfaces of bacteria, rendering them acceptable to the phagocyte. Antibodies are able to opsonize by themselves, or they can cause the complement system (see Chapter 3) to generate C3, which coats the bacterium. Phagocytes apparently possess surface Fc receptors for Ig and C3 receptors that recognize and interact with antibodies and activated C3. Because time is required for these antibodies to develop, they are of greater significance in the later stages of inflammation than in the earlier stages.

Digestion (Degranulation). When ingestion of the foreign particle is complete, cytoplasmic lysosomes (minute cell particles), which contain certain hydrolytic enzymes and peroxidase, approach the phagosome (vacuole), fuse with it, rupture, and discharge their contents into it. The mechanisms by which this phenomenon occurs are unknown. The cell then becomes degranulated as foreign materials (with the exception of inert materials) are digested. The major factors in the actual killing of bacteria within the vacuole include hydrogen peroxide and an oxidizable cofactor. Other oxygen-independent systems (e.g., alterations in pH lysozymes, lactoferrin, and the granular cationic proteins) also participate in the bactericidal process.

As a result of the release of lytic enzymes, the neutrophils die and are themselves phagocytosed by macrophages. The phagocytosis process presents no risk to the macrophage unless the ingested material is toxic or damages the lysosomal membrane, in which case the macrophage will also be destroyed.

Bacteria are not always destroyed by hydrolytic enzymes. Some may survive and eventually break out of the cell again. In this case, they may establish themselves in secondary sites within the body where they produce a secondary inflammation that again attracts neutrophils and macrophages. If the bacteria escape from secondary tissue sites, a bacteremia will develop, which can prove fatal in patients who are unresponsive to antibiotic intervention.

Other Purposes of Phagocytosis

Besides the killing of invading microorganisms, the macrophages have other important phagocytic functions. These include their ability to dispose of damaged or dying cells and to remove aging erythrocytes from the spleen. They are also involved in the removal of tissue debris from repairing wounds and in removing debris as embryonic tissues replace one another.

The mononuclear phagocytes may also be involved in the removal of cancer cells, although this activity is not well understood. Phagocytes are thought to suppress the growth of spontaneously arising tumors.

It is also postulated that the proteolytic enzymes present on the surface membranes of monocytes could be involved in tissue rejection.

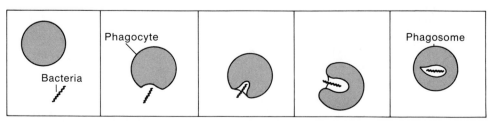

Figure 1–1. Phagocytosis (ingestion of foreign matter).

METHOD 1: SCREENING TEST FOR PHAGOCYTIC ENGULFMENT

Principle

This procedure is useful in supporting the diagnosis of impaired neutrophilic function in conjunction with clinical signs and symptoms. In principle, the test involves the combination and incubation of bacteria and phagocytes, which are then examined for the presence of engulfed bacteria.

Specimen Requirements

A minimum of 2 ml of heparinized blood (or 15 to 20 heparinized capillary tubes) is required. The specimen should be centrifuged and the test performed as soon as possible.

Reagents, Supplies, and Equipment

1. Broth culture of *Bacillus subtilis* or *Staphylococcus* coagulase (negative) species
2. Microscope slides
3. Pasteur pipettes and rubber bulb
4. 12 × 75 mm test tubes
5. Wright's stain

Procedure

NOTE: A fresh, heparinized sample of blood from a healthy volunteer should be tested in parallel with the patient's sample as a control.
1. Label two 12 × 75 mm test tubes—one as the patient's specimen, the other as the control.
2. Add four to eight drops of the buffer coat from the patient's heparinized blood and the normal control to the respectively labeled test tubes.
3. Add two to three drops of the bacterial broth culture to each tube.
4. Incubate both tubes at room temperature or 37°C for 30 minutes.
5. Place one drop of the incubated specimen on a glass slide and prepare a smear.
6. Air dry the slides.
7. Cover each smear generously with filtered Wright's stain and allow the stain to remain on the slide for at least 5 minutes.
8. Slowly add distilled water or buffer to the stain until the buffer begins to overflow the stain. Watch for the appearance of a metallic luster.
9. Gently blow on the slide to mix the stain and the buffer.
10. Allow the buffer to remain on the slide for at least 5 minutes.
11. Gently wash the stain and buffer off the slide with distilled water.
12. Air dry or carefully blot the slide between two sheets of bibulous paper.
13. Place a drop of immersion oil on each smear and examine microscopically with the oil (100 ×) immersion objective.

Interpretation

Positive—demonstration of bacterial engulfment
Negative—no bacterial engulfment
NOTE: False-negative results may be produced if the specimen is not fresh or if a coagulase-positive *Staphylococcus* specimen is used. It is important to distinguish between granules and cocci. Bacteria must also be intracellular and not extracellular for the test to be positive. The failure of phagocytosis to engulf bacteria supports the diagnosis of neutrophilic dysfunction (when taken in conjunction with the patient's signs and symptoms). It is important to realize that this is a simple screening procedure and that the presence of engulfed bacteria does not demonstrate that the bacteria have been destroyed.

Nonspecific Immunity of Body Fluids

Body fluids and secretions have long been known to possess antibacterial properties. In many instances, the action of specific antibody and complement accounts for these properties; however, additional substances that play a significant role in nonspecific defense may be present.

Natural Antibody. An antibody that is present in a host and reacts with substances with which the host has had no known contact is referred to as "natural" antibody. Three possible mechanisms have been proposed to explain their formation.

1. *Genetic.* It is possible that natural antibody production is under genetic control and, therefore,

that no antigenic stimulation of any kind is required for this production.

2. *Cross-reaction.* It has also been proposed that natural antibodies may be produced as a result of stimulation by specific antigens that have similar (but not identical) antigenic determinant groups that cross-react with the particular antigen by virtue of these chance similarities.

3. *Antigenic stimulation.* It is also possible that natural antibodies arise as the result of direct, specific antigenic stimulation—the antigens gaining access to the host by natural means. This possibility is the one that has achieved widest general acceptance.

Lysozyme. Lysozyme, an enzyme found in many types of cells, as well as in tears and saliva, has been shown to have antibacterial activity. The enzyme functions by virtue of mucolytic properties that cleave acetylamino-sugars, the backbone of both gram-positive and gram-negative bacteria. The enzyme, therefore, attacks and destroys the cell walls of susceptible bacteria. Certain basic polypeptides (with large amounts of lysine) have been shown to kill anthrax. A synergistic action of the effect of lysozyme and complement has been observed in *in vitro* studies.

Properdin. Properdin is a serum protein that exerts bactericidal and viricidal effects in the presence of the third component of complement (C3) and magnesium ions. Originally described as a naturally occurring euglobulin with a broad spectrum of activity against bacteria, evidence now suggests that the presence of minute amounts of "natural" antibody accounts for the properdin effect. Properdin, however, is indistinguishable from these antibodies by virtue of the fact that it is capable of combining with certain monomolecular antigens to activate the complement sequence at the level of the third component (see Complement Activation: The Alternative Pathway, Chapter 3).

Betalysin. The serum of many animal species (including humans) contains a heat-stable cationic substance with antibacterial activity. This substance (which is not present in plasma from the same animal) is known as betalysin. The substance is released by platelets during coagulation and probably functions through an enzymatic alteration of the cell surface of susceptible bacteria. Betalysin (also written as beta lysin) is bactericidal

for gram-positive bacteria with the exception of streptococci.

Cytokines

Interferon. Interferon (abbreviated IFN) is any of a family of glycoproteins that exert virus-nonspecific but host-specific antiviral activity by inducing the transcription of cellular genes coding for antiviral proteins that selectively inhibit the synthesis of viral RNA and proteins. Interferons also have immunoregulatory functions (inhibition of B-cell activation and antibody production enhancement of T-cell activity, and enhancement of the cytotoxic activity of natural killer (NK) cells) and can inhibit the growth of nonviral intracellular parasites. Viral infection (especially by the presence of double-stranded RNA), intracellular parasites (chlamydiae, rickettsiae), protozoa (*Toxoplasma*), bacteria (streptococci, staphylococci), and bacterial products (endotoxins) all stimulate the production of interferon.

Interferons have been divided into three groups or types, associated with specific producer cells and functions, but all animal cells are able to produce interferons, and certain producer cells (leukocytes and fibroblasts) produce more than one type.

IFN-α. This is the major interferon produced by virus-induced leukocyte cultures. The null lymphocytes are the primary producer cells, and the major activities are antiviral activity and activation of NK cells. IFN-α is also known as *leukocyte interferon.*

IFN-β. This is the major interferon produced by double-stranded RNA–induced fibroblast cultures. The primary producer cells are fibroblasts, epithelial cells, and macrophages. The major activity is antiviral activity. It is also called *epithelial-, fibroblast-,* or *fibroepithelial interferon.*

IFN-γ. This is the major interferon produced by immunologically stimulated (by mitogens or antigens) lymphocyte cultures. The T lymphocytes are the primary producers of IFN-γ, and its major activity is immunoregulation. This interferon has been implicated in aberrant expression of class II histocompatibility antigens by tissue cells (e.g., thyroid cells) that do not normally express them, leading to autoimmune disease. IFN-γ is also known as *immune interferon.*

NOTE: IFN-α and IFN-β are also known as Type

I interferon; IFN-γ is also known as Type II interferon.

Tumor Necrosis Factor (TNF). Tumor necrosis factor is the principal mediator of the host response to gram-negative bacteria and may also play a role in the response to other infectious organisms. The major source of TNF is the lipopolysaccharide (LPS)-activated mononuclear phagocyte, although antigen-stimulated T cells, activated NK cells, and activated mast cells can also secrete this protein. Interferon-γ (INF-γ), produced by T cells, augments TNF synthesis by LPS-stimulated mononuclear phagocytes. It is clear, therefore, that TNF is a mediator of both natural and acquired immunity and an important link between specific immune responses and acute inflammation.

Interleukin-1. The principal function of Interleukin-1 (IL-1), like that of TNF, is as a mediator of the host inflammatory response in natural immunity. The major cellular source of IL-1 is the activated mononuclear phagocyte. When locally produced at low concentrations, the predominant effects of IL-1 are probably immunoregulatory. When secreted in larger quantities, IL-1 enters the blood stream and exerts endocrine effects. Systemic IL-1 shares with TNF the ability to cause fever, to induce synthesis of acute phase plasma proteins by the liver, and to initiate metabolic wasting.

Interleukin-6. Interleukin-6 (IL-6) is synthesized by mononuclear phagocytes, vascular endothelial cells, fibroblasts, and other cells in response to IL-1 and, to a lesser extent, TNF. It is also made by some activated T cells. IL-6 can be detected in the circulation following gram-negative bacterial infection or TNF infusion and appears to be secreted in response to TNF or IL-1 rather than LPS itself. IL-6 causes hepatocytes to synthesize several plasma proteins, such as fibrinogen, that contribute to the acute phase response.

The Interleukin-8 Family. Members of this family are derived from antigen-activated T cells, LPS-activated or cytokine-activated mononuclear phagocytes, endothelial cells, fibroblasts (or epithelial cells), and platelets. Almost all members of this family have been shown to cause inflammation by stimulating leukocytes, the best characterized being Interleukin-8 (IL-8), which is an activating and chemotactic factor for neutrophils and, to a lesser extent, for eosinophils, basophils, and lymphocytes. Therefore, IL-8 and related cytokines may serve as the principal secondary mediators of inflammation.

Complement

Complement may be regarded as a group of nonspecific serum components that, when activated by the interaction of antigen and antibody, combine in a fixed sequence and thereby enhance the effect of antibody (see Chapter 3).

The following is a brief summary of the biologic functions of complement in immune defense:

Cytolysis. Complement mediated lysis of foreign organisms is an important defense mechanism against microbial infection. Specific humoral responses to microbes generate antibodies that bind to the organisms; these antibodies locally activate complement on the surfaces of the microbes and lead to their lysis by the formation of the "membrane attack complex." In the absence of antibody, some microorganisms may induce lysis by the activation of the alternative pathway. This mechanism may be important for preventing bacteremia by *Neisseria* bacteria. In certain pathologic conditions, the complement system may cause lysis of host cells, leading to tissue injury and disease.

Immune Adherence (C3b). Immune adherence is the covalent bonding between the cleaved form of C3 (C3b) and nearby soluble immune complexes or particulate surfaces. The portion of the C3b that does not adhere is exposed and available for binding to the receptor for C3b on human erythrocytes, B lymphocytes, monocytes, glomerular epithelial cells, or mast cells. B lymphocytes and macrophages also have receptors for C3d, and many of the cells that have receptors for C3b also have receptors for C4b. One biologic purpose for immune adherence is to facilitate the removal of soluble immune complexes. Immune adherence provides a mechanism for the soluble complexes to bind to erythrocytes, thus facilitating the removal of the complexes by the mononuclear-phagocyte system.

Immunoconglutinin. This may play a role in defense by agglutinating relatively small complexes containing bound C4, thereby making them more susceptible to phagocytosis.

Chemotactic Factors. C5a, the by-product resulting from the cleavage of C5 by either the classical or alternative pathway C5 convertase, is a potent chemotactic factor (as well as an anaphylatoxin). It induces the direct migration of neutrophils and monocytes into the area of inflammation (Hugli and Muller-Eberhard, 1978).

Anaphylatoxin. C4a, C3a, and C5a, which result from the cleavage of C4, C3, and C5, are anaphylatoxins that mediate inflammation by inducing the release of histamine from basophils and mast cells, by causing smooth muscle to contract, and by increasing vascular permeability (Hugli and Muller-Eberhard, 1978).

Kinin Activation. C2b (the fragment of C2 released during cleavage by C1s) interacts with plasmin to produce kinin-like activity. The biological activity of C2b results in smooth muscle contraction, mucous gland secretion, increased vascular permeability, and pain (Donaldson *et al.*, 1977).

Discussion. The major role of complement appears to be as an effector mechanism by which antibodies help the host eliminate foreign substances, including infectious disease agents. This is accomplished largely through the release products, such as C3a, C3b, and C5a, which contribute to the development of the inflammatory response. This is supported by the observations that congenital lack of complement is often associated with the development of certain diseases. Patients lacking C3, C3INA, C6, C7, or C8 are very susceptible to bacterial infections. The lack of certain complement components (e.g., C4 and C3) appears to be associated with a high frequency of lupus erythematosus. These observations implicate complement as an immune defense mechanism against the development of disease.

Other Nonspecific Factors

Plant extracts, the sera of invertebrates, and other body fluids of animals have been shown to have antibacterial activity. Although the properties of these substances have not been extensively studied, it is apparent that these antibacterial properties have arisen as a result of evolutionary selection rather than exposure to specific microorganisms or antigenic determinants. Several nonantibody serum proteins can also be included among these.

Accumulation of metabolic intermediaries at sites of inflammation is associated with a lowering of the pH, which has an antibacterial effect. Basic peptides and histones, which are released at the sites of inflammation by dead or dying cells, also have an antibacterial effect.

THE ACUTE PHASE PLASMA PROTEINS

Attendant to injury, the body responds by increasing the hepatic synthesis of a number of plasma proteins, resulting in an increase in the concentration of these proteins in the plasma at the site of injury. It has been suggested, as a result of experimental evidence, that these acute phase proteins play a major role in wound healing (Powanda and Moyer, 1981).

This systemic acute phase response helps to ensure survival during the period immediately following injury and must achieve the same goals as the localized inflammatory response (Kushner, 1982). This response involves the onset of fever and an increase in the granulocyte count in the blood.

The best-studied acute phase plasma proteins in humans differ considerably in the magnitude of their elevation after the onset of injury. It is on the basis of this degree of elevation that three distinct groups are classified (Table 1–1).

For further discussion, see Chapter 8.

Group	Plasma Protein	Degree of Elevation
1	Alpha$_2$-macroglobin Ceruloplasmin C3 (and other complement components)	50 per cent increase
2	Alpha$_1$-antitrypsin Fibrinogen Haptoglobin	Twofold to fourfold
3	C-reactive protein	Several hundred times

TABLE 1–1. Change in Concentration of Acute Phase Plasma Proteins Attendant to Injury

Note: The concentration of albumin usually decreases after the onset of injury.

OTHER ASPECTS OF NONSPECIFIC IMMUNITY

Nonspecific immunity is controlled by genetic factors (as evidenced by interspecies differences in susceptibility and nonsusceptibility, racial and individual differences, and certain immunologic deficiency diseases that are known to be genetically determined) and by the endocrine system (as evidenced by observations of susceptibility and nonsusceptibility influenced by hormones, adrenal hormones, thyroid hormones, sex hormones, and pineal hormones).

Certain selected diseases have been shown to affect nonspecific immunity, either through an increase or decrease in the capacity for phagocytosis and/or a diminished or increased capacity for intracellular killing of bacteria. These include diabetes mellitus, cancer, and uremia. Prematurity and burn injury may also affect nonspecific immunity in this way, as can shock, infection, and alcohol intoxication.

Nonspecific immunity can be stimulated by drugs such as endotoxin (in small doses), tuberculin, and zymosan. An increase in body temperature is also associated with an increase in metabolic function, which has a beneficial effect on nonspecific immunity. In addition, the transfusion of viable leukocytes from both normal donors and patients with chronic myelogenous leukemia is often effective in temporarily elevating the leukocyte count and thereby exerting a favorable effect on nonspecific immunity.

Nonspecific immunity has also been shown to be influenced by factors such as:

1. *Age.* The ability to respond immunologically to disease is age related, although the effects are highly variable. Incomplete development of nonspecific and specific body defenses in the unborn and newborn places these children at greater risk for developing infectious and other diseases. In contrast, 30 per cent of individuals over the age of 85 die as a result of a loss of immune defenses.

   It has been suggested that the aging process itself may involve faulty immunologic reactions. Attempts to enhance the immune system through methods such as tissue removal, cell grafting, chemical intervention, and diet may be used as an attempt to control the aging of the immune system in the future.

2. *Nutrition.* Every aspect of body defense, including phagocytosis and humoral and cellular immunity, appears to be influenced by nutritional intake. Inadequate nutrition through either the deficient or the excess intake of a particular nutrient can have detrimental effects on the immune system. In addition, errors of metabolism (either innate or acquired) that result in the inability to degrade or synthesize intermediate metabolites of a nutrient can lead to immune deficiency or dysfunction. Also, deficiencies of proteins, carbohydrates, and lipids, however caused, often result in depressed immunologic function. Finally, contaminants in foods (e.g., naturally occurring toxins of plant or animal origin such as food additives and chemicals produced during food processing or preparation) can have an adverse effect on the immune system through hypersensitivity reactions (allergies).

Besides age and nutrition, nonspecific immunity has also been shown to be influenced by such environmental and therapeutic factors as exercise and exposure, irradiation, local wound care, drugs, and anesthesia.

Psychoneuroimmunology

Psychoneuroimmunology is a relatively new scientific discipline that seeks to combine basic scientific research with psychologic and physiologic investigations on the relationship between the mind and the body with respect to body defenses. This study was prompted by observations that psychologic factors appear to be closely associated with the development of certain illnesses. It has been found, for example, that rates of illness and death tend to be higher among individuals who have recently undergone severe psychologic stress (e.g., the loss of a spouse). Immune system abnormalities have also been found in major affective disorders and in schizophrenia. On the other hand, "positive stress" may influence health in a favorable way, contributing to increased immunity and longevity. These findings are supported by the fact that hormonal and cellular changes have been detected in individuals during periods of stress, and these changes are known to affect the efficiency and function of the immune system.

JUST THE FACTS

Introduction

1. Immunology is the study of immunity.
2. *Immunity* indicates "resistance" to invasion by harmful matter.
3. A.D. 1500—Chinese inhale crusts from smallpox lesions to induce immunity. Unsuccessful.
4. 1718—Material from smallpox blisters is injected to induce immunity. Sometimes successful, but virus could be transmitted.
5. 1798—Jenner describes vaccination.
6. Almost 70 years later, Pasteur shows that heat can kill bacteria (pasteurization).
7. 1880–1900—Elie Metchnikoff elucidated the roles of phagocytosis and cellular immunity. During the same period, killed vaccines introduced, complement described.
8. 1902—Richet and Portier showed immune reaction could be damaging (anaphylaxis shown to be an immunologic reaction).
9. 1903—White and Douglas showed that acquired immunity resulted from both humoral and cellular elements and described opsonization. The term "antigen" was introduced as a result of this.
10. 1903—Arthus reaction described.
11. 1903—Von Pirquet and Schick show that diseases of skin, heart, joints, blood vessels, and kidneys as well as fever could be caused by the body's immunologic reaction to foreign protein.
12. 1920—Immunologic basis of certain allergies reported by Prausnitz and Küstner.
13. Paul Ehrlich first to use quantitative measurements of immune reactions.
14. 1928—Alexander Fleming discovers penicillin.
15. 1932—Domagk develops prontosil (antibacterial agent against *Streptococcus*). Active ingredient sulfanilamide, later found to be active against a number of organisms.
16. 1924–1926—Measurement of antigens and antibodies by precipitation described. Measurement by immunoelectrophoresis described in 1953.
17. 1952—Burton discovers hypogammaglobulinemia, which leads to dissection of the immune system into T- and B-cell systems.
18. 1944–1945—Medawar *et al.* showed that immunologic processes are involved in allograft rejection of normal organs (initiating interest in transplantation).
19. 1980–1990—Discovery of AIDS and Lyme disease. MHC shown to be important in regulation of immune response during antigen presentation.
20. Immunology has an impact on all medical disciplines.

Nonspecific Immunity

1. Immune system protects body against invasion by "non-self" substances.
2. Positive effects—natural resistance, recovery, and acquired resistance. Negative effects—rejection of life-saving organ transplant.
3. Two types of immunity recognized—natural and acquired.
4. Nonspecific (innate, natural) immunity present at birth and includes factors such as physical barrier of the skin, susceptibility and nonsusceptibility, provision of unfavorable environment for the infecting organism, flushing and capture of airborne particulate matter.
5. Innate immunity is influenced by age, nutrition, chemicals secreted by cells.
6. Innate immunity also involves inflammation, complement, phagocytosis.

Susceptibility and Nonsusceptibility

1. Certain animal species are resistant to particular disease states, others appear highly susceptible to them.
2. The phenomenon is believed to be controlled by hereditary or genetic factors.
3. The Fy^a and Fy^b (Duffy) receptors on the red cells are believed to be associated with susceptibility to malaria. Fy(a−b−) individuals appear to be resistant.
4. Susceptibility and nonsusceptibility are evident among different races of humans and can be affected by age and hormone influence.

The Epithelial Barriers

1. Skin and mucous membranes provide a physical barrier against invasion and possess active mechanisms for killing bacteria and other organisms.
2. The self-sterilizing power of the skin is achieved by desiccation, epithelial desquamation, pH, and the secretion of fatty acids with antibacterial properties.
3. The renewal of the skin's cells and the flora that inhabit the skin assist by hindering penetration by microorganisms and by helping to eliminate those that gain entry into the body.
4. Body secretions (oil of sebaceous glands, lactic acid in sweat, mucus in the nose, ear wax, urine, and feces) assist in the elimination of microorganisms.
5. The acidity and/or alkalinity of fluids in the stomach, intestinal tract, and vagina affords further protection.
6. The constant motion of cilia of the tubules protects the respiratory tract.
7. Mucosal surfaces are protected by a "slime layer" that possesses antibodies to IgA and other antimicrobial and antiviral substances.
8. Lysozyme (a bacterial enzyme that is effective in lysing certain bacteria) is present in these secretions as well as in the granules of polymorphs and macrophages and in many other body fluids.
9. The nonspecific antiviral agent "interferon," which inhibits intracellular viral replication, is synthesized by cells in response to viral infection. It is a major factor in the recovery from (rather than the prevention of) viral infections.

Inflammation

1. Inflammation is the tissue's reaction to injury and is characterized by pain, heat, redness, swelling, and sometimes loss of function.
2. Inflammation is characterized by the vascular response, the cellular responses, and by cellular proliferation and repair.

The Vascular Response

1. The primary response in acute inflammation is the localized dilation of the capillaries and venules so that more blood passes to the area of injury (termed *hyperemia*).
2. As a result of this:
   a. Plasma leaks from the vessels, making the blood more viscoid.
   b. The lubricating action of the plasmatic zone is impaired—slowing the blood flow (and sometimes stopping it in severe injury—termed *stasis*).
   c. The endothelial cells become swollen and the spaces between adjacent cells become widened, allowing plasma and cells to pass between them.
3. An exudate is formed that has a fluid and a cellular component.
4. The fluid exudate is formed as a result of increased vascular permeability, which allows the plasma proteins to leak through the vessel wall, causing the osmotic pressure effect of the plasma proteins to be lost.
5. The "ground substance" becomes more fluid, allowing the exudate to diffuse into surrounding tissues more readily, preventing an immediate rise in tissue tension. This causes pain.
6. The fluid exudate has almost the same composition as plasma and contains antibacterial substances, specific antibodies, as well as drugs and antibiotics (if present).
7. The exudate also serves to dilute irritating chemicals and bacterial toxins. The fibrinogen in the exudate is converted to fibrin, which forms a fibrin clot. The fibrin clot provides a union between severed tissues, acts as a barrier against bacterial invasion, and aids phagocytosis.

The Cellular Response

1. The defense of the body against disease states is the responsibility of the leukocyte (white cell) system.
2. There are many types of white cells, which can be divided into three general categories: granulocytes, monocytes-macrophages, and lymphocyte-plasma cells.
3. The cellular response in inflammation begins when the white cells move into the plasmatic zone and stick to the altered vessel wall.
4. The cellular exudate consists of PMNs (initially) and monocytes (in the later stages). The PMNs

are attracted into the inflamed area by chemotactic factors.

5. The neutrophil emigration may last 24 to 48 hours. They are actively phagocytic, they contain a number of biologically active macromolecules, and their active aerobic glycolysis is responsible for the formation of lactic acid, which causes pain.

6. Mononuclear cells move to the site of injury after about 4 hours and reach a peak at 16 to 24 hours (i.e., after a *single* injury).

7. Interleukin-1 (associated with fever, elevation of acute phase proteins, and infiltration of inflammatory sites by leukocytes) is stimulated by products of PMN phagocytosis and degranulation and attracts and activates other monocytes-macrophages. IL-1 also stimulates T lymphocytes to produce Interleukin-2.

8. Resolution and repair are the final stages of the inflammatory process, initiated by fibroblast proliferation. As a result:
   a. The affected area may be totally repaired.
   b. The injury may lead to the formation of an abscess with some loss of function.
   c. A granuloma may be formed (typical of delayed hypersensitivity of cell-mediated immunity).

Phagocytosis

1. Phagocytosis is the action of a specialized group of phagocytic (eating) cells that provide a defense mechanism against invasion by engulfing foreign particulate matter, which they then attempt to destroy enzymatically. (Description attributed to Elie Metchnikoff, 1907.)

Cells of the Phagocytic System

1. Polymorphonuclear leukocytes (PMNs).
2. Monocytes.

The Process of Phagocytosis

1. Initiation.
   a. Phagocytosis is initiated as a result of tissue damage.
   b. Activated phagocytes have increased surface receptors that allow for adherence to the bacterium.

2. Chemotaxis.
   a. The process in which cells tend to move in a certain direction under the stimulation of chemical substances.
   Positive chemotaxis = toward the stimulating substances.
   Negative chemotaxis = away from the stimulating substances.
   b. Leukocytes always show positive chemotaxis.
   c. Chemotactic agents include starch and certain bacteria, as well as antigen-antibody complexes, and dead tissue (when complement is present and activated). Others include formyl-methionyl-phenylalanine and LTB_4.

3. Engulfment.
   a. Engulfment is by active ameboid motion.
   b. The final structure (containing the phagocytosed particles) is known as a "vacuole" or "phagosome."
   c. The bacteria must be more hydrophobic than the phagocyte for phagocytosis to occur.
   d. Opsonins (antibodies and complement components) interact with the surfaces of bacteria, rendering them acceptable to the phagocyte.

4. Digestion.
   a. Minute cell particles that contain certain hydrolytic enzymes and peroxidase approach the phagosome, fuse with it, rupture, and discharge their contents into it.
   b. The cell becomes degranulated as foreign materials (*not* inert materials) are digested.
   c. The neutophils subsequently die and are themselves phagocytosed. Phagocytosis presents no risk to the macrophage unless the ingested material is toxic or unless it damages the lysosomal membrane.
   d. Bacteria are not always destroyed by hydrolytic enzymes. Some may survive and break out of the cell. They may then cause a secondary inflammation, which again attracts neutrophils and macrophages. If the bacteria escape from secondary tissue sites, a bacteremia will develop, which can prove fatal in patients who are unresponsive to antibiotic intervention.

Other Purposes of Phagocytosis

1. The disposal of damaged or dying cells and the removal of aging erythrocytes from the spleen.
2. The removal of tissue debris from repairing wounds.
3. The removal of debris as embryonic tissues replace one another.
4. The mononuclear phagocytes may also be involved in the removal of cancer cells.
5. The suppression of growth of spontaneously arising tumors.

Nonspecific Immunity of Body Fluids

Other substances that may play a role in nonspecific defense include:

1. "Natural" antibody. (An antibody that is present in a host and that reacts with substances with which the host has had no known contact.)
2. Lysozyme. (An enzyme found in many types of cells, as well as in tears and saliva, that has antibacterial activity.)
3. Properdin. (A serum protein that exerts bactericidal and viricidal effects in the presence of the third component of complement and magnesium ions.)
4. Betalysin. (A heat-stable cationic substance with bactericidal activity found in the serum of many animal species [including humans].)
5. Interferon. (A family of glycoproteins produced by all animal cells that exert virus-nonspecific but host-specific antiviral activity.)
6. Tumor necrosis factor. (A protein secreted by many different cells that is the principal mediator of the host response to gram-negative bacteria and may also play a role in the response to other infectious organisms.)
7. Interleukin-1. (Produced by the activated mononuclear phagocyte, which has an immunoregulatory function and exerts endocrine effects.)
8. Interleukin-6. (Synthesized by several different cells in response to IL-1 and [to a lesser extent] TNF, which causes hepatocytes to synthesize several plasma proteins.)
9. The Interleukin-8 family. (Derived from many different cells, they are the principal secondary mediators of inflammation.)
10. Complement. (A group of nonspecific serum components that enhance the effect of antibody. The biologic functions of complement in immune defense include cytolysis, immune adherence, immunoconglutinin, chemotactic factors, anaphylatoxin, and kinin activation.)

The Acute Phase Plasma Proteins

1. Attendant to injury, the body increases the hepatic synthesis of a number of plasma proteins (alpha$_2$-macroglobin, ceruloplasmin, C3, alpha$_1$-antitrypsin, fibrinogen, haptoglobin, and C-reactive protein) that are believed to play a major role in wound healing.
2. The acute phase plasma proteins differ considerably in the magnitude of their elevation after the onset of injury (see Table 1–1).

Other Aspects of Nonspecific Immunity

1. Nonspecific immunity is controlled by genetic factors and by the endocrine system.
2. Certain selected diseases and conditions have been shown to affect nonspecific immunity by increasing or decreasing the capacity for phagocytosis and/or a diminished or increased capacity for uremia.
3. Nonspecific immunity can be stimulated by drugs, by elevation in body temperature, and by the transfusion of viable leukocytes.
4. Nonspecific immunity is influenced by factors such as age, nutrition, and environmental and therapeutic factors (exercise, exposure, irradiation, local wound care, drugs, and anesthesia).

Psychoneuroimmunology

1. This is a relatively new scientific discipline that seeks to combine basic scientific research with psychologic and physiologic investigations on the relationship between the mind and the body with respect to body defenses.

Review Questions

Multiple Choice

Choose the phrase, sentence, or symbol that completes the statement or answers the question. More than one answer may be correct in each case. Answers are given at the end of this book.

1. The procedure of vaccination was originally described in 1798 by:
   (a) Pasteur
   (b) Elie Metchnikoff
   (c) Jenner
   (d) Lady Montagu
   (Introduction)

2. Alexander Fleming was the discoverer of:
   (a) anaphylaxis
   (b) penicillin
   (c) vaccination
   (d) none of the above
   (Introduction)

3. The process by which all animals resist the invasion of foreign microorganisms by natural means is known as:
   (a) natural immunity
   (b) innate immunity
   (c) acquired immunity
   (d) vaccination
   (Nonspecific Immunity)

4. The mechanisms of nonspecific immunity include:
   (a) the physical barrier of the skin
   (b) the flushing away of particulate matter that enters from the air
   (c) the development of specific antibodies
   (d) inflammation
   (Nonspecific Immunity)

5. The Duffy receptors on the erythrocyte membrane are believed to be associated with susceptibility to:
   (a) hepatitis
   (b) syphilis
   (c) malaria
   (d) all of the above
   (Susceptibility and Nonsusceptibility)

6. The self-sterilizing power of the skin is achieved by:
   (a) desiccation
   (b) pH
   (c) epithelial desquamation
   (d) the secretion of fatty acids that have antibacterial properties
   (The Epithelial Barriers)

7. The classic signs of inflammation are:
   (a) redness
   (b) swelling
   (c) heat
   (d) pain
   (Inflammation)

8. The fluid exudate in the vascular response of the inflammatory process:
   (a) is formed as a result of decreased vascular permeability
   (b) has a fluid component
   (c) has a cellular component
   (d) all of the above
   (The Vascular Response)

9. The white cells involved in the cellular response of the inflammatory process include:
   (a) granulocytes
   (b) monocytes-macrophages
   (c) lymphocyte-plasma cells
   (d) all of the above
   (The Cellular Response)

10. The emigration of mononuclear cells to the site of a single injury:
    (a) begins 16 to 24 hours after initial stimulus
    (b) reaches a peak after about 4 hours
    (c) begins about 4 hours after initial stimulus
    (d) reaches a peak at about 16 to 24 hours
    (The Cellular Response)

11. The process of phagocytosis involves the following contributing mechanisms:
    (a) chemotaxis
    (b) engulfment
    (c) degranulation
    (d) opsonization
    (The Process of Phagocytosis)

12. Other purposes of phagocytosis include:
    (a) the repairing of wounds
    (b) hemostasis
    (c) the disposal of viable cells
    (d) the removal of aging erythrocytes from the spleen
    (Other Purposes of Phagocytosis)

13. In the screening test for phagocytic engulfment:
    (a) a false-negative result may be produced if the specimen is fresh
    (b) a false-positive result may be produced if the specimen is not fresh
    (c) a false-negative result may be produced if a coagulase-positive *Staphylococcus* specimen is used

(d) the failure of phagocytosis to engulf bacteria eliminates the diagnosis of neutrophilic dysfunction
(Screening Test for Phagocytic Engulfment)

14. Lysozyme:
    (a) is an enzyme
    (b) is found in tears
    (c) is found in saliva
    (d) has antiviricidal activity
    (Nonspecific Immunity of Body Fluids)

15. Interferon-beta is also known as:
    (a) leukocyte interferon
    (b) epithelial interferon
    (c) immune interferon
    (d) none of the above
    (Nonspecific Immunity of Body Fluids)

16. The biological activity of C2b results in:
    (a) smooth muscle contraction
    (b) mucous gland secretion
    (c) increased vascular permeability
    (d) pain
    (Nonspecific Immunity of Body Fluids)

17. The acute phase plasma protein that increases several hundred times its normal concentration after the onset of injury is:
    (a) C-reactive protein
    (b) ceruloplasmin
    (c) fibrinogen
    (d) haptoglobin
    (The Acute Phase Plasma Proteins)

18. Nonspecific immunity can be affected/influenced by:
    (a) drugs
    (b) age
    (c) nutrition
    (d) none of the above
    (Other Aspects of Nonspecific Immunity)

Answer "True" or "False"

1. Louis Pasteur demonstrated that heat could kill bacteria.
   (Introduction)

2. The MHC has no role in the regulation of the immune response.
   (Introduction)

3. Innate immunity is influenced by age and nutrition.
   (Nonspecific Immunity)

4. Susceptibility and nonsusceptibility are thought to be controlled to some extent by age and nutritional factors.
   (Susceptibility and Nonsusceptibility)

5. The slime layer on mucosal surfaces has been shown to possess antibodies of the IgA class.
   (The Epithelial Barriers)

6. The inflammatory process involves a vascular response only.
   (Inflammation)

7. Activated macrophages play several roles in body defense in addition to phagocytosis.
   (Cells of the Phagocytic System)

8. The movement of cells away from a stimulating substance is known as positive chemotaxis.
   (The Process of Phagocytosis)

9. Serum opsonins interact with the surfaces of bacteria, rendering them acceptable to a phagocyte.
   (The Process of Phagocytosis)

10. The screening test for phagocytic engulfment involves the incubation of bacteria and phagocytes that are then examined for the presence of engulfed bacteria.
    (Screening Test for Phagocytic Engulfment)

11. Betalysin is released by erythrocytes during agglutination.
    (Nonspecific Immunity of Body Fluids)

12. Interferon, tumor necrosis factor, and Interleukin-1 are known as cytokines.
    (Nonspecific Immunity of Body Fluids)

13. Acute phase plasma proteins are believed to play a major role in wound healing.
    (The Acute Phase Plasma Proteins)

14. Nonspecific immunity can be stimulated by tuberculin.
    (Other Aspects of Nonspecific Immunity)

15. Humoral and cellular changes have never been detected in individuals during periods of stress.
    (Psychoneuroimmunology)

GENERAL REFERENCES

Abbas, A.K., Lichtman, A.H., and Pober, J.S.: Cellular and Molecular Immunology. Philadelphia, W. B. Saunders Company, 1991.

Arai, K., Lee, F., Miyajima, A., Miyatake, S., Aria, N., and Yokota, T.: Cytokines: Coordinators of immune and inflammatory responses. Annu. Rev. Biochem., *59:* 783–836, 1990.

Balkwill, F.R., and Burke, F.: The cytokine network. Immunol. Today, *10:* 299–304, 1989.

Beutler, B., and Cerami, A.: The biology of cachectin-TNF: A primary mediator of the host response. Annu. Rev. Immunol., 7:625–655, 1988.

DeMaeyer, E., and DeMayer-Guignard, J.: Interferons and Other Regulatory Cytokines. New York, John Wiley & Sons, 1988.

diGiovine, F.S., and Duff, G.W.: Interleukin 1: The first interleukin. Immunol. Today, *11*:13–20, 1990.

Dorland's Illustrated Medical Dictionary, 27th ed. Philadelphia,
W. B. Saunders Company, 1988.

Freeman, B.A.: Burrows Textbook of Microbiology, 27th ed.
Philadelphia, W. B. Saunders Company, 1985.

Henry, J.B.: Clinical Diagnosis and Management by Laboratory
Methods. Philadelphia, W. B. Saunders Company, 1991.

Matsushima, K., and Oppenheim, J.J.: Interleukin 8 and MCAF:
Novel inflammatory cytokines inducible by IL-1 and TNF.
Cytokine, *1*:2–13, 1989.

Sheehan, C.: Clinical Immunology; Principles and Laboratory
Diagnosis. Philadelphia, J. B. Lippincott, 1990.

Van Snick, J.: Interleukin 6: An overview. Annu. Rev. Immunol.,
8:253–278, 1990.

2
Specific Immunity

OBJECTIVES

The student shall know, understand, and be prepared to explain:
1. The concepts of specific Immunity
2. Antigens (characteristics, types, factors affecting immunogenicity, and chemical nature)
3. Antibodies, general characteristics
4. The structure of immunoglobulin
5. The general function of immunoglobulin
6. Immunoglobulin domains
7. Types of immunoglobulin, including:
    a. IgG
    b. IgM
    c. IgA
    d. IgE
    e. IgD
8. The function and characteristics of the above-mentioned immunoglobulins
9. Cells involved in specific immunity, including:
    a. The T lymphocytes
    b. The B lymphocytes
    c. NK cells
10. Other cells of the immune system, including:
    a. Monocytes and macrophages
    b. Polymorphonuclear granulocytes (neutrophils, eosinophils, basophils, and mast cells)

Introduction

Unlike nonspecific immunity, the processes of specific (or "acquired") immunity are an adaptive response to foreign antigenic stimulus, which results in the acquisition of immunologic memory and the production of antibody, which reacts *specifically* with the antigen that caused its production.

Immunity against infectious diseases may be conferred basically in two ways: (1) by actual infection or inoculation that causes the production of specific protective antibodies (known as "active" immunity), or (2) by artificial transmission of antibodies, which afford temporary protection against invading antigen (known as "passive" immunity).

In some cases, a certain degree of "cross-immunity" is afforded when there is a relationship or similarity between causative agents. In this way, immunity against one infectious agent may contribute some immunity against other infectious agents.

Several factors are involved in the *degree* of protection produced as a response to infection or inoculation. In this connection, the size of the infecting dose, the route of administration, and the type of infective agent are contributory.

Active immunity may therefore be defined as "the state of resistance developed by an individual following effective contact with foreign microorganisms or their products." Such contact may be caused by:

1. Clinical or subclinical infection.
2. The injection of live or killed microorganisms or their antigens.
3. The absorption of bacterial products (e.g., toxins).

The antibodies produced by the host in response to any of these events may take from a few days to a few weeks to develop, yet they usually persist for years, offering protection against reinfection. The agents used in active immunization are either live, killed, or attenuated (i.e., thinned: *L. attenuare* = to thin).

When foreign antigen gains entrance into the body, two types of immunologic reactions may occur. These are different but fundamentally similar mechanisms, known as humoral and cell-mediated immunity.

Humoral Immunity. Humoral immunity refers to the synthesis and release of free antibody (humoral antibody) into the blood and other body fluids. The antibody is produced by the B lymphocytes and is then capable of direct combination with and neutralization of bacterial toxins by coating bacteria to enhance their phagocytosis, and so forth.

Cell-Mediated Immunity. Cell-mediated immunity refers to the production of "sensitized" lymphocytes that take part in such reactions as the rejection of tissue transplants, the delayed hypersensitivity to tuberculin seen in patients immune to tubercule bacilli, destruction of cancer cells, and destruction of parasites. Cell-mediated immunity involves mainly the T lymphocytes and their mediators.

Note: The division of humoral and cell-mediated responses is not absolute, and the occurrence of one type of response without some involvement of the other is very rare. Certain antigens, however, tend to elicit an antibody response with a minimal cell-mediated involvement, and vice versa.

For further discussion, see Chapter 5.

ANTIGENS AND ANTIBODIES

As previously mentioned, active immunity against disease is achieved by the production of antibody (or cellular response) in the host against a specific invading foreign antigen. An antigen is, in fact, any substance that is capable of stimulating the production of antibody. Antibody, conversely, refers to a group of plasma proteins (the immunoglobulins) that are formed as a result of exposure to antigen and that react *specifically* with that particular antigen.

(Note: The outstanding characteristic of an antibody is its specificity; this implies that an antibody, once formed, is capable of reacting *only* with the antigen that elicited its production.) Stimulation with a new antigen causes the production of a new antibody. This general rule is not absolute, as in cases of "cross-immunity"—see later in this text.

Antigens (Immunogens)

An antigen is usually defined as any molecular structure that when introduced parenterally into an animal is capable of causing the production of antibodies by that animal. The antibody formed is capable of specific combination with the antigen that elicited its production. The antibodies produced are heterogenous with respect to immunoglobulin class, affinity for antigen, and specificity. At the present time, many authorities use the term *immunogen* when referring to antigen, and these terms have come to be used synonymously, although "immunogen" is the more correct term, since the term "antigen" now refers only to the ability of a substance to combine with an antibody. The immunogen therefore is correctly defined as a substance that causes a detectable immune response, and the immunogenicity of these substances is the property to induce an immune response. Therefore, when an immunogen combines with an antibody molecule, it is an antigen-antibody reaction rather than an immunogen-antibody reaction (Barrett, 1988; Goodman, 1987).

There are two major classes of immunogens:

1. Thymic-dependent antigens. These require the help of the T cells for the formation of antibody. Most immunogens are thymic dependent.
2. Thymic-independent antigens. These stimulate antibody production without interacting with T cells. Structurally, they are composed of repeating units. The response to these antigens is of the IgM class (see later in this chapter) with little or no immunologic memory generated. Lately, some investigators have found that some T-cell interaction *is* required for the production of antibody to T-cell–independent antigens, suggesting that the term *thymus efficient* might be more appropriate than *thymus independent* (Goodman, 1987).

Several terms are used when describing antigens. These terms include autologous antigen, heterologous antigen, homologous antigen, and heterophil antigen. The meanings of these terms follows:

1. *Autologous antigen.* In simple terms, this refers to one's own antigen, which, under appropriate circumstances, would stimulate the production of autoantibody. Autologous antigen is therefore synonymous with autoantigen.
2. *Heterologous antigen.* This is merely a different antigen from that used in the immunization and it may or may not react with the antibody formed, depending upon the chemical similarity to the immunizing antigen.
3. *Homologous antigen.* This refers to the antigen used in the production of antibody.
4. *Heterophil antigen.* Also known as heterogenetic antigens, these are antigens that exist in unrelated plants or animals but are either identical or so closely related that antibodies to one will cross-react with antibodies to the other.

Factors Affecting Immunogenicity

Exactly what makes a substance immunogenic is not known, although several factors are contributory.

Foreignness. It is important that an immunogen be recognized as "foreign" or "non-self" since this provokes a response to potentially harmful substances rather than the substances of the individual. The extent of the response depends on the degree of foreignness of the protein. Generally, the greater the phylogenic difference, the greater the immune response. The exact mechanisms of self–non-self recognition are not known.

Size. Antigenic substances of low molecular weight (i.e., less than 10,000) rarely stimulate the formation of antibodies and are known as *haptens*. These haptens can, however, provide antigenic specificity when coupled with a larger molecule (see further discussion, later in this chapter). High molecular weight molecules of 500,000 or greater with complex protein or polypeptide-carbohydrate structures are the best antigens. It therefore follows that the larger a molecule is, the greater the number of antigenic sites, and thus the greater the variety and quantity of antibody that will be formed.

Diversity. The immunogen molecule itself must be diverse, rather than being composed of a single amino acid or monosaccharide. This is because the entire molecule does not function as an immunoglobulin- or lymphokine-inducing structure. Instead, within each molecule, there are specific regions of limited size that function as the antigenic determinant sites, also known as *epitopes*. The number of these antigen determinant sites per molecule of antigen is referred to as the valence of the antigen. (Note: Valence, in this context, has no relationship to the ionic condition of the antigen.) It is thought that an immunogen must have at least two determinants per molecule to stimulate an antibody response. An epitope is approximately four to six amino acids or five to seven monosaccharides in length (Goodman, 1987). Aromatic amino acids such as tyrosine provide more immunogenicity than nonaromatic amino acids. The internal complexity of the molecule also contributes to immunogenicity. For example, oligosaccharides, although of sufficient size, do not have internal complexity and are poor immunogens, whereas polysaccharides, with their extensive branching, are good immunogens. Hydrophilic (moisture-absorbing) molecules are more immunogenic than hydrophobic (moisture-resisting) molecules, and hydrophilic portions of immunogens are the antigenic determinants (Barrett, 1988).

Chemical Composition and Complexity. The foreign molecule must possess a chemical structure that is unfamiliar to the host. Again, the more diverse the chemical structure, the more antigenic the molecule becomes. Proteins and carbohydrates provide the best response. Lipids and nucleic acids are weak immunogens, although under certain circumstances a response occurs (e.g., in systemic lupus erythematosus, antibodies are found against nucleic acids and nuclear proteins).

Genetic Composition. The genetic composition of the individual has recently been found to have an impact on that individual's ability to respond to an immunogen. Studies and research into the major histocompatibility complex (MHC) have been made in an attempt to understand the genetic influence on responsiveness, and it has been found that if a particular MHC antigen is not present for an immunogen, there will be no response. For example, a high response to tetanus toxoid was found in 81 per cent of individuals expressing the HLA-A9 antigen, whereas a low response to the same immunogen was found in 71 per cent of individuals expressing the HLA-A5 antigen (Sasazuki *et al.*, 1978). Other associations have also been described (Marsh *et al.*, 1981). This ability to respond is inherited as an autosomal dominant trait (see further discussion in The Immune Response, Chapter 4).

Route, Dosage, and Timing. The route, dosage, and timing of parenteral administration of the antigen are instrumental in the degree of antibody production, although the exact mechanisms for this are unclear. Generally, intravenous (into the vein) and intraperitoneal (into the peritoneal cavity) routes are effective. The intradermal (into the dermis, or skin) route offers stronger stimulus than the subcutaneous (beneath the skin) or intramuscular (into the muscle) route, although there are exceptions to this. The dose response may be partially dependent on the nature of immunogen processing (T-cell dependent or T-cell independent). Generally, the smaller the dose the less likely a response.

The Chemical Nature of Antigens

Antigens are usually large organic molecules that are either proteins, which are excellent because of their high molecular weight and structural complexity, or large polysaccharides. Lipids, on the other hand, are poor antigens because they are relatively simple and lack structural stability. (When lipids are linked to proteins or polysaccharides, however, they may function as antigens.) Nucleic acids are also poor antigens because of relative simplicity, molecular flexibility, and rapid degradation. Antinucleic acid antibodies, however, can be produced by artificially stabilizing them and linking them to an immunogenic carrier. Carbohydrates (polysaccharides) by themselves are considered too small to function as antigens. In the case of red cell blood group antigens, however, protein or lipid carriers may contribute to the necessary size, and the polysaccharides present in the form of side chains confer immunologic specificity.

Cell surface (or membrane-bound) antigens can be composed of combinations of the biochemical classes (e.g., glycoproteins or glycolipids). The HLA (histocompatibility) antigens are glycoprotein in nature and are found on the surface membranes of nucleated body cells comprising both solid tissue and most circulating blood cells (e.g., granulocytes, monocytes, thrombocytes, and lymphocytes).

ANTIBODIES

Basically, antibodies may be viewed as substances (specific glycoproteins) produced in response to antigenic (immunogenic) stimulation that are capable of specific interaction with the provoking immunogen. It is now common practice when referring to antibodies to use the general term *immunoglobulin* because of the heterogeneity in the types of molecules that can function as antibodies. This term has replaced the term "gamma globulin" because not all antibodies have γ electrophoretic mobility. In humans, five distinct structural types or "classes" of immunoglobulin have been isolated: immunoglobulin G (abbreviated IgG), IgM, IgA, IgD, and IgE.

Structure of Immunoglobulins

Each of the immunoglobulin classes has a basic structural similarity. The single structural unit consists of two sizes of peptide chain, termed "heavy" and "light" chains. A model for the basic immunoglobulin molecule was proposed by Porter in the 1950s, which showed a symmetrical, four-peptide unit, consisting of two heavy chains and two light chains linked by interchain disulfide bonds (Fig. 2–1). The number of disulfide bonds between

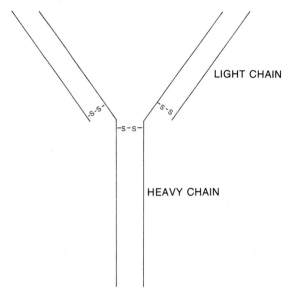

Figure 2–1. The model for the basic immunoglobulin molecule proposed by Porter.

heavy chains varies from 1 to 14 (Goodman, 1987). Only one disulfide bond joins a heavy and a light chain in most classes and subclasses. The molecule appears to be Y-shaped, the arms of the Y swinging out to an angle of 180 degrees from the horizontal.

In 1959 Porter demonstrated that treatment of IgG, which consists of a single structural unit, with the enzyme papain split the molecule into three fragments. Two of these fragments appeared to be identical and were subsequently shown to be capable of binding specifically with antigen, although they were not capable of causing agglutination or precipitation reactions. These two fragments were called *Fab* (*Fragment capable of Antigen Binding*); each is composed of one light chain and one-half of one heavy chain. The remaining fragment (in rabbit IgG) was found to crystallize upon purification and was therefore called *Fc* (*Fragment Crystalline*). This Fc fragment was found to be composed of two halves of two heavy chains and was further found to be involved in complement activation, fixation to the skin, and placental transport. Fc receptors found on other cells will bind to this region of the immunoglobulin molecule (Roitt, 1988) (Fig. 2–2).

Treatment of IgG with the enzyme pepsin results in a slightly different Fab-type fragment that not only retains the ability to bind with antigen but is also capable of causing agglutination or precipitation reactions. This fragment is known as F(ab')$_2$ because the two fragments found with papain cleavage are in this case held together by a disulfide bond. It has two antigen-binding sites and is composed of two light chains and two halves of heavy chains. If F(ab)$_2$ is treated to reduce its disulfide bonds, it breaks into two Fab fragments; further disruption of the interchain disulfide bonds in the Fab fragments demonstrates that each contains a light chain and one half of a heavy chain, called the *Fd* fragment. The remainder of the molecule is

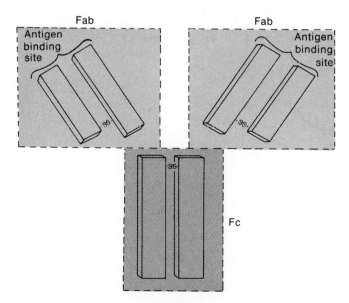

Figure 2–2. Cleavage of antibody molecule by papain.

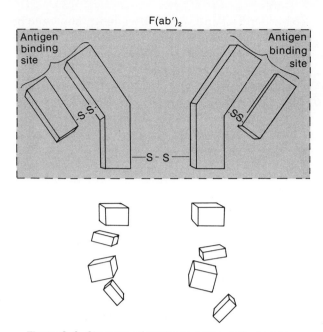

Figure 2-3. Cleavage of antibody molecule by pepsin.

split into many small fragments by pepsin digestion (Fig. 2–3).

These findings provided the following information: (1) the Fc portion of the molecule directs the *biologic activity* of the antibody molecule (e.g., placental transfer of IgG and complement fixing); (2) the Fab portion is involved in antigen binding.

Further studies of the peptide chains have been made by analysis of enzyme digestion products of myeloma proteins. In the disease known as multiple myeloma, for example, a cell making a particular immunoglobulin repeatedly divides in an uncontrolled way. The patient then possesses enormous numbers of identical cells derived as a clone from the original cell, all synthesizing the same immunoglobulin—the myeloma protein, or M-protein, which appears in the serum, often in high concentrations. Purification of the myeloma protein renders a preparation of an immunoglobulin with a unique structure.

Analysis of a number of purified myeloma proteins has revealed that the amino acid sequence of the heavy and light chains contains a "constant" region where the amino acid sequence is identical for the type and subtype, and a "variable" region, consisting of the first 110 to 120 amino acids, which varies widely between type and subtype. The variable part of the peptide chains provides specificity for binding antigen; the constant part is associated with different biologic properties, which vary from one immunoglobulin class to another (Fig. 2–4). In addition, studies of the light chains using the Bence Jones protein (found in a proportion of patients with multiple myeloma) revealed that they could be divided into two groups, called kappa (κ) and lambda (λ), which have very different amino acid sequences and are

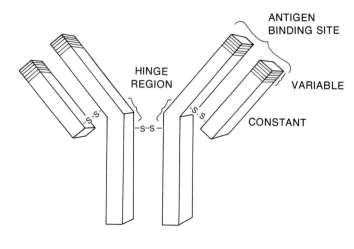

Figure 2-4. IgG molecule, showing constant and variable regions.

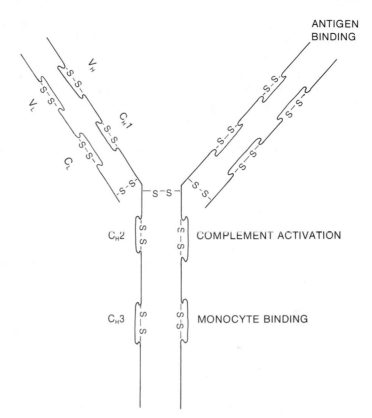

Figure 2–5. Immunoglobulin domains.

antigenically different. Whereas each immunoglobulin class is associated with a particular type of heavy chain, each myeloma protein studied thus far, whatever its class, has possessed light chains of either κ or λ specificity, but never of both together.

General Function of Immunoglobulin

For each molecule of antigen, millions of specific antibody molecules may be produced and secreted into the body fluids. Basically, the function of antibody is to neutralize toxic substances, to facilitate phagocytosis and kill microbes, and to combine with antigens on cellular surfaces and thereby cause the destruction of these cells either extravascularly (outside of the blood vessels within the mononuclear-phagocyte system) or intravascularly (within the blood vessels through the action of complement).

Immunoglobulin Domains

The four chains of the immunglobulin molecule are held together by covalent (disulfide) and non-

covalent bonds. The covalent bonds are located mainly in the hinge region (see Fig 2–4). Additional cystines form interchain disulfide bridges, and their number and position are characteristic for different classes of immunoglobulins. The internal disulfide bridges form loops in the peptide chains that are compactly folded to form globular "domains" (Edelman, 1971; Fig. 2–5) that have distinct biological properties. A light chain consists of one variable (V_L) and one constant (C_L) domain, whereas most heavy chains consist of a variable domain (V_H) and three separate constant domains (C_H1, C_H2, and C_H3). The heavy chains of IgM and IgE have an extra C_L domain.

The variable domains (variable light, V_L; and variable heavy, V_H) are responsible for the formation of a specific antigen-binding site. Studies of several myeloma Ig fragments and one intact IgG molecule through crystallization and X-ray have revealed the way in which millions of different antigen-binding sites are constructed on a common structural theme. All Ig domains have very similar three-dimensional structures based on what is now called the *immunoglobulin fold*. The variable domains each have a particular set of three hypervariable regions that are arranged in three hypervariable loops. The hypervariable loops of both the L and H variable domains are clustered together to form the antigen-binding site. The enormous variability of antigen-binding sites is achieved through changes that occur *only* in the hypervariable amino acids—without disturbing the common overall three-dimensional structure necessary for antibody function. A very small portion of the intact antibody molecule, therefore, is involved in direct antibody binding.

The C_H2 domain in IgG binds C1q, initiating the complement sequence. It is also responsible for the control of catabolic rate. The C_H3 domain is responsible for cytotropic reactions involving macrophages and monocytes, heterologous mast cells, cytotoxic killer (K) cells, and B cells.

Types of Immunoglobulin (Table 2–1)

IgG (Immunoglobulin G)

Of the major classes of immunoglobulins, IgG, which represents about 80 to 85 per cent of the total immunoglobulin, is the best known and most fully studied. It is also known as γ2-globulin and 7Sγ-globulin, the γ indicating its position in the serum electrophoretic profile, which is actually a rather broad region compared with the albumins. The 7S refers to its $S_{20,w}$ sedimentation coefficient (svedberg coefficient), a number that indicates its sedimentation rate in the analytic ultracentrifuge.

In terms of concentration, IgG occurs in amounts of 1,000 to 1,500 mg/dl of serum. This high serum level is a reflection of both the rate of synthesis and the rate of elimination of IgG. The immunoglobulin is produced at the rate of about 28 mg per kg of body weight per day and has a half-life of 21 to 23 days. IgG has a molecular weight of approximately 150,000, 2.2 to 3.5 per cent of which is in the form of carbohydrate. Most bacterial antibodies, virus-neutralizing antibodies, precipitating antibodies, hemagglutinins, and hemolysins are IgG.

The IgG molecule itself is made up of one basic structural unit known as a monomer (see Fig. 2–4), consisting of two heavy chains and two light chains, which may be κ or λ, but not both. The molecule is capable of changing its shape; free IgG is usually Y-shaped, whereas antigen-bound IgG may

TABLE 2–1. Some Biologic Properties of the Immunoglobulins					
Property	IgG	IgM	IgA	IgD	IgE
Molecular weight (approximate in d)	150,000	900,000–1,000,000	150,000–350,000	180,000	190,000
Sedimentation coefficient S_{20w}	6.7–7.0	18.0–19.0	6.6–14.0	6.9–7.0	7.9–8.0
% Carbohydrate	2.2–3.5	7–14	7.5–9.0	12–13	11–12
Normal serum concentration (approximate in mg/dl)	1,000–1,500	100–125	200–250	3	0.01–0.05
Molecular formula	$\gamma_2\kappa_2$ or $\gamma_2\lambda_2$	serum $(\mu_2\kappa_2)5\cdot J$ or $(\mu_2\lambda_2)5\cdot J$	serum $\alpha_2\kappa_2$ or $\alpha_2\lambda_2$ secretory $(\alpha_2\kappa_2)2\cdot J\cdot SC$ or $(\alpha_{2/2})_2 J\cdot SC$	$\delta_2\kappa_2$ or $\delta_2\lambda_2$	$\epsilon_2\kappa_2$ or $\epsilon_2\lambda_2$
Complement fixation (activation of classical pathway)	+	+++	−	−	−
Crosses placenta	+	−	−	−	−
Number of subclasses	4	2	2	−	−
Number of domains on heavy chains	4	5	4	4	5
Half-life (days)	21–23	5–6	5–6.5	2–8	1–5

adjust its shape to accommodate the antigen. This shape change is facilitated by the so-called hinge region, where the chains are uncoiled, allowing for some considerable flexibility (see Fig. 2–4). The reason for this shape change is not fully understood, although Edelman (1971) suggests that it may serve to expose hidden sites responsible for various functions such as complement fixation.

The latest figures, concluded from X-ray diffraction studies on human IgG molecules, give the breadth as 140Å and the length as 85Å.

So far, four subclasses of IgG have been demonstrated: IgG1, IgG2, IgG3, and IgG4. These subclasses are recognized by antisera produced in animals by injecting purified myeloma proteins and absorbing the resulting antiserum with other myeloma proteins. The average concentrations of these subclasses in normal adult serum (according to Fike, 1990) are as follows:

IgG1 = 900 mg/dl (65 to 70 per cent of the total IgG)

IgG2 = 300 mg/dl (25 per cent of the total IgG)

IgG3 = 100 mg/dl (4 to 7 per cent of the total IgG)

IgG4 = 50 mg/dl (3 to 4 per cent of the total IgG)

The number and position of the disulfide bonds vary with the IgG subclass. There are two such bonds in IgG1 and IgG4, four in IgG2 (Nisonoff *et al.*, 1975), and 15 in IgG3 (Fike, 1990; Fig. 2–6).

Differences within IgG subclasses are recognized by antisera against polymorphic antigenic determinants on γ chains. These differences constitute the Gm allotypes. There are also differences among the IgG subclasses with respect to the binding of macrophages and to the activation of complement (Table 2–2).

Most of the IgG in the serum of newborn infants is derived from the mother by placental transfer. A small amount, however, is of fetal origin, as shown by the fact that it may have the father's Gm allotype (Martensson and Fudenberg, 1965). Generally, the amount of IgG starts to increase between 3

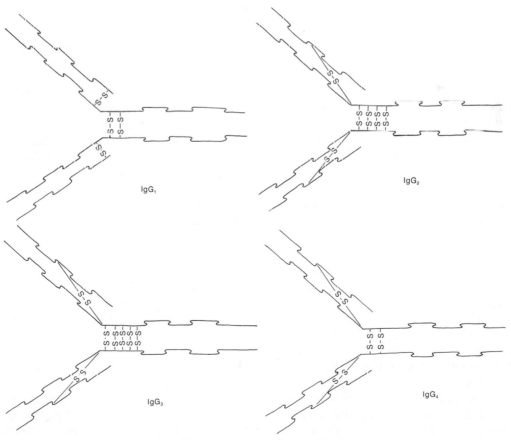

Figure 2–6. Disulfide bonding in human IgG subclasses.

TABLE 2–2. Some Characteristics of IgG Subclasses				
	IgG1	**IgG2**	**IgG3**	**IgG4**
Serum concentration (% total IgG)	65	25	6	4
Serum concentration (approximate in mg/dl)	900	300	100	50
Complement activation (classical pathway)	++	+	+++	−
Placental transfer	+	±	−	+
Reactivity with staphylococcal protein A	+	+	−	+
Gm allotypes	4	2	12	Yes
Molecular weight (approximate in d)	146,000	146,000	170,000	146,000
Number of disulfide bonds linking heavy chains	2	4	15	2
Half-life (days)	22	22	9	22

and 6 weeks after birth: antibodies are detectable at about 2 months, by which time the immunoglobulin level has reached 2 gm per l (Zak and Good, 1959). Barring any immunologic disorders, adult levels of IgG are reached in the child by the seventh year of life and remain relatively constant thereafter (Ricardo and Tomar, 1991).

IgM (Immunoglobulin M)

The IgM molecule is made up of five basic structural units in a circular arrangement (Fig. 2–7). It therefore possesses 10 heavy chains and 10 light chains. The heavy and light chains are linked to each other by disulfide (S-S) bonds in the same general manner as IgG, but there are additional disulfide bonds linking the Fc portions of alternate heavy chains to produce a molecule with a central circular portion and five radiating arms. The disulfide bonds linking the Fc portions can be broken by reducing agents (e.g., 2-mercaptoethanol [2-ME], dithiothreitol [DTT]).

The heavy chains of the IgM molecule are mu (μ) chains; the light chains, as in the case of IgG, are either κ or λ, but not both. A third type of chain, which functions in the joining or linking together of the molecule's subunits, has been termed the J (joining) chain (also found in IgA). This third chain has a molecular weight of about 15,000 and contains about 20 per cent carbohydrate. This J chain is

found invariably in association with intact IgM. The J chain is produced by IgM-secreting cells. It is an acidic glycoprotein with a high content of cysteine residues and is disulfide linked between two IgM monomers' Fc regions at the carboxyl-terminal end, where it presumably initiates the process of oligomerization.

Like IgG, the IgM molecule appears to be quite flexible in the region of the "hinge." It is capable of assuming numerous different shapes, from the fully extended form shown in Figure 2–7 to the dumpy, "crablike" form shown in Figure 2–8.

Electron micrographs of IgM molecules show them to be about 300Å in diameter—the arms being 25 to 30Å wide and 100Å long, the length of the branched sections being 55 to 70Å. The molecular weight of the molecule is 900,000 to 1,000,000; each of the five basic units has a molecular weight of about 180,000 d.

IgM is the antibody that is often first to appear after a primary antigenic stimulus, the first to appear in phylogeny (i.e., in a given species of animal), and the last to leave in senescence (the condition of growing old, i.e., deterioration). It constitutes about 10 per cent of the total immunoglobulin, with an average concentration of about 125 mg/dl. About 80 per cent of IgM is intravascular; 15 to 18 per cent is catabolized per day (Cohen and Freeman, 1960; Schultze and Heremans, 1966; Brown and Cooper, 1970). During the secondary

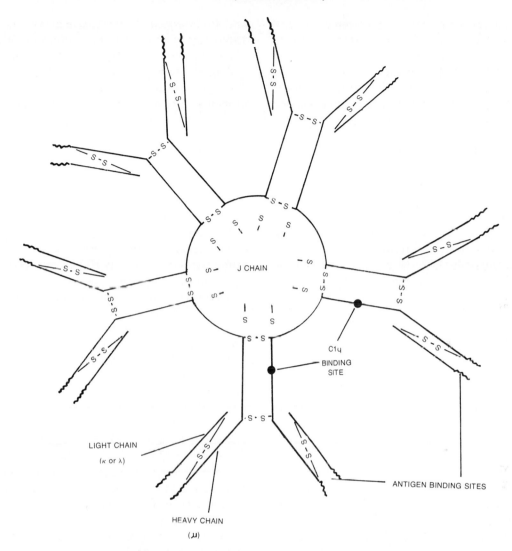

Figure 2–7. Schematic diagram of the IgM pentamer.

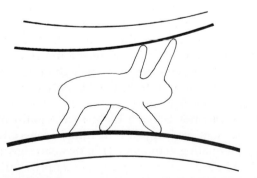

Figure 2–8. Illustration showing one of the possible shape changes of IgM.

response (i.e., the response to the second or subsequent encounter with the same foreign antigen), synthesis of IgM usually diminishes as the concentration of IgG increases.

Intact IgM is cleaved by trypsin (at 25°C) to give in succession $F(ab')_2$ (molecular weight 114,000) and Fab (molecular weight 47,000). (See Nisonoff *et al.*, 1975.)

IgM is the antibody most often formed in response to stimulus by gram-negative bacteria. The Wassermann antibodies, heterophil antibodies, rheumatoid factor, cold agglutinins, and allohemagglutinins also characteristically occur as IgM. There is some doubt as to whether all IgM molecules are capable of binding complement. The immunoglobulin is not transported across the human placenta, and therefore the concentration in cord serum is fetal in origin and measures between 5 and 10 per cent of that found in adult serum (Franklin and Kunkel, 1958; Polly *et al.*, 1962). Within 2 or 3 days of birth, the concentration of IgM starts to rise and reaches 50 per cent of adult level in 2 to 3 months and 100 per cent at about 9 months; between the ages of 9 months and 3 years, values remain at the adult level, although between the ages of 5 and 9 years, they are at the lower end of the adult range (West *et al.*, 1962).

Two IgM subclasses, IgM1 and IgM2, have been recognized, based on differences in the μ chain. A secretory form of IgM has recently been described. Its distribution in body fluids parallels that of secretory IgA.

IgA (Immunoglobulin A)

The main serum component of IgA has been found to have a sedimentation constant of from 6.6 to 14. This suggests that the molecule can be found in varying degrees of polymerization (i.e., having one or more than one structural unit). The heavy chains of the molecule are α, and the light chains, as in IgG and IgM, may be either κ or λ, but not both.

IgA exists as serum IgA and secretory IgA. These two types of IgA are not in equilibrium with each other, but are under separate control mechanisms (Goodman, 1987).

Serum IgA. The predominant portion of IgA in serum is 7S and represents only about 6 per cent of the total immunoglobulin. This is equivalent to 225 ($\pm$55) mg/dl of serum. IgA has a half-life of about 6 days (Tomasi *et al.*, 1965) and is synthesized at a rate of about 2 mg/kg of body weight per day.

Two major subclasses of human IgA, IgA1 and IgA2, are known to exist, of which IgA1 accounts for 90 per cent of the total serum IgA. IgA2 is unique in that it is completely devoid of heavy-light interchain disulfide bonding, the two chains being held together strictly by noncovalent linkages of the standard type (Jerry *et al.*, 1970). The two subclasses are therefore distinguished on the basis of antigenic differences (allotype variation in the α chain of IgA2 depends upon the presence of the antigens A2m[1] and A2m[2], whereas the α chains of IgA1 do not express allotypic variation) (Kunkel

and Prendergast, 1966; Vaerman and Heremans, 1966), as well as striking structural differences (Gray, 1970; see also Barrett, 1983).

Papain and pepsin digestion of serum IgA yields the expected Fab or F(ab')$_2$ units, but the Fc and Fc' units are difficult to isolate because of their sensitivity to further digestion by papain or pepsin. Certain bacterial proteases cleave only IgA1. Reductive cleavage to release heavy and light chains is also possible.

IgA cannot be detected in cord serum. By the age of 2 months, the amount in serum has reached about 20 per cent of the adult level (West *et al.*, 1962).

The function of serum IgA is unknown, although it may be important in antigen clearance and immune regulation. About 10 per cent of the serum IgA is in dimeric form (Ernst *et al.*, 1987).

Secretory IgA. Whereas the ratio of IgG to IgA in serum is 6:1, in the internal secretions (synovial fluid, cerebrospinal fluid, aqueous humor, and so forth) and in the external secretions (i.e., colostrum and early milk, nasal and respiratory mucus, intestinal mucus, saliva, and so forth) IgA is usually present in a much higher concentration than either IgG or IgM. In these external secretions, IgA serves as a first line of defense against microorganism invasion. It is particularly important in preventing gastrointestinal infections of the secreting glands. In contrast to IgG and IgM, the immunoglobulin is synthesized in plasma cells located primarily in the epithelial surfaces of the respiratory tract and intestine and in almost all excretory glands.

Following synthesis, some of the IgA finds its way into the systemic circulation, but most of it passes through or between the epithelial cells to be secreted. This last is known as secretory IgA (SIgA). The SIgA molecule is made up of two basic structural units (known as a "dimer") and a glycoprotein secretory component, which is linked to the respective heavy chains of the molecule by disulfide bonds and may serve to make the molecule more resistant to enzyme attacks. The J chain described in IgM is also found in SIgA and in polymeric forms of serum IgA (Fig. 2–9).

IgA does not activate the classical pathway of complement and appears to inhibit the complement-activating activity of IgG; however IgA does activate the alternate pathway of complement. IgA is not transported across the human placenta.

The functions of secretory IgA are numerous

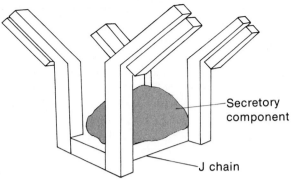

Figure 2-9. Secretory IgA (SIgA).

compared with serum IgA. Because of its unique association of the secretory component, the IgA dimer is resistant to proteolysis. The inhibitory effect on IgG complement activation (mentioned above) and the activation of the alternative pathway may both provide protection and promote inflammation. Receptors for IgA have been found on inflammatory cells. IgA may help in the destruction of bacteria and other cellular pathogens by antibody-dependent cell-mediated cytotoxicity. Secretory IgA can bind to some microorganisms, which may inhibit the ability of the microorganisms to move or to bind to the mucosal wall, preventing colonization. Individuals who are IgA-deficient have increased mucosal infections, atopy, and autoimmune diseases (Ernst *et al.*, 1987).

IgE (Immunoglobulin E)

The existence of a heat-labile antibody, originally called *reagin* (Note: This is separate and different from the reagin of syphilis) in the sera of individuals displaying various allergies was first encountered by Prausnitz and Küstner in 1921. This antibody was noted to have the following characteristics:

1. It was specific for the allergen or antigen that evoked its production.
2. It would not pass the placenta to passively hypersensitize the fetus.
3. It would not give the usual *in vitro* serologic reactions in tests such as precipitation, agglutination, complement fixation, or others associated with the heat-stable immunoglobulins.
4. On passive transfer to a normal individual, it would "fix" in the skin for several days or weeks.

Immunization of rabbits with a reagin-rich fraction prepared by DEAE cellulose ion exchange chromatography and Sephadex gel filtration resulted in an antiserum that would remove the reaginic activity of sera by serologic precipitation. Adsorption of this rabbit antiserum with the four well-known immunoglobulins did not delete the antibody from the precipitated reagin. By the extensive use of radioimmunodiffusion experiments, it was shown that reagin was in fact a new and distinct immunoglobulin; it was named IgE, the E assigned because the reagin most studied was specific for the antigen E of ragweed. IgE now refers to reagin in a general sense, and its specificity for an antigen is designated in the same way as for any other immunoglobulin.

For several years after its discovery, critical biochemical studies of the immunoglobulin were hampered by the fact that it only occurs in minute quantities in normal sera, constituting about 0.004 per cent of the total immunoglobulin, and that sera from allergic individuals with elevated IgE levels were not available for testing. The dilemma was resolved by the discovery in Sweden of a patient with a unique myeloma protein, which proved to be identical to IgE. From studies of this protein, the following data have been accumulated: IgE has a molecular weight of 190,000 and is a 7.9 to 8.0S molecule. It has a carbohydrate content of 11 to 12 per cent, and its concentration in serum is 0.01 to 0.05 mg/dl. It has a half-life of 2.5 days. Once bound to the effector cell surface by the Fc receptor, however, the half-life increases to 6 to 12 weeks (Bennich, 1974). The rate of synthesis of IgE is 2.3 μg/kg of body weight per day. There are no heavy chain subclasses of IgE, and the heavy chain has five constant domains.

Papain digestion of IgE produces several fragments, including the two Fab units and an Fc unit. In addition, a light chain fragment known as lambda C, an Fc″, and a $7S_{20,w}$ fragment are produced.

The role of IgE in allergic conditions is now clear. Hypersensitivities caused by IgE may assume any of several forms from the life-threatening anaphylactic reactions to the milder discomforts associated with food allergies. Regardless of their severity, these depend upon the presence of an IgE with a serologic specificity for the offending allergen. The combination of the allergen with IgE on the surface of mast cells and basophils releases pharmacologic agents that trigger an immediate physiologic response. (For further discussion, see Henry, 1991 [pp. 822–823]; Chen, 1990; Sheehan, 1990. See also Chapter 4 of this text.)

IgD (Immunoglobulin D)

IgD was first identified as a unique immunoglobulin in human serum in 1965 as a result of the discovery of a myeloma protein that was found to be antigenically different from other immunoglobulins. Since that time, many other examples of IgD-related myeloma proteins have been reported, although they are now known to occur in only 3 per cent of all myelomas.

IgD occurs in minute quantities in serum (3 mg/dl); therefore, the majority of chemical data available with respect to this immunoglobulin have been derived from the gamma D myeloma proteins.

IgD, like all other immunoglobulins, is made up of a basic structure of two heavy chains and two light chains. Both κ and λ light chains have been detected, although the λ-type myelomas predominate (80 per cent, compared with 20 per cent κ-type). The heavy chain of IgD, designated delta (δ), is structurally and antigenically different from the heavy chains of other immunoglobulins, although the κ and λ light chains do not differ from their kind in other immunoglobulins. The δ chain (heavy chain) has a molecular weight of 70,000 (approximately 12,000 greater than the γ chains of IgG). This additional molecular weight has led to the suggestion that the δ chain has a fourth CH unit or that the hinge region may be extended. Because of this high molecular weight of the heavy chain, IgD has an overall molecular weight of 180,000, rather than 160,000. It occurs as a 6.9 to 7.0S molecule.

Papain digestion results in the expected two Fab and one Fc fragments, but the Fc fragment is rapidly degraded further and, as such, is difficult to isolate intact.

IgD constitutes less than 1 per cent of the total immunoglobulin and contains about 12 per cent polysaccharide (all of which is attached to the heavy chain), which appears to be divided into three discrete sections, one located at the Fc-Fd interface (hinge region) and the other two in the Fc region.

IgD is synthesized at a rate of 0.4 mg/kg of body weight per day (i.e., about 100 times less than the synthetic rate of IgG) and has a half-life of only 2 to 3 days. The immunoglobulin is heat and acid labile; if stored at 56°C for 1 hour, its amount in serum is reduced by half, and, after 4 hours, only 10 per cent is recoverable. A pH of 3 denatures IgD. IgD aggregates very readily, which can change its biologic activity as well as its structure.

Very little is known about the functional importance of IgD. There is evidence, however, to suggest that IgD may be important as a membrane receptor and is synthesized early in the antigen-independent differentiation of B cells (it has been found on the surface of B cells in association with IgM) (discussed later in this chapter) (Barrett, 1988; Ernst, 1987). IgD has also been reported to have antibody activity to insulin, penicillin, nuclear antigens, and thyroid antigen.

CELLS INVOLVED IN SPECIFIC IMMUNITY

The cells involved in specific immunity include the lymphocytes and plasma cells. Lymphocytes recognize foreign antigens and/or produce antibodies; plasma cells produce antibodies.

It is generally accepted that the "parent" cell of all erythroid, myeloid, and lymphoid cellular elements is the pluripotent hemopoietic stem cell, which migrates from the yolk sac through the fetal liver, spleen, and bone marrow. From these sites, some lymphoid stem cells migrate to the thymus, where further differentiation occurs, resulting in the production of thymus-derived cells (T cells). Other lymphoid stem cells are independent of the thymus. In birds, they come under the influence of the bursa of Fabricius; in humans and other mammals, a mammalian equivalent such as the fetal liver, bone marrow, or gut-associated lymphoid tissue appears to be involved. These lymphoid stem cells differentiate to become bursa- or bone marrow-derived cells (B cells).

Both B and T lymphocytes, on appropriate stimulation by antigen, proliferate and undergo morphologic changes. The T lymphocytes become lymphoblasts, which are involved in cell-mediated reactions, and the B lymphocytes become plasma cells, which are involved in humoral antibody synthesis (Fig. 2–10).

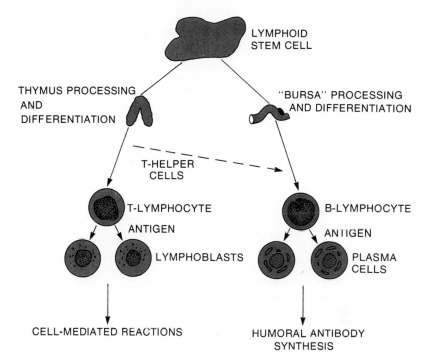

LYMPHOID
STEM CELL

THYMUS PROCESSING
AND
DIFFERENTIATION

"BURSA" PROCESSING
AND DIFFERENTIATION

T-HELPER
CELLS

T-LYMPHOCYTE

ANTIGEN

B-LYMPHOCYTE

ANTIGEN

LYMPHOBLASTS

PLASMA
CELLS

CELL-MEDIATED REACTIONS

HUMORAL ANTIBODY
SYNTHESIS

Figure 2–10. Processing and differentiation of lymphoid stem cells into immunocompetent T and B lymphocytes and further transformation and proliferation to cells of the lymphoblast and plasma cell series.

In addition to B and T lymphocytes, natural killer (NK) cells, as well as monocytes, neutrophils, eosinophils, and basophils, are also involved in the immune response. In the discussion that follows, their interaction during humoral and cell-mediated immunity is examined.

T Lymphocytes

T cells (or T lymphocytes), which represent approximately 80 per cent of the circulating lymphocytes in the peripheral blood, are associated with two types of immunologic functions, known as "effector" and "regulatory." The effector functions include the cytolysis of virally infected cells and tumor targets and the production of lymphokine. The regulatory functions include the ability to amplify or suppress other effector lymphocytes (including B and T cells).

A series of monoclonal antibodies has recently been developed that identifies the lymphocyte surface glycoproteins known as CD (cluster of differentiation) (see Table 2–3). Most circulating T cells express three of the following CD markers:

CD2: This is the sheep red blood cell (SRBC) re-

ceptor, which is the classical T-cell surface marker. When T cells are incubated with SRBC, SRBCs bind to T cells to form rosettes.

CD3: This is part of T-cell antigen-receptor complex.

CD4: This is the receptor for MHC class II molecule.

CD8: This is the receptor for MHC class I molecule.

Two subpopulations of T cells are identified in the circulation—those with the CD2, CD3, CD4 phenotype, which are associated with helper-inducer activity, and those with the CD2, CD3, CD8 phenotype, which are associated with cytotoxic or suppressor activity. It should be noted that this functional association with CD4 and CD8 (the only difference between the two subpopulations) is now believed not to be as simplistic as was once thought.

The Differentiation of T Lymphocytes

As mentioned, stem cells, or pre-T cells, arise in the bone marrow (or fetal liver) and migrate into the thymus, where they acquire developmental maturation. Bone marrow T cells do not express CD gly-

CD Designation	Molecular Weight (Kd)	Cellular Distribution	Comment	Similar Antibody Clones
CD1A	49	Thymocytes	Also expressed on Langerhans' cells in skin	OKT6, T6, Anti-Leu-6
CD2	45–50	T cells	SRBC-receptor (E-rosette receptor)	OKT11, T11, Anti-Leu-5b
CD3	19–25	T cells	Associated with T-antigen receptor	OKT3, T3, Ant-Leu-4
CD4	55–64	T-helper/inducer cells	MHC class II molecule receptor	OKT4, T4, Anti-Leu-3a
CD8	33–43	T-suppressor/cytotoxic cells	MHC class I molecule receptor	OKT8, OKT5, T8, Anti-Leu-2a
CD19	40–80	B cells		B4, Anti-Leu-12
CD20	35	B cells		B1, Anti-Leu-16
CD21	145	Mature B cells	C3d receptor	B2, Anti-CR2

TABLE 2–3. CD Markers Frequently Used to Identify T and B Cells

A more comprehensive list of CD markers and their defining monoclonal antibodies, molecular sizes, and functions can be found in Rowlands *et al.*, 1991.

coprotein, but they do contain an enzyme known as terminal deoxynucleotidyl transferase (TdT).

The earliest differentiation event is the acquisition of CD2 and CD3, which occurs in the thymic cortex. Later differentiation in the cortex is the expression of both CD4 and CD8. As the T cells move through the thymic medulla, two major events occur: (1) the development of two distinct T-cell populations, the helper-inducer T cells (CD4+) and suppressor-cytotoxic T cells (CD8+), and (2) the loss of TdT enzyme. (It is interesting to note that approximately 90 per cent of T cells die in the thymus and never enter the peripheral circulation.) The most important outcome of intrathymic differentiation is that the T cells learn to recognize self-MHC gene products. This is essential for cellular interaction in the immune responses (Osmond, 1985; Reinherz and Schlossman, 1981).

For further information regarding T-cell involvement in the immune response, see Chapter 4.

B Lymphocytes

Bone marrow-derived lymphocytes (B cells) are the precursor cells in antibody production. B-line stem cells in the bone marrow are the source of the pre-B cell. This pre-B cell, even in the animal not yet stimulated by an antigen, synthesizes IgM heavy chains (though not light chains), the globulin being confined to the cytoplasm of the cell and not secreted (as opposed to the mature B cell, which does secrete IgM and has it on its surface). It also expresses MHC class II molecules and complement receptors on the cell surface. From the bone marrow, the pre-B cell migrates to the germinal centers of the lymph nodes and spleen. As it does so, it loses some of its cytoplasmic IgM heavy chains and becomes a smaller cell with acquired surface IgM and IgD. At this stage, the B cell can be identified by the CD glycoproteins CD19, CD20, and CD21 and by surface receptors for complement components, especially C1q, C3b, C3d, and C4b, and receptors for the Fc region of IgG. The I-A and/or I-E proteins are also present in these cells.

This immature B cell differentiates into a mature B cell after antigen exposure, after which it secretes a single class of immunoglobulin molecule that is specific for a single determinant on the antigen. At the same time, there is a morphologic differentiation into a plasma cell, which is the most proficient antibody-forming cell. It should be noted that although the plasma cell contains immunoglobulin, it lacks SIg and other B-cell markers, such as Fc receptors, complement receptors, MHC class II molecules, and monoclonal antibody-defined CD glycoproteins. It is also a terminally differentiated B cell.

In the peripheral blood, approximately 5 to 15 per cent of the circulating lymphocytes are B cells, identified on the basis of their surface immunoglobulin (SIg). As mentioned, the majority of human peripheral blood B cells express both IgM and IgD; however, some B cells express IgG, IgA, or IgE. In mucosal associated lymphoid tissues, the majority of B cells express IgA as their SIg. Approximately 50 per cent of tonsillar and splenic lymphocytes are B cells.

Although B cells have many common features, they can be subdivided into major subsets on the basis of the class of immunoglobulin that they are patterned to synthesize. These are known as Bμ (IgM), Bγ (IgG), Bα (IgA), Bδ (IgD), and Bε (IgE). Within each of these subsets, further differentiation is possible, based on the type of light chain involved (κ or λ) and on the subclass of the heavy chain.

All B cells are not necessarily fixed to synthesize just one type of immunoglobulin, because class "switch" from IgM to IgG has been reported. The stimulus for this may be reexposure to antigen and assistance from T cells.

The immunoglobulin on the B-cell surface behaves as a specific receptor for antigen. The immunoglobulin has been shown to be randomly distributed over the surface of the B cell (through histochemical techniques). When antigen is added, the immunoglobulin begins to accumulate in distinct foci that further blend into one agglomerate. This is known as *lymphocyte capping*, after which there is a gradual disappearance of the antigen and the immunoglobulin as the complex moves into the interior of the cell.

Lymphocyte capping is peculiar to B cells and is not demonstrated by T cells. It signals a phase of cell differentiation into actively secreting plasma cells and memory cells, the latter of which cannot be described in cytologic terms but which are responsible for the recognition of antigen on reexposure. Plasma cells, however, are easily recognized both morphologically and functionally.

B-cell transformation into plasma cells is also stimulated by certain so-called *mitogens*, which are polyclonal in their stimulating effect (as opposed to antigen, which is characterized as monoclonal).

Polyclonal mitogens stimulate all B cells regardless of their antigen specificity, which reflects a shared ability of the mitogens to affect the plasticity of the B-cell cytoplasmic membrane in the same manner accomplished by antigen.

The most specific of the commonly used B-cell mitogens is the lipopolysaccharide (LPS), which is extracted from the cell wall of many gram-negative bacteria, where it functions as the somatic or O antigen and is an endotoxin. The lipid portion of LPS is the site of its mitogenic activity. Other mitogens for B cells include protein A (found on the surface of the bacterium *Staphylococcus aureus*), which combines with immunoglobulin on the B cell by a different mechanism than antigen but nevertheless stimulates lymphocyte transformation.

The end cell of the B-cell lineage is the plasma cell. This is about the same size as the small lymphocyte (6 to 10 μm), although not all plasma cells are the same size, and some may approach 20 μm in diameter. The nucleus for the plasma cell is in the center, and the cytoplasm, which is usually sparse in relation to that of other cells, is usually gathered at one side. The nucleus stains darkly, and the lumpy strands of chromatin give it a "cartwheel" appearance. The cytosol of plasma cells is literally filled with rough endoplasmic reticulum. This complex intracellular system consists of two serpentine, parallel membranes, which are laden with ribosomes (Fig. 2–11). The ribosomes contain considerable RNA and serve as the site of messenger RNA attachment during protein synthesis. It is here that immunoglobulin synthesis occurs.

Natural Killer (NK) Cells

The peripheral lymphocytes from nonimmunized individuals or the spleen of nonimmunized mice may also contain a population of large granular lymphocytes (LGLs) that are cytotoxic for several targets and are referred to as natural killer (NK) cells because of their wide-ranging cytotoxic abilities. These cells do not consistently express markers for B or T lymphocytes, although they do have surface IgG Fc receptors. NK cells are able to lyse virally infected cells and tumor cells without prior immunization. Unlike cytotoxic T cells, the cytolytic activity of NK cells is not MHC restricted

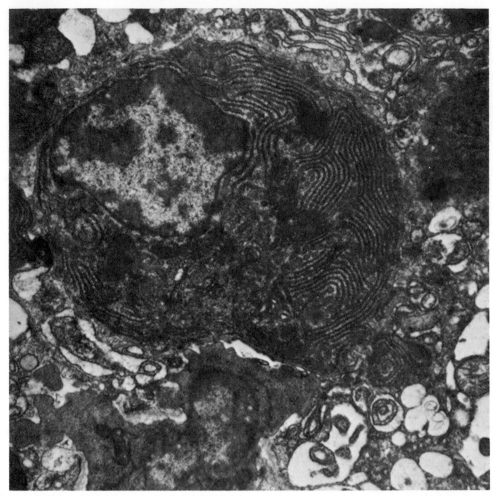

Figure 2–11. Plasma cells. (From Barrett, J. T.: Textbook of Immunology, 4th ed. St. Louis, The C. V. Mosby Company, 1983, p. 95. Courtesy of Dr. E. Adelstein.)

(i.e., they are capable of killing cells that do not have the same histocompatibility antigen on their surfaces). NK cells also play an important role in antibody-dependent cell-mediated cytolysis (ADCC) (Reinherz and Schlossman, 1981).

OTHER CELLS OF THE IMMUNE SYSTEM

Monocytes and Macrophages

Circulating monocytes, which represent approximately 4 to 10 per cent of circulating nucleated cells, are able to migrate into various tissues and become tissue macrophages. Their two main functions include the removal of particulate antigens

and the presentation of antigens to the lymphocytes. The surface markers of monocytes and macrophages are IgG Fc receptor, complement receptor, and MHC class II molecule (Reinherz and Schlossman, 1981; Platt, 1979).

Polymorphonuclear Granulocytes

The polymorphonuclear granulocytes are a heterogenous group of cells that include the neutrophils, eosinophils, and basophils. These cells are able to adhere to and penetrate the endothelial cell lining of blood vessels and migrate into surrounding tissues. They play an important role in acute inflammation (see Chapter 1).

Neutrophils. The major function of neutrophils, which represent about 70 per cent of circulating nucleated cells, is phagocytosis. This phagocytic activity is enhanced when particles (or antigens) are coated with antibody and/or complement, since Fc complement receptors are expressed on the cell surface. In this way (i.e., with the aid of complement and antibody), neutrophils play an important role in protection against extracellular microorganism infection (Reinherz and Schlossman, 1981; Platt, 1979).

Eosinophils. The major function of eosinophils is probably to kill an invading organism by releasing the granular contents of its cytoplasm to the extracellular space. For this reason, it is thought that eosinophils play an important role in protection against helminth infection. Eosinophils are triggered to release histamine and aryl sulfatase at the site of allergic response. This has the effect of inactivating the allergic mediators (e.g., histamine and slow-reacting substances of anaphylaxis), thereby dampening the allergic response.

Basophils and Mast Cells. Basophils and mast cells express Fc receptors for IgE heavy chain; therefore, IgE antibodies bind to these cells and remain stable for a long period of time. The cross-linking of the cell surface IgE by an allergen triggers the cell to release its granular contents, containing histamine and other vasoactive amines, which initiates allergic reaction.

Basophils and mast cells are indistinguishable from each other in a number of properties and functions, yet it is clear that they represent distinct cell populations.

JUST THE FACTS

Introduction

1. Specific immunity is an adaptive response to foreign antigenic stimulus that results in the production of specific antibody.
2. Immunity is conferred by actual infection resulting in antibody production (active immunity) or by artificial transmission of antibodies that give temporary protection against antigen (passive immunity).
3. Sometimes "cross-immunity" allows for immunity against one infectious agent to contribute some immunity against other infectious agents.
4. The degree of protection is determined by the

size of the infecting dose, the route of administration, and the type of infective agent.
5. Active immunity may be caused by clinical or subclinical infection, the injection of live or killed microorganisms or the antigens, and/or the absorption of bacterial toxins.
6. Antibodies may take from a few days to a few weeks to develop, yet persist for years.
7. The two types of reaction to foreign antigen invasion are humoral immunity and cell-mediated immunity.

Antigens (Immunogens)

1. An antigen is any molecular structure that, when introduced into an animal, is capable of causing the production of antibodies by that animal.
2. The term "immunogen" is correctly defined as a substance that causes a detectable immune response. The term "antigen"—though used synonymously with "immunogen"—actually refers to the ability of a substance to combine with an antibody.
3. The two major classes of immunogens are "thymic-dependent" (i.e., requiring the help of T cells for antibody formation) and "thymic independent" (or "thymus efficient," i.e., requiring minimal help of T cells for antibody formation).
4. Antigens can be autologous ("self"), heterologous (different from that used in immunization), homologous (used in antibody production), or heterophil (existing in unrelated plants or animals but cross-reacting with other antibodies).

Factors Affecting Immunogenicity

1. What makes a substance immunogenic is unknown. The contributing factors include foreignness, size, diversity, chemical composition and complexity, genetic composition, route, dosage, and timing of administration.

The Chemical Nature of Antigens

1. Antigens are either proteins or large polysaccharides.
2. Lipids are poor antigens unless linked to proteins or polysaccharides.
3. Nucleic acids are poor antigens unless linked to an immunogenic carrier.

4. Carbohydrates are too small to be antigens unless coupled to protein or lipid carriers.
5. Cell surface antigens can be composed of combinations of biochemical classes.
6. HLA antigens are glycoprotein in nature.

Antibodies

1. Antibodies are substances produced in response to antigenic stimulation that are capable of specific interaction with the provoking immunogen.
2. Antibodies are referred to as "immunoglobulins."

Structure of Immunoglobulins

1. The basic immunoglobulin molecule is a symmetrical, four-peptide unit consisting of two heavy chains and two light chains linked by disulfide bonds.
2. The number of disulfide bonds between heavy chains varies from 1 to 14.
3. Only one disulfide bond joins a heavy and a light chain (in most classes and subclasses).
4. The molecule appears Y-shaped.
5. Enzyme treatment of immunoglobulin results in the splitting of the molecule into fragments.
6. Fragmentation of immunoglobulin has revealed that the Fc portion directs the biologic activity of the molecule while the Fab portion is involved in antigen binding.
7. Heavy and light chains contain a "constant" region (where the amino acid sequence is identical for the type and subtype) and a "variable" region (the first 110 to 120 amino acids), which varies widely between type and subtype.
8. Light chains can be divided into two groups known as κ and λ.

General Function of Immunoglobulin

1. Immunoglobulins function to neutralize toxic substances, to facilitate phagocytosis and kill microbes, and to combine with antigens on cellular surfaces in order to cause the destruction of these cells.

Immunoglobulin Domains

1. Internal disulfide bridges form loops in the peptide chain, forming "domains" that have distinct biological properties.
2. Light chains have one variable and one constant domain.
3. Most heavy chains have one variable domain and three constant domains.
4. IgE light chains have an extra constant domain.
5. Variable domains are responsible for the formation of specific antigen-binding sites.
6. The C_H2 domain in IgG binds C1q and controls catabolic rate.
7. The C_H3 domain in IgG is responsible for cytotropic reactions involving macrophages and monocytes, heterologous mast cells, cytotoxic killer cells, and B cells.

Types of Immunoglobulin

1. The properties of the immunoglobulins should be studied by carefully examining Table 2–1.

IgG

1. The four subclasses of IgG are known as IgG1, IgG2, IgG3, and IgG4.
2. The number of disulfide bonds varies with the IgG subclass.
3. Differences within IgG subclasses are recognized by Gm allotypes.
4. The subclasses also differ with respect to binding of macrophages and activation of complement.
5. Most serum IgG in newborns is maternal in origin.
6. IgG starts to increase between 3 and 6 months after birth and reaches adult levels by age 7, after which it remains constant.

IgM

1. The IgM molecule is a pentamer (five basic structural units).
2. The heavy chains of IgM are mu (μ) chains, and the light chains are either κ or λ, but not both.
3. The J chain (also found in IgA) joins the molecule's subunits.

4. IgM is flexible in the region of the hinge and is capable of assuming numerous shapes.
5. IgM is the antibody first to appear after a primary antigenic stimulus, the first to appear in phylogeny, and the last to leave in senescence.
6. During the secondary response, IgM usually diminishes as the level of IgG increases.
7. Intact IgM is cleaved by trypsin.
8. IgM is the antibody most often formed in response to stimulus by gram-negative bacteria.
9. The Wassermann antibodies, heterophil antibodies, rheumatoid factor, cold agglutinins, and allohemagglutinins characteristically occur as IgM.
10. There is some doubt as to whether all IgM molecules are capable of binding complement.
11. IgM is not transported across the human placenta.
12. The concentration of IgM in cord serum is fetal in origin and measures between 5 and 10 per cent of that found in adult serum.
13. IgM has two subclasses, IgM1 and IgM2. The differences are based on differences in the μ chain.
14. A secretory form of IgM has recently been described. Its distribution in body fluids parallels that of secretory IgA.

IgA

1. The heavy chains of IgA are α; the light chains are either κ or λ, but not both.
2. IgA exists as serum IgA and secretory IgA.
3. Two major subclasses of IgA are known (IgA1 and IgA2), of which IgA1 accounts for 90 per cent of the total serum IgA. IgA2 is devoid of heavy-light interchain disulfide bonding.
4. Papain and pepsin digestion of serum IgA yields Fab or F(ab')$_2$ units. The Fc and Fc' units are difficult to isolate because of their sensitivity to further digestion by these enzymes.
5. IgA cannot be detected in cord serum.
6. The function of serum IgA is unknown.
7. In the external secretions, IgA is present in higher concentration than IgG or IgM.
8. In the external secretions, IgA serves as the first line of defense.
9. IgA is synthesized in plasma cells located primarily in the epithelial surfaces of the respi-

ratory tract and intestine and in almost all excretory glands.
10. Following synthesis, most IgA passes through or between the epithelial cells to be secreted. This is known as secretory IgA (SIgA).
11. SIgA occurs as a dimer with a secretory component and a J chain.
12. IgA does not activate the classical pathway of complement but does activate the alternative pathway.
13. The functions of secretory IgA are numerous compared with serum IgA.
14. Individuals who are IgA deficient have increased mucosal infections, atopy, and autoimmune diseases.

IgE

1. IgE was originally called "reagin."
2. IgA occurs in minute quantities in normal serum.
3. Papain digestion produces several fragments including the two Fab and an Fc unit. The other fragments are known as C, an Fc″, and a $7S_{20w}$.
4. There are no heavy chain subclasses of IgE, and the heavy chain has five constant domains.
5. IgE has a role in allergic conditions.

IgD

1. IgD occurs in minute quantities in serum.
2. IgD occurs as a monomer.
3. The heavy chain (δ) is structurally and antigenically different from the heavy chains of other immunoglobulins.
4. λ-Type light chains are more common than κ light chains.
5. Papain digestion results in two Fab fragments and one Fc fragment. The Fc is rapidly degraded further.
6. IgD is heat and acid labile.
7. Very little is known about the functional importance of IgD.

Cells Involved in Specific Immunity

1. The cells involved in specific immunity include lymphocytes, plasma cells, natural killer (NK) cells, monocytes, neutrophils, eosinophils, basophils, and mast cells.

T Lymphocytes

1. T cells represent about 80 per cent of the circulating lymphocytes.
2. T cells are associated with "effector" and "regulatory" functions.
3. T cells of phenotype CD2, CD3, CD4 are associated with helper-inducer activities.
4. T cells of phenotype CD2, CD3, CD8 are associated with cytotoxic or suppressor activities (examine Table 2–2).

B Lymphocytes

1. About 5 to 15 per cent of the circulating lymphocytes in the peripheral blood are B cells.
2. B cells are identified on the basis of their surface immunoglobulin.
3. The majority of B cells express both IgM and IgD—some express IgG, IgA, or IgE.
4. B cells can be subdivided into major subsets on the basis of the class of immunoglobulin they are patterned to synthesize.
5. All B cells are not necessarily fixed to synthesize just one type of immunoglobulin.
6. Lymphocyte capping is peculiar to B cells.
7. B-cell transformation into plasma cells can be stimulated by certain mitogens.

8. The end cell of the B-cell lineage is the plasma cell, which is an efficient antibody producer.

Natural Killer (NK) Cells

1. Large granular lymphocytes (LGLs) found in nonimmunized individuals that are cytotoxic for several targets are called natural killer (NK) cells.
2. These cells do not consistently express markers for B or T lymphocytes, although they do have surface IgG Fc receptors.
3. NK cells are able to lyse virally infected cells and tumor cells without prior immunization.
4. NK cells are not MHC restricted.
5. NK cells play an important role in ADCC.

Other Cells of the Immune System

1. Other cells of the immune system include:
   a. Monocytes and macrophages, which remove particulate antigens and present antigens to the lymphocytes.
   b. Polymorphonuclear granulocytes, which include neutrophils, eosinophils, basophils, and mast cells, and which play an important role in acute inflammation.

Review Questions

Multiple Choice

Choose the phrase, sentence, or symbol that completes the statement or answers the question. More than one answer may be correct in each case. Answers are given at the end of this book.

1. The artificial transmission of antibodies, which provide temporary protection against invading antigen, is known as:
   (a) active immunity
   (b) passive immunity
   (c) cell-mediated response
   (d) cross-immunity
   (Introduction)

2. Active immunity may be caused by:
   (a) clinical or subclinical infection
   (b) the injection of live or killed microorganisms or their antigens
   (c) the absorption of bacterial toxins
   (d) the artificial transmission of antibodies
   (Introduction)

3. The term "immunogen" refers to:
   (a) the ability of a substance to combine with antibody
   (b) a substance that causes a detectable immune response
   (c) an antibody
   (d) a substance that is capable of cross-reactivity
   (Antigens [Immunogens])

4. Factors that contribute to making a substance immunogenic include:
   (a) molecular weight
   (b) an unfamiliar chemical structure
   (c) the timing of parenteral administration
   (d) genetic composition
   (Factors Affecting Immunogenicity)

5. Antigens:
   (a) are usually large organic molecules
   (b) may be protein
   (c) may be large polysaccharides
   (d) are usually lipids
   (The Chemical Nature of Antigens)

6. The treatment of IgG with the enzyme pepsin:
   (a) results in two F(ab')₂ fragments
   (b) results in two Fab fragments and one Fc fragment
   (c) results in two Fab fragments and two Fc fragments
   (d) none of the above
   (Structure of Immunoglobulins)

7. The basic function of antibody is to:
   (a) neutralize toxic substances
   (b) facilitate phagocytosis
   (c) combine with antigen
   (d) all of the above
   (General Function of Immunoglobulin)

8. Variable domains on the immunoglobulin molecule are responsible for:
   (a) the initiation of the complement sequence
   (b) the control of catabolic rate
   (c) the formation of a specific antigen-binding site
   (d) cytotropic reactions
   (Immunoglobulin Domains)

9. IgG:
   (a) is a monomer
   (b) has a half-life of 2 to 3 days
   (c) is capable of crossing the placenta
   (d) is known to have five subclasses
   (IgG)

10. Which of the following antibodies are characteristically IgM?
    (a) Wassermann antibodies
    (b) rheumatoid factor
    (c) heterophil antibodies
    (d) cold agglutinins
    (IgM)

11. IgA:
    (a) exists only as a dimer
    (b) is detected in cord serum
    (c) is present in external secretions in higher concentration than IgG or IgM
    (d) is devoid of heavy-light interchain disulfide bonding
    (IgA)

12. IgE:
    (a) was originally called "ragweed"
    (b) constitutes 10 to 20 per cent of total immunoglobulin
    (c) has a molecular weight of 190,000
    (d) crosses the human placenta
    (IgE)

13. IgD:
    (a) is heat and acid labile
    (b) occurs in large quantities in serum
    (c) has a molecular weight of 160,000
    (d) is denatured at a pH of 7
    (IgD)

14. The cells involved in specific immunity include:
    (a) T cells
    (b) B cells
    (c) A cells
    (d) all of the above
    (IgA)

15. T cells with the phenotype CD2, CD3, CD4 are associated with:
    (a) helper-inducer activity
    (b) cytotoxic activity
    (c) suppressor activity
    (d) none of the above
    (T Lymphocytes)

16. B lymphocytes:
    (a) constitute approximately 90 per cent of the circulating lymphocytes in the peripheral blood
    (b) are bone-marrow–derived lymphocytes
    (c) can be identified by the CD glycoproteins CD19, CD20, and CD21
    (d) synthesize IgG only
    (B Lymphocytes)

17. Natural killer (NK) cells:
    (a) have surface IgG Fc receptors
    (b) express markers for B or T lymphocytes
    (c) are MHC restricted
    (d) are not MHC restricted
    (Natural Killer [NK] Cells)

18. Other cells of the immune system include:
    (a) monocytes
    (b) macrophages
    (c) neutrophils
    (d) eosinophils
    (Other Cells of the Immune System)

Answer "True" or "False"

1. When an immunogen combines with an antibody molecule, this would most correctly be termed an immunogen-antibody reaction.
   (Antigens [Immunogens])

2. An antigen used in the production of antibody is termed a "homologous" antigen.
   (Antigens [Immunogens])

3. One of the factors that contribute to the immunogenicity of a substance is the size of the substance.
   (Factors Affecting Immunogenicity)

4. HLA antigens are glycoprotein in nature.
   (The Chemical Nature of Antigens)

5. All antibodies have gamma electrophoretic mobility.
   (Antibodies)

6. Treatment of IgG with the enzyme "pepsin" results in two Fab fragments and two Fc fragments.
   (Structure of Immunoglobulins)

7. The variable domains of the immunoglobulin molecule are responsible for the formation of a specific antigen-binding site.
   (Immunoglobulin Domains)

8. The C_H2 domain in IgG binds C1q, initiating the complement sequence.
   (Immunoglobulin Domains)

9. The immunoglobulin that has the highest molecular weight is IgA.
   (Types of Immunoglobulin)

10. IgG is the only immunoglobulin to cross the placenta.
    (Types of Immunoglobulin)

11. The T cells that are associated with helper-inducer activity have the phenotype CD2, CD3, CD4.
    (T Lymphocytes)

12. B lymphocytes can be identified by the CD glycoproteins CD19, CD20, and CD21.
    (B Lymphocytes)

GENERAL REFERENCES

Abbas, A.K., Lichtman, A.H., and Pober, J.S.: Cellular and Molecular Immunology. Philadelphia, W. B. Saunders Company, 1991.

Dorland's Illustrated Medical Dictionary, 27th ed. Philadelphia, W. B. Saunders Company, 1988.

Freeman, B.A.: Burrows Textbook of Microbiology, 27th ed. Philadelphia, W. B. Saunders Company, 1985.

Henry, J.B.: Clinical Diagnosis and Management by Laboratory Methods. Philadelphia, W. B. Saunders Company, 1991.

Sheehan, C.: Clinical Immunology: Principles and Laboratory Diagnosis. Philadelphia, J. B. Lippincott, 1990.

Walter, J.B.: An Introduction to the Principles of Disease, 2nd ed. Philadelphia, W. B. Saunders Company, 1982.

3

Complement

OBJECTIVES

The student shall know, understand, and be prepared to explain:
1. A general overview of the activities of complement
2. The components of complement (nomenclature)
3. Complement activation by the classical pathway
4. The effects of complement activation
5. Complement activation by the alternative pathway
6. Biologic functions associated with complement activation
7. The destruction of complement *in vitro*
8. The role of complement in disease states, specifically:
   a. Rheumatologic diseases
   b. Infectious diseases
   c. Renal diseases
   d. Dermatologic diseases
   e. Hematologic diseases
9. The clinical significance of complement deficiency
10. The diseases associated with complement component deficiency
11. The measurement of complement components by hemolytic assays (The CH_{50} total hemolytic complement assay)
12. The measurement of individual complement components. General principles involving:
    a. Functional assays
    b. Immunoassays

Introduction

The term *complement* refers to a complex set of 14 distinct serum proteins (nine components), each of which can be isolated. The general properties of complement, which serve to distinguish it from the immunoglobulins and other serum proteins and their activities, are as follows:

1. Complement plays a role in the cytolytic destruction of cellular antigens by specific antibodies, although not all cellular antigens are susceptible to dissolution by complement and immunoglobulins. In general, those cells that are naturally most fragile (white blood cells, erythrocytes, thrombocytes, and gram-negative bacteria) are the most susceptible to immune cytolysis, whereas yeasts, molds, many gram-positive bacteria, most plant cells, and even

most mammalian cells resist complement-mediated cytolysis.

2. Complement activity in antigen-antibody reactions is destroyed by heating sera to 56°C for 30 minutes (see further discussion later in this chapter).

3. IgM and IgG are the only immunoglobulins that react with complement. The subclasses of IgG are not equally potent in this respect. IgG4 fails to operate with the complement system, and IgG3 is the most active in this regard (when compared with the other IgG subclasses). IgA, IgD, and IgE do not function with complement.

4. Provided that the immunoglobulin is of the proper class, complement is bound to all antibody-antigen complexes. This fixation occurs even when complement is not required to display the serologic reaction being studied (e.g., precipitation or agglutination). The classical pathway of complement activation (see later discussion) is initiated by the binding or fixation of complement by complexes of antigen and antibody.

5. Complement is found in all mammalian sera and in the sera of most lower animals, including birds, fish, amphibia, and sharks (elasmobranches). There is no increase in complement levels, which constitute about 10 per cent of the total globulins, as a result of immunization.

6. Complement from one species will usually react with immunoglobulins of another species from the same taxonomic order and can therefore be considered a nonspecific serologic reagent. Interaction decreases as the taxonomic position of the two species becomes more distant.

7. Portions of the complement system contribute importantly to chemotaxis, opsonization, immune adherence, anaphylatoxin formation, virus neutralization, and other physiologic functions.

8. Complement can be activated by nonserologic reactions (e.g., the properdin activation—see Complement Activation: The Alternative Pathway, later in this chapter). In these alternative pathways, complement activation is initiated by complex polysaccharides or enzymes.

9. Complement is a complex of nine major components that act in consort with one another. All nine of these components are required for "classical" activation, whereas only six (i.e., exclusive of the first three) are required in the properdin activation pathway (see later discussion).

The discovery of complement is credited to Pfeiffer (1894) and resulted from his studies on experimental cholera infections in guinea pigs, although a heat-labile protective activity of blood had been described earlier and named "alexin" by Buchner.

Pfeiffer's experiments were confirmed in 1898 by Bordet, who also described immune hemolysis following the mixture of red blood cells with specific antibody and alexin. The term *complement* was proposed by Ehrlich at approximately the same time. The term *complement*, which means something that completes or makes perfect, was considered more meaningful than the term *alexin*, which means to ward off, and has therefore persisted.

Bordet and Gengou (1901) formulated the complement fixation test (described in Chapter 17), which, until recently, was the standard serologic test for the diagnosis of syphilis. Because of his many contributions to the understanding of immunity and complement, Bordet received the Nobel Prize in Medicine in 1919.

THE COMPONENTS OF COMPLEMENT (NOMENCLATURE)

As previously mentioned, there are nine basic components in the classical activation sequence of complement. These components are numbered sequentially from C1 to C9. The individual peptide chains of these proteins are designated by Greek letters (e.g., C3α, C3β, C4β, and C4γ) in keeping with the biochemical system for identifying the subunit peptides that have a quarternary structure.

When a peptide chain is fragmented by proteolysis, the resulting cleavage peptides are denoted by lower-case arabic letters (e.g., C3a, C3b, C4a, and C4b). These difficult letter systems are important, because they carry a particular meaning (e.g., C3a and C3b *arise* from C3α and therefore refer to different things and cannot be used interchangeably. If a fragment loses activity as a result of further proteolysis, the letter i is added to indicate inactivation (e.g., C3b$_i$ or iC3b)

When a complement component is activated, a horizontal bar over the designation for the protein is usually used, although this practice is gradually losing its popularity. Under this system, C1 becomes C̄1 when it acquires esterase activity; when referring to specific fragments, the appropriate letters are used (e.g., C̄4b2a). Note: The bar over the designation is now more commonly being used to indicate single components or multicomponent complexes that have enzymatic activity (Gaither and Frank, 1991).

Recent studies of the alternative (properdin) pathway of complement activation have revealed several additional serum proteins that function with the "later" components of activation (i.e., those that follow C3 in the classical pathway). At lease five additional proteins participate in the alternative pathway, and these have recently acquired their own nomenclature. Under this system, there is factor B (formerly known as C3 proactivator), factor D (formerly known as C3 proactivator convertase), C3b,Bb (the C3 activator), cobra venom factor (CVF), and P (properdin factor). This raises the number of proteins in the complement system to 14—9 classical pathway molecules plus 5 alternative pathway molecules.

To these 14 molecules, all of which are present in normal serum, must be added those serum proteins that modulate complement-derived activities. These include C1 inhibitor (C1INH), BIH (H), C3b inactivator (I), C4-binding protein (C4BP), anaphylatoxin inactivator, MAC (membrane attack complex) inhibitor, and C3 nephritic factor (NF).

If plasmin, Hageman's factor, Hageman's factor fragments, and other molecules are included, the total number of proteins that participate in the complement system can be extended beyond these. The complement system, therefore, can be viewed as a highly complex system that involves more than 25 molecules whose biologic activities are numerous and closely coordinated.

COMPLEMENT ACTIVATION: THE CLASSICAL PATHWAY

The activation of complement is often referred to as the complement "cascade," which begins when the C1 molecule is activated by certain reactions. From that point, the components C4, C2, and C3 participate (in that order rather than in straight numerical sequence), followed by the remaining molecules C5 to C9, terminating in cytolysis of certain cellular elements whose antigens initiated the sequence.

C1: The Recognition Unit

C1, the first component of complement, is a macromolecule with a molecular weight of approximately 600,000 and a sedimentation coefficient of 18 (Table 3–1). In its associated form, it is a trimolecular complex, held together by calcium ions (Ca^{++}). Removal of calcium (by the use of chelating compounds such as ethylenediaminetetraacetic acid [EDTA]) causes C1 to dissociate into three subunits; restoration of calcium causes the reassociation of C1 into trimeric form. The presence of calcium therefore can be regarded as essential for the integrity of the complex.

The three subunits of C1 are called C1q, C1r, and C1s and are different in size and in chemical properties (see Table 3–1). The C1q molecule is by far the largest (molecular weight 410,000) and can be easily viewed under the electron microscope, where it appears as six "globes" held on slender

Characteristic	C1q	C1r	C1s	C2	C3	C4	C5	C6	C7	C8	C9
Serum concentration (μg/ml)	150	50	50	15	1250	400	80	60	55	55	60
Sedimentation coefficient ($S_{20/w}$)	11.2	7.5	4.5	4.5	9.5	10.0	8.7	5.5	6.0	8.0	4.5
Molecular weight	410,000	83,000	83,000	110,000	180,000	206,000	180,000	130,000	120,000	150,000	79,000
Number of peptide chains	18	2	1		2	3	2	1	1	3	1
Electrophoretic position	γ_2	β	α	β_1	β_2	β_1	β_1	β_2	β_2	γ_1	α

TABLE 3–1. Characteristics of the Complement Components

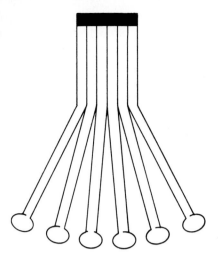

Figure 3–1. The C1q molecule.

shafts that fuse into a common base (Fig. 3–1). These globes are believed to act as the recognition units that bind to the Fc region of the complement-activating IgM and IgG immunoglobulins. This is believed to occur in the C_H2 domain of IgG and IgM. For C1q to initiate the cascade, it must attach to *two* Fc fragments. With IgG-coated cells, therefore, two antibody molecules, each of which can contribute only one Fc fragment, must bind to adjacent antigen sites. It appears that if the IgG molecules are attached to nonadjacent fits, the Fc pieces

are too far apart to initiate complement activation. IgM, however, has five Fc pieces, and therefore one molecule of this immunoglobulin is independently capable of causing complement to be bound. IgA, IgD, and IgE do not bind C1q and therefore cannot initiate the complement cascade.

The other two subunits, C1r and C1s, are similar molecules, each composed of a single peptide chain with a molecular weight approaching 83,000 (see Table 3–1), and contain about 7 to 9 per cent of their protein weight in polysaccharide. C1r is a beta globulin and a proteolytic zymogen (or proenzyme) in its native state. It tends to self-associate to form a dimer (which probably explains why the molecular weight of C1r is frequently given as 160,000 to 180,000). C1s, which is an alpha globulin, is also a proteolytic zymogen (proenzyme) when free. Once bound to C1r, it develops esterase activity.

The exact mechanisms of C1r and C1s activation remain uncertain, although it has been suggested that their incorporation into antigen-antibody complexes creates a susceptibility to a naturally existing serum protease such as plasmin or thrombin (Fig. 3–2).

C4: The Activation Unit

Once the C1 complex is attached, the esterolytic site on C1s activates the next complement compo-

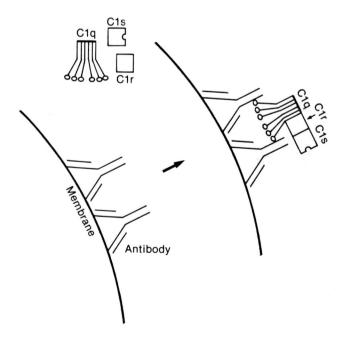

Figure 3–2. Fixation and activation of the first component of complement (C1).

nent, C4 (Fig. 3–3). C4 is a beta globulin with a molecular weight of 206,000, which originates from a pro C4 (molecular weight 210,000), synthesized by macrophages. In human serum, its serum concentration of 400 μg/ml is second only to the serum concentration of C3. The molecule itself consists of three peptide chains, C4α, C4β, and C4γ, which are joined by disulfide bonds. The "attack" of C1s on C4 takes place in the α chain and releases C4a, a so-called subunit of C4. This C4a subunit, which has a molecular weight of about 8000, is released and appears to play no further part in the complement sequence; however, it has been recognized as an anaphylatoxin, which is able to bind to mast cells and cause them to discharge their cytoplasmic granules. The remainder of the molecule is known as C4b (molecular weight about 198,000). This subunit will attach to receptors on erythrocyte surfaces, bacterial cell membranes, and other antigens. It does not attach to C1 on the antigen-antibody complex (Fig. 3–4).

C2: The Second Activation Unit

C2 is also activated by C1s, although probably only after the C1s-C4 interaction has taken place.

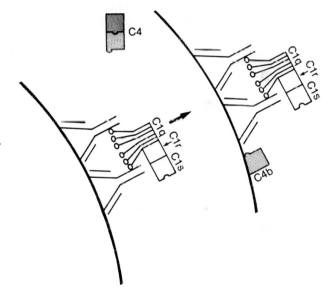

Figure 3–3. Fixation and activation of C4.

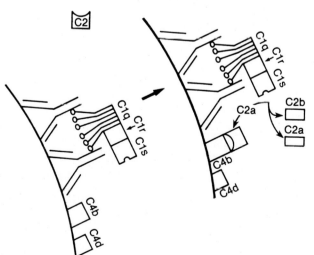

Figure 3–4. Fixation and activation of C4.

C2 is a beta₁ globulin with a molecular weight of 110,000 and occurs in small quantities in serum (15 µg/ml being recorded as the average level). C2 binds with C4b and is cleaved by C1s into C2a and C2b subunits. These subunits have molecular weights of 70,000 and 30,000, respectively. C2b is very labile and will decay with a half-life of 10 minutes if not bound to C4b. The role of C2b is uncertain at this time, but C2a is known to bind to C4b in the presence of magnesium to form C42, a proteolytic enzyme known as C3 convertase.

C3: The Third Activation Unit

C3 is the complement component that is most abundant in serum (1250 µg/ml; see Table 3–1). It is a beta₂ globulin (B$_{IC}$ globulin) with a molecular weight of 180,000 and originates from pro C3, secreted by macrophages. C3 consists of two polypeptide chains, α and β, joined by a number of disulfide bonds (Fig. 3–5). C3 convertase hydrolyzes a peptide bond in the α chain to produce C3a, a peptide with a molecular weight of 8,900, which is an anaphylatoxin. The remainder of the molecule is known as C3b, and it is this subunit that attaches to $\overline{C4b2a}$.

Factor I (working in collaboration with factor H) produces two splits in the α chain of C3b, but the bits of α remain covalently bonded to the β chain (Harrison and Lachman, 1980; Sim *et al.*, 1981). The resulting product is called C3b$_i$ (i.e., inactive, indicating the inability to bind to factor B, although

one property, the ability to react with conglutinin, is concurrently gained). Further enzymatic cleavage of C3b$_i$ gives rise to the fragments C3c, C3d, and C3e. It is not clear whether the cleavage of C3de to C3d and C3e occurs physiologically in the circulation; in cold agglutinin disease, the red cells are coated with C3de and not with C3d alone (Lachmann and Pangburn, 1981).

Similarly, C4b is cleaved in two places by factor I in the presence of C4b-binding protein, first to C4b$_i$ and subsequently to C4c and C4d (Nagasawa *et al.*, 1980).

The new complex, $\overline{C4b,2a,3b}$, is known as C5 convertase, which, like C3 convertase, relies on C2a for its enzymatic activity (Fig. 3–6).

C5: The First Membrane Attack Unit

The next component of complement to become involved in the activation cascade is C5, which, in many respects, is like C3 (see Table 3–1). C5 is a beta₁ globulin with a molecular weight of 180,000, and like C3, it is derived from a precursor molecule (in this case pro C5), secreted from macrophages. C5 is also structurally similar to C3, being composed of two peptide chains, α and β, linked by disulfide bonds (Fig. 3–7). C5 convertase (activated C4b,2a,3b complex) cleaves C5 into two subunits, C5a and C5b. C5a is released into the body fluids, where, as anaphylatoxin II, it acts as a mediator of inflammation and as a chemotaxin for granulo-

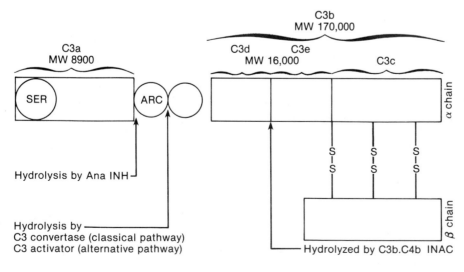

Figure 3–5. The peptide structure of C3. Activation of C3 follows peptide bond cleavage in the alpha-chain by C3 convertase or C3 activator. The anaphylatoxic split product, C3a, is inactivated by removal of its carboxyl terminal arginine by Ana INH. C3b is converted to C3i by C3b.C4b INAC hydrolysis and removal of C3d. (From Barrett, J. T.: Textbook of Immunology, 4th ed. St. Louis, The C. V. Mosby Company, 1983.)

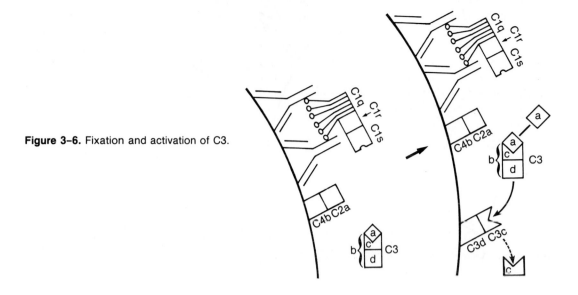

Figure 3-6. Fixation and activation of C3.

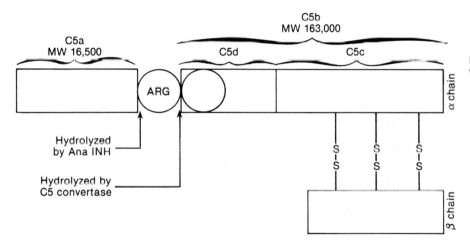

Figure 3-7. The peptide structure of C5.

cytes. C5b, which remains after the removal of C5a, can be further degraded into C5c and C5d, the biologic roles of which are not known. Intact C5b, which attaches to the earlier complement components and to a specific receptor on the cell surface, serves as the activator of C6 and C7 and, therefore, is the first element in the membrane attack complex (Fig. 3–8).

C6 and C7: The Second and Third Membrane Attack Units

Very little is known about C6 and C7 except that both are beta$_{IC}$ globulins (beta$_2$ globulins) with molecular weights of about 125,000 (see Table 3–1).

C6 has a human serum concentration of 60 μg/ml; the level of C7 is 55 μg/ml. C5b cleaves C6 into C6a and C6b. Both C6b and C7 appear to bind to C5b by absorption (Fig. 3–9). The difficulty in obtaining further information about C6 and C7 is probably due to the ease with which they associate with C5 in a trimolecular complex.

C8 and C9: The Final Membrane Attack Units

The next molecule to become involved in the complement cascade is C8, which is composed of three peptide chains, C8α, C8β, and C8γ, two of which are covalently linked to each other (C8γ and

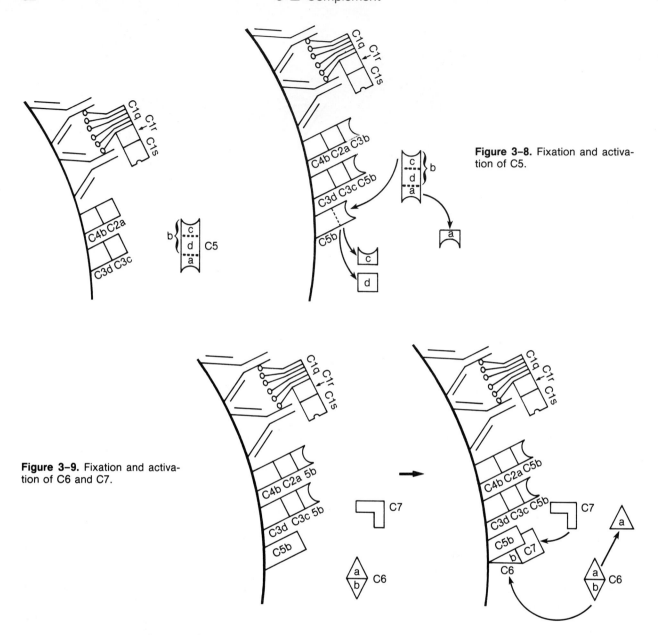

Figure 3–8. Fixation and activation of C5.

Figure 3–9. Fixation and activation of C6 and C7.

C8α) by disulfide bonds, and a third (C8β), which is not covalently joined to the other two. C8 is inserted into the membrane and disrupts it. This disruption of the membrane appears to be irreversible, although the presence of C9 is apparently important in the formation of the membrane defect.

The final complement molecule to interact in the cascade is C9, which is an alpha globulin with a molecular weight of about 79,000. C9 appears to enhance the activity of C8 (Fig. 3–10).

THE EFFECTS OF COMPLEMENT ACTIVATION

The most significant effect of complement activation on sensitized erythrocytes (i.e., those combined with specific antibody) or sensitized gram-negative bacteria is the cytolysis of the cell carrying the antigen. The C5 to C9 complex inserts into the lipid bilayer membrane where it forms a transmembrane protein channel. The exact causative force for

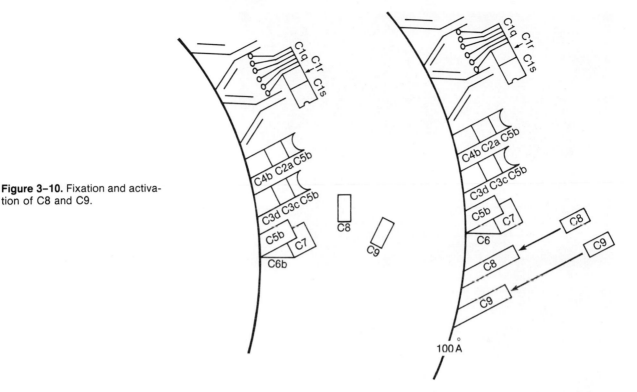

Figure 3–10. Fixation and activation of C8 and C9.

the attendant lysis continues to evade identification, although it can be assumed that the disturbance of the lipid bilayer allows for the free exchange of ions as well as water molecules across the membrane. The influx of Na^+ and H_2O would then lead to a disruption of osmotic balance, producing cell lysis. The protein channel is funnel-shaped, being larger in diameter on the exterior surface than on the interior surface.

In the absence of C9, cells will still undergo lysis, although at a slower rate. When C9 is added, "holes" can be observed on the surfaces of the cells (Humphrey and Dourmashkin, 1965; Fig. 3–11). These holes have been observed in all cells (e.g., red cells, Krebs' ascites tumor cells, bacteria) lysed by the action of complement and have been observed on pseudomembranes formed by the absorption of serum lipids onto a carbon-coated surface; they are also observed when cells are lysed by certain other agents (e.g., saponin; Humphrey and Dourmashkin, 1969). The diameter of these holes is about 80 to 100 μm (8 to 10 nm) and they appear to be about the same size (100Å) regardless of the causative antibody (Rosse *et al.*, 1966).

It is interesting to note that the holes do not pen-

etrate the membrane and, therefore, should more correctly be described as "erosions" on the membrane. These erosions can be erased with lipid solvents. How they contribute to rapid cell lysis is not known. (See also Biologic Functions Associated with Complement Activation, later in this chapter.)

COMPLEMENT ACTIVATION: THE ALTERNATIVE PATHWAY

The alternate complement activation pathway was originally described by Pillemer *et al.* (1954), who discovered that cell wall preparations from yeast or zymosan would activate complement. This activation was related to the newly discovered serum globulin properdin and became known as the "properdin pathway." Since that time, it has been discovered that many complex polysaccharides will activate this alternative pathway (e.g., liposaccharides, bacterial capsules, teichoic acids from bacterial cell walls, insulin, dextran). At least four serum proteins function in the alternative pathway that do not contribute to the classical pathway. These are factor B, factor D, properdin (factor P), and initiating factor (IF).

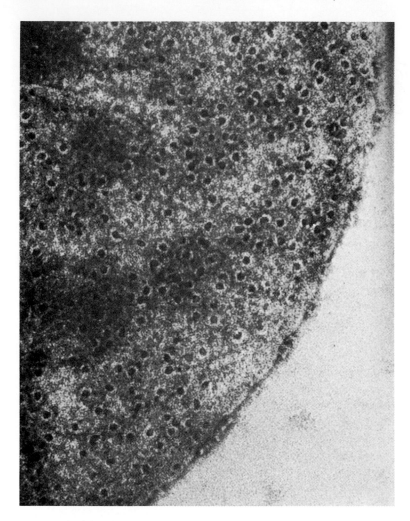

Figure 3–11. Multiple lesions in the cell wall of *Escherichia coli* bacterium caused by the interaction with IgM antibody and complement. Magnification × 400,000. (Courtesy of Drs. R. Dourmashkin and J. H. Humphrey.)

The activation of the alternative pathway is believed to be the end result of interactions of the proteins mentioned above. The mechanisms are not fully understood. A major step is the conversion of factor B to an active form, $B\overline{b}$, capable of cleaving C3 in a manner similar to that of $C\overline{42}$ in the classical pathway. Factor D is responsible for cleaving B into $B\overline{b}$. This action requires the presence of native C3 and magnesium. Once C3 is converted to C3b, both C3b and $B\overline{b}$ form a complex (C3 convertase on the surface of the initiator). C3b is a more efficient promoter of the conversion of B to $B\overline{b}$ than is native C3, so that the C3b generated by this mechanism accelerates the conversion of more B to $B\overline{b}$ and thus of C3 to C3b. Properdin participates in this pathway by binding to $C\overline{3bB\overline{b}}$, thereby preventing the spontaneous decay of this complex. This complex can then activate the rest of the complement system.

The alternative pathway, therefore, proceeds to the C3 activator stage without the participation or consumption of C1, C4, or C2 (Bitter-Suerman *et al.*, 1972). Once the activator splits C3a from C3, the activation sequence proceeds to C9 in the same way as in the classical pathway.

BIOLOGIC FUNCTIONS ASSOCIATED WITH COMPLEMENT ACTIVATION

The large number of proteins involved in the complement system and the complexities of their interaction, plus the fact that two separate mechanisms have evolved for the activation of the complement system, suggest that several important biologic activities are associated with this system. Many of these functions (which do not include cell

TABLE 3–2. Properties of the Complement-Derived Peptides

Protein	Source	Molecular Weight	Biologic Activity	Released By
C2b	C2	37,000	Unknown	$C\overline{1s}$
C3a	α chain of C3	8,900	Anaphylatoxic	C3 convertase and C3 activator
C4a	α chain of C4	9,000	Anaphylatoxic	$C\overline{1s}$
C5a	α chain of C5	11,000	Anaphylatoxic and chemotactic	C5 convertase

From Barrett, J. T.: Textbook of Immunology. St. Louis, The C. V. Mosby Co., 1983.

lysis) are not known. Table 3–2 lists the most widely accepted biologic functions of complement components and complement fragments. Although many of these are self-explanatory, it should be mentioned that anaphylatoxic factors cause mast cells to degranulate and release their various mediators in the absence of cytotoxicity. The opsonic properties of the complement proteins appear to depend upon the presence of specific receptors on the surfaces of phagocytic cells. Foreign materials with opsonically active fragments on their surfaces interact with these receptors, leading first to membrane adherence and, as a second step, to phagocytosis.

The control of the biologic properties of these complement fragments is the responsibility of specific serum protein inhibitors such as C1 esterase inhibitor (which destroys the enzymatic activity of activated C1); C3b inactivator destroys the integrity of the opsonically active protein C3b. An inactivator of cell-bound C6 is also known to exist, as is an inactivator of the vasoactive material anaphylatoxin, which destroys the activity of C3a and, to a lesser extent, C5a.

THE DESTRUCTION OF COMPLEMENT *IN VITRO*

Complement components can be destroyed *in vitro* in the following ways:

Anticoagulants. As previously mentioned, ionized calcium (Ca^{++}) is required for the integrity of C1 and is therefore required for the activation of complement via the classical pathway. Similarly, ionized magnesium (Mg^{++}) is required for the formation of the C3 convertase of both the classical

and alternative pathways (i.e., C42 and C3b,Bb, respectively). Because of this, all chelators of Ca^{++} and Mg^{++} (also written as Ca^{2+} and Mg^{2+}) will inhibit complement activity. For example, the addition of 2 mg of Na_2H_2EDTA to 1 ml of serum completely blocks the activation of complement.

The anticoagulant heparin is also anticomplementary and in sufficient quantities will completely inhibit the cleavage of C4 by activated C1.

Heating. The heating of serum to 56°C for 30 minutes completely activates C1 and C2. C4 is also damaged (although to a lesser extent) (Bier *et al.*, 1945; Heidelberger and Mayer, 1948). Factor B of the alternative pathway is inactivated by heating to 50°C for 20 minutes.

Normal Serum Inhibitor. Serum normally contains an inhibitor of activated C1, which does not interfere with the conversion of C1 to activated C1 but directly inhibits the action of activated C1 by binding to and removing activated C1s and C1r from the activated C1qrs complex.

Storage. On storage, serum regularly becomes anticomplementary—preliminary observations suggest that the alteration may principally affect C4.

COMPLEMENT IN DISEASE STATES

In the majority of disease states, complement functions normally in producing inflammation and tissue damage. In those cases in which complement plays a role in the development of disease, it is often being activated by an irregular antibody, immune complex for foreign material. The activity of a disease state can often be followed by assessing the level of one or another complement component (see Measurement of Complement Components, later in this chapter).

In addition to the role of complement components in disease states, there is now considerable interest in the detection of decay products in various body fluids. In this respect, C3 decay products have been found in the sera of patients with primary biliary cirrhosis, rheumatoid arthritis, and lupus erythematosus. Because this area is currently under active investigation, it is probable that this list will grow rapidly.

The following is a brief review of the levels of complement in various disease states. The reader interested in more detailed information is referred to the list of general references at the end of this chapter.

Rheumatologic Diseases

Systemic Lupus Erythematosus. In systemic lupus erythematosus (SLE), circulating immune complexes activate complement and are deposited in a variety of tissue sites, leading to tissue damage. It has been suggested that the activity of the disease can be followed by the determination of C3 and C4 levels. As mentioned, C3 decay products have also been found in the sera of patients with this disease.

Rheumatoid Arthritis. Depressed levels of complement have been shown to exist in rheumatoid arthritis as well as in a number of other rheumatologic diseases. Normal or elevated serum complement levels are found in juvenile rheumatoid arthritis and in most patients with adult-onset rheumatoid arthritis. Depressed CH_{50} and cleavage products of C3 and properdin factor B are thought to represent intra-articular activation in the synovial fluid of almost all patients with seropositive rheumatoid arthritis. This is not true of fluids obtained from patients with degenerative arthritis (Hunder, 1977).

Others. Normal or elevated serum complement levels are also found in patients with paledromic arthritis, pseudogout, gout, Reiter's syndrome, and gonococcal arthritis. Depressed CH_{50} and cleavage products of C3 and properdin factor B are also thought to represent intra-articular activation in the synovial fluid of many patients with SLE, pseudogout, gout, Reiter's syndrome, and gonococcal arthritis.

Infectious Diseases

Patients with gram-negative septicemia and certain fungal diseases (e.g., cryptococcal septicemia) are often depleted of C3 and components of the alternative pathway of complement activation. It is now known that patients with HB_SAg-positive infectious hepatitis may have an early fall in serum C3, which later returns to normal. This may be associated with signs of immune complex disease (e.g., arthralgia). Complement also appears to play a similar role in a number of parasitic infections, including malaria. In patients with vivax malaria, C1, C4, and C2 may be depressed; in addition to these, C3 may be depressed in falciparum malaria.

Renal Diseases

Michael (1974) reported that complement is of key importance in glomerular damage in a variety of the glomerulonephritides. This is usually demonstrated through the deposition of C3 and/or other components in the vicinity of the glomerular basement membrane. Many patients will show activation of the alternative pathway on serum analysis. In interstitial and tubular disease, the role of complement is less clear, although it is believed by some investigators that complement may also have some function in these disorders.

Dermatologic Diseases

Complement is believed to play a role in the ongoing tissue damage in a variety of dermatologic illnesses, including pemphigus vulgaris, bullous pemphigoid, and herpes gestationis. Serum complement levels are usually normal or elevated in these chronic inflammatory states, and the importance of complement is suggested by immunofluorescent analysis of tissue biopsies and by studies of blister fluid.

Hematologic Diseases

Complement plays an important role in opsonization of erythrocytes in many types of autoimmune hemolytic anemia, leading to their clearance by the cells of the mononuclear-phagocyte system. It should be noted, however, that even in those cases in which complement is clearly involved, complement levels are usually normal. Complement is of particular importance in the clearance of cells coated with IgM cold agglutinins of anti-I specificity. In paroxysmal nocturnal hemoglobinuria (PNH), the patient's red cells and other blood cell elements develop a membrane defect that renders them susceptible to complement-mediated lysis. This acquired cellular defect is associated with cytotoxicity and clearance due to activation of the alternative pathway by the cell membrane.

CLINICAL SIGNIFICANCE OF COMPLEMENT DEFICIENCY

The complement system is significant both in the diagnosis of disease and in the understanding of pathophysiology of several human disease states (Table 3–3). Reduced amounts of serum complement activity have been reported in a variety of disease states (e.g., systemic lupus erythematosus [SLE], glomerulonephritis, acute glomerulonephritis, acute serum sickness, advanced cirrhosis of the liver). Other diseases (e.g., obstructive jaundice, thyroiditis, acute rheumatic fever, rheumatoid arthritis) are associated with elevated serum complement concentrations.

Inadequate amounts of various components of the complement system (including the inhibitors and inactivators that regulate the activation cascade) may arise from genetic conditions in which the component is not synthesized at all or is produced at subnormal levels. It is also possible that the molecule may be synthesized normally, yet may be defective in some structural way, rendering it functionally inert. A deficiency of one of the complement proteins may also be produced by hypercatabolism (i.e., an increased rate of breakdown or degradation), and this may be difficult to distinguish from activation of the molecule, particularly if only a late-acting component is involved.

The elevation of complement levels has been reported in a number of conditions, yet the significance of this observation is not clear. The most likely explanation is simply overproduction.

In the case of genetic disorders, the absence of the complement component follows simple mendelian inheritance patterns and is inherited as an autosomal recessive trait. Therefore, patients who are heterozygous tend to have half the normal

TABLE 3–3. Diseases Associated with Complement Deficiency

Deficient Component	Associated Diseases
C1q	Sex-linked agammaglobulinemia Hypocomplementemic urticarial vasculitis Severe combined immunodeficiency SLE-like syndrome Increased susceptibility to bacterial infection
C1r	Upper respiratory tract disease Chronic kidney disease SLE-like syndrome
C1s	SLE-like syndrome Increased susceptibility to bacterial infection
C1sINH	Hereditary angioneurotic edema
C4	SLE Glomerulonephritis Pyogenic infection
C2	SLE Dermatomyositis Repeated infectious disease Chronic renal disease Autoimmune disease Increased susceptibility to bacterial infection
C3	Recurrent pyogenic infections SLE-like syndrome Poststreptococcal glomerulonephritis Pyogenic infections
C3b inactivator	Recurrent pyogenic infections Urticaria
C5	SLE *Neisseria* infections
C5 dysfunction	Leiner's disease Gram-negative skin and bowel infections
C6	*Neisseria* infections SLE Raynaud's phenomenon Sclerodema-like syndrome Vasculitis
C7	*Neisseria* infections SLE Raynaud's phenomenon Sclerodactyly Telangiectasia
C8	*Neisseria* infections Xeroderma pigmentosa SLE-like syndrome
C9	*Neisseria* infections
Properdin	Pyogenic infections
Factor D	Pyogenic infections

levels and patients who are homozygous have little or no detectable complement component activity.

Deficiencies involving every component of the classical activation sequence are known. The majority of these patients present with one or another manifestation of autoimmune disease. The role of complement deficiency in the development of these diseases is not yet clear, although it has been hypothesized that autoimmunity may be a manifestation of chronic viral illness, and, if complement aids in viral neutralization, an interruption of those pathways of activation may promote chronic viral infection.

The deficiency of complement components has an effect on complement activation, as summarized in Table 3–4.

C1q Deficiency

Human deficiency of C1q was originally reported in 1961, and many other examples have been added since that time. Most of these cases have been associated with a sex-linked agammaglobulinemia, hypocomplementemic urticarial vasculitis, or severe combined immunodeficiency. C1q deficiency is frequently associated with a loss of B and T lymphocytes (and therefore with depressed levels of IgG in the circulation); therefore it is difficult to recognize any single defect associated with it. C1q deficiency has also been described in patients with an SLE-like syndrome and increased susceptibility to bacterial infection (Wara *et al.*, 1975).

C1r Deficiency

Normal C1q levels have been noted in those few individuals in whom markedly depressed levels of C1r have been detected. All of these patients had extensive medical histories, revealing multiple episodes of upper respiratory tract disease, chronic kidney disease, or a lupus erythematosus (LE)-like syndrome.

C1s and Activated C1s INH Deficiency

Patients with C1s deficiency may have a loss of almost 50 per cent of their C1s. Very little is known about the association of C1s deficiency and human health, although several of the individuals studied

TABLE 3–4. Complement Activation Abnormalities Associated with Complement Component Deficiencies

Complement Activation Abnormality	Deficient Component
Defective classical pathway activation	C1q, C1r, C1s, C4, C2
Defective classical/alternative pathway activation	C3
Defective alternative pathway activation	Properdin, factor D
Defective MAC formation	C5, C6, C7, C8, C9

had an LE-like syndrome and an increased susceptibility to bacterial infection (Day *et al.*, 1973).

Activated C1s INH deficiency, however, is clearly associated with hereditary angioneurotic edema (HANE). This disease is transmitted as an autosomal dominant deficiency in which the subjects average 31 µg/ml of activated C1s INH, compared with 180 µg/ml for normal individuals.

C4 Deficiency

Decreased C4 levels accompanied by elevated anti-DNA and ANA titers confirm a diagnosis of SLE. C4 deficiency has also been associated with glomerulonephritis and pyogenic infection. C4 deficiency, however, has been recognized as an autosomal recessive characteristic. The homozygous condition reveals absolutely no C4, whereas in the heterozygous state, up to 30 per cent of the normal values were observed. The alternative complement pathway is intact in C4-deficient individuals and may be their major source of protection against bacterial and viral infections.

C2 Deficiency

This is the most common of the human complement deficiencies; more than 40 cases, revealing both heterozygous and homozygous origins, have been described. The heterozygous individuals have 30 to 70 per cent of the normal C2 levels, whereas the homozygous C2-deficient individuals range below 4 per cent of normal values, based on hemolytic assays. The frequency of hypersensitive disease such as LE and dermatomyositis and repeated infectious disease exceeds that which would be expected on the basis of random distribution in C2-deficient individuals. Patients with C2 deficiency have chronic renal disease and antibody directed against DNA. C2 deficiency has been associated with HLA-A25, HLA-B18, and HLA-DR2. Approximately half of the individuals with decreased C2 have autoimmune disease; the other half appear normal but are susceptible to bacterial infection.

C3 Deficiency

Many C3-deficient individuals are recorded in the medical literature, yet only one individual is known to have total C3 deficiency (2.5 µg/ml of serum compared with a normal level of 1,250 µg/ml). Five other children in the same family plus the mother had about half-normal C3 levels. The patient had experienced a considerable number of infections, which emphasizes the critical role of C3 not only in linking the classical and alternative pathways but also in immune adherence, opsonization, and chemotaxis, all of which are important disease functions.

Two forms of C3 deficiency exist: type I and type II. In type I, C3 is probably deficient as a result of a deficiency of C3 inactivator. Type II C3 deficiency is the type reported in the individual just described (Alper *et al.*, 1973). This patient's decreased level of C3 was found to be associated with increased destruction and decreased synthesis.

Patients with poststreptococcal glomerulonephritis and pyogenic infections have extremely decreased levels of C3.

C5 Deficiency

Familial C5 dysfunction has been described in patients presenting with failure to thrive, diarrhea, seborrheic dermatitis, and susceptibility to infection with bacterial organisms (Miller and Nilsson, 1970). In three examples of C5 dysfunction, the C5 level, as determined immunochemically, was normal but hemolytic titrations of complement could detect no C5. A depression of phagocytic activity, which could be restored to normal with human C5, was noted in these individuals. The higher incidence of infectious disease in these patients is related to this loss of phagocytic activity.

In the case of C5 dysfunction (Leiner's disease) patients are predisposed to skin and bowel infec-

tions, characterized by eczema. In these patients, C5 levels are normal, but the C5 component fails to promote phagocytosis.

C6, C7, C8, and C9 Deficiency

Human C6 deficiency has been described in four individuals who lacked hemolytically or immunochemically active C6. The patients and siblings of these individuals had half-normal serum levels of C6. C6 deficiency appears to be associated with increased susceptibility to *Neisseria* infections, as well as SLE, Raynaud's phenomenon, scleroderma-like syndrome, and vasculitis.

Several patients have been described who are deficient in C7, which is associated with severe bacterial infections caused by *Neisseria* species, SLE, Raynaud's phenomenon, sclerodactyly, and telangiectasia. C8 deficiency is also associated with *Neisseria* infections and with SLE-like syndrome and xeroderma pigmentosa. C9 deficiency is also associated with *Neisseria* infections.

Other Deficiencies

Deficiencies of properdin and factor D, which result in defective alternative pathway activation, are associated with pyogenic infections.

MEASUREMENT OF COMPLEMENT COMPONENTS

Hemolytic Assays

Hemolytic assay provides a crude screening test for complement activity in human serum. The test uses sheep erythrocytes coated with antierythrocyte antibody. Hemolysis of the sheep erythrocytes is measured spectrophotometrically as the absorbance of released hemoglobin and can be directly related to the number of red blood cells lysed. For clinical purposes, measurement of total hemolytic activity of serum is taken at 50 per cent of the hemolysis level. The CH_{50} is an arbitrary unit that is defined as the quantity of complement necessary for 50 per cent lysis of red cells under rigidly standardized conditions of red blood cell sensitization with antibody. These results are expressed as the reciprocal of the serum dilution giving 50 per cent hemolysis.

Both the classical activation components and terminal complement components are measured during this reaction. Low levels of complement confirm complement activation (or degradation *in vitro*). The test is useful in:

1. screening for genetic deficiencies of the complement system,
2. diagnosing hereditary angioneurotic edema,
3. monitoring the progress of patients with immune complex disease.

Elevations in total hemolytic activity are associated with acute inflammatory conditions, leukemia, Hodgkin's disease, sarcoma, and Behçet's disease. Decreases in complement level occur in a variety of conditions, including congenital defects, liver disease, nutritional imbalance, and hypocatabolism. In addition, complement fixation can result from the presence of tissue or cell-bound immune complexes, or when circulating immune complexes are displayed. Bound immune complexes can be associated with chronic glomerulonephritis, rheumatoid arthritis, hemolytic anemia, and graft rejection. Circulating immune complexes are characteristically associated with SLE, acute glomerulonephritis, subacute bacterial endocarditis, and cryoglobulinemia.

METHOD 1: CH₅₀ TOTAL HEMOLYTIC COMPLEMENT ASSAY

The technique described here is intended for use with the kit provided by Sigma Diagnostics, Sigma Chemical Co., St Louis, Missouri.

Materials

The Kit Contains:

1. Sheep red blood cells sensitized with antisheep antibodies suspended in buffer, pH 7.3, with stabilizer. Sodium azide is added as a preservative. Store at 2 to 6°C.
2. Reference standard CH_{50}. This is a lyophilized human serum containing a known CH_{50} value. The total hemolytic complement activity is indicated on the label. Store the dry vials at −20°C. Immediately before use, reconstitute the contents of the vial by adding 0.3 ml of deionized water. Mix gently until dissolution is complete. Any remaining solution should be stored (within 30 minutes) at −70°C (or in liquid nitrogen). If such storage is not available, discard the remaining contents of the vial.
3. CH_{50} low activity control and CH_{50} high activity control. These should be reconstituted and stored in exactly the same way as for the reference standard (see 2, above). The controls should be treated in exactly the same manner as the test specimen. The total hemolytic activity should be within approximately 10 per cent of the value indicated on the vials.

Additional Materials Required (Not Provided with Kit):

1. Refrigerated centrifuge.
2. Spectrophotometer and cuvettes.
3. Pipetting device capable of accurately delivering 0.005 ml (5 μl).
4. Timer.

Collection and Preparation of Specimens

1. At least 2 ml of clotted blood is required. The specimen should be allowed to clot at room temperature, then separated by centrifugation at 4°C.
2. Remove the serum from the clot and keep at 4°C.
3. Commence testing immediately. If this is not possible, store the serum at −70°C. Hemolysis renders a specimen unsuitable for testing.

Procedure

Allow the sheep red blood cells to warm to room temperature before use. Immediately before use, resuspend the cells by repeated inversions.

1. For each test sample and control, label one tube of sheep cells. Label one tube for the Reference Standard and one tube Lysis Control (spontaneous lysis).
2. Pipette 0.005 ml of test sample, controls, or reference standard into the appropriately labeled tube. No sample is added to the lysis control.
3. Mix all tubes by repeated inversion.

4. Incubate the tubes at room temperature (18 to 26°C) for 60 minutes (± 5 minutes).
5. Mix the contents of the tubes again by repeated inversion.
6. Centrifuge all tubes at approximately $600 \times g$ for 10 minutes.
7. Transfer the supernatant fluid to a cuvette.
8. Read absorbance of the supernatant at 415 nm within 15 minutes after centrifugation. Zero the instrument using a water blank. Read and record the absorbance of the Lysis Control (Control). Zero the instrument using the Lysis Control as a blank. Read and record the absorbance value of the Reference Standard (Standard) and of each test specimen and the controls (Specimen).

Interpretation

The CH_{50} value of each specimen or control is calculated as follows:

CH_{50} value of the specimen $=$

$$\frac{Specimen}{Standard} \times CH_{50} \text{ value of standard}$$

Discussion

The absorbance value of the lysis control when read against water at 415 nm should be less than 0.15 using a spectrophotometer with a 1 cm light-path. If the (Control) exceeds 0.15, the assay results are not valid and the test must be repeated.

Plasma must not be used in the assay.

The test has various limitations, as follows:

1. Results of the test, which are a quantitative value, represent the functional total hemolytic complement activity. Values achieved with this method can be used to determine the presence of abnormal whole complement levels but cannot identify the abnormal component.
2. The measurement of total CH_{50} hemolytic activity cannot exclude all acquired or congenital abnormalities of individual components.
3. The procedure must be taken as an aid to diagnosis and not as diagnostic in itself.

THE MEASUREMENT OF INDIVIDUAL COMPLEMENT COMPONENTS

In order to establish that a deficiency of some complement molecule exists, it is necessary to have a reliable method of quantitating the individual components or the whole complement system. At the present time, accurate methods are available for measuring all of the nine classical pathway components, most of the alternative pathway components, and several enzymes and inhibitors that regulate the complement system. Many of these methods, however, are still considered to be research techniques and are not available routinely. This discussion will be confined to techniques that do not require a laboratory skilled in complement research for their performance. Two types of techniques are in use: those that measure the complement proteins as antigens in serum, and those that measure the functional activity of the components.

Functional Assays

Functional complement assays can be considered to be both sensitive and precise tools for measuring the activity of a complement component. Some of these methods can be used to quantitate activity at the molecular level, whereas others express complement components in arbitrary titration units. The level of activity is measured by using pure preparations of each component added sequentially to antibody-coated erythrocytes until the step is reached in the activation sequence just prior to addition of the component to be measured. The test sample is then added, and the degree of hemolysis is related to the presence of later-acting components. This test is described in detail by Rapp and Borsos (1970). The disadvantages of functional assays are that they are complex and time-consuming and require relatively highly purified reagents, which are costly when compared to those required for immunochemical tests.

Immunoassays

Immunochemical assays (i.e., antigenic) are generally simpler to perform than those for evaluating functional activity.

These antigenic assays are highly specific and require fewer specialized reagents and considerably less time. The reagents that are required are commercially available, either serum or plasma can be used, and the commonly available methods of freezer storage (i.e., − 20°C) are sufficient. It should be noted, however, that antigenic assays have the disadvantage of not being able to provide information on the activity of a component because they may detect degradation products as well as functionally active components. Also, in general, antigenic assays are not as sensitive as functional assays and may not detect the presence of a complement component in certain body fluids whose presence *can* be shown by its functional activity. The sensitivity of assays depends to some extent upon the strength of the antisera used, and, with usual assays, as little as 1 to 10 μg/ml of a protein antigen can be measured. It should also be noted that, whereas antisera to many of the complement proteins are available commercially (e.g., C1q, C4, C3, C5, properdin factor B, C1 inhibitor), the others are not generally available except as research reagents.

JUST THE FACTS

Introduction

1. "Complement" refers to 14 distinct serum proteins, 9 components.
2. Complement plays a role in the cytolytic destruction of cellular antigens by specific immunoglobulins.
3. Not all cellular antigens are susceptible to complement-mediated cytolysis.
4. IgM and IgG react with complement (IgG subclasses vary in this respect).
5. Complement is bound to all antigen-antibody complexes.
6. Complement is found in the sera of mammals, lower animals, birds, fish, amphibia, and sharks.
7. Complement from one species will usually react with immunoglobulins from another species from the same taxonomic order. This interaction decreases as the taxonomic position of the two species becomes more distant.
8. Complement contributes to chemotaxis, opsonization, immune adherence, anaphylatoxin formation, virus neutralization, and other physiologic functions.
9. Complement can be activated by nonserologic reactions.

The Components of Complement (Nomenclature)

1. The components of complement are numbered C1 to C9.
2. The individual peptide chains of these proteins are designated by Greek letters.
3. Fragments are designated by lower-case arabic letters (e.g., C3a).
4. The letter i is added to indicate inactivation (e.g., $C3b_i$ or iC3b).
5. Activation is sometimes indicated by a horizontal bar over the designation. This is more commonly used to indicate enzymatic activity.
6. At least five additional proteins participate in the "alternative" pathway.
7. Several proteins that modulate complement-derived activities have been isolated.

Complement Activation: The Classical Pathway

1. Complement activation (classical pathway) begins with C1 activation.
2. From this point, C4, C2, C3, and C5 to C9 participate (in that order).

C1: The Recognition Unit

Note: Study Table 3–1 for characteristics of the complement components.
1. C1 is a trimolecular complex (molecular weight 600,000) held together by Ca^{++}.
2. The three subunits are called C1q, C1r, and C1s.
3. C1q must attach to two Fc fragments to initiate the sequence.
4. The exact mechanism of C1r and C1s activation remains uncertain.

C4: The Activation Unit

1. C1s activates C4, which releases C4a and C4b.
2. C4a plays no further part in the complement sequence.
3. C4b attaches to receptors on erythrocyte surfaces, bacterial cell membranes, and other antigens. It does not attach to the antigen-antibody complex.

C2: The Second Activation Unit

1. C2 is activated by C1s, though probably only after the C1s-C4 interaction has taken place.
2. C2 occurs in small quantities in serum.
3. C2 binds with C4b and is cleaved by C1s into C2a and C2b.
4. C2b is labile and decays rapidly. Its role is uncertain.
5. C2a binds to C4b in the presence of magnesium to form C42 (a proteolytic enzyme known as C3 convertase).

C3: The Third Activation Unit

1. C3 is the most abundant complement component in serum.
2. C3 is split by C3 convertase into C3a and C3b.
3. C3b attaches to activated C4b2a.
4. Factor I (with factor H) splits the α chain of C3b. The resulting product is $C3b_i$ (indicating the inability to bind with factor B). The ability to react with conglutinin is concurrently gained.
5. Enzymatic cleavage of $C3b_i$ produces C3c, C3d, and C3e.
6. The complex is activated C4b,2a,3b (C5 convertase), which relies on C2a for its enzymatic activity.

C5: The First Membrane Attack Unit

1. C5 convertase cleaves C5 into two subunits, C5a and C5b.
2. C5a is released into the body fluids where, as anaphylatoxin II, it acts as a mediator of inflammation and a chemotaxin for granulocytes.
3. C5b can be further degraded into C5c and C5d.
4. Intact C5b attaches to earlier complement components and to a specific receptor on the cell surface.
5. C5b activates C6 and C7.

C6 and C7: The Second and Third Membrane Attack Units

1. C5b cleaves C6 into C6a and C6b.
2. Both C6b and C7 appear to bind to C5b by absorption.
3. C6 and C7 associate easily with C5 in a trimolecular complex.

C8 and C9: The Final Membrane Attack Units

1. C8 is inserted into the cell membrane and disrupts it irreversibly.
2. C9 appears to enhance the activity of C8.

The Effects of Complement Activation

1. The most significant effect of complement activation is cytolysis of the cell carrying the antigen.
2. In the absence of C9, cells undergo lysis at a slower rate.
3. With C9, holes are observed on the surfaces of cells.
4. These holes appear to be about the same size regardless of the causative antibody.
5. The holes do not penetrate the membrane but are more like "erosions," which can be erased with lipid solvents. How they contribute to cell lysis is not known.

Complement Activation: The Alternative Pathway

1. Many complex polysaccharides will activate the alternative pathway.
2. At least four serum proteins (factor B, factor D, properdin [P], and initiating factor [IF]) function in the alternative pathway.
3. The alternative pathway proceeds to the C3 activator stage without the participation or consumption of C1, C4, or C2.
4. Once C3 has been split to form C3a, the activation sequence proceeds to C9 in the same way as the classical pathway.

Biologic Functions Associated with Complement Activation

1. Several biologic activities are associated with the complement system. (Study Table 3–2.)
2. The control of biologic properties of the complement fragments is the responsibility of specific serum protein inhibitors.

The Destruction of Complement In Vitro

1. Complement is destroyed in vitro by anticoagulants, heating, normal serum inhibitors, and storage.

Complement in Disease States

1. Complement has a role in certain rheumatologic diseases (SLE, rheumatoid arthritis, and others), infectious diseases, renal diseases, dermatologic diseases, and hematologic diseases.

Clinical Significance of Complement Deficiency

1. Study Table 3–3.

Measurement of Complement Components

1. Complement activity in human serum is routinely screened using hemolytic assay (CH_{50} total hemolytic complement assay).
2. Individual complement components are measured using functional assays and imunoassays.

Review Questions

Multiple Choice

Choose the phrase, sentence, or symbol that completes the statement or answers the question. More than one answer may be correct in each case. Answers are given at the end of this book.

1. Complement:
   (a) plays a role in the cytolytic destruction of cellular antigens by specific antibodies
   (b) is activated by IgE
   (c) is found in all mammalian sera
   (d) cannot be activated by nonserologic reactions
   (Introduction)

2. The number of major complement components that participate in the classical activation pathway is:
   (a) 6
   (b) 14
   (c) 9
   (d) 25
   (Introduction)

3. Which of the following immunoglobulins does not function with complement?
   (a) IgA
   (b) IgM
   (c) IgG3
   (d) IgE
   (Introduction)

4. The order of activation of the first four components of complement in the classical pathway is:
   (a) C1, C2, C3, C4
   (b) C1, C3, C4, C2
   (c) C1, C4, C2, C3
   (d) C1, C4, C3, C2
   (Complement Activation: The Classical Pathway)

5. The three subunits of C1 are called:
   (a) C1q, C1r, C1s
   (b) C1r, C1s, C1t
   (c) C1a, C1b, C1c
   (d) C1qr, C1rs, C1st
   (C1: The Recognition Unit)

6. Of the three subunits of C1:
   (a) C1q is the largest
   (b) C1q is the smallest
   (c) C1r has the highest molecular weight
   (d) C1s is the largest
   (C1: The Recognition Unit)

7. The C4 molecule consists of:
   (a) six peptide chains
   (b) four peptide chains
   (c) three peptide chains, joined by hydrogen bonds
   (d) three peptide chains, joined by disulfide bonds
   (C4: The Activation Unit)

8. C2:
   (a) is a $beta_1$ globulin
   (b) has a molecular weight of 110,000
   (c) occurs in small quantities in serum
   (d) is cleaved by C1s into C2a and C2c subunits
   (C2: The Second Activation Unit)

9. The most abundant complement component in serum is:
   (a) C1
   (b) C2
   (c) C3
   (d) C4
   (Table 3–1)

10. The complement component C5:
    (a) has a molecular weight of 180,000
    (b) is composed of two peptide chains

(c) is structurally similar to C1
(d) is an α globulin
(C5: The First Membrane Attack Unit)

11. In the absence of C9:
(a) cells do not undergo lysis
(b) cells undergo lysis at an accelerated rate
(c) cells undergo lysis at a slower rate
(d) "holes" are not observed on the cell surface
(The Effects of Complement Activation)

12. The alternative pathway of complement activation:
(a) was originally known as the "properdin" pathway
(b) involves the complement components C1 to C9
(c) is the same as the classical pathway
(d) involves at least four serum proteins that do not contribute to the classical pathway
(Complement Activation: The Alternative Pathway)

13. Complement components can be destroyed in vitro by:
(a) anticoagulants
(b) heating to 37°C for 30 minutes
(c) normal serum inhibitor
(d) long-term storage
(The Destruction of Complement In Vitro)

14. C1q deficiency is associated with:
(a) SLE-like syndrome
(b) sex-linked agammaglobulinemia
(c) Neisseria infections
(d) all of the above
(C1q Deficiency)

15. The most common of the human complement deficiencies is:
(a) C1q deficiency
(b) C4 deficiency
(c) C2 deficiency
(d) C3 deficiency
(Clinical Significance of Complement Deficiency)

Answer "True" or "False"

1. The subclasses of IgG are equally potent in their ability to react with complement.
(Introduction)

2. If a complement fragment loses its activity, the letter i is added to indicate inactivation.
(The Components of Complement [Nomenclature])

3. The C1 complex is held together by calcium ions.
(C1: The Recognition Unit)

4. For C1q to initiate the complement cascade, it must attach to two Fab fragments.
(C1: The Recognition Unit)

5. The C4a subunit attaches to C1 on the antigen-antibody complex.
(C4: The Activation Unit)

6. C2a binds to C4b in the presence of magnesium to form C42.
(C2: The Second Activation Unit)

7. C6 and C7 associate easily with C5 in a trimolecular complex.
(C6 and C7: The Second and Third Membrane Attack Units)

8. The function of C9 appears to be to enhance the activity of C8.
(C8 and C9: The Final Membrane Attack Units)

9. The "holes" in the cell surface caused by C9 penetrate the cell membrane.
(The Effects of Complement Activation)

10. Properdin participates in the alternative pathway by binding to activated C3bBb.
(Complement Activation: The Alternative Pathway)

11. The anticoagulant heparin inhibits the cleavage of C4 by activated C1.
.(The Destruction of Complement In Vitro)

12. C3 decay products are not found in patients with systemic lupus erythematosus.
(Rheumatologic Diseases)

13. Complement is of particular importance in the clearance of cells coated with IgM cold agglutinins of anti-I specificity.
(Hematologic Diseases)

14. A deficiency of the C5 complement component results in defective MAC formation.
(Table 3–4)

15. Deficiencies of every component of the classical activation sequence are known.
(Clinical Significance of Complement Deficiency)

16. Plasma may be used in the CH_{50} total hemolytic complement assay.
(Method 1: CH_{50} Total Hemolytic Complement Assay)

17. Antigenic assays are not as sensitive as functional assays in the measurement of individual complement components.
(Immunoassays)

GENERAL REFERENCES

Abbas, A.K., Lichtman, A.H., and Pober, J.S.: Cellular and Molecular Immunology. Philadelphia, W. B. Saunders Company, 1991.

Baron, E.J., and Finegold, S.M.: Bailey and Scott's Diagnostic Microbiology, 8th ed. St Louis, C. V. Mosby Company, 1990.

Bellanti, J.A.: Immunology III. Philadelphia, W. B. Saunders Company, 1985.

Dorland's Illustrated Medical Dictionary, 27th ed. Philadelphia, W. B. Saunders Company, 1988.

Freeman, B.A.: Burrows Textbook of Microbiology, 27th ed. Philadelphia, W. B. Saunders Company, 1985.

Henry, J.B.: Clinical Diagnosis and Management by Laboratory Methods. Philadelphia, W. B. Saunders Company, 1991.

Mollison, P.L., Engelfriet, C.P., and Contreras, M.: Blood Transfusion in Clinical Medicine, 8th ed. Oxford, Blackwell Scientific Publications, 1987.

Sheehan, C.: Clinical Immunology: Principles and Laboratory Diagnosis. Philadelphia, J. B. Lippincott, 1990.

Walter, J.B.: An Introduction to the Principles of Disease, 2nd ed. Philadelphia, W. B. Saunders Company, 1982.

4

The Immune Response

Introduction

When foreign antigen gains entry into the body, several important changes may be initiated, collectively known as the *immune response,* which result in the elimination of the alien antigen. A remarkable feature of this phenomenon is the ability of the adult mammal to distinguish between its own antigens (known as "self" antigens) and those of external or foreign origin (known as "non-self" antigens). This means that, as a general rule, antibody is *selectively* produced in response to foreign substances, yet it is not produced to antigens that are recognized as "self."

The immune response is presumed to have been

67

evolved by animals as a means of self-protection in a world teeming with microorganisms; yet, whereas the self–non-self response is selective, the reaction to foreign substances is not, and antibodies are formed regardless of whether or not these substances are bacterial products.

Under certain circumstances, these antibodies can react with foreign material if it is reintroduced and can produce severe damage to tissue components (the phenomenon known as *hypersensitivity*). It is evident that the immune response is not only concerned with immunity to infection but that it is also involved in many disease processes, and, under certain circumstances, it *causes* hypersensitivity (see further discussion later in this chapter).

As previously mentioned, the immune response results in the formation of antibodies, these being either immunoglobulins or cell-bound.

GENETIC CONTROL OF THE IMMUNE RESPONSE

Certain antibodies, which were found to react with antigens expressed on leukocytes, were discovered in multitransfused individuals and multiparous women in the 1950s. The antigens (because they were expressed on leukocytes) were called human leukocyte antigens (HLAs). Although this name has been retained, the region of the genome, now known to be the most genetically diverse of all regions, was named the major histocompatibility complex (MHC). The MHC has been found to be important in transplantation, disease associations, differentiation of individuals (e.g., paternity testing), and, more recently, the regulation of the immune response during antigen presentation (Schwartz, 1987).

The Antigens of the MHC

Ten distinct genetic areas are located in the major histocompatibility complex, which occupies a position on the short arm of chromosome number 6. These genetic areas are named HLA-A, -B, -C, -E, -D/DR, -DQ, -DP, -DN, -DO, and [C2, C4, and Bf] (Fig. 4–1), and each gene yields a specific antigen product.

There are three *classes* of gene products that arise out of this gene complex:

Class I Antigens. These are cellular proteins made up of a single glycoprotein chain (molecular weight 44,000) and include the HLA-A, -B, and -C antigens. Most of the protein is on the outer surface of the cell membrane (281 of the total 338 amino acids), but a small portion passes through the cell membrane (25 amino acids) and into the interior of the cell (32 amino acids). A second protein, known as β_2 microglobulin, is loosely associated with class I antigens. These antigens are found on all nucleated cells, and some remnants have been found on red cells (Issitt, 1985). The class I antigens are those that are recognized in graft rejection (Schwartz, 1987).

Class II Antigens. These are also cellular proteins but are composed of two glycoprotein chains, (α–molecular weight 34,000 d) and (β–molecular weight 29,000 d), and include the HLA-D/DR, -DQ, and -DP antigens. The α and β chains are located next to each other on the cell membrane but are not covalently bound. They function together, however, since both chains are transmembrane. Each glycoprotein chain is encoded in the MHC locus, and multiple alleles exist for different α and β chains. One gene codes for the α chain and three different genes code for the β chain. The same α chain is shared by all HLA-DR molecules; this

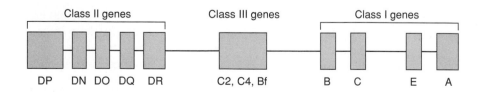

Figure 4–1. The ten genetic areas of the major histocompatibility complex (MHC).

chain can combine with any β chain. There are two α and two β chain genes for the DP and DQ subregions. It is believed that the α chain of one subregion can combine only with the β chain of the same subregion. Class II antigens are not found on nucleated cells but are restricted to immunocompetent cells, particularly B cells and macrophages. These antigens are important for antigen presentation and interactions between immunocompetent cells.

Class III Antigens. These are considered to be minor MHC antigens. They are mainly proteins secreted by cells and are complement components C2, C4 (which activate C3 in the classical pathway), and factor B (which activates C3 by the alternative pathway). The polymorphism of these antigens is less than that of the class I and class II antigens.

The Role of the MHC in Regulating the Immune Response

The fact that the MHC has a role in regulating the immune response is evidenced by MHC restriction. This occurs when a lymphocyte population can be activated only in the presence of an antigen and an MHC molecule. For example CD8-positive cells (cytotoxic T cells) will respond only if a viral antigen is associated with a class I MHC antigen on a virally infected cell. The viral antigen plus the class I antigen on the target cell are recognized by the CD3 and CD8 receptors, respectively, on the surfaces of cytotoxic T cells. The class I antigen alone or the virus alone on a virally infected cell will not cause a response.

In the case of a viral antigen being associated with a class II MHC antigen, the response will involve a CD4-positive cell (a T-helper cell). The CD3

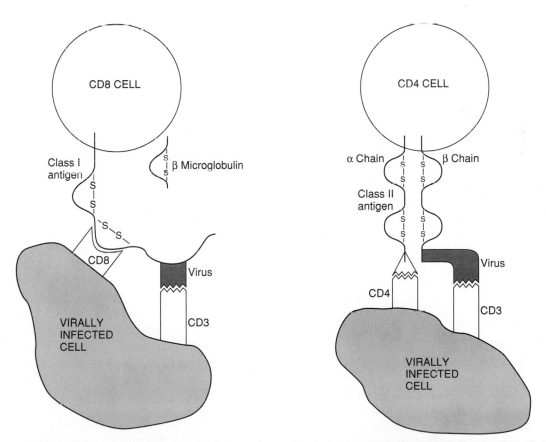

Figure 4–2. Reaction of class I and class II MHC antigens with virally infected cells. (Modified from Fike, D.J.: Major histocompatibility complex. In Sheehan, C.: Clinical Immunology: Principles and Laboratory Diagnosis. Philadelphia, J. B. Lippincott, 1991.)

and CD4 receptors on the helper cells recognize the viral antigen plus the class II antigen (Fig. 4–2). It is believed that the lymphocyte is activated by a signal that results from the CD3 molecule interaction (Roitt, 1988).

THE FORMATION OF IMMUNOGLOBULIN

The immune response, following the entry of foreign antigen into the body, is preceded by a period of antigen elimination, after which a primary response occurs, or, if the antigen has been encountered previously, a secondary response occurs.

Antigen Elimination

If foreign antigen is injected intravenously, three phases of antigen removal are easily detected:

The First Phase. This takes about 10 to 20 minutes if particulate antigens are used and represents the time required for equilibrium of the antigen to occur within tissues and fluids. Almost 90 per cent of the antigen is removed from the circulation in the first passage through the liver, lung, and spleen through extensive phagocytosis. Soluble antigens are not removed from the blood quite as quickly because of their slower pinocytic uptake by cells. If the antigen is aggregated, it is removed faster, indicating that size is important in phagocytosis and pinocytosis.

The Second Phase. This is a gradual catabolic degradation and removal process, which continues over a period of 4 to 7 days and represents the gradual enzymatic hydrolysis and digestion of the antigen. The limits of this period are regulated by the enzymatic capability of the host for the particular type of substrate that the antigen represents. In hosts that fail to produce antibody (i.e., become tolerant to the antigen), this phase is extended for several weeks and represents the last phase of antigen elimination.

The Third Phase. In the final phase of antigen elimination, there is, once again, accelerated removal of antigen. The phase is sometimes known as the immune elimination segment and is the result of the newly formed antibody molecules combining with the antigen, enhancing phagocytosis, digestion, and removal. The absolute removal of all antigen, however, may take many months or even years (Fig. 4–3).

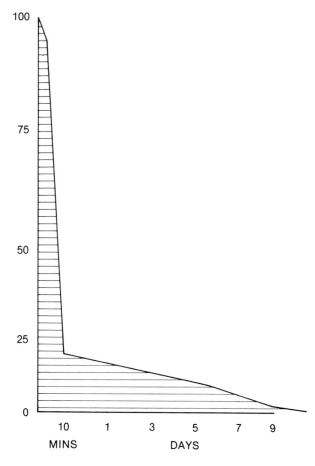

Figure 4–3. The antigen elimination curve. (From Barrett, J. T.: Textbook of Immunology, 4th ed. St. Louis, The C. V. Mosby Company, 1983, p. 142.)

The Primary Response

Following the first injection of antigen, there is a lag of several days before antibody is detected in the serum. This latent period (also known as the "induction" period) varies from several hours to several days, depending upon the kind of antigen involved, the amount of antigen given, the route of administration, the species of animal and its health, and the sensitivity of the test used to detect the antibody. On the average, antibody usually appears from the fifth to the tenth day after injection of antigen.

It should be noted that the latent period is *not* a reflection of the amount of time it takes for antibody production to begin at a cellular level. In fact, when antibody-forming cells are removed from an immunized animal, antibody synthesis can be detected within 20 minutes after exposure to the antigen. Because only a few cells are involved in antibody production at this time, it may take several days before the antibody is detectable in the serum. Another consideration is that the first antibody molecules to appear in the serum may find residual antigen still in the circulation and may combine with it, making the detection of the antibody difficult by usual serologic tests. These antigen-antibody complexes are secreted rapidly, so that the first evidence of *free* antibody is not until a few days after the first antibody molecules are liberated into the serum. In this way, very large injections of antigens may tend to extend the latent period.

At the end of the latent period, the primary antibody response becomes visible. The titer of the antibody gradually increases over a period of a few days to a few weeks, reaches a plateau, and then begins to drop. The general shape of the primary response curve is that of the typical sigmoid curve, with an extended decay phase. A typical primary response curve is given in Figure 4–4, although it should be noted that the exact shape of the curve will be dictated by the variables already stated.

The first immunoglobulin class to appear in the primary antibody response is IgM, followed by the production of IgG.

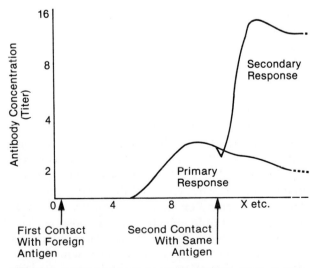

Figure 4–4. Primary and secondary response to foreign antigen.

The Secondary Response

After second (or subsequent) exposure to a foreign antigen, the response of the host differs dramatically from that of the primary response. At first, there is a sharp drop in the amount of circulating antibody because it is complexing with the newly injected antigen. Immediately thereafter (usually within 2 or 3 days under normal conditions and circumstances), the level of antibody in the blood increases markedly. This increase continues for several days, and ultimately the titer of the antibody far surpasses that attained in the primary response. The secondary response is also known as the memory, anamnestic, or booster response. It is as though the host is now primed for that particular antigen and is able to respond to it in an accelerated way (see the discussion that follows).

All of the variables that affect the primary response also to some extent affect the secondary response. Although the latent period is briefer, there is a heightened titer, and the duration of detectable antibody in the blood is extended.

It should be noted that the rapid response seen is not the result of the release of *stored* antibody, but rather the result of bulk synthesis of the new antibody. This has been proved through experiments with radiolabeled amino acids that were injected at the same time as the antigen. When the antibody was studied after a few days, it was found to be heavily labeled with isotope, indicating recent production.

There is no time limit for the secondary response—it may be induced at any time after the primary response, even many years later when the primary titer has dropped to zero. If the secondary response is nearer to the time of the primary response, however, it is usually more striking than it would be after several years.

The secondary response may be repeated many times until the physiologic limit of the host reaction to the involved foreign antigen is reached. This may not occur until three to five booster injections of the antigen have been given.

The secondary response may be induced by cross-reactive antigens. The degree of response in these cases can be correlated with the similarity of the two antigens—the more alike they are, the better the response is likely to be.

In some cases, so-called negative anamnesis may

occur. This can result from the treatment of the immunized host, which may cause lysis or hyperplasia of the antibody-forming cells. It should be noted, however, that the response in these cases is usually minimal.

After the secondary response, the decrease in antibody titer seems to be more gradual than it is after the primary response. This is probably the result of two factors:

1. More cells are involved in antibody production in the secondary response. If some of these cells are long-lived and continue to function, antibody will be formed over a longer period of time after the secondary response than after the primary response.
2. The antiserum in the secondary response is quantitatively different from that of the primary response, containing more IgG, which has a half-life of 25 to 35 days. The primary antiserum is relatively rich in IgM, which has a half-life of only 8 to 10 days. IgG has been referred to as the "memory component," implying that IgM anamnesis does not occur. This is true in a relative sense only, because secondary IgM levels are in fact somewhat greater than primary IgM levels.

When soluble antigens or autocoupling haptens are used for reactivation of the immunoglobulin, a certain danger exists in that a proportion of the antibody produced after the primary antigenic exposure has the capacity to fix to tissue cells, and these cell-bound antibodies can attach to the injected antigen while still attached to the tissue cells. In some cases, this *in vivo* cell-bound antigen-antibody reaction can trigger a set of reactions that may be lethal to the host. This syndrome is known as anaphylactic shock and, under certain conditions, may be considered a hazard to reimmunization. (See further discussion under Hypersensitivity, this chapter.)

The secondary response, as previously mentioned, occurs as a result of "immunologic memory," carried by the small lymphocytes. This means that the small lymphocytes retain information regarding the challenging antigen. Immunologic memory can be transferred from one animal to another. Small lymphocytes from a rat that has already given a primary response to an antigen challenge can be injected into another rat with no previous contact with that antigen. Subsequent challenge with the antigen to the recipient rat results in a secondary-type response, with rapid production of high-strength antibodies.

THE EFFECTS OF IMMUNOGLOBULIN *IN VIVO*

Immunity

The primary effect of immunoglobulin *in vivo* is to provide immunity for the host against reinfection. In the case of most infective agents, antibodies that are produced in response to infection are directed against the antigenic components of the organism itself and are called *antibacterial, antiviral,* or *antifungal* antibodies. In general, since the organisms have many antigenic determinants, antibodies are produced that have different specificities.

Some of these antibodies play a protective role against reinfection (i.e., provide immunity), whereas others appear to have no protective activity. These nonprotective antibodies, through their detection in the blood, are, however, useful in diagnosis (e.g., in cases of typhoid fever or secondary syphilis; see Chapter 6).

Active immunization is carried out through the injection of a suspension of the invasive organism (either living or dead) or through the injection of a *toxoid* (i.e., a chemically altered preparation of bacterial toxin). In addition, passive antibacterial immunity can be achieved by injecting human or animal sera containing specific antibodies, although the discovery of potent antibiotics has made the use of such sera unnecessary. Passive immunization against *viral* infections, however, still has a useful role (e.g., anti-measles serum is used to prevent very young children from contracting this infection).

Antibacterial antibodies provide immunity to infection in a variety of ways—some may act as opsonins and aid phagocytosis, others activate complement and lead to lysis of the organism. The activation of complement also releases factors such as C3b, for example, which acts as an opsonin. The spread of infection is limited by anaphylatoxins and chemotactic factors, which augment the inflammatory response, or by agglutinins, although the role of the latter in this is probably minor.

Globulin antibodies are generally named according to the nature of the test used to detect them (e.g., antitoxin, precipitin), although some antibodies are capable of performing several functions, depending upon the conditions under which they are examined. For example, diphtheria toxin, which is capable of neutralizing toxin in an *in vivo* experiment, is rightly known as an "antitoxin"; *in vitro*, however, it can produce a precipitin with its corresponding antigen and can, in this instance, be called a "precipitin." Some antibodies (e.g., those directed against certain red cell antigens) produce agglutination in the absence of complement (agglutinins) and lysis when complement is fixed (lysin).

Hypersensitivity

While the immune response is primarily of *benefit* to the host, it is now clear that it may also have negative effects (e.g., tissue damage). This is known as *hypersensitivity* (Table 4–1). The mechanisms of tissue damage resulting in hypersensitivity have been divided into four categories: Type I (anaphylactic); Type II (cytotoxic); Type III (immune-complex disorders); and Type IV (delayed hypersensitivity).

Anaphylaxis (Type I Hypersensitivity). This type of reaction is also known as immediate hypersensitivity, because the reaction occurs within minutes of contact with the antigen or allergen. The effector cells involved in allergic response are circulating basophils or tissue mast cells that are sensitized by the cytotropic antibody, IgE, the immunoglobulin being bound to the cell surface by way of Fc receptors. Upon subsequent exposure to the allergen, these sensitized cells are triggered to release vasoactive amines (contained in their cytoplasmic granules) that produce allergic symptoms. The extent of allergic response is dependent partly on the size of the allergen (small allergens may not have sufficient numbers of epitopes to facilitate the essential Fc receptor cross-linking to trigger a basophil or mast cell, whereas a larger molecule may not be able to diffuse across the mucosal surface to reach the sensitized effector cells). Exposure to allergens can be through inhalation, absorption from the digestive tract, or direct skin contact. The extent of allergic response is also partly influenced by the port of entry of the allergen. A bee sting, for example, introduces the allergen into the circulation, causing a systemic anaphylaxis, whereas an inhaled allergen can cause respiratory symptoms (e.g., rhinitis and asthma). The various clinical conditions (asthma, eczema, hay fever) are collectively known as "atopy" because they share many common features.

There is evidence of a strong hereditary linkage associated with allergy (Marsh *et al.*, 1981). About 5 to 10 per cent of the population become sensitized when exposed to airborne allergens.

The Mediators of Allergic Response. The mediators of allergic response can be divided into two categories:

Preformed Mediators

Histamine. Histamine causes contraction of the bronchioles and smooth muscle of blood vessels, increases capillary permeability, and increases mucous gland secretion in the airway. The mediator is

Type	Reaction	Antibody	Clinical Examples
I	Anaphylactic	IgE	Asthma, hay fever, helminth infestation
II	Cytotoxic	IgG, IgM	Antibacterial antibodies, autoimmune disease (Hashimoto's thyroiditis, antigastric antibodies in pernicious anemia, hemolytic anemia, etc.), viral disease prevention
III	Immune complex	IgG, IgM	Serum sickness, glomerulonephritis, and immune-complex disease
IV	Delayed hypersensitivity	Sensitized lymphocytes	Tuberculin skin test (also fungal skin tests, Frei antigen, etc.), rejection of allografts or xenografts, "resistance" to viral disease

TABLE 4–1. Types of Clinical Hypersensitivity

Modified from Raphael, S. S.: Lynch's Medical Laboratory Technology, 4th ed. Philadelphia, W. B. Saunders Co., 1983.

stored in the granules. It can be released within 1 to 2 minutes after the reaction of allergen and antibody and has an activity duration of about 10 minutes.

Eosinophil Chemotactic Factor of Anaphylaxis. This preformed mediator is released during degranulation. It stimulates eosinophils to migrate to the site of an antigen-antibody reaction. Eosinophils are involved in phagocytosis and disposal of antigen-antibody complexes, and they release the enzymes histamine and arylsulfatase, which dampen the allergic reaction caused by allergic mediators.

Newly Synthesized Mediators. After the effector cells (basophils and mast cells) are triggered, the newly synthesized mediators are derived from membrane lipid. Arachidonic acid is liberated by the action of phospholipid A or phospholipase C and diacylglycerol lipase. The freed arachidonic acid is then processed by one of two metabolic pathways: the cyclooxygenase (prostaglandin synthetase) pathway, which leads to prostaglandin D_2 production, or the 5-lipoxygenase pathway, which leads to leukotriene production.

Prostaglandin D_2 causes vasodilation and increased vascular permeability. This results in erythematous wheal and flare reaction (the same clinical symptoms seen with histamine). The prostaglandin D_2 effect can persist for as long as 2 hours.

Leukotrienes C_4, D_4, and E_4 cause erythema and wheal formation. They also cause bronchospasm when inhaled. Their bronchoconstrictive potency is 30 to 1000 times that of histamine. Leukotrienes C_4 and D_4 have also been shown to stimulate mucous secretion by human airway tissue.

Cytotoxic (Type II Hypersensitivity). This type of reaction is manifested by the production of antibodies that are capable of destroying cell surface molecules or tissue components. The antibodies, which are IgG or IgM, bind to the cell-bound antigen, which can result in the activation of complement and destruction of the cell (cytolysis). Erythrocytes, leukocytes, and platelets can be lysed by this process. Examples of cytotoxic reactions include hemolytic reactions to blood transfusion (immediate or delayed), nonhemolytic reactions (febrile reactions, reactions to platelet transfusions, reactions to plasma constituents, allergic and anaphylactoid reactions, anaphylactic reactions [anti-IgA]), and immune hemolytic anemias, such as

hemolytic disease of the newborn. Tissue damage may be mediated by accelerated clearance of the antibody-sensitized target cells by the mononuclear phagocytic system, blockade of normal cellular function because of antibody binding to the target cells, complement-mediated lysis of the target cells, or the damage of innocent bystander cells or tissue by the lysosomal enzymes released by the neutrophils present at the site of antigen-antibody reactions.

Cytotoxic reactions involving transfusion are of most interest to the immunohematologist, and therefore details of these reactions will not be given here. The interested student is referred to the list of general references given at the end of this chapter for more detailed information.

Cytotoxic antibodies to tissue components frequently cause inflammatory responses, leading to hematuria, renal failure, and hemoptysis. A classic example of this is Goodpasture's syndrome.

Immune-Complex Reactions (Type III Hypersensitivity). Certain types of antibodies (predominantly IgG and IgM) have the ability to combine with their corresponding antigens to form complexes that can activate complement. The deposition of these circulating immune complexes in tissues causes inflammation. This results in the liberation of chemotactic factors and polymorphs, which are attached to the complexes and release damaging lysosomal enzymes. Localized immune complex formation can also result in Type III hypersensitivity. Inflammation of the joint seen in rheumatoid arthritis is an example. Examples in which these immune complexes produce disease include the Arthus reaction, chronic immune-complex disease, and serum sickness.

The Arthus Reaction. If subcutaneous injections of an antigen are given to an animal on a weekly basis, progressively more severe local reactions are observed. Swelling and redness appear within 1 hour, and hemorrhage and necrosis develop over the next few hours. The pathogenesis is as follows:

1. The injected antigen diffuses into the vessel walls and encounters the specific IgG that is present in the blood.
2. The antigen-antibody complexes activate complement in the vessel wall.
3. Polymorphs accumulate and release their lysosomal enzymes.

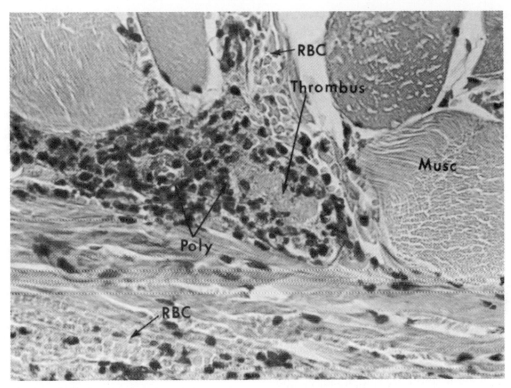

Figure 4–5. The Arthus reaction in a rabbit. This section is from the subcutaneous tissues and includes striated muscle (Musc). The blood vessel in the center is sectioned obliquely and shows occlusion of its lumen by thrombus. Its walls are heavily infiltrated by polymorphs (Poly), many of which are degenerating. Free red cells (RBC) in the tissues bear witness to the severity of vascular damage ($\times$ 550). (From Walter, J. B.: An Introduction to the Principles of Disease, 2nd ed. Philadelphia, W. B. Saunders Company, 1982, p. 127.)

4. The cell wall is damaged, and thrombosis follows (Fig. 4–5).

The Arthus reaction is believed to be the explanation for some types of vasculitis in humans, such as that seen in gonococcal septicemia.

Chronic Immune-Complex Disease. A number of naturally occurring diseases are believed to be caused by deposits of immune complex and complement in the tissues (e.g., systemic lupus erythematosus [SLE], serum sickness, acute diffuse glomerulonephritis, rheumatic fever, rheumatoid arthritis, and periarteritis nodosa). These diseases show some or all of the features of arthritis, carditis, glomerulonephritis, and vasculitis.

Serum Sickness. Serum sickness can occur in individuals who have had no previous contact with the offending antigen (primary serum sickness) or in those who have been previously sensitized with the offending antigen (accelerated serum sickness). In both cases, the pathogenesis is the same, although the onset of symptoms is more immediate in accelerated serum sickness.

Pathogenesis. Following the injection of a large dose of antigen, antibody is produced, which enters the blood stream in increasing amounts over a period of days (in the primary syndrome) or as soon as a few hours (in the accelerated syndrome). If the antigen is still circulating by the time that there is a sizable amount of circulating antibody, antigen-antibody complexes are formed and are rapidly eliminated by the activity of the mononuclear-phagocyte system. The complexes are deposited on a sensitive membrane such as beneath the glomerular endothelium, skin, and joints. Complement is then activated, polymorphs accumulate, and inflammatory products that cause tissue damage are released. In both the primary and accelerated syndromes, there may be production of IgE as well as IgM and IgG, and, in these instances, anaphylactic symptoms may occur. The syndrome is characterized by fever, joint pains, and urti-

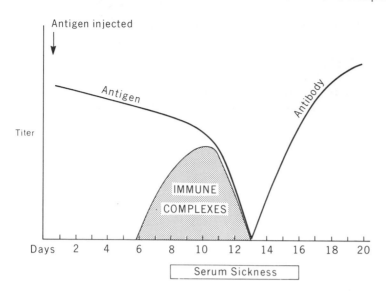

Antigen injected

Antigen

Antibody

Titer

IMMUNE
COMPLEXES

Days   2   4   6   8   10   12   14   16   18   20

Serum Sickness

Figure 4–6. A graph showing changes in antigen and antibody titer during serum sickness. (From Walter, J. B.: An Introduction to the Principles of Disease, 2nd ed. Philadelphia, W. B. Saunders Company, 1982, p. 147.)

carial eruptions, which occur within the time limits given.

The course of the illness is variable, depending upon the type, extent, and severity of the lesions that may involve the joints (arthritis), kidney (glomerulonephritis), heart (myocarditis), and skin (vasculitis). In general, as immune complexes are catabolized, the symptoms of the illness subside and free antibody appears in the blood (Fig. 4–6).

Serum sickness provoked by drugs forming haptens with body protein antigens (e.g., penicillin, streptomycin) is well known.

Cell-Mediated Reactions (Type IV Hypersensitivity). See later in this chapter under Hypersensitivity in Cell-Mediated Immunity.

CELL-MEDIATED IMMUNITY

Cell-mediated immunity is probably a factor in immunity to all infections, but it is of particular importance with respect to infections with viruses, fungi, and acid-fast bacillary infections such as tuberculosis and leprosy.

The presence of cell-bound antibody is, like the humoral immune response, associated with either immunity to infection or hypersensitivity. Neither cellular immunity nor hypersensitivity, however, can be transferred to another animal by transferring serum; it can only be affected by the transfer of lymphocytes.

There is no simple way to measure or assess cell-mediated immunity; only the response to challenging infection can reveal its presence.

THE EFFECTORS OF THE CELL-MEDIATED IMMUNE RESPONSE

The effectors of the cell-mediated immune response involve primarily cytotoxic T lymphocytes (with antibody playing a subordinate role), which destroy targets by direct cell contact, and soluble mediators, collectively known as *cytokines*, which have direct cytolytic activity or enhance the cytolytic activity of the effector cells. In addition, macrophages and natural killer (NK) cells are involved in the response, as is an effector mechanism that involves antibodies and cells for target destruction, known as antibody-dependent cell-mediated cytolysis (ADCC).

Cytotoxic T Cells (T_C). These cells are capable of destroying target cells without antibody involvement, although *direct* cell contact is required. This contact is achieved by the T-cell receptor, which binds to the target antigen, and the MHC molecule on the target cell surface, which leads to target cell swelling and destruction. This killing activity can be repeated with the T_C moving from one cell to another. The main function of these cells is to eliminate virally infected host cells. They are CD8-positive cells with MHC class I restriction. A second type of T_C, found in patients undergoing graft rejection or in the tumor-infiltrating lymphocytes, is CD4 positive and MHC class II restricted (Roitt, 1985).

Macrophages. Macrophages play a dual role in the cell-mediated immune response; they present antigen to the T cells during the induction phase and become activated in response to lymphokines during the effector phase. Lymphokines modulate the functions of macrophages. For example, macrophage migration inhibition factor (MIF) inhibits the migration of macrophages so that they are retained at the site of antigen response. In addition, macrophage activation factor (MAF) enhances their microbicidal and tumoricidal activities. It is important to note that the biologic activities are not antigen specific. Lymphokines produced by the T cells sensitized to one antigen may activate macrophages that will destroy the sensitized antigens as well as other unrelated targets (Roitt, 1985).

Natural Killer Cells. Natural killer cells do not express T- or B-cell markers; however, they consistently express Fc receptors on the cell surface. They are capable of killing virally infected cells or neoplastic cells without previous sensitization. The cellular activities are modulated by lymphokines. IL-2, for example, stimulates their proliferative activities, and their cytolytic activities are enhanced by interferon (Roitt, 1985; Lazarus and Baines, 1985; MacDougall *et al.*, 1986).

Antibody-Dependent Cell-Mediated Cytolysis (ADCC). The phenomenon by which effector cells with cytolytic activity and Fc receptors are able to lyse antibody-coated target cells is known as antibody-dependent cell-mediated cytolysis. The antibody involved is usually IgG, which is directed against viral or tumor antigens on the target cell surface. The antigen specificity in this cytolytic activity therefore resides in the antibody molecule. The effector cells are poorly defined. NK cells probably play an important role—however, any Fc receptor-positive cell (including macrophages, monocytes, and neutrophils) has the potential to be an effector cell (Roitt, 1985).

Cytokines. Cytokines are protein molecules that, in effect, transmit messages between cells. The primary biologic activities of cytokines are regulation of cell growth and regulation of cellular differentiation. Cytokines that are produced by lymphocytes are known as *lymphokines;* those produced by monocytes are known as *monokines.*

Lymphokines are primarily produced by activated T cells. Their activities are as follows:

IL-2. This is a T-cell growth factor that induces proliferation of antigen-activated T cells and enhances the cytolytic activities of NK cells.

IL-3. This lymphokine supports the growth of pluripotential stem cells of the hematopoietic system.

Granulocyte-Macrophage Colony-Stimulating Factor. This lymphokine affects hematopoiesis by inducing the growth of hematopoietic cells that are differentiated and committed to becoming granulocytes or macrophages.

IL-4. This is also known as B-cell growth factor 1. It is produced by activated T cells and stimulates proliferation of antigen-activated B cells.

B-Cell Growth Factor 2. This induces differentiation of proliferating B cells into antibody-secreting plasma cells.

MIF and MAF. These regulate macrophage function (see Macrophages, above).

Gamma Interferon. This lymphokine enhances the cytolytic activities of NK cells and the activation of macrophages.

Two well-known monokines are IL-1, which stimulates IL-2 receptor expression and IL-2 synthesis by antigen-activated T cells, and tumor necrosis factor (TNF), which has direct cytolytic activity against tumor cells (Le and Vilcek, 1987).

The MHC Restriction of T-Cell Antigen Recognition

In general, T cells recognize antigens *in association with* MHC molecules. T cells are generally not stimulated by free or soluble antigens. T_H cells are known to be MHC class II restricted, and T_C cells are known to be MHC class I restricted. This is logical in view of the fact that cytotoxic T cells eliminate virally infected cells and therefore need to recognize the antigen in conjunction with the MHC class I molecule, which is widely distributed on all nucleated cells in the host, whereas T_H cells are regulatory and therefore need to recognize antigens, which are limited to cells of the immune system (i.e., MHC class II molecules).

The Activation of T Cells

Activation of an effector T cell requires three signals—antigenic stimulation, IL-1, and IL-2. The sequence is as follows:

1. A macrophage or other antigen-presenting cell presents the antigen and provides IL-1.
2. A T_H cell recognizes the antigen (in conjunction with an MHC class II molecule on the antigen-presenting cell surface). During the cell contact, the antigen-presenting cell may receive a signal or signals from the T_H cell and releases IL-1. IL-1 promotes the IL-2 receptor expression or IL-2 synthesis by the T cells. Only T cells that are already sensitized by the antigen can respond to IL-1.
3. An effector T cell that is sensitized by the antigen and stimulated by IL-1 expresses IL-2 receptors. In the presence of IL-2, it undergoes blast transformation, cell division, and differentiation. The effector T cells may be cytotoxic or lymphokine-producing T cells.

Hypersensitivity in Cell-Mediated Immunity

Cell-mediated hypersensitivity is also known as Type IV, or *delayed hypersensitivity* (see Table 4–1). It is mediated by cells; circulating antibody and complement are not involved. Many reactions to immunologic insult involve both cellular and humoral components; those that may be used as examples of this type of response include the tuberculin skin reaction (described below), contact sensitivity, and granulomatous hypersensitivity.

Type IV hypersensitivity is mediated by soluble factors (lymphokines) released by the sensitized T lymphocytes. The lymphokines have biologic activities affecting various cell types (as described above). The reaction is generally controlled by normal control mechanisms. In the hypersensitive individual, however, multiple antigenic challenges can lead to the ulceration and necrosis of the lesion. Symptoms usually develop over a 24- to 48-hour period (after antigen exposure) and peak within 72 hours. Histologic examination shows mononuclear infiltration, which is characteristic.

The Tuberculin Skin Reaction (the Koch Phenomenon). If tubercle bacilli are injected into a normal guinea pig, a nodule appears at the site of injection after an incubation period of 10 to 14 days, followed by ulceration. The bacilli spread to local lymph nodes, and finally they reach the blood stream, resulting in the death of the animal within 6 to 12 weeks. The injection of more tubercle bacilli into a different site in the same animal infected 4 to 6 weeks previously elicits a completely different response: the nodule appears within 1 or 2 days, ulcerates, and then heals, and the bacilli tend not to spread to local lymph nodes. The details of this second type of response were introduced at the end of the 19th century by Robert Koch, who produced a crude filtrate of a broth culture of *Mycobacterium tuberculosis* called *old tuberculin*, which, although valueless as a therapeutic agent (the purpose for which it was originally introduced), was nevertheless found to be of value as a diagnostic tool. Koch's old tuberculin has now been replaced by the purified protein derivative of tuberculin (PPD). When given intradermally in considerable dilution (1:1,000 to 1:10,000) in 0.1-ml amounts, an area of induration of 5 mm or more in diameter at the site of injection surrounded by erythema observed after 48 hours is considered a positive response in individuals who have a hypersensitivity to tuberculoprotein (i.e., those who have been sensitized by previous or present tuberculosis). The test is known as the *tuberculin* or *Mantoux test.* It should be noted that this test, although indicative of sensitization, does not indicate the clinical activity of the disease. The exact relationship between skin sensitivity and the level of cellular immunity is not clear, but it is likely that such a relationship exists.

Other skin tests used similarly include histoplasmin, coccidioidin, blastomycin, and the Frei test.

The characteristics of the Koch phenomenon are:

1. The reaction is delayed, taking at least 12 hours to develop. This is unlike other types of hypersensitivity reactions, which generally take only a few minutes.
2. There is an accumulation of lymphocytes and macrophages (giving a *mild* inflammatory reaction) rather than polymorphs at the site of insult.
3. The reaction is not mediated by histamine (or by any other mediators of acute inflammation) and is not blocked by antihistaminic drugs.

4. Immunoglobulins are not involved in the reaction.
5. The sensitivity to a particular antigen may be transferred from a sensitive to an insensitive individual by the transfer of T lymphocytes but not by the transfer of serum. If T lymphocytes are transferred, passive hypersensitivity persists for as long as the injected cells live in the new host, and, in some way, the transplanted cells alter the new host's own lymphocytes, so that these also take part in the delayed type of skin reaction that is subsequently elicited. Not only living cells but also *extracts* of lymphocytes from responsive individuals can be used to transfer delayed hypersensitivity through the action of a substance known as *transfer factor,* which is one of the lymphokines. The action of this substance is not fully understood; it is evidently very potent, however, because a single injection can bestow hypersensitivity on a recipient for many months.

Cell-mediated immune reactions are of great importance in the transplantation of tissues, in immunity to viral diseases, in forms of contact sensitivity (i.e., systemic sensitization through direct skin contact with the antigen [e.g., poison ivy and poison oak]) (Diaz and Provast, 1987), and in autoimmune disease (see Chapter 14). Cell-mediated immune reactions are also important in granulomatous hypersensitivity, which results from the persistent presence of microorganisms within the macrophages that the cell is unable to destroy. This is seen in tuberculosis, in leprosy and sarcoidosis, and in autoimmune disease (see Chapter 14).

IMMUNOGLOBULIN DEFICIENCY DISEASES

The immunoglobulin deficiency diseases can be considered under three headings: (1) the primary immunodeficiency syndromes, (2) the secondary immunodeficiency syndromes, and (3) the acquired immunodeficiency syndrome.

Primary Immunodeficiency Syndromes. The primary immunodeficiencies are those conditions in which, as a primary hereditary condition, the cellular, humoral, or both immune mechanisms are deficient. At one extreme, therefore, there may be agammaglobulinemia or dysgammaglobulinemia in which one or several immunoglobulins are absent because of B-cell deficiency—or, at the other extreme, thymic dysplasia will produce T-cell deficiency with lack of cell-mediated immune mechanisms. In the Wiskott-Aldrich syndrome, combined deficiencies occur in which deficiency of immunoglobulin(s) is combined with loss of cell-mediated responses.

Primary immunodeficiencies should also, for the sake of completeness, include disorders of phagocyte functions, such as Chédiak-Higashi syndrome, and a group of derangements of the complement system, discussed in Chapter 3.

Secondary Immunodeficiency Syndromes. The secondary immunodeficiencies result from involvement of the immunogenic system in the course of another disease. Such diseases include tumors of the lymphoid system involving B or T cells (causing inadequate function), as well as hematologic disorders in which phagocytes are quantitatively or qualitatively deficient (e.g., leukemia). Protein-losing conditions (e.g., nephrotic syndrome) deplete the body of immunoglobulins. In addition, patients with diabetes mellitus and renal failure exhibit diminished resistance to infection by a mechanism that is poorly understood.

Immunologic function is also affected by drugs (e.g., cortisone and cytotoxic agents) as well as by x-irradiation used in cancer therapy. In contrast, many drugs are used therapeutically as immunosuppressives, particularly in transplant surgery, glomerulonephritis, and so forth.

Acquired Immunodeficiency Syndrome. See Chapter 13.

THE IMMUNE RESPONSE: FUNCTIONAL ASPECTS

The functions of the immune response are as follows:

Recognition. Since, as previously mentioned, an individual does not generally produce antibodies to antigens regarded as self, it follows that a mechanism must exist for recognizing an antigen as foreign. Moreover, the system must have a memory so that the same antigen can be recognized after reexposure. Morphologically, the small lymphocytes are the "recognition" cells, which *initiate* the immune response, and as such are termed *immunologically competent cells.*

Processing. Subsequent to recognition as foreign, an antigen's determinants must be processed in such a way that a *specific* antibody can be produced. The macrophages are believed to perform this function, because they ingest antigen and appear to release factors that act on the antibody-producing cells.

Production. The final phase of the immune response is the production of antibody, which involves the synthesis of a range of specific proteins as well as the formation of immune lymphocytes. This manufacturing system must be regulated in some way so that the immune response can be discontinued when the antigen stimulation is withdrawn.

Certain theories have been postulated to explain the production of antibody, both in terms of the role played by the antigen and the extraordinary specificity of the antibodies.

The *instructive theory,* proposed in 1930, postulated that antigens play an instructive role, acting as molds or templates during antibody synthesis. The primary drawback to this theory is that it assumes that antigen remains in the body throughout the period of antibody production (an assumption for which there is little direct evidence because the immune response is responsible for their rapid elimination). In addition, it is difficult to imagine how a protein molecule (or its determinants) could modify the synthesis of a specific globulin in a cell, although this has been explained through the theory that contact with antigen produces a *permanent* modification of the antibody-producing cell. The explanation is still unsatisfactory, however, because it suggests a change of a self-replicating nature being handed down to the progeny of the cells for many generations.

The *selective theory (germ line theory),* formulated in 1960, postulated that cells exist in the adult that are capable of mounting an immune response against *any* non-self antigen that the host is likely to encounter. The antigen *selects* these cells and stimulates them to grow and produce antibody, thereby determining the quantity of antibody produced, but not its specificity.

The *somatic mutation theory,* in contrast, postulated that during embryonic development, many somatic mutations in the immunologically compe-

tent cells result in the formation of a *range* of cells that are capable of mounting an immune response for any encountered antigen. In adults, such contact stimulates growth of these cells, thus producing bodies of cells or "clones" (the name given to a group of cells of like hereditary constitution that has been produced asexually from a single cell; gr. *klon* = a cutting used for propagation). As the size of the clone increases, so does the intensity of antibody production.

If somatic mutation occurs so frequently, obviously cells are produced that can manufacture antibody against all possible antigens, and, inevitably, some mutations will result in cells capable of forming antibodies against the embryo's own developing tissues. The fact that this does not occur lends support to the theory that some mechanisms must exist, activated during embryonic development, for the destruction of these so-called *forbidden clones,* so that any antigen present in the embryo is recognized as self and that at birth no cells are present that are capable of producing antibody to it.

Recent studies have offered insight into the mechanism for the generation of antibody diversity through an understanding of structure and gene rearrangements of the antibody gene families.

The genes for antibody are located on three different chromosomes; the heavy chain genes are on chromosome number 14, the λ light chain genes are on chromosome number 22, and the κ light chain genes are on chromosome number 2. The V_H region is encoded by three genes that are transcribed into three polypeptide segments—V_H, D, and J_H. The V_L region is encoded by two genes that are transcribed into two polypeptide segments—V_L and J_L. These are known as the V genes (variable-segment genes) of the heavy and light chains. Many different genes exist for *each* V gene, and therefore a B cell is provided with an enormous library of genes from which the appropriate combination of V genes can be selected for V_H and V_L synthesis.

The process of V-gene recombination occurs very early in the development of the B cell, allowing for the emergence of B-cell populations that are extremely diverse and able (collectively) to recognize an unlimited number of antigens. The lack of *precision* in the joining of recombining genes provides even greater diversity (known as *junctional diversity*). Finally, the high mutation rates of V genes contribute to even greater diversity.

The combination of these three facts (gene recombination, junctional diversity, and V-gene mutation) allows the immune system to respond to an unlimited number of antigens with remarkable specificity.

IMMUNOLOGIC TOLERANCE

Immunologic tolerance refers to the situation in which, under certain conditions or circumstances, a foreign antigen fails to elicit the formation of antibody in the recipient. The terms *immunologic nonresponsiveness* and *immune paralysis* are synonymous with immunologic tolerance.

Studies of immune tolerance stem from the work of Owen (1945), who made the observation that dizygotic twin cattle (i.e., nonidentical), which shared the same placental circulation and whose circulations were thereby linked (known as chimerism), progressed through life with appreciable numbers of each other's red cells in their blood. Conversely, if they had not shared the same circulation, red cells from one twin injected into the other rapidly provoked an immune response. On the basis of this information, Burnet and Fenner (1941) postulated that an animal would be tolerant toward antigens encountered during embryonic life. This was considered the basis whereby the antigens indigenous to the body (i.e., self antigens) were recognized and therefore did not provoke immune responses, whereas foreign antigens (i.e., non-self antigens) did. This hypothesis was put to the test by Billingham *et al.* (1953), who injected embryonic mice with adult cells and showed that after birth the infant mice were tolerant toward skin from the same adult donors.

Tolerance can also be induced using soluble antigens. For example, rabbits injected at birth with bovine serum albumin fail to make antibodies on later challenge with this protein. Other immunogens that induce a state of tolerance include bacteria and tissue cells (Barrett, 1988).

It is now realized that tolerance can be induced in the adult as well as in the neonate. T cells are involved in tolerance at low antigen levels, whereas both B and T cells are made unresponsive at high antigen dose.

B-cell tolerance can be induced by the following:

Clonal Abortion. This occurs when an immature B cell is exposed to a low concentration of antigen and the maturation of that B cell is arrested so that it may not respond to that antigen on subsequent exposure.

Clonal Exhaustion. This occurs when a B cell is repeatedly exposed to T-independent antigens. All mature B cells expressing the receptor for this antigen are already antibody-producing cells—therefore no additional antigen binding and antibody production can occur (Roitt, 1985).

Functional Deletion. This occurs when T_H cells are not present to help T-dependent antigens, thereby not allowing B cells to mature into antibody-producing cells. This type of tolerance occurs in cases of high antigen dose where there are too few B cells to respond to such a dose.

Antibody-Forming Cell Blockade. This mechanism has a low ability to induce tolerance. It occurs when antigen binds to all receptors and thereby inhibits immunoglobulin secretion.

T-cell tolerance can be induced by:

Clonal Abortion. As with immature B cells, immature T cells may also be clonally aborted. When the immature T cell is exposed to low antigen concentration, its maturation is arrested so that the T cell may not respond to that antigen on subsequent exposure.

Functional Deletion. This may occur when one T-cell subset becomes tolerant to an antigenic determinant and fails to stimulate a functional B cell to produce antibody.

T-cell Suppression. This occurs when suppressor T cells actively suppress other T-cell subsets or B cells (Roitt, 1985).

B- and T-cell tolerances differ with respect to the time taken to become tolerant of (e.g., T-dependent antigens may tolerate T cells found in the spleen and thymus within hours of challenge but require up to 4 days to tolerate adult splenic B cells) the required dosage (B-cell tolerance requires a considerably higher level of antigen than that required for T-cell tolerance) and the duration of the state of tolerance, which is dependent on the mechanism by which tolerance was induced, and, to some extent, on the persistence of the antigen.

The ability of the body not to respond to autologous antigens is known as *self-tolerance*. While some B cells are normally present in an individual that recognize autologous antigens, they are inactive because of the lack of antigen recognition by T-helper cells (this would be an example of functional deletion) (Roitt, 1985).

AUTOIMMUNITY

As previously stated, under normal conditions and circumstances, an individual does not produce antibodies to antigens regarded as "self." In certain cases, however, the mechanisms that prevent their formation may break down, giving rise to the production of "self-antibodies," or *autoantibodies*, which are directed against the individual's own tissues.

There are, theoretically, three circumstances under which autoantibodies are produced:

1. If the antigenicity of tissue proteins is altered due to *degenerative lesions* (i.e., following necrosis of tissue, such as in skin burns) or the attachment of a hapten (in which case the antibodies are directed against the hapten rather than against the normal tissue proteins).
2. If a tissue antigen is anatomically isolated from the immunologically competent cells (and therefore not recognized as self), the release of this antigen into the tissues following injury or disease results in the formation of autoantibodies.
3. If a self protein is no longer recognized due to altered reactivity of the immune mechanism. This last condition is known to occur in cases of lymphocytic leukemia. In cases such as this, autohemolysins are sometimes produced, giving rise to a hemolytic anemia.

Autoantibodies may be immunoglobulin or cellular. The immunoglobulin might be of any class and may be *organ specific* (i.e., directed against a determinant present in one organ) or *non–organ specific* (i.e., directed against DNA, mitochondria, and immunoglobulin determinants).

Further discussion of autoantibodies and autoimmune diseases can be found in Chapter 14.

JUST THE FACTS

Introduction

1. The changes that are initiated when foreign antigen gains entry into the body are collectively known as the "immune response," which results in the elimination of the alien antigen through the formation of antibodies.
2. Antibody is selectively produced in response to foreign substances ("non-self") but is not produced to antigens recognized as "self."
3. The reaction to foreign substances is not selective.

Genetic Control of the Immune Response

1. The MHC is the most genetically diverse region of the genome.
2. Antigens on human leukocytes are called HLAs.
3. The MHC is important in transplantation, disease associations, paternity testing, and the regulation of the immune response during antigen presentation.

The Antigens of the MHC

1. Class I antigens include HLA-A, -B, and -C. These antigens are found on all nucleated cells.
2. Class II antigens include HLA-D/DR, -DQ, and -DP. These antigens are restricted to immunocompetent cells, particularly B cells and macrophages.
3. Class III antigens are complement components C2, C4, and factor B, which activate complement via the classical (C2, C4) or alternative (factor B) pathway.

The Role of the MHC in Regulating the Immune Response

1. The role of MHC regulation of the immune response is evidenced by MHC restriction.
2. The combination of viral antigen and class I antigen activates cytotoxic T cells.
3. The combination of viral antigen and class II antigen activates T-helper cells.

The Formation of Immunoglobulin

Antigen Elimination

1. There are three phases of antigen removal.
2. During the first phase, almost 90 per cent of the antigen is removed in the first passage through the lung, liver, and spleen through extensive phagocytosis.
3. Soluble antigens are not removed quite as quickly.
4. Aggregated antigen is removed faster.
5. The second phase is a gradual catabolic degradation and removal process through enzymatic hydrolysis and digestion.
6. The phase may extend for several weeks if the host fails to produce antibody.
7. The third phase is the production of antibody, which enhances phagocytosis, digestion, and removal. Absolute removal, however, may take years.

The Primary Response

1. On the average, antibody usually appears in the serum from the fifth to tenth day after the injection of antigen.
2. Antibody synthesis in the antibody-forming cells can be detected within 20 minutes of exposure to antigen.
3. After the latent period, the titer of the antibody rises, reaches a plateau, and then begins to drop.
4. The first immunoglobulin class to appear is IgM, followed by the production of IgG.

The Secondary Response

1. Introduction of the same antigen for a second time promotes a secondary response. This differs from a primary response in that:
   a. The latent period is shorter.
   b. The circulating antibody reaches higher titer.
   c. IgG is the predominant immunoglobulin.
   d. The antibody response tends to persist for a longer period of time.

The Effects of Immunoglobulin *in Vivo*

Immunity

1. The primary effect of immunoglobulin *in vivo* is to provide immunity for the host against reinfection.
2. Antibodies that have no protective role are useful in diagnosis.
3. Active immunity can be achieved through the injection of antigen.
4. Passive immunity can be achieved by injecting specific antibodies.
5. Globulin antibodies are generally named according to the nature of the test used to detect them (e.g., antitoxin, precipitin, etc.).

Hypersensitivity

1. The negative effect of the immune response (e.g., tissue damage) is known as hypersensitivity.
2. There are four categories of hypersensitivity.
3. Type I (anaphylaxis, immediate) has the following characteristics:
   a. The reaction occurs within minutes of contact.
   b. The effector cells are circulating basophils or tissue mast cells sensitized by IgE.
   c. The sensitized cells (after subsequent exposure to the allergen) are triggered to release vasoactive amines, which produce allergic symptoms.
   d. The extent of the response is party dependent on the size of the allergen and the port of entry.
   e. Exposure can be through inhalation, absorption, or direct skin contact.
   f. There is a possible hereditary linkage associated with allergy.
   g. The mediators of allergic response are preformed mediators (histamine and eosinophil chemotactic factor) and newly synthesized mediators (prostaglandin D_2 and leukotrienes C_4, D_4, and E_4).
4. Type II (cytotoxic) has the following characteristics:
   a. Manifested by the production of antibodies.
   b. The antibodies (IgG or IgM) bind to cell-bound antigen, which can activate complement and destroy the cell.

c. Erythrocytes, leukocytes, and platelets can be destroyed by this process.

d. Examples are hemolytic transfusion reactions, nonhemolytic transfusion reactions, hemolytic disease of the newborn.

e. Tissue damage can be manifested by several factors.

f. Cytotoxic antibodies to tissue components can cause inflammation leading to hematuria, renal failure, and hemoptysis.

5. Type III (immune-complex reactions) has the following characteristics:

a. Antibodies (IgG and IgM) combine with corresponding antigens to form complexes that activate complement.

b. Complexes are deposited in tissues, causing inflammation.

c. Chemotactic factors and polymorphs are released, attach to complexes, and release damaging lysosomal enzymes.

d. Examples include the Arthus reaction and chronic immune-complex disease (serum sickness).

6. Type IV (cell-mediated). See below.

Cell-Mediated Immunity

1. Cell-mediated immunity is particularly important with respect to viruses, fungi, and acid-fast bacillary infections (tuberculosis, leprosy).

The Effectors of the Cell-Mediated Immune Response

1. The effectors of the cell-mediated immune response are:

a. Cytotoxic T cells, whose main function is to eliminate virally infected host cells.

b. Macrophages, which present antigen to the T cells (induction phase), and become lymphokine activated (effector phase).

c. Natural killer cells, which kill virally infected cells or neoplastic cells.

d. Cytokines, which transmit messages between cells.

2. The phenomenon by which effector cells are able to lyse antibody-coated target cells is known as antibody-dependent cell-mediated cytolysis (ADCC).

The MHC Restriction of T-Cell Antigen Recognition

1. T_C cells are MHC class I restricted.
2. T_H cells are MHC class II restricted.

The Activation of T Cells

1. Activation of an effector cell requires:
a. Antigenic stimulation.
b. IL-1 production.
c. IL-2 production.

Hypersensitivity in Cell-Mediated Immunity

1. This is Type IV hypersensitivity.
2. It is mediated by cells (antibody and complement are not involved).
3. Type IV hypersensitivity is modulated by lymphokines. The reaction is usually controlled by normal control mechanisms.
4. Multiple antigenic challenges in the hypersensitive individual lead to allergic symptoms.
5. The tuberculin skin reaction is an example of Type IV hypersensitivity.
6. Cell-mediated immune reactions are important in:
a. Tissue transplantation.
b. Immunity to viral diseases.
c. Contact sensitivity.
d. Granulomatous hypersensitivity.
e. Autoimmune disease.

Immunoglobulin Deficiency Diseases

1. The primary immunodeficiency syndromes include those conditions in which, as a primary hereditary condition, the cellular, humoral, or body mechanisms are deficient.
2. The secondary immunodeficiencies result from the involvement of the immunogenic system in the course of another disease.
3. Acquired immunodeficiency syndrome (AIDS) is discussed in Chapter 13.

The Immune Response: Functional Aspects

1. The functional aspects of the immune response include:
a. The recognition of the antigen as foreign.

b. The processing of the antigen to produce specific antibody.

c. The production of antibody.

2. The theories postulated to explain the diversity of antibody include the instructive theory, the selective theory (germ line theory), and the somatic mutation theory.

3. Specificity of antibodies is now explained in terms of the combination of gene recombination, junctional diversity, and V-gene mutation.

Immunologic Tolerance

1. This refers to the situation in which a foreign antigen fails to elicit the formation of antibody. The mechanisms of immune tolerance include:

   a. Chimerism.

   b. Fetal exposure to antigen.

   c. B-cell tolerance (clonal abortion, clonal exhaustion, functional deletion, and antibody-forming cell blockade).

   d. T-cell tolerance (clonal abortion, functional deletion, T-cell suppression).

2. B- and T-cell tolerances differ with respect to time taken to become tolerant, required dosage of antigen, and duration.

3. The ability of the body not to respond to autologous antigens is known as self-tolerance.

Autoimmunity

1. Autoantibodies are produced:

   a. If the antigenicity of tissue proteins is altered due to degenerative lesions or the attachment of a hapten.

   b. If a tissue antigen is anatomically isolated from immunologically competent cells.

   c. If a self protein is no longer recognized due to altered reactivity of the immune system.

2. Autoantibodies may be immunoglobulin or cellular.

3. The immunoglobulin might be of any class and may be organ specific or non–organ specific.

Review Questions

Multiple Choice

Choose the phrase, sentence, or symbol that completes the statement or answers the question. More than one answer may be correct in each case. Answers are given at the end of this book.

1. As a general rule, antibodies:
   (a) are selectively produced in response to foreign substances
   (b) are produced to self antigens
   (c) are not produced to self antigens
   (d) can produce severe damage to tissue components upon reintroduction of foreign material.
   (Introduction)

2. The Class II antigens of the MHC:
   (a) are found on all nucleated cells
   (b) are restricted to immunocompetent cells
   (c) are complement components
   (d) are cellular proteins
   (The Antigens of the MHC)

3. If a viral antigen is associated with a class I MHC antigen on a virally infected cell, this will cause a response by:
   (a) cytotoxic T cells
   (b) T-helper cells
   (c) a class II MHC antigen

   (d) none of the above
   (The Role of the MHC in Regulating the Immune Response)

4. The first phase of antigen elimination:
   (a) takes about 10 to 20 minutes if particulate antigens are used
   (b) results in almost 90 per cent of the antigen being removed from the circulation
   (c) continues over a period of 4 to 7 days
   (d) is also known as the immune elimination segment
   (Antigen Elimination)

5. The primary antibody response:
   (a) results in the production of IgG antibodies
   (b) is faster than the secondary immune response
   (c) results first in the production of IgM antibodies
   (d) none of the above
   (The Primary Response)

6. After second (or subsequent) exposure to a foreign antigen:
   (a) there is an immediate sharp drop in the amount of circulating antibody
   (b) an anamnestic response occurs
   (c) IgG antibody is predominant

(d) All of the above
(The Secondary Response)

7. An antibody that is capable of neutralizing toxin is known as:
   (a) an antitoxin
   (b) an agglutinin
   (c) a lysin
   (d) a precipitin
   (Immunity)

8. Type I hypersensitivity is known as:
   (a) cytotoxic hypersensitivity
   (b) immediate hypersensitivity
   (c) anaphylaxis hypersensitivity
   (d) cell-mediated hypersensitivity
   (Hypersensitivity)

9. Cytotoxic hypersensitivity is seen in:
   (a) hemolytic transfusion reactions
   (b) hemolytic disease of the newborn
   (c) febrile transfusion reactions
   (d) all of the above
   (Hypersensitivity)

10. Which of the following is/are not involved in the cell-mediated immune response?
    (a) cytotoxic T cells
    (b) macrophages
    (c) complement
    (d) natural killer cells
    (The Effectors of the Cell-Mediated Immune Response)

11. T$_H$ cells are:
    (a) MHC class I restricted
    (b) MHC class II restricted
    (c) MHC class I and class II restricted
    (d) none of the above
    (The MHC Restriction of T-Cell Antigen Recognition)

12. Cell-mediated hypersensitivity is mediated by:
    (a) cells
    (b) circulating antibody
    (c) complement
    (d) all of the above
    (Hypersensitivity in Cell-Mediated Immunity)

13. Cell-mediated immune reactions are of great importance in:
    (a) granulomatous hypersensitivity
    (b) tissue transplants
    (c) immunity to viral diseases
    (d) contact sensitivity
    (Hypersensitivity in Cell-Mediated Immunity)

14. In the primary immunodeficiency syndromes:
    (a) the cellular mechanisms may be deficient
    (b) the humoral mechanisms may be deficient
    (c) the cellular and humoral mechanisms may be deficient

(d) only the humoral mechanism is deficient
(Immunoglobulin Deficiency Diseases)

15. The genes for antibody are located on:
    (a) chromosome number 1
    (b) four different chromosomes
    (c) three different chromosomes
    (d) chromosomes number 14, 22, and 2
    (The Immune Response: Functional Aspects)

16. B-cell tolerance can be induced by:
    (a) clonal abortion
    (b) functional deletion
    (c) T-cell suppression
    (d) clonal exhaustion
    (Immunologic Tolerance)

17. Autoantibodies:
    (a) may be of any immunoglobulin class
    (b) may be immunoglobulin or cellular
    (c) may be non–organ specific
    (d) are antibodies that are produced to self antigens
    (Autoantibodies)

Answer "True" or "False"

1. The immune response to foreign substances is not selective.
   (Introduction)

2. The MHC is involved in the regulation of the immune response during antigen presentation.
   (Genetic Control of the Immune Response)

3. The class III antigens of the MHC are complement components that activate C3.
   (The Antigens of the MHC)

4. Class I MHC antigens associated with a viral antigen on a virally infected cell will cause CD4-positive cells to respond.
   (The Role of the MHC in Regulating the Immune Response)

5. The final phase of antigen elimination involves the combining of antigen with antibody.
   (Antigen Elimination)

6. The latent period in the primary response is also known as the "induction" period.
   (The Primary Response)

7. The secondary response occurs as a result of immunologic memory, carried out by the small lymphocytes.
   (The Secondary Response)

8. All antibodies serve to protect the host against reinfection.
   (Immunity)

9. Approximately 60 per cent of the population becomes sensitized when exposed to airborne allergens.
(Hypersensitivity)

10. The Arthus reaction is an example of Type III hypersensitivity.
(Hypersensitivity)

11. The cytolytic activities of natural killer cells are stimulated by IL-2.
(The Effectors of the Cell-Mediated Immune Response)

12. IL-1 is referred to as a monokine.
(The Effectors of the Cell-Mediated Immune Response)

13. Three signals are required of the activation of a T cell: antigenic stimulation, IL-1, and IL-2.
(The Activation of T Cells)

14. Histologic examination of the lesion produced in Type IV hypersensitive individuals shows mononuclear infiltration.
(Hypersensitivity in Cell-Mediated Immunity)

15. Drugs have no effect on immunologic function.
(Immunoglobulin Deficiency Diseases)

16. Junctional diversity refers to the lack of precision in the joining of recombining genes.
(The Immune Response: Functional Aspects)

17. Tolerance cannot be induced by soluble antigens.
(Immunologic Tolerance)

18. Autoantibodies are never directed against a determinant present in only one organ.
(Autoimmunity)

GENERAL REFERENCES

Abbas, A.K., Lichtman, A.H., and Pober, J.S.: Cellular and Molecular Immunology. Philadelphia, W. B. Saunders Company, 1991.

Baron, E.J., and Finegold, S.M.: Bailey and Scott's Diagnostic Microbiology, 8th ed. St Louis, C. V. Mosby Company, 1990.

Bellanti, J.A.: Immunology III. Philadelphia, W. B. Saunders Company, 1985.

Dorland's Illustrated Medical Dictionary, 27th ed. Philadelphia, W. B. Saunders Company, 1988.

Freeman, B.A.: Burrows Textbook of Microbiology, 27th ed. Philadelphia, W. B. Saunders Company, 1985.

Henry, J.B.: Clinical Diagnosis and Management by Laboratory Methods. Philadelphia, W. B. Saunders Company, 1991.

Sheehan, C.: Clinical Immunology: Principles and Laboratory Diagnosis. Philadelphia, J. B. Lippincott, 1990.

Walter, J.B.: An Introduction to the Principles of Disease, 2nd ed. Philadelphia, W. B. Saunders Company, 1982.

5

The Antigen-Antibody Reaction *in Vitro*

OBJECTIVES

The student shall know, understand, and be prepared to explain:
1. The fundamental reaction between antigen and antibody
2. Types of immunologic reactions
3. The specificity and sensitivity of immunologic tests
4. The principles of the following immunologic tests:
   a. Precipitation, to include double diffusion, radial immunodiffusion, countercurrent immunoelectrophoresis, immunoelectrophoresis, immunofixation, and rocket electrophoresis
   b. Agglutination, to include direct agglutination, viral hemagglutination, passive and reverse passive agglutination, antiglobulin techniques, and the agglutination inhibition reaction
   c. Reactions involving complement, to include the complement fixation test and the immune adherence reaction
   d. Neutralization of toxins and viruses
   e. Fluorescent antibody reactions, to include the direct technique, the indirect technique, the complement staining technique, and the inhibition technique
   f. Immunoassays, to include radioimmunoassay and enzyme linked immunoassays
   g. Titration
   h. Nephelometry, to include procedure, light source, and limitations
   i. Cellular assay procedures, to include the reagents used and applications in the clinical laboratory

Introduction

The fundamental reaction between antigen and corresponding antibody is simply one of *combination*, followed by secondary or tertiary reactions (see Types of Immunologic Reactions, below).

There are several types of reaction of antigen-antibody complexes *in vitro*. Each will be considered here in turn, but first it is necessary to study the basic reaction, the simple combination of antigen and antibody both *in vivo* and *in vitro*, known as *sensitization*.

Sensitization. An antigen and its specific antibody possess complementary corresponding structures that enable the antigenic determinants to come into very close apposition with the binding site on the antibody molecule where the two are held together by weak intermolecular bonds, believed to include opposing charges on ionic groups, hydrogen bonds, hydrophobic (nonpolar) bonds, and Van der Waals forces. This is not a covalent bond and, in fact, is about one tenth as powerful as a covalent bond.

The antigen-antibody reaction, which is reversible in accordance with the law of mass action, may be written thus:

$$\text{Free Ag} + \text{Ag (hapten)} \underset{k_2}{\overset{k_1}{\rightleftharpoons}} \text{AbAg (hapten)}$$

where k_1 is the rate constant for the forward reaction and k_2 is the rate constant for the reverse action.

According to the law of mass action (see Hughes-Jones, 1963):

$$\frac{\text{(AgAb)}}{\text{(Ab)} \times \text{(Ag)}} = \frac{k_1}{k_2} = K$$

where (Ab), (Ag), and (AgAb), respectively, are the concentrations of antibody, antigen, and antigen-antibody (the combined product) and K is the equilibrium or association constant, which can be looked upon as a measure of the "goodness of fit" of the antibody to the corresponding antigen. The value of K is ultimately dependent upon the strength of the antigen-antibody bonds, and, because all antisera contain populations of antibody molecules with a variety of binding strengths, the K value of the serum for any specific reaction is the measure of the *average* binding strength of all antibody populations present.

At equilibrium, the rates of association and dissociation are constant, so that the amount of complex that forms equals the amount of complex that dissociates. The net charge in the concentration of complex, therefore, is zero. The ratio of these two rate constants is the affinity constant K_A, and is specific for each antibody-hapten pair:

$$K_A = \frac{\text{Association rate}}{\text{Dissociation rate}} = \frac{k_1}{k_2}$$

The ratio of the concentration of the complex compared with the product of the concentrations of free antibody and free antigen (hapten) is called the affinity constant:

$$K_A = \frac{\text{Ab-Ag (hapten complex)}}{\text{(Free Ab) (Free Ag (hapten))}}$$

The higher the equilibrium constant, the more will be the amount of antibody combining with antigen at equilibrium. Assuming that a certain minimum number of antibody molecules must be bound to each red cell (for example) for agglutination to occur, the ratio of (AgAb) to (Ag) at equilibrium should be as high as possible. In practical terms this means that a high ratio of serum to cells increases test sensitivity.

It should be noted that while *affinity* relates to the strength of an antibody-hapten or antibody-epitope bond, the term *avidity* relates to the overall bonding between multivalent antibodies and antigens. Antibody *specificity* is defined by the antigen that induced its production, as opposed to *cross-reactivity*, in which a second, structurally similar antigen can bind to the antibody.

TYPES OF IMMUNOLOGIC REACTIONS

Antigen-antibody tests can be classified as *primary, secondary,* or *tertiary,* according to whether the test is dependent merely upon the interaction between the antigen and its corresponding antibody or whether it is based on a secondary manifestation such as precipitation, flocculation, agglutination, complement fixation, and so on, following the primary interaction. Tertiary manifestations occur as *biologic* reactions (i.e., the biologic effects of complement activation, such as opsonization, phagocytosis, chemotaxis).

Primary Reactions. The primary reaction can be viewed simply as the specific recognition and combination of the antigen with the binding site of its corresponding antibody. In general, primary tests are more sensitive than secondary or tertiary tests and are not dependent upon the variables that control the latter (discussion follows). The quantitative tests that involve the primary reaction include immunofluorescence, radioimmunoassay, and immunoenzymatic assays. In general, these tests require either a purified antigen or an antibody preparation; a technique to quantitate the antigen or antibody with the use of a radioisotope, enzyme, or fluorescent label; or a method to separate the antigen-antibody complex from free antibody or antigen in solution.

Secondary Reactions. The secondary reactions are the conformation of the amino acid chain resulting from interchain hydrogen bonding. These include precipitation in solution or in gel, direct agglutination or hemagglutination (i.e., involving erythrocytes or other particles coated with antigen or antibody), and complement fixation.

Tertiary Reactions. The tertiary reactions involve the folding of polypeptide chains through hydrophobic and hydrogen bonds. These include phagocytosis, opsonization, chemotaxis, immune adherence, and cellular degradation.

At a basic level, antibody molecules are considered to be capable of recognition, binding, and complexing with specific antigen, yet many variables exist within the confines of this basic concept, because not all antigens or antibodies are subject to the same type of behavior. The reaction of specific IgG with a hapten antigen, for example, usually produces the complexes $(hapten)_2 = (antibody)_1$. Further, in the case of multivalent protein antigens, complexes of varying sizes may be formed in proportion to the antigen and antibody concentrations. Immune complexes of varying sizes have varying degrees of solubility; their ability to localize along vascular basement membrane and fix complement *in vivo* is responsible for a wide range of immune complex-mediated hypersensitivity diseases. As will be clear from this, the application and understanding of immunologic tests involve a knowledge of this variability, in terms of type, specificity, affinity, antibody and antigen concentration, and, finally, of biologic activity.

Quaternary Reactions. These involve the association of polypeptide subunits to form one protein.

THE SPECIFICITY AND SENSITIVITY OF IMMUNOLOGIC TESTS

As knowledge has accumulated with respect to the variation of behavior of different antibodies, a broad spectrum of different immunologic methods

Table 5–1. Relative Sensitivity of Immunologic Tests Involving Secondary Manifestations of Antigen-Antibody Reactions

Immunologic Test	Minimum of Antibody N (μg) Detectable or Needed for Reaction
Precipitation	
Tube precipitation	0.1
Immunodiffusion	0.1–0.3
Agglutination	
Qualitative	0.5
Quantitative	0.2–0.1
Hemagglutination, passive	0.001
Hemagglutination-inhibition	0.001
Coombs' reaction	0.01
Complement fixation	0.05

From Henry, J. B. (ed.): Clinical Diagnosis and Management by Laboratory Methods, 18th ed. Philadelphia, W. B. Saunders Company, 1991, p. 850.

has been developed, some of which are considerably more sensitive than others. Antigen-antibody binding assays, for example, are sensitive in the nanogram to picogram per milliliter range, whereas the agar gel test for α_1 fetoprotein is in the range of 3,000 ng/ml. These varying levels of sensitivity are well illustrated by the different tests for hepatitis B-associated surface antigen (HbsAg; Chapter 7). The agar gel diffusion test, for example, is 10 times *less* sensitive than the cross electrophoretic or electroimmunodiffusion methods and 10,000 times less sensitive than the radioimmunoassay procedure. The relative sensitivity of immunologic tests involving secondary manifestations of antigen-antibody reactions with respect to the minimum amount of antibody detectable or needed for reaction is given in Table 5–1.

The variation in standardization and specificity of immunologic methods is a common problem. This is because certain antibodies that have a high affinity and are potent may give unwanted cross-reactions, whereas weak antisera may be specific but not sensitive. False reactions (i.e., those caused by factors other than those expected or desired) are also a problem in this respect.

PRECIPITATION

Precipitation involves the interaction of antigen with antibody in "correct" proportions, resulting in

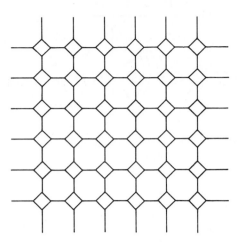

Figure 5–1. The lattice hypothesis: antigen (◊) bound to antibody (—) to form a lattice.

a visible precipitate. The soluble antigens used in the precipitin reaction are solutions of molecules, which are usually protein or carbohydrate in nature. The antibodies can be either polyclonal or monoclonal. The simplest form of the precipitin reaction would be the layering of antigen in solution over a small volume of antiserum. Precipitation occurs at the interface of the two reagents, forming a ring.

A concept of the reaction between antigen and antibody resulting in precipitation was described by Marrack (1938). This concept, sometimes known as the *lattice hypothesis,* is based on the fact that antibody has more than one valence and therefore may be found with antigen to form a coarse "lattice" (Fig. 5–1).

This reaction is influenced by the quantities of antigen and antibody present. To understand the events that occur, one must assume that an antibody molecule has only two reactive sites, whereas antigens have multiple sites that can react with antibody. When a relatively small amount of antigen is added to an excess of antibody, all the valences of the antigen are satisfied, and complexes are formed that are composed of much antibody and little antigen (Fig. 5–2,*1*). As increasing amounts of antigen are added to the same amount of antibody, the proportions change (Fig. 5–2,*2*) until a point of optimal proportion is reached (Fig. 5–2,*3*). This point is known as the *equivalence zone.* Further addition of antigen would shift the reaction into the area of antigen excess (Fig. 5–2, *4* and *5*). The largest amount of precipitate is found at the equivalence zone, and excess of either reactant may produce false-negative results (Fig. 5–3). The reaction is rarely used now, but it can provide a fairly good quantitative estimate of the amount of antigen or antibody in an unknown; the equivalence zone of the unknown is determined and compared with that of a standard.

It should be noted that a so-called prozone phenomenon is sometimes observed, in which an antibody apparently reacts more strongly when it is diluted than when it is undiluted. The phenomenon has often been attributed to lack of optimal proportions between antigen and antibody, although according to Wiener (1970), it may actually occur in one of two ways:

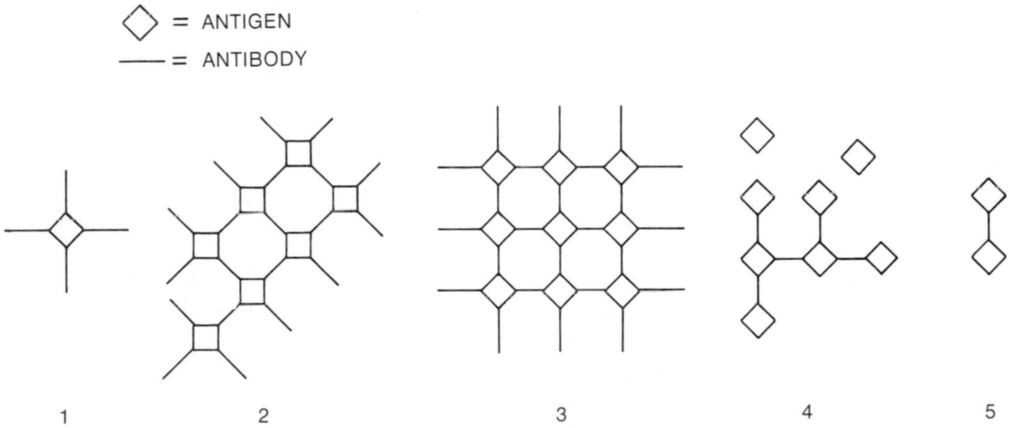

◊ = ANTIGEN

—— = ANTIBODY

1	2	3	4	5

Figure 5–2. The lattice hypothesis. *1,* Antibody excess—all valences of antigen satisfied; *2,* moderate antibody excess; *3,* optimal proportions; *4,* antigen excess; *5,* extreme antigen excess—both valences of antibody satisfied. (Modified from Pauling, L.: The theory of the structure and process of formation of antibodies. J. Am. Chem. Soc. 62:2643, 1940.)

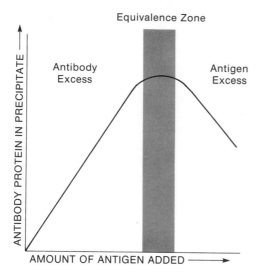

Figure 5–3. Precipitation curve with a constant amount of antibody.

1. It may be due to the use of fresh serum containing complement. This can be proven by inactivating the serum and retitrating, whereupon the prozone disappears.
2. It may be due to the presence of both IgM (agglutinating) and IgG (blocking) antibodies in the same serum. This prozone will disappear if the tests are carried out in a high-viscosity medium (e.g., human AB serum, bovine albumin) in place of saline.

Types of Reactions

The precipitin reaction is of practical use in the laboratory when it takes place in agar gel or other semisolid media through which soluble molecules can diffuse. The location and density of the precipitin bands in the reaction are determined by differences in the concentration and rates of diffusion of the different molecules. This allows for easier identification of multiple components in mixtures of antigens and antibodies. Thus, a preparation containing several antigens will give rise to multiple precipitation lines (Fig. 5–4), whereas a preparation containing only one antigen will give rise to one precipitation line with its corresponding antibody (Fig. 5–5). Note that when reagents are present in optimal proportions, the precipitation line formed will generally be concave to the well containing the reactant of higher molecular weight,

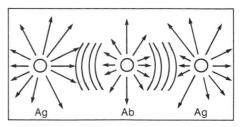

Figure 5–4. A test sample containing several antigens, giving rise to several precipitation lines.

whether it be antigen or antibody. This is caused by the slower diffusion rate of larger-sized molecules.

Double Diffusion

The double-diffusion technique (also referred to as the Ouchterlony technique) was the first method used in establishing the relationship of HB$_S$Ag to type B hepatitis. It is known as "double" diffusion because both antigen and antibody diffuse. If the well size and shape, distance between wells, temperature, and incubation time are optimal, this diffusion results in a visible precipitate at the point of equivalence perpendicular to the axis line between the wells, which is then compared with the reaction of standard antigen and specific antibody (of known concentration) in a comparison test. The concentration and rate of diffusion of antigen and antibody will determine the location of the band (e.g., antibody excess will cause the band to be located nearer the antigen well). If two antigens are present in the solution that can be recognized by the antigen, two precipitin bands form independently (Fig. 5–6). This results in three basic reaction patterns: identity, nonidentity, and partial identity.

Identity. The identity reaction is revealed when the lines of precipitation come together on the

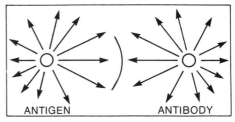

Figure 5–5. A precipitation test showing a single antigen and its corresponding antibody, resulting in a single line of precipitation.

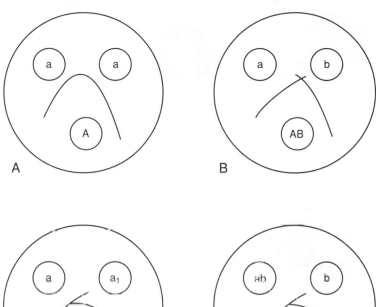

Figure 5–6. Precipitation pattern of Ouchterlony type of immunodiffusion (double diffusion).

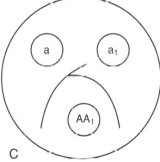

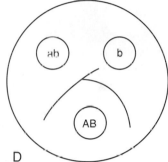

plate, forming a smooth curve (Fig. 5–6,*A*). This indicates that the antibody is precipitating identical antigen specificities in each preparation. It does *not* mean that the antigens are identical (although they may be)—they are only revealed to be identical as far as the antibody can distinguish the difference.

Non-Identity. The non-identity reaction is revealed when the precipitation lines cross one another (Fig. 5–6,*B*). They intersect (cross) because they have no antigenic determinants in common.

Partial Identity. The partial identity reaction is revealed when the precipitation lines merge with spur formation (Fig. 5–6,*C*), which indicates that the antigens are not identical but do possess common determinants.

Note: A *reaction of inhibition* occurs when antigens carry unrelated determinants and the antibody contains separate antibody components (Fig. 5–6,*D*).

Antibodies associated with autoimmune disorders (e.g., rheumatoid arthritis, systemic lupus erythematosus, systemic sclerosis, Sjögren's syndrome, and vasculitis) can be identified using dou-

ble diffusion. The technique has the limitation of being only semiquantitative (the thickness of a band only *suggests* increased or decreased levels of antibody) and is subject to several sources of error (e.g., caused by irregular patterns due to overfilling of wells, irregular well punching, nonlevel incubation, gel drying, overheating, inadequate time for diffusion, or antibody degradation due to bacterial or fungal contamination). It should also be noted that, considering the lattice theory, antigen or antibody excess may yield false-negative results. This may be partially overcome by using several concentrations of both antigens and antibodies, so that the combination will be in the zone of equivalence.

Radial Immunodiffusion (RID)
(Fig. 5–7)

This single-diffusion method can be used for the quantitation of immunoglobulins and other serum proteins, including complement components. The antiserum is always in the gel, so if immunoglobu-

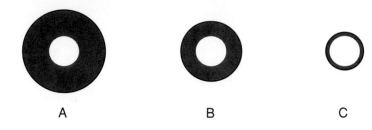

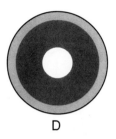

Figure 5–7. The ring patterns of radial immunodiffusion. A, B, and C are normal; D is an example of double precipitin rings.

lins are quantitated, the immunoglobulin is the antigen. This technique may be used when the nature of a protein is not readily differentiated by standard electrophoretic procedures.

The technique involves the addition of antiserum (which should be monospecific, highly specific, and of excellent precipitating ability) to a liquified gel, which is poured into a plate and allowed to solidify by cooling to room temperature. The antigen solution is added to wells cut into the agar. The antigen diffuses in all directions from the well, and precipitation occurs in a ring surrounding the well in the zone of equivalence. While the precipitin ring is enlarging, the log of the antigen concentration is approximately proportional to the diameter of the endpoint, and the area (square of the diameter) varies directly with the concentration.

Two principal RID methods have been developed:

The Fahey (Kinetic Diffusion) Method. In this method (Fahey, 1965) the diameter of the precipitin rings is measured at 18 hours. The logarithm of the concentration of the standards is proportional to the diameter of the precipitin ring. Using semilogarithmic paper, the y-axis is the analyte concentration and the x-axis is the diameter of the ring, including the well diameter. A high concentration, a normal concentration, and a low concentration are generally used as standards. If these three points do not fall in a straight line, then a line is drawn from point to point. The analyte concentration of the patient and control sera may be read from the graph

The Mancini (Endpoint Diffusion) Method. In this method (Mancini, 1965) the antigen is allowed to diffuse fully to achieve maximal precipitation. The amount of time needed varies according to the molecular weight and concentration of the protein being measured. A maximal ring diameter is obtained in about 24 hours by IgG in normal concentration and in 50 to 72 hours by IgM in normal concentration. The concentration of the antigen is plotted on linear graph paper on the y-axis, and the diameter squared (D^2) of the precipitin ring is plotted on the x-axis. The relationship between the concentration of the standards and the square of the diameter of the precipitin rings is the line of best fit. The concentration of the unknown sera is read from this graph.

Sources of error include:

1. Over- or underfilling of the wells
2. Spilling the patient's serum on the gel
3. Nicking the side of the well when filling
4. Improper incubation time and temperature
5. Specimen contamination

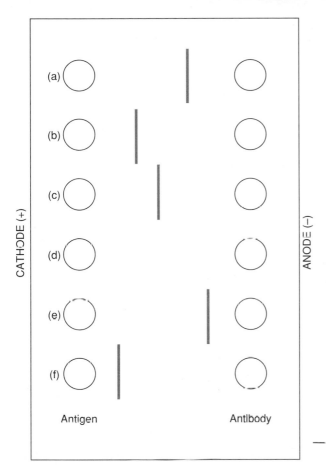

CATHODE (+)　　　　ANODE (−)

Antigen　　　　　Antibody

Figure 5–8. Countercurrent electrophoresis. If the precipitin line is closer to the antibody well, a higher concentration of antigen is indicated. If the precipitin line is closer to the antigen well, a higher concentration of antibody is indicated. A precipitin line in the middle (c) indicates equal concentrations of antigen and antibody. Sample (d) has no antigen present.

Countercurrent Immunoelectrophoresis (CIEP)

In this method, gel is poured onto a plate and cooled. Two columns of wells are cut, with the antigen in one well and the antibody in the other. The plate is placed in an electric field (which shortens the time required to produce precipitation). At pH 8.6, the antigen migrates toward the anode and the antibody migrates toward the cathode. Precipitation occurs at equivalence (Fig. 5–8).

CIEP can be semiquantitative if serial dilutions are used. The serial dilution of an antigen causes the precipitin line to move closer to the antibody well as the concentration of antigen increases (provided that the concentration of antibody is kept constant).

If the concentration of antibody is serially diluted (keeping the concentration of antigen constant), higher concentrations of antibody will move the precipitin line toward the antigen well.

CIEP is useful in the detection of autoantibodies, antibodies to infectious agents, and certain microbial antigens (A.M. Johnson, 1986; Roitt, 1988).

Sources of error include:

1. The reversal of wells so that the current is applied in the wrong direction
2. Improper pH of the buffer
3. Insufficient electrophoresis time
4. Prozone or postzone
5. Wells that are not parallel

Immunoelectrophoresis

This is a useful procedure for the identification of monoclonal proteins, including free κ and λ chains. The procedure utilizes both electrophoresis and double diffusion. The principle of the method is as follows: Under an electrical current, antigen migrates through a gel medium (e.g., agar; Fig. 5–9).

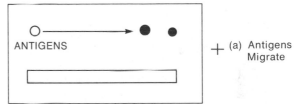

ANTIGENS

− 　　　　 + (a) Antigens Migrate

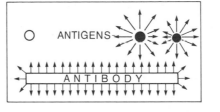

ANTIGENS

ANTIBODY

(b) Antibody Added to Trough: Migration Through Gel

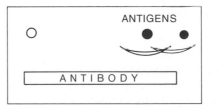

ANTIGENS

ANTIBODY

(c) Precipitation Arcs Formed

Figure 5–9. The principle of immunoelectrophoresis.

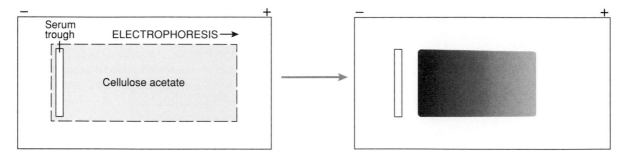

Figure 5–10. Immunofixation.

The current is then stopped. A trough is cut in the agar and filled with antibody. A precipitin arc is then formed. Because antigen (theoretically at a point source) diffuses rapidly and antibody from a trough diffuses with a plane front, the reactants meet in optimal proportions for precipitation along the arc. The arc is closest to the trough at a point where antigen is in highest concentration. This technique may be used in two-dimensional or multidimensional forms; antigens are then separated on the basis of their electrophoretic mobility. A normal control serum is performed simultaneously so that the two may be compared.

This procedure is relatively insensitive to the antigen and antibody ratios. It has been used for the detection of free light chain proteins and as a screening procedure to detect immunoglobulin classes. It may also be used to identify urine proteins. The procedure is semiquantitative (since the size of the arc is an indication of the amount of immunoglobulin present). The shape and position of precipitin arcs can provide clues as to the monoclonality of a protein.

It should be noted that prolonged diffusion will result in artifacts, especially at the anode and cathode. Also, marked antibody excess may result in multiple concentric arcs that could be mistaken for multiple antigen reactions.

Immunofixation Electrophoresis (IFE)

In the IFE technique (Fig. 5–10), a cellulose acetate strip impregnated with antiserum is placed over the separate proteins after serum, urine, or cerebrospinal fluid are electrophoresed. Diffusion of the antiserum into the gel occurs rapidly, resulting in precipitation of antigen-antibody complexes.

The cellulose acetate strips are then removed and the precipitin bands are stained. The staining area identifies the location of the specific protein as it would be found in routine protein electrophoresis.

Compared with immunoelectrophoresis, the immunofixation technique is more sensitive to the antigen and antibody ratios. Serum dilution is quite often necessary to produce the reaction. Urine and cerebrospinal fluid have to be concentrated to be in the line of equivalence (urine about 25 times and cerebrospinal fluid about 50 to 100 times). When applying the cellulose acetate to the gel, care should be taken to ensure the absence of air bubbles, since these would hamper diffusion and may result in a precipitation reaction being missed.

Rocket Electrophoresis

The rocket (or Laurell) technique (Fig. 5–11) is used to quantitate antigens other than immunoglobulins. The antiserum is incorporated into the agar, and the unknown antigen is placed in the well and electrophoresed. As the antigen migrates through the gel, it combines with antibody, and precipitation occurs along the lateral boundaries in the shape of a rocket. The total distance of antigen migration and precipitation is directly proportional to the antigen concentration.

AGGLUTINATION

Agglutination reactions are similar to precipitin reactions except that the union of antibody occurs with suspended particulate antigens rather than with soluble antigens. Both types of reactions have lattice formation, which is influenced by the num-

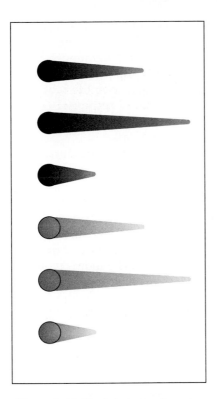

Figure 5–11. Rocket electrophoresis.

ber of antigenic determinants and is subject to prozone and postzone. The particles involved are cells (bacteria, yeast, erythrocytes) or latex particles, which, in general, are large enough for direct observations. When these antigens combine with their specific antibodies, aggregation (or clumping) of the particles is seen. This occurs in two phases: (1) specific antigen-antibody binding and (2) lattice formation. If one of these reactants is of known specificity, the clumping may be used for the identification of the corresponding reactant. The procedure may be performed with the slide, tube, or microtiter technique. Slide tests are rapid, with most procedures requiring only 2 to 3 minutes of rotation at room temperature. Tube techniques generally require longer incubation times (from 15 minutes to overnight) and may be incubated at 4°C, at 20°C (room temperature), or at 37°C (body temperature). Microtiter techniques are generally adaptations of test tube procedures. They have the advantage of using less of the patient sample and less reagent.

Several factors influence the reaction, including elevation or decrease of temperature, motion (shaking, stirring, centrifugation), pH, and the class of antibody (IgM, because of their large size and five basic structural units, are able to bind up to five antigens, whereas IgG are poor agglutinins and often require special conditions in order to produce agglutination).

Agglutination results are usually quantitative (i.e., they indicate the presence of an antigen or antibody, but do not indicate the amount), although the reaction can also be used as a semiquantitative test with doubling dilutions of antisera. The strength of the antibody (i.e., the "titer") is then used as the reciprocal of the highest dilution that gives a distinctly positive reaction (see Titration, later in this chapter).

Agglutination results from the cross-linking of the cells or particles by antibody molecules, although antibody-induced changes in the electrical charge may also be important.

The range of usefulness of the agglutination reaction has been considerably extended in recent years. This was made possible by the observation that erythrocytes can absorb various polysaccharides and that after treatment with tannic acid (acting as a mordant), they can also absorb many protein antigens (i.e., in passive hemagglutination).

In addition, polystyrene latex suspensions have become available, and the latex particle agglutination test has become a useful tool for the detection of rheumatoid factor and is helpful in the diagnosis of rheumatoid arthritis (see Chapter 14). Passive agglutination tests can also be used for the detection of soluble antigen. In the agglutination inhibition test, antiserum is first combined with antigen, and then the indicator red cells or latex particles coated with the same antigen are added. Inhibition indicates the presence of both antigen and specific antibody.

Types of Agglutination Reaction

The major types of agglutination reaction include the following:

Direct Agglutination. This uses antigens found naturally on the surface of cells (e.g., erythrocytes or bacteria). Direct agglutination of red cells (known as hemagglutination) may be used to detect ABO and Rh antigens. The test may also be used to detect antibodies to infectious agents (e.g., the cold agglutinin test for the detection of antibodies to

Mycoplasma pneumoniae, which react with the I antigens on red cells) and heterophil antibodies (using the antigens found on horse, sheep, or beef red blood cells). Direct agglutination is also used with the involvement of bacterial natural antigens, which demonstrate recent infection by measuring the titer of antibody against a specific species of bacteria. Finally, direct agglutination can be used to detect febrile antibodies (e.g., the Widal test, which uses *Salmonella* bacteria to detect antibodies in typhoid and paratyphoid fevers). In most cases, however, direct agglutination lacks sensitivity and specificity with respect to febrile antibodies, and therefore other procedures are most often recommended (Nicols and Nakamura, 1986; Stansfield, 1981).

Viral Hemagglutination. Viral hemagglutination occurs when a virus (e.g., rubella or influenza) agglutinates red blood cells by binding to receptors on the red blood cell surface. The test most often used in this connection is the viral hemagglutination inhibition test, which inhibits the virus from agglutinating the erythrocytes and in that way reveals its presence.

Passive and Reverse Passive Agglutination. In passive agglutination, the antigen is attached (coated) to a particulate "carrier." If antibody is attached to a particulate carrier, the technique is referred to as reverse passive agglutination. The carriers currently used are charcoal, latex particles, gelatin particles, and erythrocytes. These carriers differ in their ability to bind a high concentration of antigen or antibody, and therefore certain carriers are more suited to certain tests. Passive agglutination procedures can be used to detect the nontreponemal antibody in syphilis, rheumatoid factor, rubella antibody, and thyroglobin antibody. Latex particles and red cells may also be used to detect antigen in the reverse passive agglutination technique. The technique is used to detect C-reactive protein.

Antiglobulin Techniques. These tests are generally used in the immunohematology laboratory. In principle, erythrocytes have a net negative charge and therefore repel one another. Since IgG molecules are small and cannot link one antigen-binding site on one erythrocyte to another antigen-binding site on a second erythrocyte, the lattice is not formed and the reaction (i.e., the binding of antigen to antibody) is not visible. To overcome this spatial deficiency, anti-human IgG (antiglobulin reagent) is added, which bridges the gap between the cells. This anti-human immunoglobulin reagent, produced by injecting rabbits with purified γ chains and then harvesting the rabbit anti-human IgG after the immune response, can be used in fluorescence immunoasssays, radioimmunoassays, and enzyme immunoassays.

There are two specific procedures by which the antiglobulin test can be done. The direct antiglobulin test is used when an *in vivo* attachment of a red cell antibody to an individual's red cells has occurred (e.g., in hemolytic disease of the newborn, autoimmune hemolytic anemia, hemolytic transfusion reactions, and, in the case of drugs, binding to red cell membranes). The indirect antiglobulin test is used in the immunohematology laboratory to determine compatibility between donor and recipient (i.e., to ensure that no irregular antibodies are present in the patient's serum that may hinder the success of a transfusion of blood cells).

Agglutination Inhibition Reaction. This two-step agglutination inhibition procedure can be used with direct or passive agglutination but is not appropriate to detect the presence of an antigen. In the first step, soluble antigen in the patient's sample is incubated with known antibody reagent. If the soluble antigen is present, a reaction will take place but will not be visible. In the second step, the particulate antigen (either a natural antigen or a red cell or latex particle with antigen attached) is added. If the antigen was present in the patient sample, there is no free antibody to attach to the particulate antigen—agglutination is therefore inhibited, which represents a positive test. If agglutination occurs, the test is negative. This procedure is used to detect human chorionic gonadotropin in serum or urine and the presence of soluble A, B, and H substances in body fluids.

REACTIONS INVOLVING COMPLEMENT

Complement components can be quantitated immunologically when the component reacts with monospecific antisera. The functional ability of the complement cascade can be measured by lysing red blood cells.

Functional assays and the principle of comple-

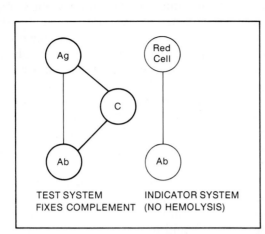

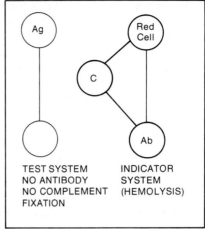

Figure 5-12. The complement fixation test.

ment component assays are discussed in Chapter 3 of this text, along with the decrease or increase of complement components in various disease states.

The Complement Fixation Test

The complement fixation test is based on the fact that when an antigen combines with an antibody in the presence of complement, the complement is "fixed" by the antigen-antibody complex and is unable to react with cells sensitized with other antigen-antibody complexes. As an indicator of the presence of "unfixed" complement, erythrocytes sensitized with specific antibodies are used. Lysis of these erythrocytes indicates the presence of unfixed complement; alternatively, the lack of hemolysis indicates that the complement has reacted with the test antigen-antibody complex (Fig. 5-12).

The test is of limited usefulness because it is applicable to IgM antibodies only and because other assays give comparable or better sensitivity while being easier to perform. In addition, the antigen must be free of "anticomplementary" activity. The test is useful, however, in viral, rickettsial, and fungal serology. Diseases that may be diagnosed by complement fixation are Rocky Mountain spotted fever, herpes simplex infection, and influenza.

Immune Adherence Reaction

Another reaction involving complement is the immune adherence reaction, although this too is of limited usefulness. This reaction is based on the fact that, following the primary specific antigen-antibody reaction, the antigen-antibody complex develops an ability to adhere to particles such as erythrocytes, silica, starch granules, and bacteria. Early *in vitro* tests of this phenomenon revealed that complement was an essential part of the reaction. Practically speaking, the test has little application in the clinical laboratory, although it has been successfully used for the antigenic differentiation of species of trypanosomes and leptospires and for the diagnosis of trypanosomiasis and syphilitic infection.

NEUTRALIZATION OF TOXINS AND VIRUSES

Neutralization tests can be useful when neither precipitation nor agglutination succeeds in demonstrating an antigen-antibody reaction. Moreover, in work with viral agents, neutralization is a useful technique. One should note that the neutralization of toxins or viruses is the essence of a major protective mechanism in several disease states (e.g., diphtheria, tetanus).

The principle of the test is simple. In the case of viruses, a dose of virus known to be lethal to a test animal is mixed with the serum to be tested for antibody against the virus. The mixture is injected into the test animal, which is observed for reaction. If the lethal dose fails to kill the test animal, neutralizing antibody is known to be present in the test serum. In the case of toxins, an individual who has been exposed to toxin-producing bacteria is injected with antitoxin. The toxin-antitoxin reaction *in vivo* then protects the recipient by neutralizing the toxin. This toxin-inactivating ability of antiserum can be assayed by observing the *in vivo* neutralization of the toxin in laboratory animals. Failure to protect the animal means that the test serum has no protective antibodies against the particular toxin. Antitoxin potency can also be measured by precipitation and by flocculation techniques *in vitro*. The Schick test for the detection of antibody to diphtheria toxin and the Dick test for the detection of antibody to scarlatinal toxin are examples of *in vivo* toxin neutralization.

FLUORESCENT ANTIBODY REACTIONS (IMMUNOFLUORESCENCE)

Immunofluorescence was first developed almost 30 years ago by Coons (1956, 1958, 1961), yet its true value and potential have only recently been exploited. The technique involves the study of antigens in tissue sections by the use of specific antibody that has been labeled with color and is applied over a section of tissue so that a microprecipitate is formed at the site of the antigen. The fluorescent dye usually used, fluorescein isocyanate or isothiocyanate, is linked with serum antibody and yields a blue-green fluorescent substance, which is detected in a fluorescent microscope when illuminated with ultraviolet light.

The simplest application of the technique, using a single treatment with labeled antibody and a subsequent wash in physiologic buffer saline to remove the excess of uncombined labeled antibody, is known as the *single-layer* or *direct* technique. The purpose of the technique is to identify unknown antigen by using known fluorescein-labeled antibody. It consists of exposing the unknown antigen to the known labeled antibody and washing and examining the mixture with the fluorescent microscope (Fig. 5–13).

The method has been used for the identification of foreign antibodies in tissues (e.g., particulate viruses and their soluble antigens and bacteria, protozoa, and fungal antigens).

Several modifications of this technique exist, including the following:

Indirect or Double-Layer Technique. This procedure is used for the detection of antibody in unknown sera. Unlabeled antibody is exposed to antigen, and this is followed by the addition of labeled antiglobulin sera, directed against the globulin of the species used in the initial exposure. Fluorescence in this case indicates that the reaction between the antigen, the unknown antibody, and the labeled antiglobulin has taken place (Fig. 5–14).

Complement Staining Technique. This procedure is similar to the indirect procedure except that the antiglobulin conjugate is directed against the species supplying the complement. The main advantage of this technique over the indirect method is that a single conjugate (e.g., anti–guinea-pig complement) may be used to test the serum from any species. The test procedure is as follows:

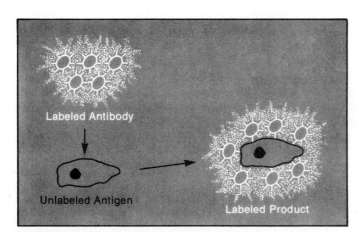

Figure 5–13. Single-layer (or "direct") fluorescent antibody procedure.

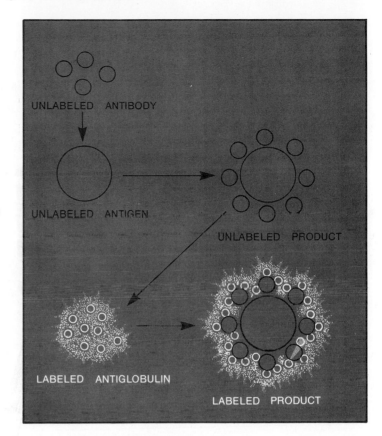

Figure 5–14. Indirect (or double-layer) fluorescent antibody procedure.

1. Heat-inactivated unknown antibody and a fixed amount of guinea-pig complement are added simultaneously to known antigen.
2. After incubation and washing, labeled antibody (anti–guinea pig complement) is added and the mixture is incubated again.

Fluorescence indicates that a reaction has occurred between the unknown antibody and the antigen, resulting in the fixation of complement to the complex, and that a subsequent reaction has occurred between the guinea-pig complement and the anti–guinea-pig complement (Fig. 5–15).

Inhibition Technique. The inhibition technique is based on the procedure of blocking specific antigen-antibody reactions by initial exposure to a different aliquot of homologous antibody. In this way, unlabeled antibody is added to antigen, saturating the antigen. Subsequently, labeled antibody is added. No fluorescence is seen, and the test remains nonreactive because no antigen sites remain to react with the labeled antibody (Fig. 5–16).

IMMUNOASSAYS

"Immunoassay" is a general term that refers to many techniques performed in the clinical laboratory. They can be non-labeled or labeled reagent assays. Examples of non-labeled immunoassays are immunoprecipitin methods, agglutination methods, and light-scattering techniques for the detection of antigen-antibody complexes by equilibrium or kinetic approaches.

The original technique of using antigen-coated cells or particles in agglutination techniques can be considered the original method for labeling components in immunoassays. Any substance that will complex to another substance is referred to as a *ligand*. In laboratory immunoassays, the ligand is the substance to be measured. It could be an antigen combining with antibody, a hormone combining with a transport protein, or a drug combining with an antibody. In a ligand assay, one reactant is labeled so that the amount of binding can be monitored. The types of labels include those that are radioactive or nonradioactive (e.g., enzymes and

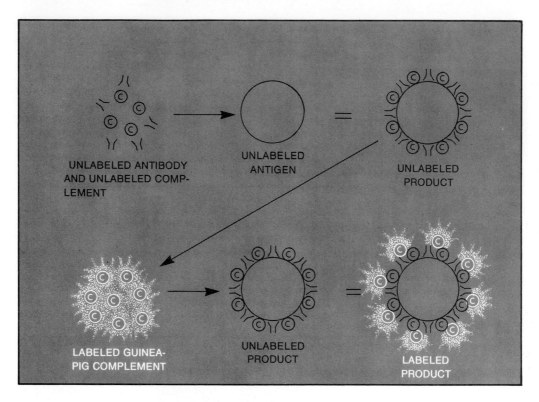

Figure 5–15. Complement staining technique.

fluorescent molecules). The assay is named according to the attached label. Radioimmunoassay uses a radioactive label, enzyme immunoassay uses an enzyme label, chemiluminescent assay uses a light-emitting label, and fluorescence immunoassay uses a fluorescent label. The many methods available utilize either monoclonal or polyclonal antibodies or binding proteins to capture the ligand. They can be qualitative or quantitative, and reactions may be designed to occur in the soluble or solid phase.

Radioimmunoassay (RIA)

The radioimmunoassay method is widely used. The concentration of antigen or antibody in serum samples is measured with the use of radioisotopes. If antibody concentration is being measured, the radioactive-labeled antibody competes with the patient's unlabeled antibody for binding sites on a known amount of antigen. When all three components are present in the system, an equilibrium exists.

The general procedure for radioimmunoassay is as follows:

1. The antigen in saline is incubated on a microplate or in a test tube. Small quantities of antigen become absorbed onto the plastic surface, and, following incubation, free antigen is washed away. The plate is then blocked with an excess of an irrelevant protein that prevents any subsequent binding of protein.
2. Test antibody is added, which binds to the antigen. Unbound proteins are washed away, and the antibody is detected by a radiolabeled ligand. Unbound ligand is then washed away, and the radioactivity of the plate or tube is counted on a gamma counter.

As the amount of test antibody increases, the counts per minute rise from a background level through a linear range to a plateau. Antibody titers can only be detected correctly within the linear range. The plateau binding rate is usually 20 to 100 times the background count. A reduction in radioactivity of the antigen-antibody complex compared with the radioactive counts measured in the control test with no antibody is used to quantitate the amount of patient antibody bound to the antigen.

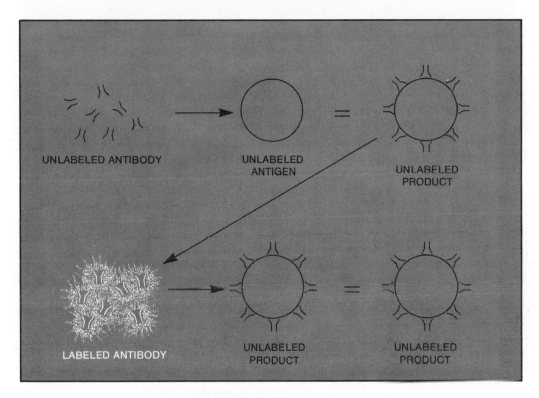

Figure 5–16. Inhibition technique.

A slight modification of the standard radio-immunoassay (antigen or allergen is covalently bound to a cellulose disc rather than noncovalently to a radioimmunoassay plate) allows the procedure to measure antigen-specific IgE where the ligand is a labeled anti IgE antibody. The modification permits the high sensitivity necessary to bind small quantities of IgE present in serum by having much more antigen. The procedure is known as the *radio-allergosorbent test.*

In addition, the *radioimmunosorbent test* is a competition radioimmunoassay for total serum IgE. In this procedure, the plate is sensitized with anti-IgE, and increasing amounts of labeled IgE are added to the plate to determine the maximum amount of IgE that the plate can bind. A quantity of labeled IgE equivalent to approximately 80 per cent of the plateau binding is chosen. The amount of labeled IgE is mixed with the serum containing the IgE to be tested. The test IgE competes with the labeled IgE. Therefore, the more IgE that is present in the test serum, the less the amount of labeled IgE that binds.

The radioimmunoassay is extremely sensitive and has the ability to detect trace amounts of antigen or antibody. In addition, the technique allows for a large number of tests to be performed in a relatively short period of time. The major disadvantage is the hazard and the instability of isotopes.

Enzyme-Linked Immunoassays (ELISA)

These are rapidly supplementing and at times replacing radioimmunoassays and immunofluorescence for the identification of specific antibody. In fact, the principle of ELISA is similar to that of immunofluorescence in that a purified enzyme is linked in a stable manner to a specific antibody.

Horseradish peroxidase and alkaline phosphatase are two commonly used enzymes in the ELISA technique, although other enzymes can be used. The requirements of the utilized enzyme with respect to the technique are as follows:

1. The enzyme activity should be easily detectable either by a cytochemical method or by a change in absorbance at a specific wavelength.

2. For cytochemical uses the enzyme substrate should not be readily diffusible; in fact, it is preferable if a precipitate results from the reaction.

3. In tissue work, it is useful if the optimal pH of the enzyme is at or close to neutral.

4. The enzyme should not affect tissue structure.

5. The active enzyme should be available in pure form because if it is not, immunoglobulins could be labeled with "inactive" materials and could decrease the sensitivity and specificity of the reaction.

6. Enzyme activity is often decreased when enzymes are bound to antibodies, but this activity should not be abolished.

7. The enzyme must be stable for storage purposes.

8. A small enzyme is less likely to interfere with antigen-antibody reactions by steric hindrance and is more likely to penetrate tissue.

In performing ELISA techniques, there should be no natural substrates in tissue or in the clinical specimen.

Two main ELISA methods have been used for toxicology, viral antibody studies, electron microscopy, and light microscopy for the identification of antigens and antibodies: namely, the enzyme-conjugate method and the so-called unlabeled–antibody-enzyme method. The enzyme-conjugate method is considered to be less sensitive than radioimmunoassay or immunofluorescence, sensitivity being lost by the preparation of the conjugate and competition from unlabeled immunoglobulins. The unlabeled–antibody-enzyme method, which usually utilizes soluble enzyme–anti-enzyme complexes, is considered to be more specific and is more sensitive, the sensitivity being gained by saturation of all the tissue antigen sites with specific antibody and allowing little excess enzyme or anti-enzyme in the mixture (Sternberger, 1974).

ELISA methods can be automated, are stable, and do not carry the potential hazards of radioisotopes. Tissue preparations do not fade as they do with fluorescent work, and light microscopy may be used.

TITRATION

In clinical serology, the titer of a substance refers to the number of antibody molecules per unit volume of the original serum. This gives an indication of the antibody concentration in a patient's serum. The titer is read at the highest dilution of serum that gives a reaction with antigen. For example, if the last tube showing a reaction contains a volume of 1 ml and the serum in this tube is 1 part in 1,000 parts, the titer is given as 1,000 units per milliliter.

NEPHELOMETRY

Nephelometry (or turbidimetry), based on the classic antigen-antibody precipitin reaction first described by Heidelberger and Kendall (1935), is the photometric measurement of the quantity of cloudiness or turbidity in a solution caused by suspended particles. The interaction of light with the particles in solution causes the light to be transmitted through the solution and be absorbed, reflected, or scattered by the particles. The technique is now routinely used to quantitate specific proteins such as immunoglobulins, complement components, and immune complexes, and has been found to provide great advantages over the standard techniques of radial immunodiffusion and immunoelectrophoresis because it is accurate, precise, fast, easy to perform, and fully automated.

The procedure of nephelometry is based on the reaction of the protein being assayed and a specific antiserum. Protein in a patient's specimen reacts with specific nephelometric antiserum to human proteins and forms insoluble complexes. When light is passed through the suspension, the incident light is scattered. The scattered light can be detected with a photodiode. The amount of scattered light is proportional to the number of insoluble complexes and can be quantitated by comparing the unknown patient values with standards of known protein concentration.

The interaction of antigen and antibody in solution depends on many factors, most important of which is their relative concentrations (as given by the Heidelberger curve). If antibodies are present in excess, a proportional relationship exists between the antigen and the resulting signal. If the antigen overwhelms the quantity of antibody, the measured signal drops. The reaction conditions are optimized through the addition of antiserum into the cuvette, which initiates the antigen-antibody binding reaction, and a short period of slow complex formation is reflected in the slow increase of light scattering. Rapid scatter intensity follows because of acceleration in the immunoprecipitin formation. The amount of scattered light reaches a plateau and falls off when the precipitin starts to aggregate and settle out of solution. The rate of increase of scattering and the height of the plateau reached are directly related to the antigen concentration and the dilution of antiserum. Nephelometry, which is based on the antigen-antibody reaction rate and the plateau stage, is used for kinetic and endpoint assays, respectively, to measure the antigen concentrations in patients' specimens.

The light source used in nephelometry is an infrared high-performance laser emitting device (LED), which produces a light beam of high colinearity at a wavelength of 840 nm. Because an entire solid angle is measured after convergence of this light via a lens system, an intense measuring signal is available when the primary beam is blocked off. Light scattered in the forward direction in a solid angle to the primary beam ranges between 13 and 24 feet and is measured by silicone photodiode with an integral amplifier. The electrical signals are digitalized and compared with reference curves and then converted into protein concentrations.

In the immunoprecipitation reaction, the time to reach plateau light scattering may vary from a few minutes to 1 hour, depending on reaction conditions. In general, an initial blank measurement is taken 10 seconds after the reaction components have been mixed. A second measurement is taken 6 minutes later, and, after subtraction of the original (1 second) blanking value, a calculation is made against the multiple-point or single-point calibration in a computerized program.

Like all other immunoassays, nephelometry is subject to interferences and limitations caused by:

1. Spurious light scattering due to dust particles, endogenous particles such as lipoprotein, or intrinsic specimen turbidity
2. Nonspecific side reactions and precipitation of macromolecules in samples
3. Freezing and thawing of samples, which may cause protein denaturation or aggregation of immunoglobulins, resulting in high sample blank value or background light scattering

CELLULAR ASSAY PROCEDURES

Cell function may be assessed using a variety of test procedures. These include:

Flow Cell Cytometry. In this method a large number of cells pass through an aperture, where they are exposed to light or electric current to generate a signal that is measured. The test uses specific antibody to detect cell markers and is used to assess the number of T_H, T_S, and B lymphocytes as well as natural killer (NK) cells, granulocytes, and other cells.

Latex Bead Ingestion. This technique uses latex beads to assess monocyte number.

Lymphocyte Transformation. This technique uses mitogen or specific antigen to determine the ability of a lymphocyte to respond to a stimulus.

Mixed-Lymphocyte Culture. This technique uses recipient and donor lymphocytes to detect compatibility or incompatibility with respect to HLA-D antigen. The test is also used to detect HLA-D antigens using patient lymphocytes.

Migration Inhibition. This technique uses monocytes and granulocytes to determine the ability of the lymphocyte to produce chemotactic factors.

Microcytotoxicity. This technique is used to detect HLA-A, -B, -C and -DR antigens and/or HLA antibodies.

Cell-Mediated Monocytolysis. This technique uses tumor cells to determine the ability of monocytes to kill cells.

Antibody-Dependent Cell-Mediated Cytotoxicity (ADDC). This technique uses tumor cells or cells containing bacteria to determine the ability of NK cells to lyse other cells.

Lympholysis. This technique uses a labeled target cell to determine the ability of cytotoxic T cells to lyse cells.

Boyden Chamber. This technique uses a chemotactic agent to determine the ability of neutrophils to respond to a chemotactic agent.

Phagocytosis. This procedure uses *Escherichia coli* polysaccharide with oil red O stain to determine the ability of neutrophils to phagocytize.

Nitroblue Tetrazolium Test. This test uses nitroblue tetrazolium to determine the ability of neutrophils to effect intracellular kill.

Additional information regarding these tests can be obtained by referring to the list of general references at the end of this chapter.

JUST THE FACTS

Introduction

1. The fundamental reaction between antigen and corresponding antibody is one of combination, followed by secondary or tertiary reactions.
2. Antigens and specific antibodies possess complementary corresponding structures that enable the antigenic determinants to come into very close apposition with the binding site on the antibody molecule.
3. Antigen and specific antibody are held together by weak intermolecular bonds (opposing charges on ionic groups, hydrogen bonds, hydrophobic bonds, and Van der Waals forces).
4. "Affinity" refers to the strength of an antibody-hapten or antibody-epitope bond.
5. "Avidity" refers to the overall bonding between multivalent antibodies and antigens.
6. "Specificity" is defined by the inducing antigen. This is opposed to "cross-reactivity," in which a second, structurally similar antigen can bind to the antibody.

Types of Immunologic Reactions

1. The "primary" reaction is the recognition and combination of antigen with the corresponding binding sites of its antibody.
2. The "secondary" reaction is the conformation of the amino acid chain resulting from interchain hydrogen bonding.
3. The "tertiary" reaction involves the folding of polypeptide chains through hydrophobic and hydrogen bonds.
4. The "quarternary" reaction involves the association of polypeptide subunits to form one protein.

The Specificity and Sensitivity of Immunologic Tests

1. Different immunologic methods vary in their sensitivity. This can cause problems because:
   a. Certain high-affinity, potent antibodies may give unwanted cross-reactions (false reactions).
   b. Weak antisera may be specific but not sensitive, which also may result in false reactions.

Precipitation

1. Precipitation involves the interaction of antigen and antibody in optimal proportions, resulting in a visible precipitate.
2. A concept of the reaction is based on the lattice hypothesis.

Types of Reactions

1. The types of precipitation reaction (methods) include:
   a. *Double diffusion,* in which both antigen and antibody diffuse. The technique detects antibodies associated with autoimmune disorders, and is semiquantitative.
   b. *Radial immunodiffusion,* which involves the Fahey and Mancini methods (which differ in incubation times). The technique is used for the quantitation of immunoglobulins and other serum proteins, including complement components.
   c. *Countercurrent immunoelectrophoresis (CIEP),* which involves two columns of wells. The technique is useful in the detection of autoantibodies, antibodies to infectious agents, and certain microbial antigens.
   d. *Immunoelectrophoresis,* which utilizes both electrophoresis and double diffusion. The procedure is useful for the identification of monoclonal proteins including free κ and λ chains and urine proteins, and as a screening procedure to detect immunoglobulin classes. The procedure is semiquantitative.

Immunofixation

1. Immunofixation is more sensitive to antigen and antibody ratios than immunoelectrophoresis.

2. Dilution is often necessary to produce the reaction.

Rocket Electrophoresis

1. This technique is used to quantitate antigens other than immunoglobulins.

Agglutination

1. Agglutination has many similarities to precipitation.
2. The particles involved are cells or latex particles.
3. Agglutination may be used to detect either antigen or antibody.
4. The test may be performed on slides, in tubes, or on microtiter plates.
5. Temperature, motion, pH, and class of antibody influence the agglutination reaction.
6. Agglutination reactions are quantitative or semi-quantitative.

Types of Agglutination Reaction

1. The major types of agglutination reaction include direct agglutination, viral hemagglutination, passive and reverse passive agglutination, antiglobulin techniques, and the agglutination inhibition reaction.

Reactions Involving Complement

1. The tests involving complement have been discussed in Chapter 3.
2. The complement fixation test is of limited usefulness, but has been used in viral, rickettsial, and fungal serology.
3. The immune adherence reaction is also of limited usefulness, but has been used successfully for the antigenic differentiation of species of trypanosome and leptospires and for the diagnosis of human trypanosomiasis and of syphilitic infection.

Neutralization of Toxins and Viruses

1. Neutralization tests are used when neither precipitation nor agglutination succeeds in demonstrating an antigen-antibody reaction.
2. Neutralization of toxins or viruses is the essence

of a major protective mechanism in several disease states.
3. The Schick test and the Dick test are examples of *in vivo* toxin neutralization.

Fluorescent Antibody Reactions
(Immunofluorescence)

1. Immunofluorescence involves the study of antigens in tissue sections through the use of specific antibody that has been labeled with color and is applied over a section of tissue so that a microprecipitate is formed at the site of the antigen. A fluorescent dye is linked with serum antibody and yields a blue-green fluorescent substance that is detected in a fluorescent microscope.
2. Modifications of the technique include:
   a. The direct technique.
   b. The indirect or double-layer technique.
   c. Complement-staining technique.
   d. Inhibition technique.

Immunoassays

1. Immunoassays can be non-labeled or labeled reagent assays.
2. Non-labeled assays include immunoprecipitin methods, agglutination methods, and light-scattering techniques.
3. Labeled assays are named according to the attached label.
4. Methods utilize either monoclonal or polyclonal antibodies or binding proteins.
5. They can be qualitative or quantitative and can occur in the soluble or solid phase.
6. Radioimmunoassays use radioactive labels (isotopes). They are sensitive and have the ability to detect trace amounts of antigen or antibody. The technique is rapid and a large number of tests can be performed in a short period of time. The major disadvantage is the hazard and instability of isotopes.
7. Enzyme-linked immunoassays (ELISA) are similar to immunofluorescence techniques in that a purified enzyme is linked in a stable manner to a specific antibody. There are many requirements for the utilized enzyme with respect to the technique. Two main methods are used: the enzyme-

conjugate method and the unlabeled-antibody–enzyme method.

8. ELISA methods can be automated, are stable, and do not carry the potential hazard of radioisotopes. Tissue preparations do not fade as they do in fluorescent work, and light microscopy can be used.

Titration

1. A titer refers to the number of antibody molecules per unit volume of the original serum, giving an indication of antibody concentration.
2. A titer is read as the highest dilution of serum that gives a reaction with antigen.

Nephelometry

1. Nephelometry is the photometric measurement of the quantity of cloudiness or turbidity in a solution caused by suspended particles, measured by scattered light.
2. The technique is used to quantitate specific proteins (immunoglobulins, complement components, and immune complexes).
3. Limitations of the procedure include spurious light scattering, nonspecific side reactions, and freezing and thawing of specimens.

Cellular Assay Procedures

1. Cell function may be assessed using a variety of test procedures, including flow cell cytometry, latex bead ingestion, lymphocyte transformation, mixed-lymphocyte culture, migration inhibition, microcytotoxicity, cell-mediated monocytolysis, ADCC, lympholysis, Boyder chamber test, phagocytosis, and the nitroblue tetrazolium test.

Review Questions

Multiple Choice

Choose the phrase, sentence, or symbol that completes the statement or answers the question. More than one answer may be correct in each case. Answers are given at the end of this book.

1. Antigen and specific antibody are held together by weak intermolecular bonds, believed to include:
   (a) Van der Waals forces
   (b) hydrophilic bonds
   (c) opposing charges on ionic groups
   (d) all of the above
   (Introduction)

2. The quantitative tests that involve the primary antigen-antibody reaction include:
   (a) direct agglutination
   (b) hemagglutination
   (c) complement fixation
   (d) immunofluorescence
   (Types of Immunologic Reactions)

3. The agar gel diffusion test:
   (a) is more sensitive than the radioimmunoassay procedure
   (b) is less sensitive than the cross-electrophoretic method

   (c) is more sensitive than electroimmunodiffusion
   (d) is equally as sensitive as the radioimmunoassay procedure
   (The Specificity and Sensitivity of Immunologic Tests)

4. In the precipitation test, the largest amount of precipitate is found:
   (a) at the equivalence zone
   (b) in the area of antigen excess
   (c) in the area of antibody excess
   (d) none of the above
   (Precipitation)

5. When reagents are present in optimal proportions in a precipitation reaction, the precipitation line will generally be:
   (a) concave to the well containing the reactant of higher molecular weight
   (b) convex to the well containing the reactant of higher molecular weight
   (c) concave to the well containing antigen, regardless of molecular weight
   (d) concave to the well containing antibody, but only if the antibody is of lower molecular weight
   (Types of Reaction)

6. In double diffusion, when the lines of precipitation come together on the plate forming a smooth curve, this indicates:
   (a) that the antigens are not identical
   (b) that the antigens have no antigenic determinants in common
   (c) that the antibody is precipitating identical antigen specificities in each preparation
   (d) none of the above
   (*Double Diffusion*)

7. In the Fahey method, the diameter of the precipitin rings is measured at:
   (a) 2 hours
   (b) 18 hours
   (c) 50 to 72 hours
   (d) 3 days
   (*Radial Immunodiffusion*)

8. Countercurrent immunoelectrophoresis:
   (a) is a quantitative procedure
   (b) is a semiquantitative procedure if serial dilutions are used
   (c) is useful in detecting autoantibodies
   (d) works best when the wells are not parallel
   (*Countercurrent Immunoelectrophoresis*)

9. Immunoelectrophoresis:
   (a) utilizes both electrophoresis and double diffusion
   (b) is extremely sensitive to the antigen and antibody ratios
   (c) may be used to identify urine proteins
   (d) is a semiquantitative procedure
   (*Immunoelectrophoresis*)

10. Agglutination reactions are influenced by:
    (a) temperature
    (b) pH
    (c) centrifugation
    (d) the class of antibody involved
    (*Agglutination*)

11. Direct agglutination techniques may be used to detect:
    (a) the nontreponemal antibody of syphilis
    (b) ABO and Rh antigens
    (c) febrile antibodies
    (d) all of the above
    (*Types of Agglutination Reaction*)

12. Diseases that may be diagnosed by complement fixation are:
    (a) Rocky Mountain spotted fever
    (b) herpes simplex infection
    (c) influenza
    (d) all of the above
    (*Reactions Involving Complement*)

13. Immunofluorescence has been used for the identification of:
    (a) particulate viruses and their soluble antigens
    (b) bacteria

(c) protozoa
(d) fungal antigens
(*Fluorescent Antibody Reactions [Immunofluorescence]*)

14. Radioimmunoassay:
    (a) is an extremely insensitive technique
    (b) has the ability to detect trace amounts of antigen or antibody
    (c) involves the use of radioisotopes
    (d) all of the above
    (*Immunoassays*)

15. Nephelometry is routinely used to quantitate:
    (a) immunoglobulins
    (b) complement components
    (c) immune complexes
    (d) all of the above
    (*Nephelometry*)

16. The microcytotoxicity test is used to:
    (a) assess monocyte number
    (b) determine the ability of monocytes to kill cells
    (c) detect HLA-A, -B, -C and -DR antigens
    (d) determine the ability of neutrophils to phagocytize
    (*Cellular Assay Procedures*)

Answer "True" or "False"

1. A high ratio of serum to cells decreases test sensitivity.
   (*Introduction*)

2. The precipitation reaction is an example of a secondary antigen-antibody test.
   (*Types of Immunologic Reactions*)

3. Antigen-antibody binding assays are less sensitive than the agar gel test for α_1-fetoprotein.
   (*The Specificity and Sensitivity of Immunologic Tests*)

4. The precipitation reaction is not influenced by the quantities of antigen and antibody present.
   (*Precipitation*)

5. In the precipitation reaction, a preparation containing several antigens will give rise to multiple precipitation lines.
   (*Types of Reaction*)

6. When precipitin lines cross one another, they have no antigenic determinants in common.
   (*Double Diffusion*)

7. If the wells in countercurrent immunoelectrophoresis are reversed, this will have no effect on the accuracy of the test.
   (*Countercurrent Immunoelectrophoresis*)

8. The shape and position of the precipitin arcs in immunoelectrophoresis can provide clues as to the monoclonality of a protein.
   (*Immunoelectrophoresis*)

9. The immunofixation technique is less sensitive to the antigen and antibody ratios than immuno-electrophoresis.
(Immunofixation)

10. The Laurell technique is used to quantitate antigens other than immunoglobulins.
(Rocket Electrophoresis)

11. The agglutination reaction is not subject to prozone or postzone.
(Agglutination)

12. Rabbit anti-human IgG can be used in radio-immunoassays.
(Types of Agglutination Reaction)

13. Complement components can be quantitated immunologically when the component reacts with monospecific antisera.
(Reactions Involving Complement)

14. The Schick test is an example of *in vivo* toxin neutralization.
(Neutralization of Toxins and Viruses)

15. ELISA methods cannot be performed with light microscopy.
(Immunoassays)

16. A titer gives an indication of the antigen concentration in a patient's serum.
(Titration)

17. Nephelometry is the photometric measurement of the quantity of cloudiness or turbidity in a solution caused by suspended particles.
(Nephelometry)

18. Flow cell cytometry can be used to assess granulocyte number.
(Cellular Assay Procedures)

GENERAL REFERENCES

Abbas, A.K., Lichtman, A.H., and Pober, J.S.: Cellular and Molecular Immunology. Philadelphia, W. B. Saunders Company, 1991.

Baron, E.J. and Finegold, S.M.: Bailey and Scott's Diagnostic Microbiology, 8th ed. St Louis, C. V. Mosby Company, 1990.

Bellanti, J.A.: Immunology III. Philadelphia, W. B. Saunders Company, 1985.

Dorland's Illustrated Medical Dictionary, 27th ed. Philadelphia, W. B. Saunders Company, 1988.

Freeman, B.A.: Burrows Textbook of Microbiology, 27th ed. Philadelphia, W. B. Saunders Company, 1985.

Henry, J.B.: Clinical Diagnosis and Management by Laboratory Methods. Philadelphia, W. B. Saunders Company, 1991.

Sheehan, C.: Clinical Immunology; Principles and Laboratory Diagnosis. Philadelphia, J. B. Lippincott, 1990.

Walter, J.B.: An Introduction to the Principles of Disease, 2nd ed. Philadelphia, W. B. Saunders Company, 1982.

6

Syphilis

OBJECTIVES

The student shall know, understand, and be prepared to explain:

1. A brief history of the origin of syphilis
2. The morphology of *Treponema pallidum*
3. The metabolism of *T. pallidum*
4. The syphilis antigens: Wassermann, treponemal
5. The stages of syphilis and their correlation with test results
6. The antibodies in syphilis, specifically:
   a. Development
   b. The production of immunity
7. The treatment of syphilis and its correlation with test results
8. Syphilis and blood transfusion
9. A description of neurosyphilis
10. A description of congenital syphilis
11. The diseases related to syphilis, specifically:
    a. Yaws
    b. Pinta
    c. Bejel
    d. Rabbit syphilis
12. The principles of the laboratory tests for syphilis
13. The methods of syphilis testing, including:
    a. The Venereal Disease Research Laboratory slide test with serum and spinal fluid
    b. The fluorescent treponemal antibody absorption test with serum
    c. The dark-field microscopic examination of *T. pallidum*
    d. The rapid plasma reagin card test on serum
    e. The unheated serum reagin test on serum
    f. The *T. pallidum* immobilization test
14. A brief description of the principles of other tests for syphilis

Introduction

Two schools of thought exist regarding the origin of syphilis. The first of these, often referred to as the "pre-Columbian theory," states that syphilis was present in Europe prior to the voyage of Columbus, but was not recognized as such, was confused with other diseases (e.g., leprosy), or was present in a milder form than is seen today. Hudson (1963) and others believe that the disease probably first appeared in the tropics (Central Africa) as a condition closely resembling the present day treponematoses, such as yaws, and was eventually introduced into other parts of the world by travelers and traders. The fact that the treponemes of syphilis and yaws are morphologically indistinguishable, that both respond to the same treatment, and that the same blood tests are reactive in both diseases are points in support of the pre-Columbian theory.

The second school of thought, sometimes referred to as the "Columbian theory," states that syphilis was endemic in Haiti (then called Hispaniola) and was subsequently contracted and carried to Europe by Columbus's crew. In 1494, King Charles VIII of France beseiged Naples and shortly after the fall of the city syphilis became widespread in the army and throughout Italy. The disease was later given its name through a poem "Syphilis sive Morbus Gallicus," written by Fracastorius in 1530, although at the time of the Naples seige, the Italians called it the "French disease" and the French called it the "Italian disease." The English, by contrast, called it the "Spanish disease," and medical literature of the day called it "the great pox" or "the evil pox."

As will be obvious, neither the Columbian theory nor the pre-Columbian theory is entirely satisfactory. The conclusion that a previously endemic disease could so suddenly become epidemic is as difficult to believe as the theory that the disease spread so rapidly from a single port of entry. What is certain is that the disease became the subject of medical literature in the closing years of the 15th century, the first mention being in an edict issued by the Diet of Worms on October 7, 1495. In 1497 mercury was being advocated as treatment for the disease by at least two physicians, Widmann and Gilino, and in 1498 the first major book about syphilis was written by Francisco Lopez de Villalobos.

For centuries, no specific etiology was assigned to syphilis. Many early writers who were also astrologists blamed the disease on a malignant alignment of the stars and planets. Later, syphilis, along with certain other diseases, was ascribed to a lack of balance between the humors of the body. The bacteriologic era of medicine, heralded by the work of Pasteur, Koch, Loffler, and others, stimulated a search for the cause of the disease. Numerous bacteria were reported as causal, but the critical experiments resisted confirmation or repetition.

The five-year period from 1905 to 1910 produced, through numerous discoveries, the important contributions to the modern age of syphilis management. In 1905, Schaudinn and Hoffman of Hamburg discovered that syphilis was caused by a spirochete that they called *Spirochaeta pallida*. The same workers later changed the name to *Treponema pallidum*, but, because the original name had been widely used, both were regarded as correct. A year later, Wassermann, Neisser, and Bruck (1906) described a diagnostic blood test (Wassermann test). As this knowledge developed, so did the methods of treatment. In 1909 Ehrlich of Frankfurt produced "606," or "salvarsan," an organic arsenic preparation that was effective when given intravenously. The term *606* was applied because it was Ehrlich's 606th experiment with drugs of this group. The generic name is *arsphenamine*. Some years later, Ehrlich produced neoarsphenamine, which was even more effective. Intramuscular injection of bismuth was proposed as treatment by Sazerac and Levaditi in 1921, as a less toxic and more effective substitute for mercury.

With little doubt, the greatest single therapeutic advance in the history of infectious diseases was the discovery of penicillin by Sir Alexander Fleming. Soon after the discovery of the antibiotic in 1943, John Mahoney in New York reported remarkable results obtained with penicillin in the treatment of four patients with primary syphilis. The healing of lesions was little short of miraculous. Other workers soon confirmed Mahoney's findings, and within a short period of time penicillin had completely replaced all other forms of treatment for all phases of the disease. Even now, almost 50 years later, penicillin remains the drug of choice in treatment of the disease.

The prevalence of syphilis is not known with certainty. In the United States, the total number of cases reported each year has fluctuated since the early 1960s, with 33.7 cases per 100,000 population reported in 1976, compared with just over 70 cases per 100,000 population in the mid-1940s. In 1974, almost 40 million people were tested for syphilis, and 1.2 million had positive reactions (Blount and Holmes, 1975). Congenital syphilis has decreased by almost 90 per cent since 1950, and the mortality rate has dropped from about 1 case per 100,000 in 1967 to just over 0.1 per cent in 1975, although this statistic may be unreliable owing to the fact that in deaths reportedly due to other causes, syphilis may have been a contributing factor.

The incidence of the disease remained relatively steady during the years 1955 to 1958; it increased from 113,894 cases in 1958 to a peak of 126,245 cases in 1962 and then declined to 71,761 cases in 1976. In 1977, 9.4 cases per 100,000 population were reported. This increased to 14.6 cases per 100,000 population in 1982 and then decreased to 14.1 cases per 100,000 in 1983. In 1987, the number of reported cases of primary and secondary syphilis increased by 25 per cent over the total reported for 1986 (Centers for Disease Control, Atlanta, Georgia, 1988). By 1990, the number of cases reported was 134,225 (Centers for Disease Control, Atlanta, Georgia, 1991). These data can only be regarded as relative because the vast majority of cases (possibly as high as 70 to 80 per cent) are not reported. A problem that has also recently surfaced in the epidemiology of the disease is the disproportionately high number of cases in homosexual or bisexual males. A study conducted in England, Scotland, and Wales in 1971 revealed that 42 per cent of the males reported to have primary or secondary syphilis were homosexual. A similar study in the United States revealed that 34 per cent of males with syphilis were either homosexual or bisexual, an increase of 10 per cent over the level reported in 1969.

MORPHOLOGY OF *TREPONEMA PALLIDUM*

Treponema pallidum (subspecies *pallidum*) is a member of the order Spirachaetales and the family Treponemataceae and the genus *Treponema*. This family contains three genera: *Borrelia*, *Treponema*, and *Leptospira*. The genus *Treponema* contains four principal species of pathogenic organisms: *T. pallidum* (responsible for human syphilis), *T. pertenue* and *T. carateum* (the etiologic agents for yaws and pinta, respectively), and *T. cuniculi* (responsible for rabbit syphilis).

The morphologic characteristics of *T. pallidum* can be studied microscopically. The usual method used in clinical tests is that of dark-field (or dark-ground) illumination, although both the phase-contrast and the electron microscopes have been used.

T. pallidum is seen microscopically as a close-coiled, thin, regular spiral organism varying in length from 6 to 15 µ and consisting of 8 to 24 coils (Figs. 6–1 and 6–2). The width of the spiral is seldom more than 0.25 µ. Electron microscopic studies have revealed the anatomic structure of the cell, which presents as an axial bundle surrounded by a number of spirally wound filaments that, when they have become detached from the axial bundle, have been misinterpreted as flagella (Ovčinnikov and Delektorsij, 1966, 1968). There is probably a periplast or capsular structure. Evidence suggests that *T. pallidum* multiplies by transverse fission and that the active phase of this probably occurs about every 30 hours.

In aqueous media, young treponemes spin vigorously around their long axis in an apparently useless type of motion. In more viscous media, however, they achieve sufficient traction to propel themselves. In tissues, they show remarkable flexi-

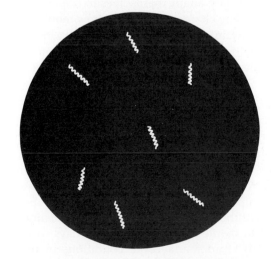

Figure 6–1. Microscopic view of *T. pallidum* (diagrammatic).

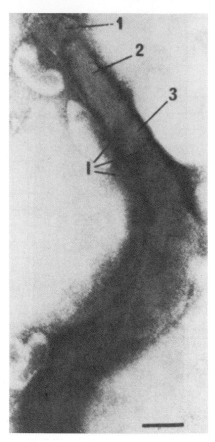

Figure 6–2. Electron micrograph of *T. pallidum* (Nichol's strain). (From Hovind-Hougen, K.: Acta Pathol. Microbiol. [Scand.] 255:1, 1976. Reproduced in Braude, A. I.: Medical Microbiology and Infectious Diseases. Philadelphia, W. B. Saunders Company, 1981, p. 491.)

bility as they adapt themselves to the intracellular spaces. The characteristic corkscrew motility is produced by internal periplasmic flagella located between the outer membrane and the periplasmic cylinder (body) of the spirochete (Johnson, 1986).

METABOLISM OF *TREPONEMA PALLIDUM*

Outside the host, *T. pallidum* is extremely susceptible to a variety of physical and chemical agents that rapidly bring about its destruction. Suspensions of the organism, however, have remained viable and motile for periods up to 15 days when kept at 35°C under anaerobic conditions in medium containing serum albumin, glucose, carbon diox-

ide, pyruvate, cysteine, glutathione, and serum ultrafiltrate.

The metabolic capabilities of the cultivable treponemes show some variation, although for all of them, nutritional requirements are complex. They require and use glucose (or other fermentable carbohydrate) as a primary energy source, as well as multiple amino acids, purines, and pyrimidines. Many strains also need biocarbonate and one or more coenzymes. All require at least one exogenously supplied fatty acid; for some oral strains, a short-chain acid is sufficient, but others require one or more acids of 16 to 18 carbon chains.

T. pallidum has not been recovered in blood, serum, or plasma stored at 4°C for more than 48 hours, although organisms may remain alive for up to 5 days in tissue specimens removed from diseased animals. Suspensions of treponemes frozen at −70°C or lower in the presence of glycerol or other cryoprotective agents, however, can be kept viable for years.

Very little is known about the interaction between *T. pallidum* and the human host. It is believed that both humoral and cell-mediated immune responses are involved. Antitreponemal anticardiolipin antibodies are produced, an inflammatory response (which involves lymphocytes, plasma cells, and macrophages) is initiated, immune complexes are formed, and the organism is walled off in lesions. The disease then enters a latency or "remission" stage (Baseman, 1983).

ANTIGENS

The Wassermann Antigen

In the original form of the Wassermann test an extract of liver containing many treponemes from human fetuses with congenital syphilis was used as antigen. The specific ligand involved, however, was later found to be present in extracts of normal liver and other mammalian tissues. Subsequently, the ligand was isolated from cardiac muscle and identified as a phospholipid, diphosphatidyl glycerol, which was called *cardiolipin*.

Cardiolipin is a normal constituent of host tissue; therefore, a theory arose that the development of the antibody represented an autoimmune response (a theory supported by the fact that the Wassermann antibody—anticardiolipin—appears in other disorders, e.g., lupus erythematosus). Free cardiolipin, however, is a hapten and must be bound to a suitable carrier to be antigenic. The lipid composition of cultivable treponemes depends to a considerable extent upon the lipids in the growth medium; therefore it is possible that pathogenic treponemes growing *in vivo* have access to a plentiful supply of this phospholipid, which could be incorporated into the treponeme, the microbial cell being a foreign carrier and the bound cardiolipin serving as the immunogenic determinant.

The Treponemal Antigens

In the treponemes, two classes of antigen have been recognized, those restricted to one or more species and those shared by many different spirochetes.

The only well-studied treponemal component is a protein that is found in most treponemes, both saprophytic and pathogenic species. This antigen, once widely used in a diagnostic test for syphilis, was first obtained from the Reiter treponeme, a spirochete reputed to be a cultivable, nonvirulent variant of *T. pallidum*. In its purest form, it is a macromolecule associated with RNA. This antigen (or a very similar protein) is present in many indigenous treponemes of the human alimentary tract and many individuals acquire weak, low-level "natural" antibodies to it.

THE STAGES OF SYPHILIS (CORRELATION WITH TEST RESULTS)

Syphilis in humans is ordinarily transmitted by sexual contact. In the infected male, the offending *T. pallidum* organisms are either present in lesions on the penis or discharged from deeper genitourinary sites along with the seminal fluid. In infected females, the lesions are commonly located in the perineal region or on the labia, vagina wall, or cervix. In approximately 10 per cent of cases, the primary infection is extragenital, usually in or about the mouth.

Primary (or Early) Stage

T. pallidum appears to enter the skin only through small breaks, although, like all other spirochetes, it is capable of passing through intact mucous membranes, after which it is carried by the blood stream to every organ of the body. Multiplication of the organism at the site of entrance results, within as few as 10 and as many as 60 days, in the development of a characteristic primary inflammatory lesion known as a *chancre* (Fig. 6–3).

The chancre usually begins as a papule (a small, circumscribed, solid elevation of the skin) and then breaks down to form a superficial ulcer with a clean, firm base. The chancre in males may occur on any part of the external genitalia, the most common site being the coronal sulcus of the penis. It may also occur inside the urethra (the so-called intrameatal chancre), in which case the only symptom may be scanty serous urethral discharge. In females the primary chancre may occur on the labium majus or minus, at the fourchette, on the clitoris, near the urethral orifice, on the cervix uteri or (rarely) the vaginal wall, or on the vulva (in which case it can be associated with considerable edema of the labia).

The primary chancre persists for 1 to 5 weeks

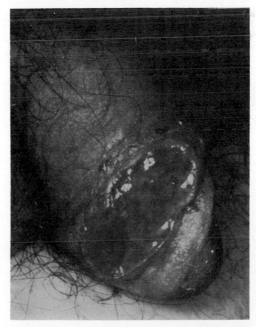

Figure 6–3. Typical primary chancre in the early stage of syphilis.

and then heals spontaneously. During this stage, the serum in 30 per cent of cases becomes serologically active after 1 week; in 90 per cent of cases, it becomes reactive after 3 weeks. Serum tests for syphilis usually give positive results between the first and third weeks after the appearance of the chancre. Fewer than 10 per cent of cases show a positive reaction by the fifth day. The reagin titer (see later in this chapter) increases rapidly during the first 4 weeks and then remains stationary for approximately 6 months.

Secondary Stage

The secondary stage of syphilis usually occurs from 6 to 8 weeks after the appearance of the primary chancre. In about one third of cases this systemic secondary stage appears before the chancre disappears and is usually characterized by a generalized rash, which often involves the mucous membranes (Fig. 6–4).

During the secondary stage, lesions may develop in the eyes, joints, or central nervous system. These secondary lesions, particularly in the mucous membranes, contain large numbers of spirochetes and, when located on exposed surfaces, are highly contagious. As with primary syphilis, these lesions subside spontaneously after 2 to 6 weeks.

In the secondary stage, serologic tests for syphilis are invariably positive.

Note: In some cases (albeit rarely), the primary and secondary stages of syphilis go unnoticed, the first signs and symptoms of the disease being the late (or tertiary) lesions.

The Late Latent Stage

Generally after the second year of infection, syphilis enters the late stage, which is usually contagious. The stage begins with a period of latency, in which there are no clinical signs or symptoms of the disease, the only indication of infection being positive serologic tests. This latent stage may last for many years, or even for the rest of the patient's life, with the patient dying from causes unrelated to syphilis.

After an infection has persisted for more than 4 years, it is rarely communicable except between mother and fetus.

Tertiary Stage

The first lesions of the tertiary stage of syphilis are usually seen from 3 to 10 years after the primary stage (or later). The lesions, known as *gummata*, are usually located on the skin, mucous membranes, subcutaneous and submucous tissue, bones, joints, muscles, and ligaments. When gummata are located on the skin or bones, they cause relatively little trouble. Serious manifestations,

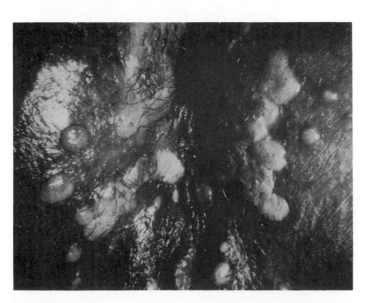

Figure 6–4. Lesions of secondary syphilis (anal area).

however, usually result when these lesions are present in the nervous system (causing general paralysis or tabes dorsalis), in the cardiovascular system (causing, in many cases, aortic aneurysm), and in the eyes (where they may cause permanent blindness).

In about one fourth of untreated cases, the tertiary stage is asymptomatic and is recognized only by serologic tests. Note that occasionally the primary and systemic lesions heal so completely that even the serologic tests become nonreactive.

ANTIBODIES IN SYPHILIS

Development

Individuals infected with *T. pallidum* respond immunologically by producing both specific and nonspecific antibodies. The specific antibodies are directed against the pathogenic *T. pallidum;* the nonspecific antibodies are directed against the protein antigen group common to pathogenic spirochetes. The antibodies against the group antigen in cases of primary syphilis are fixed with IgG and IgA. Specific antitreponemal antibodies in early or untreated early latent syphilis are predominantly IgM, although the same immunoglobulin is reported to be present in only 23 per cent of sera from patients with untreated late latent syphilis. This early immune response to infection is rapidly followed by the appearance of IgG antibodies, which soon become predominant. The largest elevations in IgG levels are seen in the secondary stage. Between the secondary and the early latent stage, total IgG does not appear to decrease significantly, but basic IgG does. This suggests a closer relationship of the fluctuations in the number of treponemes with basic IgG levels than with total IgG levels. Nonspecific IgA antibodies increase significantly during the course of untreated syphilis.

Production of Immunity

Immunity to *T. pallidum* develops in the course of syphilis both in rabbits and in humans. Some immunity can be detected in rabbits with experimental syphilis just 3 weeks after infection with the organism. Resistance to reinfection increases to a maximum approximately 3 months after infection.

Termination of the disease within the first 3 months by penicillin therapy renders the individual susceptible to reinfection.

Attempts to induce immunity against experimental infection in rabbits by means of *T. pallidum* vaccine have been made by a number of investigators, some reporting failure and others reporting success.

Protective immunity against syphilis can be induced by vaccines containing nonviable *T. pallidum* or certain cultivable nonpathogenic treponemata. The need for high-volume dosage and the difficulties in the production of sufficient quantities of *T. pallidum*, however, hamper the general use of vaccines. The comparatively easily cultivable nonpathogenic treponemata would be a preferable source of vaccine, but further study is required to determine the true effectiveness of these preparations in conferring protective immunity.

It is possible that there is no *complete* immunity to *T. pallidum*. Studies have shown that active lesions may be brought under control and animals may be resistant to rechallenge with *T. pallidum*, but the host is not able to rid itself of the infecting organism, which persists in the lymph nodes. Human subjects have been found to be resistant to rechallenge with *T. pallidum* during latency, although observations have shown that they have not succeeded in eradicating the infecting organism.

TREATMENT OF SYPHILIS (CORRELATION WITH TEST RESULTS)

If a patient infected with *T. pallidum* is adequately treated before the appearance of the primary chancre, it is probable that the serologic tests will remain nonreactive. If treatment is given before the appearance of reagin (i.e., the seronegative primary stage), the serologic tests also usually give no reaction. After the appearance of reagin (i.e., the seropositive primary stage), the serologic tests usually become nonreactive 6 months after treatment. Note: Reagin is an anti-cardiolipin antibody, a nonspecific treponemal antibody formed during *T. pallidum* infection. This is not the same as the IgE antibody (the reagin of allergy); see discussion under IgE in Chapter 2.

In the secondary stage of the disease, serologic

tests usually become nonreactive within 12 to 18 months after treatment. After the secondary stage, however, treatment has variable effects on serologic test results; yet, as a general rule, the sooner treatment is given, the more marked will be the serologic response.

If the patient is treated 10 years or more after the onset of the disease, the serologic tests can be expected to change little, if at all.

In about 10 per cent of cases, patients who receive adequate treatment during the primary or secondary stage of syphilis fail to exhibit a decrease or reversion of serologic test results and show reactive test results indefinitely. These patients are said to be "seroresistant" or "Wassermann-fast." This phenomenon may be due to the continued presence of reagin, indicating a definite immune response or persistent foci of infection. Neurosyphilis is frequently associated with seroresistance in both the early and late stages. In cases of a persistently reactive serologic test, spinal fluid should be examined to determine whether the disease has been controlled.

Individuals who are allergic to penicillin are usually treated with tetracycline, with the exception of pregnant women, who are treated with erythromycin because tetracycline has been shown to have adverse effects on the human fetus (US Department of Health and Human Services, 1985). Studies have shown that the Nichols strain of *T. pallidum* can accept penicillinase-producing plasmids (Wilcox and Guthe, 1966). This may cause changes in antibiotic therapy for syphilis infection in the future.

SYPHILIS AND BLOOD TRANSFUSION

Syphilis may be transmitted by blood transfusion when very fresh blood is used. Blood stored at 4°C for 4 days or more, however, is unlikely to transmit syphilis, because *T. pallidum* is unable to survive under these conditions. In most cases, since the primary routine tests on blood donations take several days to complete, the causative organism is usually dead before transfusion is given. In addition, a serologic test for syphilis is standard procedure for all blood donations; therefore, the disease is rarely a problem.

NEUROSYPHILIS

Neurosyphilis is syphilis of the central nervous system. In all types of neurosyphilis, the essential changes are the same: obliterative endarteritis, usually of the terminal vessels, with associated parenchymatous degeneration, which may or may not be sufficient to produce symptoms.

Neurosyphilis is divided into the following groups, depending upon the type and degree of central nervous system lesions present:

Asymptomatic Neurosyphilis. The patient is usually seen because of a reactive serologic test for syphilis. There are no signs or symptoms indicative of central nervous system involvement; however, examination of the cerebrospinal fluid, obtained by lumbar or cisternal puncture, reveals an increase in cells and total protein, a positive reagin test, and an abnormal colloidal-gold test.

Meningovascular Neurosyphilis. There are definite signs and symptoms of nervous system damage, resulting from cerebrovascular occlusion, infarction, and encephalomalacia with focal neurologic signs. The cerebrospinal fluid is always abnormal, with an increase in cells and total protein and a positive reagin test. In this type of neurosyphilis, usually meningeal or vascular involvement is seen.

Parenchymatous Neurosyphilis. This type of neurosyphilis presents as paresis (incomplete paralysis) or tabes dorsalis (degeneration of the dorsal columns of the spinal cord and of the sensory nerve trunks, with wasting.)

1. The signs and symptoms of paresis may be myriad, although they are always indicative of widespread parenchymatous damage. Personality changes range from minor to psychotic, and frequently there are focal neurologic signs. Serologic blood tests are reactive, and the cerebrospinal fluid is invariably abnormal.
2. Tabes dorsalis: The spinal fluid in tabes dorsalis gives abnormal findings in 90 per cent of cases; the serum is reactive in 75 per cent of cases. Signs and symptoms include primary posterior column degeneration with ataxia (failure of muscle coordination), areflexia (absence of reflexes), paresthesias (abnormal sensations, e.g., burning, prickling), bladder disturbances, impotence, and often lightning pains. Gastric or ab-

dominal "crises" frequently begin with vomiting (which may result in serious electrolyte imbalance) and severe abdominal pain. Trophic joint changes result from loss or impairment of the sensation of pain; the knee joint is most commonly involved, and severe degeneration is common. Syphilitic optic atrophy is also frequently seen.

The signs and symptoms of paresis and tabes dorsalis frequently coexist in the same patient (so-called taboparesis).

CONGENITAL SYPHILIS

Congenital syphilis is acquired during fetal life from the maternal circulation through the placental passage of *T. pallidum* from the 18th week of gestation onward. This is more likely to occur when the mother is suffering from early syphilis, particularly the primary or secondary stage, rather than late syphilis. Adequate treatment of the mother before the 18th week of pregnancy prevents infection of the fetus. Because penicillin will cross the placenta in adequate amounts, treatment of the mother after the 18th week of pregnancy will also cure the infected fetus.

The clinical manifestations of congenital syphilis may be divided into early, late, and the stigmata. Ordinarily, the division between the early and late stages of the disease is placed at the second year of life. Many of the lesions of the first two years of life are infectious and resemble those of secondary syphilis in the acquired form of the disease. The late lesions, appearing from the third year onward, are mostly of the gummatous type and are non-infectious. The stigmata are the scars or deformities resulting from early or late lesions that have healed.

DISEASES RELATED TO SYPHILIS

Yaws

Treponema pertenue, the organism that causes the tropical disease known as yaws, is virtually indistinguishable from *T. pallidum* (Fig. 6–5). In fact, the only difference in the diseases produced by these organisms is the character of the lesions. Both the primary and the secondary lesions of yaws are

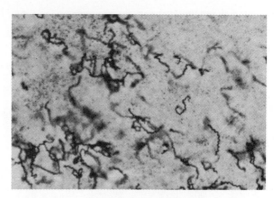

Figure 6–5. *Treponema pertenue* in biopsy specimen. Krajian-Erskine silver impregnation stain. (From Freeman, B. A.: Textbook of Microbiology, 22nd ed. Philadelphia, W. B. Saunders Company, 1985, p. 800.)

more persistent than those of syphilis, and unlike in syphilis, scar formation develops at the site of the secondary infection. The lesions are granulomatous or wart-like, with a granular surface similar to that of a raspberry; hence the name *frambesia* (also known as papillomas; Fig. 6–6). The tertiary stage is characterized by nodular or ulcerative necrosis (gummas of skin and subcutaneous tissue), gummas and subperiosteal thickening of the long bones, and plantar hyperkeratosis (Fig. 6–7). Nasopalatal destructive lesions (gangosa), destruction of joints (particularly the interphalangeal joints), and mobile soft-tissue nodules near the joints (juxta-articular nodes) occur commonly in yaws and are also seen in bejel (discussed later in this chapter). The healed ulcerative lesions leave thin depigmented scars and sometimes severe disfigurement (Fig. 6–8).

In general, yaws is not as grave a disease as syphilis, because it rarely involves the viscera, and congenital yaws is very uncommon. The disease occurs in the tropics, where the combination of high temperature and humidity promotes the persistence of open skin lesions and thus facilitates nonvenereal transmission by direct contact.

Yaws responds dramatically to treatment with penicillin, often requiring only a single long-acting injection.

Pinta

The causative organism of the disease known as pinta is *Treponema carateum*, which, like *T. pertenue*, is morphologically indistinguishable from

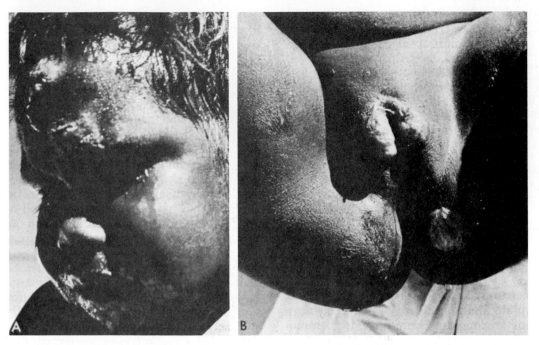

Figure 6–6. Secondary yaws: papillomas of face, genitalia, and buttocks. (From Braude, A. I.: Medical Microbiology and Infectious Diseases. Philadelphia, W. B. Saunders Company, 1981, p. 1616.)

T. pallidum (Fig. 6–9). Pinta is a nonvenereal disease endemic in Central and South America, which usually occurs in childhood and is contracted through skin contact. Serologic tests are reactive as in cases of syphilis.

The initial lesion in pinta is commonly found on the legs. It starts as a papule but soon forms a

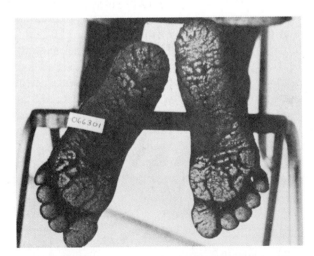

Figure 6–7. Tertiary yaws: plantar hyperkeratosis. (From Braude, A. I.: Medical Microbiology and Infectious Diseases. Philadelphia, W. B. Saunders Company, 1981, p. 1616.)

circular, scaly patch known as a *pintid*. A papular, annular papular, or papulosquamous rash then appears on the limbs and face after an interval of several months. Many years later, lesions of the face, hands, and feet produce atrophy and depigmentation.

Pinta is a relatively mild chronic disease with a good prognosis. Lawton-Smith *et al.* (1971) investigated 11 cases of late pinta in Venezuela and found no ocular or neurologic abnormalities except in one patient with pinta and bilateral interstitial keratitis.

Penicillin is effective in treatment, especially in the early stages.

Bejel

Bejel is probably a variety of nonvenereal syphilis. It has been studied by Hudson (1958) and Csonka (1952). Usually no primary lesion is seen. Secondary lesions consist of generalized papular, annular papular, and papulosquamous eruptions. Perineal and genital condylomata and mucous patches are common. After a latency period, tertiary lesions may be observed in subcutaneous tissue, skin, and bones. The nasopharynx and larynx are often involved. The nervous system, cardiovas-

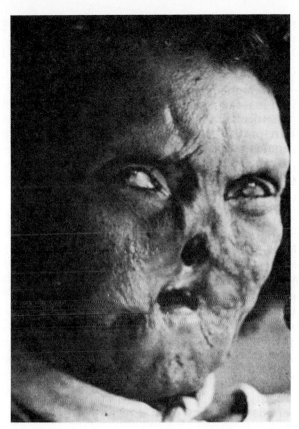

Figure 6–8. Tertiary yaws: facial scarring following gangosa. (From Braude, A. I.: Medical Microbiology and Infectious Diseases. Philadelphia, W. B. Saunders Company, 1981, p. 1618.)

cular system, and other viscera are not involved, however, and there is no evidence of transmission *in utero.*

Differentiation from syphilis is made on clinical grounds. The causative organism (treponeme) is indistinguishable from *T. pallidum* and is sometimes referred to as *T. pallidum II* or *T. pallidum endemicum* to distinguish it from *T. pallidum* of venereal syphilis. Serologic tests for syphilis are positive in cases of bejel.

Penicillin is effective in treatment unless contraindicated by allergy.

Rabbit Syphilis

Rabbit syphilis is a natural venereal infection of rabbits, producing minor lesions of the genitalia. The causative organism is morphologically identical to the spirochete of syphilis and is known as

Treponema cuniculi. Rabbits with this disease do not give positive Wassermann reactions and do not develop antibodies that immobilize *T. cuniculi.*

SEROLOGIC TESTS FOR SYPHILIS

Principles

Infection of humans with *T. pallidum* provokes in the host a complex antibody response. Serologic tests for syphilis are based on the detection of one or more of these antibodies. No "ideal" single test is available at present, and although more than 200 procedures have been described, only a few are routinely used. Host antibodies are of two known types: (1) non-treponemal antibodies, or reagin, which react with lipid antigens; and (2) treponemal antibodies, which react with *T. pallidum* and closely related strains.

Reagin Tests for Syphilis. In the course of certain diseases, including syphilis, a substance appears in the serum of affected patients that has the properties of an antibody. The substance is known as "reagin," and it possesses the ability to combine with colloidal suspensions of lipoids extracted from animal tissue (most commonly beef heart), which then clump together to form visible masses, a process known as *flocculation.* After combining with reagin, the lipoidal particles have the power to fix complement.

An example of an easily performed reagin test is the Venereal Disease Research Laboratory (VDRL)

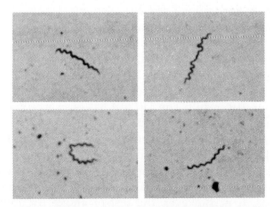

Figure 6–9. Various forms of *Treponema carateum.* Krajian-Erskine silver impregnation stain. (From Freeman, B. A.: Textbook of Microbiology, 22nd ed. Philadelphia, W. B. Saunders Company, 1985, p. 802.)

slide test, which can be used quantitatively and qualitatively for detecting reagin in serum and cerebrospinal fluid (see later in this chapter for test procedure). Other reagin tests include the rapid plasma reagin (RPR) test of Portnoy *et al.* (1957), which uses the incorporation of chlorine chloride to modify the basic VDRL antigen and allows for the testing of plasma without preliminary heating. An extension of this principle is seen in the plasmacrit (PCT) test of Andujar and Mazurek (1959), the unheated serum reagin (USR) test described by Portnoy and Carson (1960), the rapid plasma reagin (RPR) (circle) card test (Portnoy, 1963), and the automated reagin test of McGrew *et al.* (1968), developed by the VDRL in 1970. Commercial reagents have been developed and evaluated for other rapid reagin tests that are designed to react at a level comparable to the VDRL test (Caputo, 1975; March *et al.*, 1974).

It should be noted that reagin is part of the gamma globulin portion of serum and is probably present in small quantities in normal sera. These quantities, however, are insufficient to give positive results with standard test procedures.

Treponemal Tests for Syphilis. Nelson (1948) showed that the serum of patients with syphilis contains an antibody that is distinct from reagin and that, in the presence of complement, inhibits the normal movement of virulent treponemes of syphilis. On the basis of this information, a test was developed by Nelson and Mayer (1949) called the *Treponema pallidum* immobilization (TPI) test. The organisms are extracted from lesions in experimentally infected rabbits and incubated with syphilitic serum and guinea pig complement. Under these conditions, the organisms lose their motility. If 50 per cent or more of the treponemes are immobilized, the test is regarded as positive. If fewer than 20 per cent are immobilized, the test is negative. The range 20 to 50 per cent represents an area of "doubtful" result. The TPI test has been accepted as the treponemal test of reference, but it is not useful in assessing therapy, because once the secondary stage is past, the test is likely to remain positive for the rest of the patient's life, regardless of treatment, and it does not distinguish between the treponematoses. It is, however, the test of choice for spinal fluid, especially for detecting neurosyphilis when reagin tests give nonreactive or equivocal results.

Since 1949 efforts have been made to develop

similar techniques for routine laboratory use. Tests using killed *T. pallidum,* such as the *Treponema pallidum* complement fixation (TPCF) test, have failed to satisfy this goal in terms of simplicity and cost. The so-called Reiter protein complement fixation (RPCF) test is more satisfactory, however. This test uses a protein fraction derived from the cultivable Reiter treponeme, which shares a common group antigen with *T. pallidum* and other treponemes (Wallace and Harris, 1967). The complement fixation test is used with Reiter protein antigen substituted for nonspecific antigen.

Another treponemal test is the fluorescent treponemal antibody absorption (FTA-ABS) test described by Hunter *et al.* (1964). In this technique, a drop of a suspension of dead *T. pallidum* (Nichols virulent stain) serves as antigen. The suspension is dried and fixed on a slide, and diluted patient's serum is added. If antibody is present, the treponemes become coated with a layer of antibody globulin, detectable by the addition of fluorescein isothiocyanate-labeled antihuman immunoglobulin, which unites with the bound globulin and fluoresces when examined by dark-ground illumination under ultraviolet light.

By this method, an antibody specific for *T. pallidum* and other allied pathogenic treponemes and a group-reactive antibody that reacts with both pathogenic and commensal treponemes are detected. This group antibody, present in most normal sera in low concentrations, becomes increased with syphilis infection. By dilution of the serum in a heated culture filtrate of Reiter treponemes (sorbent), the group antibody is theoretically "blocked," and the specific antibody is then free to unite with the treponemal antigen. This is the basis of the FTA-ABS test (Hunter *et al.,* 1964), which has proved extremely sensitive, especially in cases of primary syphilis, and has been shown to have good specificity. False-positive reactions, however, have been noted in patients with balanitis and in those with lupus erythematosus. The FTA-ABS test can also be used to detect different immunoglobulin classes by using monospecific conjugates. This is of practical value in the differentiation of neonatal syphilis from passive transfer of maternal antibody because IgM does not cross the placenta.

The *Treponema pallidum* hemagglutination (TPHA) test (Garner and Clark, 1975) is also extremely sensitive and has the advantage of being easy to perform. The antigen used is a suspension of formolized tanned sheep red cells sensitized with an ultrasonicate of virulent *T. pallidum*. Serum is added to an absorbing diluent to remove cross-reacting antibodies, and sensitized cells are added. Unsensitized cells added to a second tube serve as a control. The tubes are allowed to stand at room temperature. A positive result is revealed by the gradual agglutination of the sensitized cells; the unsensitized cells (control) form a compact button at the bottom of the tube.

The direct fluorescent antibody (DFA) test is another useful test for syphilis that has distinct advantages over dark-field examination of chancre fluid for treponemes. Of particular advantage is the fact that dried slides can be saved or mailed to a reference laboratory for testing or examination.

NOTES ON SEROLOGIC TESTS FOR SYPHILIS

1. When testing a sample for syphilis, the following should be noted:
   a. More than one screening test should be performed if results are found to be positive, to guard against false-positive results.
   b. There is no serologic test that will differentiate syphilis from other treponemal infections (e.g., yaws, bejel).
   c. False-positive results may be the result of:
      i. Human error or contaminated specimens.
      ii. Variations from the normal (a few patients produce an excess of reagin, giving a positive reagin test, in which case treponemal tests must be performed).
      iii. Diseases allied to syphilis (e.g., yaws).
      iv. Biologic reactions associated with infections or recent immunizations. These are usually "acute" and last no longer than a few months. "Chronic" false-positive results are seen in cases of leprosy.
2. In the interpretation of serologic tests for syphilis, the following factors should be taken into account:
   a. Geographic area or country of origin. Diseases related to syphilis, whose causative organisms are indistinguishable from *T. pallidum*, can result in misdiagnosis.
   b. Ability of the patient to produce reagin or treponemal antibodies.
   c. Stage of the illness.
   d. Previous antibiotic therapy.
   e. Manner in which serologic tests are performed.
   f. Various conditions that may cause biologic false-positive results (discussed earlier).

Negative Reactions

The technologist should keep in mind that a negative serologic test for syphilis may indicate, besides the fact that the patient does not have syphilis, any of the following:

1. The infection is too recent to have produced antibodies that give reactions.
2. The test has been rendered *temporarily* nonreactive by consumption of alcoholic fluids prior to testing.
3. The test is *temporarily* nonreactive because of treatment.
4. The disease is latent or inactive.
5. The patient has not produced protective antibodies because of immunologic tolerance.
6. Inferior technique.

Weakly Reactive Results

Weakly reactive results may be due to:

1. Very early infection.
2. Lessening of the activity of the disease after treatment.
3. Biologic false-positive reaction.
4. Inferior technique.

Positive Results

Positive results usually indicate that the patient has syphilis. The technologist should keep in mind, however, that such results could be due to inferior technique or may be biologic false-positive results.

Control of Serologic Tests for Syphilis

Control sera of graded reactivity should be included each time serologic testing procedures are performed. For the nontreponemal flocculation test with serum and spinal fluid, the antigen suspension should be controlled daily. The results obtained should reproduce the established reactivity pattern: With unacceptable results, testing should be delayed until optimal reactivity has been established. This can be done by preparing another antigen suspension, correcting temperature (room temperature should be 23°C to 29°C), adjusting equipment, and so on. For the FTA-ABS test, control sera should be included in each test run. Results should be considered invalid if controls are unacceptable.

Control sera of graded reactivity for nontreponemal and treponemal test procedures are obtainable from commercial sources or may be prepared from individual sera (or pooled sera) after testing. High-titer reactive serum may be used for spinal fluid controls.

Quality control of reagents obtained from commercial sources is also important. Chemicals and distilled water should be of high quality and should always be used according to the manufacturer's directions.

METHOD 1: VENEREAL DISEASE RESEARCH LABORATORY (VDRL) SLIDE TEST WITH SERUM

Materials

1. Mechanical rotator—adjustable to 180 rpm, circumscribing a circle ¾ inch in diameter on a horizontal plane.
2. Slides—2 inch × 3 inch, with 12 paraffin or ceramic rings approximately 14 mm in diameter. (Note: If glass slides with ceramic rings are used, the rings must be high enough to prevent spillage when rotated; they must be cleaned so that serum will spread to the inner surfaces of the ceramic rings; they must be discarded if the ceramic rings begin to flake off.)
3. Ring maker to make paraffin rings approximately 14 mm in diameter.
4. Slide holder for 2 inch × 3 inch microscope slides.
5. 18-, 19-, and 23-gauge hypodermic needles.
6. Syringe—Luer-type, 1 or 2 ml.
7. 30-ml, round, glass-stoppered, narrow-mouthed bottles, approximately 35 mm in diameter, with flat interbottom surfaces. (Note: Bottles with convex interbottom surfaces are unsatisfactory.)

Reagents

1. VDRL antigen: Antigen for this test is a colorless, alcoholic solution containing 0.03 per cent cardiolipin, 0.9 per cent cholesterol, and a sufficient amount of purified lecithin to produce standard reactivity (usually 0.21 per cent ± 0.01 per cent). Before being put into use, each lot of antigen must be serologically standardized by comparison with an antigen of known reactivity. Antigen lots, once controlled, are stored in the dark at either refrigerator (6°C to 10°C) or room temperature in screw-capped (Vinylite liners) bottles or hermetically sealed glass ampules. At these temperatures, the components of the antigen remain in solution. Formation of a precipitate indicates changes resulting from factors such as evaporation or additive materials contributed by pipettes. Such ampules should be discarded.
2. 1.0 per cent buffered saline solution, prepared by adding 0.5 ml of formaldehyde (neutral, reagent-grade); 0.093 gm $Na_2HPO_4 + 12H_2O$; 0.170 gm KH_2PO_4; and 10.0 gm NaCl to 1,000 ml of distilled water. This solution yields potentiometer readings of pH 6.0 ± 0.1 and is stored in screw-capped bottles. (Note: When an unexplained change in test reactivity occurs, the pH of the buffered saline should be checked to determine whether this is a contributing factor. Saline with pH outside the acceptable range should be discarded.)
3. 0.9 per cent saline, prepared by adding 900 mg of dry sodium chloride (A.C.S.) to each 100 ml of distilled water.

Preparation of Antigen Suspension

1. Pipette 0.4 ml of buffered saline to the bottom of a 30-ml round glass- or screw-capped bottle.
2. Add 0.5 ml of antigen directly onto the saline while rotating the bottle on a flat surface gently and continuously. The antigen should be taken from the lower half of a 1.0-ml pipette graduated to the tip and it should be added drop by drop at a speed that allows 0.5 ml of antigen to be added every 6 seconds. The pipette tip should remain in the upper third of the bottle, and rotation should not be vigorous enough to splash the saline onto the pipette. The proper speed of rotation is achieved when the center of the bottle

circumscribes a 2-inch-diameter circle approximately three times per second.

3. Blow the last drop of antigen from the pipette without allowing the pipette to touch the saline.
4. Continue the rotation of the bottle for 10 seconds.
5. Add 4.1 ml of buffered saline from a 5.0-ml pipette.
6. Place the top on the bottle and shake from the bottom to the top and back approximately three times per second.
7. The antigen suspension is now ready for use and may be kept for 1 day. Each time the suspension is used, it should be mixed gently. Do not mix the suspension by forcing it back and forth through any syringe or pipette; this may cause the breakdown of particles and loss of reactivity.

Testing Accuracy of Antigen Emulsion Delivery Needles

Because it is of primary importance that the proper amounts of reagents be used, the needles used should be checked daily. For the slide quantitative test on serum (described later in this chapter), dispense the antigen suspension from a syringe fitted with an 18-gauge needle without bevel that will deliver 60 drops (± 2 drops) of antigen suspension per milliliter when the syringe and needle are held vertically.

For the slide quantitative test on serum, two tests are required. The first is performed with a 19-gauge needle without bevel that will deliver 75 drops (± 2 drops) of antigen suspension per milliliter when the syringe and needle are held vertically; the second is performed with the 23-gauge needle (with or without bevel) that will deliver 100 drops (± 2 drops) of *saline* per milliliter when the syringe and needle are held vertically.

Needles that do not meet these specifications should be adjusted and calibrated or discarded.

Preliminary Testing of the Antigen Suspension

1. Test the control sera of graded reactivity (i.e., reactive, weakly reactive, or nonreactive) using the slide quantitative test (described later).

2. Reactions with control sera should reproduce the established reactivity pattern. The nonreactive serum should show complete dispersion of antigen particles. Unsatisfactory antigen suspensions or pools of antigen suspensions should not be used.

Preparation of Serum for Testing

1. Heat clear serum obtained from centrifuged clotted blood in a 56°C water bath for 30 minutes before testing (to destroy complement).
2. Examine the serum when it is removed from the water bath, and recentrifuge it if it is found to contain particle debris.
3. If serum is allowed to remain untested for 4 hours or more after original heating, reheat for 10 minutes at 56°C before testing.
4. When tested, the serum must be at room temperature.

Procedure (VDRL Qualitative Test on Serum)

1. Pipette 0.05 ml of heated serum into one ring of a paraffin-ringed or ceramic-ringed slide. (Glass slides with concavities, wells, or glass rings are not recommended for this test.)
2. Add one drop ($^1/_{60}$ ml) of antigen suspension onto each serum with an 18-gauge needle and syringe.
3. Rotate the slides for 4 minutes on a mechanical rotator that describes a ¾-inch-diameter circle when set at 180 rpm.
4. Read tests microscopically with a 10× ocular and a 10× objective immediately after rotation.

Reading and Reporting of Results

At 100× magnification, the antigen particles appear as short rod forms. Aggregation of these particles into large or small clumps is interpreted as degrees of reactivity. Read as follows:

No clumping (or slight roughness) : Nonreactive
Small clumps : Weakly reactive
Medium or large clumps : Reactive

Note: A *prozone reaction* is occasionally encountered. This type of reaction is demonstrated when complete or partial inhibition of reactivity occurs with undiluted serum; maximal reactivity is obtained only with diluted serum. This prozone reaction may be so pronounced that only a weakly reactive (or "rough" nonreactive) result is produced in the qualitative test by a serum that is strongly reactive when diluted. Therefore, it is recommended that any serum producing a weakly reactive (or "rough" nonreactive) result in the qualitative test be retested with the quantitative procedure before a report of the VDRL slide test is released. When a reactive result is obtained on some dilution of a serum that produced only a weakly reactive (or "rough" nonreactive) result before dilution, the test should be reported as reactive, and the qualitative titer should be reported.

Procedure (VDRL Slide Quantitative Test on Serum)

1. Prepare a 1:8 dilution of the serum under test by adding 0.1 ml of the serum to 0.7 ml of 0.9 per cent saline by using a 0.2-ml pipette graduated in 0.01-ml subdivisions.
2. Mix thoroughly, and allow the pipette to stand in the dilution until all dilutions are prepared (if more than one serum is to be tested).
3. Using this pipette, transfer 0.04 ml, 0.02 ml, and 0.01 ml of the 1:8 serum dilution into the fourth, fifth, and sixth paraffin rings, respectively.
4. Blow out the remaining serum dilution into the dilution tube.
5. With the same pipette, transfer 0.04 ml, 0.02 ml, and 0.01 ml of *undiluted* serum into the first, second, and third paraffin rings, respectively.
6. Add two drops (0.01 ml per drop) of 0.9 per cent saline to the second and fifth rings of each serum with a 23-gauge needle and a syringe.
7. Add three drops (0.01 ml per drop) of 0.9 per cent saline to the third and sixth rings of each serum with a 23-gauge needle and syringe.
8. Rotate the slides gently by hand for about 15 seconds to mix the serum and saline.
9. Add one drop (^{1}/75 ml) of antigen suspension to each ring with a 19-gauge needle and a syringe.
10. Rotate the slide for 4 minutes at 180 rpm.
11. Read the test microscopically immediately after rotation.

Reading and Reporting of Results

1. The result of the reaction between the serum and the antigen is read as either reactive or nonreactive.
2. Definite clumping of the antigen particles is reported as reactive; no clumping or slight roughness of antigen particles is reported as nonreactive.

The highest dilution exhibiting a reaction is considered the "endpoint." Weakly reactive reactions are not counted as significant in reporting an endpoint titer; therefore, if a serum shows positive reactions at dilutions of 1:2 and 1:4, weakly reactive reactions at 1:8, and no reaction at higher dilutions, the test is reported as "reactive 1:4." A serum that exhibits a reactive reaction in the undiluted serum *only* is reported as "reactive, undiluted only."

METHOD 2: VENEREAL DISEASE RESEARCH LABORATORY (VDRL) SLIDE TEST WITH SPINAL FLUID

Materials

1. Antigen suspension (prepared as described for the VDRL slide test with serum; see p. 124)
2. 1.0 per cent buffered saline (prepared as described for the VDRL slide test with serum; see p. 124)
3. 10.0 per cent unbuffered saline
4. 0.9 per cent unbuffered saline
5. Slides (agglutination)—1¼ × 3 inches, with 12 concavities, each measuring 16 mm in diameter and 1.75 mm in depth

Preparation of "Sensitized Antigen Suspension"

1. Add one part of 10 per cent saline to one part of VDRL slide test suspension.
2. Mix by gently rotating the bottle or inverting the tube, and allow to stand at least 5 minutes but not more than 2 hours before use.

Testing Accuracy of Antigen Suspension Delivery Needles

For the slide quantitative and qualitative tests on spinal fluid, dispense sensitized antigen suspension from a syringe fitted with a 21- or 22-gauge needle, which will deliver 100 drops (± 2 drops) per milliliter when the syringe and needle are held vertically. Needles not meeting this criterion should be adjusted and calibrated before use or discarded.

Procedure (VDRL Slide Qualitative Test on Spinal Fluid)

Note: Tests should be performed within the temperature range of 23°C to 29°C because slide flocculation tests for syphilis are affected by room temperature and below room temperature the test reactivity is decreased.

1. Pipette 0.05 ml of spinal fluid into one concavity of an agglutination slide.
2. Add one drop (0.02 ml) of sensitized antigen suspension to each spinal fluid with a 21- or 22-gauge needle.
3. Rotate slides for 8 minutes on a mechanical rotator at 180 rpm.
4. Read tests microscopically with a low-power objective, at 100× magnification. Record as follows:

Definite clumping or flocculation of antigen
particles : Reactive
Complete dispersion of antigen particles, no
agglutination or flocculation : Nonreactive

Procedure (VDRL Quantitative Test on Spinal Fluid)

Note: Quantitative tests are performed on all spinal fluids found to be reactive in the qualitative test.

1. Prepare spinal fluid dilutions as follows: Pipette 0.2 ml of 0.9 per cent saline into each of five or more tubes. Add 0.2 ml of unheated spinal fluid to tube 1, mix well, and transfer 0.2 ml to tube 2. Continue mixing and transferring 0.2 ml from one tube to the next until the last tube is reached. The dilutions are 1:2, 1:4, 1:8, and so forth.
2. Test each spinal fluid and undiluted spinal fluid as described for the qualitative procedure.
3. Report results in terms of the highest dilution of spinal fluid giving a positive reaction.

METHOD 3: FLUORESCENT TREPONEMAL ANTIBODY ABSORPTION (FTA-ABS) TEST WITH SERUM

Materials

1. Incubator—adjustable for 35°C to 37°C
2. Dark-field fluorescent microscope assembly
3. Bibulous paper
4. Diamond-point pencil (optional)
5. Template—used as a guide for cutting circles of 1.0 cm inside diameter on glass slides (optional)
6. Slide board or holder
7. Moist chamber: Place moistened paper inside a convenient cover fitting and slide board
8. Loop—immersion, low-fluorescence, non-drying
9. Microscope slides—1 inch × 3 inch, fronted end, approximately 1 mm thick
10. Cover slips—No. 1, 22 mm square
11. Dish—staining, glass, or plastic, with removable slide carriers
12. Glass rods—approximately 100 mm × 4 mm, both ends fire polished

Reagents

1. *Treponema pallidum* antigen: The antigen for this test is a suspension of *T. pallidum* (Nichols strain) extracted from rabbit testicular tissue, containing a minimum of 30 organisms per high dry field. The antigen may be stored at 6°C to 10°C or may be processed by lyophilization. Lyophilized antigen is also stored at 6°C to 10°C and is reconstituted for use according to directions when needed. Any antigen that becomes contaminated with bacteria or does not give the appropriate reactions with control sera must be discarded.
2. FTA-ABS test sorbent: This is a standardized product prepared from cultures of Reiter treponemes. It may be purchased in lyophilized or liquid state and should be stored according to the manufacturer's directions.
3. Fluorescein-labeled antihuman globulin (conjugate): this should be of proven quality for the FTA-ABS test. Each new lot of conjugate should be tested to ensure its dependability with re-

spect to working titer and to verify that it meets the criteria concerning nonspecific staining and standard reactivity. The lyophilized conjugate should be stored at 6°C to 10°C. Rehydrated conjugate should be dispensed in not less than 0.3-ml quantities and should be stored at −20°C or lower. For practical purposes, a conjugate with a working titer of 1:400 or higher may be diluted 1:10 with sterile phosphate-buffered saline (containing Merthiolate in a concentration of 1:5,000) before storage. When conjugate is thawed for use, it should not be refrozen but should be stored at 6°C to 10°C. It may then be used as long as acceptable reactivity is obtained with test controls. If a change in FTA-ABS test reactivity is noted in routine testing, the conjugate should be retitered to determine whether this is the contributing factor.

4. Phosphate-buffered saline (PBS), pH 7.2 ± 0.1: The solution is prepared as follows. To each liter of distilled water add:
   a. 7.65 gm NaCl
   b. 0.724 gm Na_2HPO_4
   c. 0.21 gm KH_2PO_4
   Several liters may be produced and stored in large Pyrex (or equivalent) or polyethylene bottles. The pH of the solution should be 7.2 ± 0.1. PBS outside this range should be discarded.
5. Tween-80: To prepare PBS containing 2 per cent Tween-80, heat the two reagents in a 56°C water bath. To 98 ml of PBS, add 2 ml of Tween-80 (by measuring from the bottom of the pipette). The 2 per cent Tween-80 solution should be pH 7.0 to 7.2 and should be checked periodically because the solution may become acid. Store at refrigerator temperature, and discard if a precipitate forms or if the pH moves out of the acceptable range.
6. Mounting medium, consisting of one part PBS, pH 7.2, plus 9 parts glycerin (reagent quality).
7. Acetone (A.C.S.).

Preparation of *Treponema pallidum* Antigen Smears

1. Mix the antigen suspension well with a disposable pipette and rubber bulb, drawing the suspension into and expelling it from the pipette at least 10 times to break the treponemal clumps and to ensure an even distribution of trepo-

nemes. To ensure that treponemes are adequately dispersed before making slides for the FTA-ABS test, check by dark-field examination. Additional mixing may be required.
2. Cut two circles of 1 cm inside diameter with a diamond-point pencil on clean slides. Wipe the slides with clean gauze to remove loose glass particles. Slides with pre-etched circles are also satisfactory for this test.
3. Smear one loopful of *T. pallidum* antigen evenly within each circle by using a standard 2-mm, 26-gauge platinum wire loop. Allow to air dry for 15 minutes.
4. Fix the smears in acetone for 10 minutes, and allow them to air dry thoroughly. Not more than 60 slides should be fixed with 200 ml of acetone. Store the acetone-fixed smears at a temperature of −20°C or lower. Fixed, frozen smears can be used indefinitely provided that satisfactory results are obtained with controls. Antigen smears should not be thawed and refrozen.

Preparation of Sera

Test and control sera should be heated at 56°C for 30 minutes before testing. Previously heated test sera should be reheated for 10 minutes at 56°C on the day of testing.

Note: Bacterial contamination or excessive hemolysis may render specimens unsuitable for testing.

Controls

Control sera from commercial sources should be stored and controlled according to the manufacturer's directions. Include the following controls in each test run:

1. Reactive (4+) control. Reactive serum or a dilution of reactive serum should demonstrate strong (4+) fluorescence when diluted 1:5 in PBS and only slightly reduced fluorescence when diluted 1:5 in sorbent. Prepare as follows:
   a. Using a 0.2-ml pipette and measuring from the bottom, add 0.05 ml of reactive control serum to a tube containing 0.2 ml of PBS. Mix well—at least eight times.
   b. Using a 0.2-ml pipette and measuring from the bottom, add 0.05 ml of sorbent. Mix well—at least eight times.
2. Minimally reactive (1+) control. Dilutions of reac-

tive serum demonstrating the *minimal* degree of fluorescence are reported as "reactive" for use as a reading standard. The reactive (4+) control serum may be used for this control when diluted in PBS according to directions.

3. Nonspecific serum controls. A nonsyphilitic serum known to demonstrate at least 2+ nonspecific reactivity in the FTA test at a dilution of PBS of 1:5 or higher should be used. Prepare as follows:
   a. Using a 0.2-ml pipette and measuring from the bottom, add 0.05 ml of nonspecific control serum to a tube containing 0.2 ml of PBS. Mix well—at least eight times.
   b. Using another 0.2-ml pipette and measuring from the bottom, add 0.05 ml of nonspecific control serum to a tube containing 0.2 ml of sorbent. Mix well—at least eight times.
4. Nonspecific staining controls:
   a. Antigen smear treated with 0.03 ml of PBS.
   b. Antigen smear treated with 0.03 ml of sorbent. Controls 1, 3, and 4 are included for the purpose of controlling reagents and test conditions. Control 2 (minimally reactive control serum) is included as the reading standard (Table 6–1).

Check Testing of New Lots of Reagents

Each new lot of reagents should be tested in parallel with a standard reagent giving satisfactory results before being placed into routine use.

TABLE 6–1. Control Pattern Illustration

	Reaction*
Reactive control	
a. 1:5 PBS dilution	R4+
b. 1:5 sorbent dilution	R(4+ to 3+)
Minimally reactive (1+) control	R1+
Nonspecific serum controls	
a. 1:5 PBS dilution	R(2+ to 4+)
b. 1:5 sorbent dilution	N
Nonspecific staining controls	
a. Antigen, PBS, and conjugate	N
b. Antigen, sorbent, and conjugate	N

*R = reactive; N = normal. Test runs in which these control results are not obtained are considered unsatisfactory and should not be reported.

Procedure

1. Identify the previously prepared slides by numbering the frosted end with a lead pencil (see preparation of *T. pallidum* antigen smears).
2. Number the tubes to correspond with the sera and control sera being tested, and place in racks.
3. Prepare controls—reactive (4+), minimally reactive (1+), and nonspecific control serum dilutions as already described.
4. Pipette 0.2 ml of sorbent into a test tube for each test serum.
5. Using a 0.2-ml pipette and measuring from the bottom, add 0.05 ml of the heated serum into the appropriate tube, and mix at least eight times. Note: The interval between preparing serum dilutions and placing them on the antigen smears should not exceed 30 minutes.
6. Cover the appropriate antigen smears with 0.03 ml of the reactive (4+), minimally reactive (1+), and nonspecific control dilutions.
7. Cover the appropriate antigen smears with 0.03 ml of the PBS and 0.03 ml of the sorbent for "nonspecific" staining controls a and b, respectively.
8. Cover the appropriate antigen smears with 0.03 ml of the test serum dilutions.
9. Place in a moist chamber to prevent evaporation.
10. Place the moist chamber in an incubator at 35°C to 37°C for 30 minutes.
11. Rinsing procedure: Place the slides in slide carriers and rinse slides with running PBS for about 5 minutes, then place the slides in a staining dish containing PBS for 5 minutes. Agitate the slides by dipping them in and out of the PBS at least 10 times. Again, place the slides in a staining dish containing *fresh* PBS for 5 minutes, and agitate by dipping them in and out at least 10 times. Rinse the slides in running distilled water for about 5 seconds.
12. Blot the slides *gently* with bibulous paper to remove all water drops. Alternatively, shake off excess water, place the slides on a clean towel, and then dry them with a hair dryer (not hot air).
13. Dilute the conjugate to its working titer in PBS containing 2 per cent Tween-80.
14. Place approximately 0.03 ml of diluted conju-

TABLE 6–2. Method of Recording Intensity of Fluorescence

Reading	Intensity of Fluorescence	Report
2+ to 4+	Moderate to strong	Reactive (R)
1+	Equivalent to minimally reactive (1+) control	Reactive (R)
Less than 1+	Weak but definite, less than minimally reactive (1+) control	Borderline (R)
—	None or vaguely visible	Nonreactive (N)

gate on each smear. Spread uniformly with a glass rod to cover the entire smear.

15. Repeat steps 9, 10, 11, and 12.
16. Mount the slides immediately by placing a small drop of mounting medium on each smear and applying a cover slip.
17. Examine slides as soon as possible. If a delay is unavoidable, slides may be placed in a darkened room and read within 4 hours.
18. Read microscopically, using an ultraviolet light source and a high-power dry objective. A combination of BG 12 exciting filter, not greater than 3 mm in thickness, and OGI barrier filter (or their equivalents) has been found to be satisfactory for routine use.
19. Check the nonreactive smears by using illumination from the tungsten light source in order to verify the presence of treponemes.
20. Using the minimally reactive (1+) control slide as the reading standard, record the intensity of fluorescence of the treponemes as shown in Table 6–2.

Note: All specimens with intensity of fluorescence of 1+ or less should be retested. When a specimen initially read as 1+ is retested and subsequently read as 1+ or greater, the test is reported as "reactive." All other test results on retest are reported as "borderline." It is not necessary to retest nonfluorescent (nonreactive) specimens (Table 6–3).

TABLE 6–3. The FTA-ABS Reporting Scheme

Test Reading	Repeat	Report*
4+		R
3+		R
2+		R
1+	1+ or greater	R
	1+, less than 1+, or negative	B
Less than 1+	1+, less than 1+, or negative	B
		N

*R = reactive; B = borderline; N = nonreactive.

Borderline Results

A report should accompany each borderline result, stating that the result cannot be interpreted as reactive or nonreactive. If the result is found the *first* time the specimen is submitted from a particular patient, a new specimen should be requested for retesting. On subsequent occasions, the laboratory should suggest a careful review of the patient's history and findings, because it will be on these criteria that diagnosis will be based.

METHOD 4: DARK-FIELD MICROSCOPY EXAMINATION OF *TREPONEMA PALLIDUM*

Materials

1. Dark-field microscope assembly. This is an ordinary microscope equipped with the following:
   a. Mechanical stage
   b. Dark-field condenser
   c. 10× ocular(s)
   d. Low-power objective (10×)
   e. High dry objective (40 to 45×)
   f. Oil-immersion objective fitted with a funnel stop or equipped with a built-in iris diaphragm to lower the numerical aperture of the objective below that of the condenser. Preferably, the microscope should be *parafocal* (i.e., when objectives are changed, the correct focus is maintained).
2. Illuminator—preferably external with iris diaphragm and a 100-watt bulb. Internal microscope base illuminators are satisfactory when connected to a rheostat transformer.
3. Microscope slides—1 × 3 inches, frosted ends
4. Cover glass—size No. 1, 22 × 22 mm square
5. Oil-immersion, nondrying
6. Lens paper
7. Lens cleaner

8. Forceps, cover glass
9. Applicator sticks
10. Surgical gloves—rubber or plastic
11. Gauge—2 × 2 inch square, sterile
12. Saline—physiologic, sterile
13. Scalpel
14. Loop—bacteriologic
15. Pipette—capillary, disposable, sterile
16. Bulb—rubber, 1- or 2-ml capacity
17. Speculum—bivalve
18. Clamp—Kelly or hemostat
19. Alcohol—70 per cent, or iodine solution
20. Syringe—1- or 2-ml, sterile
21. Needles—20- and 23-gauge, sterile

Collection and Submission of Specimens

Careful specimen collection for dark-field examination is especially important because the objective is to obtain serous fluid that is rich in *T. pallidum* and as free as possible of red blood cells and tissue debris, which may obscure the treponemes. The lesion should be thoroughly cleansed to remove tissue debris and superficial spirochetal flora, such as the larger *Borrelia*-like organisms and the smaller indigenous treponemes (e.g., *T. genitalis*). When collecting specimens, the technologist should use rubber gloves and take *all necessary precautions to avoid accidental infection*. Remove any scab or crust covering the lesion; cleanse with a gauze pad wet with tap water or physiologic saline. (Note: Do not use antiseptics or soap because of the potential anti-treponemal effect.) Dry the area; abrade the lesion with a dry gauze pad to provoke slight bleeding and exudation of the tissue fluid. As oozing occurs, wipe away the first few drops containing red blood cells, and await the appearance of relatively clear serous exudate. If necessary, apply pressure at the base of the lesion or apply a suction cup over the lesion to promote the appearance of tissue fluid. Ideally, the specimen should be obtained from the depths of the lesion rather than from its surface because of the greater likelihood of finding motile treponemes. For direct examination, apply clean cover glasses or slides to the oozing lesion, or use a bacteriologic loop to transfer the fluid from the lesion to glass slides. Flatten the cover glass evenly on the side with the blunt end of an applicator stick to remove air bubbles, and examine immediately.

(Note: It may be necessary to examine several slides before treponemes are found.)

Lesions of early syphilis that are not manifest but are suspected necessitate special management. In the female, lesions of the cervix and vaginal vault present special problems for the collection of satisfactory material for dark-field examination. With visualization provided by a bivalve speculum, remove all cervical or vaginal discharge of an interfering nature. Cleanse the lesion with physiologic saline, dry it, and abrade it as before (in this instance, by rubbing with a gauze pad held by a Kelly clamp). As the bleeding stops and serous exudate appears, obtain the material for a bacteriologic loop.

Lesions of the skin, even in the fading stage, merit examination. Materials can be obtained by making a small linear incision, by scraping with a sharp scalpel (or the side of the bevel of a hypodermic syringe by using it as a knife edge), or by injection of a drop or two of sterile saline in the base of the lesion with a small-gauge hypodermic needle and syringe. Mucous membrane lesions (patches) usually present no problem except in the mouth, where other treponemes that are almost identical morphologically to *T. pallidum* and have the same motility may be present as part of the indigenous flora (e.g., *T. microdentium*).

If it proves impossible to find treponemes after several examinations, a sample from the regional lymph node may be obtained, particularly if the node is palpable. The skin over the node should be sterilized by swabbing with iodine and alcohol or some other suitable agent. Rinse a sterile 20-gauge needle and 2-ml syringe with sterile saline, and allow a few drops of saline to remain in the needle. Hold the node firmly, and insert the needle well into the node. The ability to manipulate the node freely with the needle top is a good indication that the capsule has been pierced. Leaving the needle in place, carefully detach the syringe, draw a small amount of air (approximately 0.1 ml) into it, and reattach it to the needle. Inject the residual saline into the node, macerate the tissue by gently manipulating the needle in various directions, and aspirate as much material as possible. Discharge the aspirated material onto slides for immediate examination. (Note: This procedure should be done by a physician.)

Dark-field examination should be accomplished immediately, either by bringing the patient to the microscope or by bringing the microscope to the patient. Any appreciable delay in examination of the specimen may result in questionable findings because of reduced or complete loss of motility of the treponemes.

Adjustment of the Microscope for Dark-Field Examination

Dark-field illumination is accomplished by blocking out the central rays of light with an opaque stop in the dark-field condenser and reflecting peripheral rays from the side to the upper surface of the microscope side. The only direct rays of light entering the objective are those reflected from the surface of an object in the field. The object appears bright against a dark background.

1. Align the microscope and the illuminator. The external illuminator should be 6 to 20 inches in front of the plane (or flat) side of the microscope mirror.
2. Adjust the iris diaphragm on the front of the illuminator to a diameter of about 20 mm.
3. Using a piece of paper placed across the mirror surface, adjust the illuminator so that the image of the filaments of the light bulb is shown in sharp focus on the central area of the plane side of the mirror. This is done with the focusing knob on the light housing or by moving the housing backward and forward.
4. Remove the paper, and adjust the angle of the mirror to direct the light beam into the bottom of the condenser.
5. Raise the substage containing the condenser to its maximal height. The top of the condenser should be just slightly below the level of the stage. Adjust the height by rotating the top of the condenser clockwise to lower and counterclockwise to raise.
6. Lower the substage slightly, and place 2 or 3 drops of immersion oil on the top of the condenser.

    To complete the microscope adjustment and to verify the adjustment before examination of patient material, prepare a suspension of gingival scrapings in a drop of saline on a slide and mount with a cover slip. Proceed as follows:
7. Place the slide on the stage, and center the specimen over the condenser and the bottom of the slide (with care to avoid trapping air bubbles).

9. Rotate the objective turret to center the 10× objective over the specimen.
10. Bring the specimen into focus by using the coarse adjustment knob.
11. Center the light in the field by adjusting the mirror or by rotating the two centering screws located at the base of the condenser.
12. Focus the condenser by raising or lowering the substage until the smallest diameter of the circular area of intense light is seen.
13. Recheck the centering of the light, and adjust if necessary.
14. Rotate the objective turret, and center the high dry (40 to 45×) objective over the specimen.
15. Using the fine adjustment knob, bring the specimen into focus.
16. Open the iris diaphragm on the light until the entire field is illuminated.

Examination of Specimens

1. Place the slide to be examined under the microscope, and adjust the microscope if necessary.
2. Search the entire specimen methodically for spiral organisms having morphology and motility characteristics of *T. pallidum.*
3. If a suspected organism is seen, center it in the field with the mechanical stage for examination with the oil-immersion objective.
4. Rotate the objective turret halfway so that a *small* drop of immersion oil can be placed on the cover glass.
5. Continue rotation of the turret until the oil-immersion objective is in place over the specimen and in contact with the oil on the cover glass.
6. Examine the organism carefully for identification; focus with the fine adjustment knob only.
7. If organisms are found that have the characteristic morphology and motility of *T. pallidum,* make a positive report. (Note: Do not make the negative report until a careful and exhaustive search of several slides has been made.)

Care should be taken to ensure that the organism seen is, in fact, *T. pallidum.* This can be accomplished only after experience with identification. Practically speaking, *T. pallidum,* as opposed to other spiral organisms, is usually uniform in size, shape, and motility. In contrast, *Borrelia*-like organisms are usually mixed with many other spiral and bacterial types, so that any one preparation will contain spiral forms of various sizes, shapes, and motilities. Experience in this case is the best teacher. In general, though, *T. pallidum* is a thin, tightly wound, rigid, spiral organism exhibiting little flexibility, and does not move rapidly from place to place. Any coarsely wound spiral organism exhibiting great flexibility and rapidly moving from place to place, therefore, is *not T. pallidum*.

Interpretation

The demonstration of treponemes with characteristic morphology and motility of *T. pallidum* constitutes a positive diagnosis of syphilis in either the primary, secondary, early congenital, or infectious relapse stages, regardless of the results of serologic testing. In primary syphilis, it may be possible to identify the etiologic agent and to diagnose the disease before the serologic tests become reactive.

Failure to find the organism does not rule out the diagnosis of syphilis. In addition to meaning that the lesion is not syphilitic, negative results of dark-field examination may mean that (1) a sufficient number of organisms were not present to be detected, (2) the patient has received antitreponemal drugs locally or systemically, (3) the lesion is "fading" or approaching natural resolution or disappearance, or (4) the lesion is one of late syphilis.

When negative results are obtained, the dark-field examination should be repeated on at least 3 different days, and serologic follow-up should be continued for about 4 months—at weekly intervals for the first month and every 2 weeks thereafter—before the possibility of syphilis is ruled out.

METHOD 5: RAPID PLASMA REAGIN (RPR) (CIRCLE) CARD TEST ON SERUM

Materials

All equipment and supplies necessary to perform the RPR (circle) Card Test are contained in a kit supplied by Hynson, Westcott, and Dunning, Inc., Baltimore, Maryland, with the exception of controls, the rotating machine, and the humidifier cover.
1. The kit contains the following:
   a. RPR Card Test antigen. This cardiolipin is similar to that prepared for the unheated serum reagin test (Method 6). It also contains a suspension of especially prepared charcoal particles that allows the test to be read macroscopically. The antigen should be stored according to the manufacturer's directions (usually 2°C to 8°C), in which case the unopened ampule will have a shelf life of at least 12 months from the date of manufacture. Once the ampule has been opened, it usually remains stable for about 3 months and should not be used after the expiration date on the sample. Each new lot of antigen suspension should be carefully compared with an antigen suspension of known reactivity before being placed into routine use.
   b. 20-gauge needle without bevel
   c. Plastic dispensing bottle
   d. Plastic-coated cards—each with 10 18-mm circle spots
   e. Dispenstirs—0.05 ml per drop
   f. Capillary pipettes—0.05-ml capacity
   g. Rubber bulbs
   h. Stirrers
2. Rotating machine—adjustable or fixed at 100 rpm, circumscribing a ¾-inch diameter circle on a horizontal plane.
3. Humidifier cover—any convenient cover containing a moistened pan may be used to cover the cards during rotation.
4. Pipettes (optional)—these may be used in place of Dispenstirs or capillary pipettes:
   0.2-ml, graduated in 0.01-ml subdivisions
   0.5-ml, graduated in 0.01-ml subdivisions
   1.0-ml, graduated in 0.01-ml subdivisions

Testing the Accuracy of Delivery Needles

The 20-gauge disposable needle without bevel should be checked each day by placing the needle on a 2-ml syringe or a 1-ml pipette, filling it with antigen suspension, and counting the number of drops delivered in 0.5 ml when the needle is held in a vertical position. The needle is considered satisfactory if 60 drops ± 2 drops are obtained in 1.0 ml. A needle not meeting this specification should be discarded.

Preliminary Testing of Antigen Suspension

1. Attach the needle hub to the tapered fitting on the plastic dispensing bottle. Shake the antigen ampule to resuspend the antigen particles, snap the ampule neck at the break line, and withdraw all of RPR Card Test antigen into the dispensing bottle by suction, collapsing the bottle and using it as a bulb. Shake the dispenser gently before each series of antigen drops is delivered.
2. Test the control sera of graded reactivity each day as described under Procedure, below. Serum controls can be obtained from the daily test runs or from individual donors.
3. Use only those suspensions that have given the designated reactions with the controls.

Preparation of Serum

1. Centrifuge the blood specimen at room temperature at a force that is sufficient to separate the serum from the cells (generally 1,500 to 2,000 rpm for 5 minutes).
2. Retain the serum in the collection tube.
3. Serum is tested without heating but should be at 23°C to 29°C at the time of testing.

Procedure

1. Place 0.5 ml of unheated serum on an 18-mm circle of the test card, using a Dispenstir, a 0.05-ml capillary pipette with attached bulb, or a serologic pipette.
2. Spread the serum with the Dispenstir (inverted, using the closed end) or a stirrer (broad end) to fill the entire circle. (Note: Be careful not to scratch the card surface.)
3. Add exactly one drop ($1/60$ ml) of the RPR Card Test antigen suspension to each test area containing serum. Do not stir.
4. Place the card on the rotator, and cover with the humidifier cover.
5. Rotate for 8 minutes at 100 rpm.
6. Read the tests without magnification immediately after rotation. The card may be briefly rotated or tilted by hand if necessary to differentiate nonreactive from minimally reactive results.

7. Report the results as follows:
       Small to large clumps : Reactive (R)
   No clumping, or slight
                       roughness : Nonreactive (N)
   Note: Specimens giving any degree of clumping should be subjected to further serologic study, including quantitation.
8. Upon completion of tests, remove the needle, rinse in water, and air dry. Do not wipe the needle; this removes the silicone coating. Recap the dispensing bottle, and store in the refrigerator.

METHOD 6: UNHEATED SERUM REAGIN (USR) TEST ON SERUM

Materials

1. Centrifuge—angle head, Sorvall SS-2, type "XL" or equivalent
2. Tachometer
3. Cotton gauze
4. Rotating machine—adjustable to 180 rpm, circumscribing a circle ¾ inch in diameter on a horizontal plane
5. Tubes—stainless steel, 50-ml capacity, without flange
6. Ring maker—to make paraffin rings approximately 14 mm in diameter
7. Slide holder for 2 × 3 inch microscope slides
8. Hypodermic needle—18-gauge, without bevel
9. Syringe—Luer type, 1- or 2-ml
10. Bottles—30-ml, round, glass-stoppered, narrow-mouth, approximately 35 mm in diameter with *flat* interbottom surface
11. VDRL antigen
12. VDRL buffered saline
13. Phosphate (0.02M) Merthiolate (0.2 per cent) solution—prepared by dissolving 1.42 gm Na_2HPO_4, 1.36 gm KH_2PO_4, and 1.00 gm Merthiolate in distilled water to a final volume of 500 ml. The pH of the solution should be 6.9. It should be stored in the dark at room temperature and may be used, thus stored, for a period of 3 months.
14. Chlorine chloride solution (40 per cent)—prepared by dissolving the entire contents of a 250-gm bottle of chlorine chloride in distilled water to a final volume of 625 ml

15. EDTA (0.1M)—prepared by dissolving 3.72 gm EDTA ([ethylenedinatrilo] tetra-acetic acid disodium salt) to a volume of 100 ml in distilled water. This solution may be used for 1 year.
16. Resuspending solution, prepared as follows:
    EDTA (0.1M) 1.25 ml
    Chlorine chloride (40 per cent) 2.5 ml
    Phosphate (0.02M) Merthiolate (0.2 per cent) 5.0 ml
    Distilled water 1.25 ml
    Note: This solution should be prepared each time antigen suspensions are made.

Preparation of Antigen Suspensions

1. Prepare antigen suspensions as for the VDRL slide tests (see Method 1).
2. Centrifuge measured amounts of the antigen suspension into stainless steel tubes in an angle centrifuge at room temperature at 200 g for 15 minutes (start timing when centrifuge *reaches* desired speed). From 5 to 30 ml may be centrifuged in a single centrifuge tube.
3. Locate the sediment, and decant supernatant fluid by inverting the tube away from the side containing the sediment. While holding the tube in an inverted position, wipe the inside with cotton gauze without disturbing the sediment.
4. Resuspend with a volume of resuspending solution equal to that of the original volume of antigen suspension that was centrifuged.
5. If more than one centrifuge tube is used, combine all solutions in a bottle, stopper tightly, and shake gently for a few seconds to obtain an even suspension. This is the completed antigen suspension.
6. Each new lot of antigen suspension should be compared with an antigen suspension of known reactivity before use. Store the antigen suspension at 3°C to 10°C, at which it will remain stable for at least 6 months.

Testing Accuracy of Delivery Needles

The 18-gauge needle without bevel should be checked each day by placing it on a syringe, filling it with antigen suspension, and counting the number of drops delivered in 1.0 ml when the needle is held in a vertical position. The needle is considered satisfactory if 45 drops (± 1 drop) are obtained from 1 ml of antigen suspension. A needle that does not meet this specification should be discarded.

Preliminary Testing of Antigen Suspension

Withdraw only sufficient antigen suspension from the stock bottle for 1 day's testing, and return the stock bottle to the refrigerator. The antigen suspension should be kept at room temperature for not less than 30 minutes before it is used.

Test control sera of graded reactivity every day as described under Procedure, below. Serum controls can be obtained from the daily test runs or from individual donors.

Use only those suspensions that give satisfactory results with controls.

Preparation of Serum

1. Centrifuge the blood specimen at room temperature at a force sufficient to separate the serum from the cellular elements (usually 1,500 to 2,000 rpm for 5 minutes).
2. Retain the serum in the original collection tube.

Procedure

Note: Serum and USR antigen suspensions should be at 23°C to 29°C at the time of testing.
1. Pipette 0.05 ml of unheated serum from the original collection tube into one ring of a paraffin-ringed glass slide.
2. Add one drop ($1/45$ ml) of antigen suspension onto each serum sample.
3. Rotate slides on the rotating machine at 180 rpm for 4 minutes.
4. Read tests microscopically with a 10× ocular and a 10× objective immediately after rotation.
5. Report the results as follows:
   Medium and large clumps : Reactive (R)
   Small clumps : Weakly reactive (W)
   No clumping or very slight roughness : Nonreactive (N)
   Note: Specimens giving any degree of clumping should be subjected to further serologic study, including quantitation.

THE *TREPONEMA PALLIDUM* IMMOBILIZATION (TPI) TEST

The TPI test has undergone extensive clinical and laboratory evaluation and has been accepted as the treponemal test of *reference* (i.e., it is the standard test against which all other treponemal tests are evaluated). The test, however, has certain limitations:

1. It requires live treponemes from infected animals and is difficult to perform.
2. It does not distinguish the various treponematoses (i.e., yaws, pinta, bejel).
3. It cannot distinguish between active and latent infection.
4. It cannot be used as an index of therapeutic response.
5. It fails to detect early syphilis.
6. It is ineffective when the patient is on antibiotics.

On the positive side, the test is the one of choice for spinal fluids, especially for detecting neurosyphilis when reagin tests give nonreactive or equivocal results.

Briefly, the test involves the mixing of live, actively motile *T. pallidum* extracted from the testicular chancre of a rabbit and complement. The mixture is incubated in an atmosphere of 5 per cent CO_2 and 95 per cent N_2 and is then observed with a dark-field microscope to determine the proportion of treponemes immobilized relative to the controls. Sera causing immobilization are called TPI positive.

Perhaps the greatest value of the test is in confirming syphilis or ruling out biologic false-positive reactions; yet only a few research laboratories currently perform the test. This is primarily because of the exacting nature of the procedure, the fact that it is not well standardized, and the fact that few laboratories wish to maintain "cultures" of live *T. pallidum*.

OTHER TESTS FOR SYPHILIS

The *T. pallidum hemagglutination test* (TPHA, or, when microtechniques are used, the MHA-TP) is a fairly recent addition to syphilis serology. In the test, tanned sheep red cells are coated with antigen from the Nichols strain of *T. pallidum,* and the serum is absorbed with sorbent similar to that in the FTA-ABS test. A positive reaction is considered to be due to serum antibodies specific for syphilis. The test is simple, rapid, and reproducible and is available in a kit form from Amos Division, Miles Laboratories, Inc., Elkhart, Indiana. Studies have shown that the MHA-TP test is comparable to the FTA-ABS test in all categories of syphilis except the primary stage, in which the MHA-TP is less reactive than either the FTA-ABS or the VDRL tests. In general, however, the MHA-TP is highly specific and can be considered a satisfactory substitute for the FTA-ABS test. The chief advantages of MHA-TP when compared with FTA-ABS are its simplicity and economy. The reagents and equipment are less expensive, and the procedure technically lends itself to automation. In this regard, it can be used as a highly specific screening test. Furthermore, the reading of the test is less subjective, and quality control is significantly easier.

A third hemagglutination assay is the *hemagglutination treponemal test for syphilis* (HATTS). This test, like the TPHA test, uses gluteraldehyde-stabilized turkey erythrocytes, whereas the MHA-TP test uses tanned formalin-fixed sheep erythrocytes.

The sensitivity and specificity of these tests are virtually identical and the choice of one over another as a confirmatory test is purely a matter of user preference.

The *enzyme-linked immunosorbent assay* (ELISA) methodology is also being applied to syphilis serology. In this test, tubes coated inside with *T. pallidum* antigen are incubated with dilute serum from patients. The tubes are washed, and enzyme-labeled antihuman immunoglobulin is added. The amount of enzyme (commonly, alkaline phosphatase) activity is measured by adding substrates to the tube and measuring the reaction product formed. The principles of the ELISA technique are discussed in Chapter 5.

JUST THE FACTS

Introduction

1. The "pre-Columbian theory" states that syphilis was present in Europe prior to the voyage of Columbus.

2. Some believed that the disease first appeared in Central Africa and was carried by travelers and traders.
3. The "Columbian theory" states that syphilis was endemic in Haiti (Hispaniola) and was carried to Europe by Columbus's crew.
4. Neither the pre-Columbian nor the Columbian theory is entirely satisfactory.
5. In 1495 the disease was first mentioned in the medical literature.
6. In 1497 mercury was advocated as treatment.
7. In 1905 the causative spirochete was discovered and named *Spirochaeta pallida*. Later, the name was changed to *Treponema pallidum*.
8. In 1906 the Wassermann test was described.
9. Several treatments were advocated, including salvarsan (606) (known as arsphenamine), neoarsphenamine, and bismuth.
10. In 1943 penicillin was found to be a miraculous cure.
11. The prevalence of syphilis has fluctuated over the years. In 1990 there were 134,225 cases in the United States. About 30 to 40 per cent of cases were found in homosexual or bisexual males.

Morphology of *Treponema pallidum*

1. *Treponema pallidum* is a member of the order Spirachaetales, the family Treponemataceae, and the genus *Treponema*.
2. The family contains three genera: *Borrelia*, *Treponema*, and *Leptospira*.
3. The genus *Treponema* contains four principal species of pathogenic organisms, *T. pallidum, T. pertenue, T. carateum,* and *T. cuniculi.*
4. *T. pallidum* is a close-coiled, thin, regular spiral organism, from 6 to 15 μ in length and consisting of 8 to 24 coils.
5. The organism is believed to multiply by transverse fission.
6. In aqueous media, young treponemes spin vigorously around their long axis in an apparently useless type of motion. In viscous media, they propel themselves.

Metabolism of *Treponema Pallidum*

1. Outside the host, *T. pallidum* is susceptible to a variety of physical and chemical agents that rapidly bring about its destruction.

2. Under anaerobic conditions in various media, the organism can remain viable and motile for up to 15 days at 35°C.
3. Treponemes have complex nutritional requirements.
4. *T. pallidum* has not been recovered in blood, serum, or plasma stored at 4°C for more than 48 hours.
5. Treponemes can be kept viable when frozen (−70°C) for years.
6. Both humoral and cell-mediated immune responses are involved in the interaction between *T. pallidum* and the human host. Antibodies are produced, there is an inflammatory response, immune complexes are formed, and the lesion is walled off. The disease then enters the latency stage.

Antigens

The Wassermann Antigen

1. The antigen used in the Wassermann test is cardiolipin.
2. Free cardiolipin is a hapten and is bound to the microbial cell in order to be antigenic.
3. The microbial cell is the foreign carrier and the bound cardiolipin is the immunogenic determinant.

The Treponemal Antigens

1. In the treponemes, two classes of antigens have been recognized: those restricted to one or more species and those shared by many different spirochetes.
2. The Reiter treponeme (reputed to be a cultivable, nonvirulent variant of *T. pallidum*) can be used as antigen.

The Stages of Syphilis (Correlation with Test Results)

1. Syphilis is ordinarily transmitted by sexual contact.
2. In males, *T. pallidum* organisms are present in lesions on the penis or discharged from deeper genitourinary sites along with the seminal fluid.
3. In females, the lesions are commonly located in

the perineal region or on the labia, vaginal wall, or cervix.

4. The primary infection is extragenital (usually in or about the mouth) in 10 per cent of cases.

Primary (or Early) Stage

1. *T. pallidum* enters the skin through small breaks, but can pass through intact mucous membranes where it is carried by the blood stream to every organ of the body.
2. A chancre develops at the site of entrance within 10 to 60 days.
3. The primary chancre persists for 1 to 5 weeks, then heals.
4. Serum tests for syphilis usually become positive between the first and third week after the appearance of the chancre.

Secondary Stage

1. This usually occurs 6 to 8 weeks after the chancre appears—in one third of cases, it occurs before the chancre disappears.
2. Symptoms are generalized rash (often involving mucous membranes) and lesions in eyes, joints, or central nervous system.
3. Secondary lesions contain large numbers of spirochetes. When located on exposed surfaces, they are highly contagious.
4. The lesions subside spontaneously after 2 to 6 weeks.
5. Serologic tests are invariably positive.
6. Sometimes (rarely) primary and secondary stages go unnoticed.

The Late Latent Stage

1. This occurs after about the second year of infection.
2. The disease is contagious during this stage.
3. There are no clinical signs or symptoms.
4. Serologic tests are positive.
5. This stage may last for years or even for the rest of the person's life.
6. After 4 years the disease is rarely communicable, except between mother and fetus.

Tertiary Stage

1. Lesions are usually seen from 3 to 10 years after primary stage (or later).
2. Lesions (gummata) are usually located on skin, mucous membranes, subcutaneous and submucous tissue, bones, joints, muscles, and ligaments.
3. Lesions are serious when present in the nervous system, the cardiovascular system, and the eyes.
4. In about one fourth of untreated cases, this stage is asymptomatic.
5. Serologic tests are usually positive—occasionally negative (one fourth of untreated cases).

Antibodies in Syphilis

Development

1. Infected individuals produce specific and nonspecific antibodies.
2. Specific antibodies are directed against pathogenic *T. pallidum*.
3. Nonspecific antibodies are directed against the protein antigen group common to pathogenic spirochetes.
4. Specific antibodies in early or untreated early latent syphilis are predominantly IgM. In late latent stage, only 23 per cent are IgM.
5. Levels of IgG antibodies are elevated during secondary stage.
6. Total IgG remains constant during secondary and early latent stages—basic IgG decreases.
7. Nonspecific IgA antibodies increase significantly during the course of untreated syphilis.

Production of Immunity

1. Immunity develops to a maximum about 3 months after infection.
2. Termination of the disease by treatment renders the individual susceptible to reinfection.
3. Attempts to induce immunity in rabbits have been successful in some reported cases.
4. Vaccines are available but are not used generally because of high-volume dosage requirements.
5. It is possible that there is no *complete* immunity to *T. pallidum*.

Treatment of Syphilis (Correlation with Test Results)

1. If treatment occurs before the appearance of the chancre or before the appearance of reagin, serologic tests remain nonreactive.
2. After the appearance of reagin, tests become negative after 6 months.
3. In the secondary stage, treatment results in non-reactive tests within 12 to 18 months. About 10 per cent of patients show reactive tests indefinitely.
4. After the secondary stage, treatment has variable effects on serologic test results.
5. If treatment occurs 10 years or more after infection, serologic test results do not change.
6. For penicillin-allergic patients, tetracycline is the drug of choice.
7. Pregnant women should be treated with erythromycin.
8. The Nichols strain of *T. pallidum* can accept penicillinase-producing plasmids—this may cause a change in future antibiotic therapy.

Syphilis and Blood Transfusion

1. Blood stored for 4 days or more at 4°C is unlikely to transmit syphilis.
2. Serologic tests for syphilis are standard for all blood donations.

Neurosyphilis

1. This is syphilis of the central nervous system.
2. There are three groups of neurosyphilis:
   a. Asymptomatic neurosyphilis. There are no signs or symptoms, but there are reactive serologic tests.
   b. Meningovascular neurosyphilis. There are signs and symptoms, with either meningeal or vascular involvement.
   c. Parenchymatous neurosyphilis. This presents as paresis (incomplete paralysis) or tabes dorsalis (degeneration of the dorsal columns of the spinal cord and of the sensory nerve trunks with wasting).

Congenital Syphilis

1. Congenital syphilis is acquired from the mother during fetal life.

2. *T. pallidum* crosses the placenta from the 18th week of gestation onward.
3. Congenital syphilis is more likely to occur if the mother has early (primary or secondary) syphilis rather than late syphilis.
4. Adequate treatment of the mother before the 18th week of pregnancy prevents infection.
5. Treatment of the mother after the 18th week of pregnancy will also cure the fetus because penicillin will cross the placenta.
6. The lesions of the first 2 years of life are infectious and resemble those of secondary syphilis in the acquired form of the disease.
7. Late lesions, appearing from the third year onward, are mostly of the gummatous type and are noninfectious.
8. The stigmata are the scars or deformities resulting from early or late lesions that have healed.

Diseases Related to Syphilis

1. Causative organisms are:
   a. Yaws—*Treponema pertenue*
   b. Pinta—*Treponema carateum*
   c. Bejel—*Treponema pallidum II* or *Treponema pallidum endemicum*
   d. Rabbit syphilis—*Treponema cuniculi*
2. All organisms are indistinguishable morphologically from *T. pallidum.*
3. All diseases respond to penicillin treatment.
4. Diseases are distinguished on the basis of clinical manifestations and the appearance and location of lesions.
5. Serologic tests for syphilis are reactive (Wassermann nonreactive in rabbit syphilis).
6. Special characteristics are:
   a. Yaws—occurs in tropics—not as grave a disease as syphilis—rarely involves the viscera—congenital yaws uncommon
   b. Pinta—nonvenereal—endemic in Central and South America—usually contracted in childhood through skin contact—primary lesion found on the legs
   c. Bejel—probably a variety of nonvenereal syphilis—no primary lesions
   d. Rabbit syphilis—venereal infection of rabbits—minor lesions of genitalia—no antibodies that immobilize organism

Serologic Tests for Syphilis

1. Serologic tests for syphilis are based on the detection of one or more of the antibodies produced.
2. There is no single ideal test.
3. There are two known types of host antibodies:
   a. Reagin antibodies (non-treponemal), which react with lipid antigens
   b. Treponemal antibodies, which react with *T. pallidum* and closely related strains
4. Reagin tests include VDRL slide test, rapid plasma reagin test (RPR), plasmacrit test (PCT), unheated serum reagin test, rapid plasma reagin (RPR) circle card test, and automated reagin test.

Note: Reagin is present in normal serum; quantities are insufficient, however, to give positive results with standard test procedures.

5. Treponemal tests include *Treponema pallidum* immobilization test (TPI), *Treponema pallidum* complement fixation (TPCF) test, Reiter protein complement fixation (RPCF) test, fluorescent treponemal antibody test, fluorescent treponemal antibody absorption (FTA-ABS) test, *Treponema pallidum* hemagglutination (TPHA) test, direct fluorescent antibody (DFA) test.

Notes on Serologic Tests for Syphilis

The student should study this section in the text which is written in point form.

Review Questions

Multiple Choice

Choose the phrase, sentence, or symbol that completes the statement or answers the question. More than one answer may be correct in each case. Answers are given at the end of this book.

1. Which of the following pathogenic organisms is responsible for human syphilis?
   (a) *Treponema parridum*
   (b) *Treponema pallidum*
   (c) *Treponema pertenue*
   (d) *Treponema cuniculi*
   (Introduction)

2. The genera of the family Treponemataceae include:
   (a) *T. pallidum*
   (b) Borrelia
   (c) *T. cuniculi*
   (d) Treponema
   (Morphology of Treponema pallidum)

3. Under anaerobic conditions and in appropriate medium, *T. pallidum* can be kept viable and motile at 35°C for:
   (a) 4 hours
   (b) up to 24 hours
   (c) up to 72 hours
   (d) up to 15 days
   (Metabolism of Treponema pallidum)

4. In human syphilis, the primary infection is extragenital in approximately:
   (a) 10 per cent of cases
   (b) 1 per cent of cases
   (c) 50 per cent of cases
   (d) 99 per cent of cases
   (The Stages of Syphilis)

5. The primary chancre in human syphilis appears at the site of entrance of *T. pallidum* within:
   (a) 10 to 60 days of contact
   (b) 3 months of contact
   (c) 1 day of contact
   (d) 90 days of contact
   (Primary [or Early] Stage)

6. The secondary stage of syphilis usually occurs:
   (a) from 6 to 8 weeks after infection
   (b) 2 weeks after infection
   (c) from 6 to 8 weeks after the appearance of the chancre
   (d) 10 years after infection
   (Secondary Stage)

7. During the late latent stage of syphilis:
   (a) serologic tests are usually negative
   (b) serologic tests are positive
   (c) there are no clinical signs or symptoms
   (d) the chancre is still present
   (The Late Latent Stage)

8. The lesions of the tertiary stage of syphilis are usually located on the:
(a) skin
(b) mucous membranes
(c) muscles
(d) bones, joints, and ligaments
(Tertiary Stage)

9. Specific antitreponemal antibodies in early or untreated early latent syphilis are predominantly:
(a) IgG
(b) IgM
(c) IgA
(d) IgE
(Antibodies in Syphilis—Development)

10. Immunity to *T. pallidum:*
(a) develops in the course of syphilis both in rabbits and in humans
(b) can be detected in rabbits with experimental syphilis just 3 weeks after infection with the organism
(c) can be induced by vaccines containing nonviable *T. pallidum.*
(d) is probably never complete
(Production of Immunity)

11. If treatment is given in a case of syphilis that is in the seropositive primary stage, the serologic tests usually become nonreactive after:
(a) 1 month
(b) 6 months
(c) 5 years
(d) 2 to 3 weeks
(Treatment of Syphilis)

12. Blood stored at 4°C for 4 days or more:
(a) is unlikely to transmit syphilis
(b) is likely to transmit syphilis
(c) provides an ideal environment for *T. pallidum*
(d) should be retested for the presence of *T. pallidum* immediately before transfusion
(Syphilis and Blood Transfusion)

13. Neurosyphilis:
(a) is syphilis of the central nervous system
(b) may be asymptomatic
(c) usually involves obliterative endarteritis
(d) all of the above
(Neurosyphilis)

14. Congenital syphilis:
(a) is acquired through the placental passage of *T. pallidum* from the sixth week of gestation onward
(b) is more likely to occur when the mother has late syphilis
(c) cannot be prevented by treatment of the mother after the 18th week of gestation.
(d) none of the above
(Congenital Syphilis)

15. The organism *T. cuniculi* causes the disease known as:
(a) pinta
(b) yaws
(c) bejel
(d) rabbit syphilis
(Diseases Related to Syphilis)

16. Which of the following are categorized as "reagin tests" for syphilis?
(a) VDRL slide test
(b) TPHA test
(c) RPR (circle) card test
(d) FTA-ABS test
(Serologic Tests for Syphilis: Principles)

17. When testing a sample for syphilis:
(a) more than one screening test should be performed if results are found to be positive
(b) false-positive results may result from diseases that are related to syphilis
(c) the results may be inaccurate due to the fact that the patient has been recently immunized
(d) the differentiation of syphilis from other treponemal infections is not a problem
(Notes on Serologic Tests for Syphilis)

18. A negative serologic test for syphilis may indicate:
(a) that the infection is too recent to have produced antibodies that give reactions
(b) that the test could be temporarily nonreactive because of the consumption of alcoholic beverage by the patient prior to testing
(c) that the disease is latent
(d) that the patient has not produced protective antibodies because of immunologic tolerance
(Notes on Serologic Tests for Syphilis)

19. When testing a specimen for syphilis, weakly reactive results may be due to:
(a) very early infection
(b) lessening of the activity of the disease after treatment
(c) biologic false-positive reaction
(d) biologic false-negative reaction
(Notes on Serologic Tests for Syphilis)

Answer "True" or "False"

1. The spirochete discovered to cause human syphilis was originally named *Spirochaeta pallida.*
(Introduction)

2. In aqueous media, young treponemes achieve sufficient traction to propel themselves.
(Morphology of Treponema pallidum)

3. The interaction between *T. pallidum* and the human host is believed to involve both humoral and cell-mediated responses.
(Metabolism of Treponema pallidum)

4. Cardiolipin is a normal constituent of host tissue.
   (The Wassermann Antigen)

5. *T. pallidum* is not capable of passing through intact mucous membranes.
   (Primary [or Early] Stage)

6. During the secondary stage of syphilis, serologic tests are usually negative.
   (Secondary Stage)

7. After four years, syphilis infection is communicable between mother and fetus.
   (The Late Latent Stage)

8. In about one fourth of untreated cases of syphilis, the tertiary stage is asymptomatic.
   (Tertiary Stage)

9. Nonspecific IgA antibodies increase significantly during the course of untreated syphilis.
   (Antibodies in Syphilis—Development)

10. A pregnant woman who is allergic to penicillin should be treated with tetracycline.
    (Treatment of Syphilis)

11. Serologic tests for syphilis are reactive in asymptomatic neurosyphilis.
    (Neurosyphilis)

12. Treatment of a mother suffering from syphilis with penicillin after the 18th week of gestation will also cure the fetus.
    (Congenital Syphilis)

13. The organisms for yaws, pinta, bejel, and rabbit syphilis are easily distinguishable morphologically from *T. pallidum*.
    (Diseases Related to Syphilis)

14. The Reiter protein complement fixation test is an example of a reagin test for syphilis.
    (Serologic Tests for Syphilis: Principles)

15. Control sera should be included with serologic testing procedures for syphilis only when the test is found to be nonreactive.
    (Notes on Serologic Tests for Syphilis)

GENERAL REFERENCES

Baron, E.J., and Finegold, S.M.: Bailey and Scott's Diagnostic Microbiology, 8th ed. St Louis, C. V. Mosby Company, 1990.

Freeman, B.A.: Burrows Textbook of Microbiology, 27th ed. Philadelphia, W. B. Saunders Company, 1985.

Henry, J.B.: Clinical Diagnosis and Management by Laboratory Methods. Philadelphia, W. B. Saunders Company, 1991.

Sheehan, C.: Clinical Immunology; Principles and Laboratory Diagnosis. Philadelphia, J. B. Lippincott, 1990.

7

Viral Hepatitis

OBJECTIVES

The student shall know, understand, and be prepared to explain:
1. A brief description of hepatitis
2. The hepatitis viruses
3. Hepatitis A with respect to:
   a. Hepatitis A virus (HAV)
   b. Antibodies to HAV
   c. Serologic tests for HAV
4. Hepatitis B, with respect to:
   a. Hepatitis B virus (HBV)
   b. Markers for HBV
   c. Subtypes of HBsAg
   d. Antibodies to HBsAg
   e. Incidence of hepatitis B
   f. Transmission of hepatitis B
   g. Clinical signs and symptoms of hepatitis B
   h. Protection against HBV by antibody
   i. HBV vaccine
5. Non-A, non-B hepatitis, with respect to:
   a. Incidence of non-A, non-B hepatitis
   b. Transmission of non-A, non-B hepatitis
   c. Clinical signs and symptoms of non-A, non-B hepatitis
   d. Serologic tests for non-A, non-B hepatitis
   e. Hepatitis C virus (HCV)
6. Delta hepatitis, with respect to
   a. General characteristics
   b. The hepatitis delta virus (HDV)
   c. Antibodies to HDV
   d. Transmission of HDV
   e. Clinical signs and symptoms of delta hepatitis
   f. Treatment
7. The serologic detection of hepatitis markers, including:
   a. The serologic detection of anti-HAV
   b. The serologic detection of HBsAg
8. Practical considerations in hepatitis testing
9. The serologic methods used in hepatitis testing, specifically:
   a. Ouchterlony double diffusion
   b. Counterelectrophoresis

c. Rheophoresis
d. Complement fixation
e. Reversed passive latex agglutination
f. Reversed passive hemagglutination
g. Radioimmunoassay
h. Enzyme-linked immunoassay
10. The serologic detection of anti-HBs
11. The serologic detection of HBcAg and anti-HBc
12. The serologic detection of HBeAg and anti-HBe
13. Serologic tests in delta hepatitis

Introduction: Hepatitis

Hepatitis is a generic term referring to an inflammation of the liver. The term, however, is more generally used to refer to the clinical, laboratory, and/or histologic effects of liver injury, whether or not inflammation is present.

The vast majority of cases of hepatitis are the result of damage to the liver cells (hepatocytes), caused by viruses, bacteria, fungi, parasites, drugs, toxins, or physical agents such as heat, hyperthermia, radiation, and so forth, or by excessive alcohol intake, although some cases are idiopathic—no etiology is identified. Some hepatocytes are affected much more severely than others, and a certain proportion are irreversibly injured. In non-fatal cases, the lost hepatocytes are usually replaced by the regeneration of new cells. The term *fulminant hepatitis* is applied when the number of hepatocytes destroyed is so great that too few remain to maintain basic liver function (i.e., hepatic failure).

The morphologic changes that occur in the liver vary with the cause of hepatitis. Generally, the hepatocytes show nonspecific evidence of injury, with cell swelling (called *ballooning degeneration* when severe) and necrosis—either as eosinophilic bodies (acidophil bodies) or as small cytoplasmic fragments of ruptured hepatocytes.

Because of the many different causes of hepatitis, wherever possible the term should be qualified with an etiologic modifier (e.g., viral hepatitis, alcoholic hepatitis, radiation hepatitis). This chapter will be confined to the study of viral hepatitis.

The Hepatitis Viruses

Although many viruses may cause hepatitis, the terms *viral hepatitis* and *acute viral hepatitis* are generally used only to refer to cases caused by specific hepatotropic viruses. These include hepatitis A virus (HAV), hepatitis B virus (HBV), non-A, non-B hepatitis virus (NANB), and delta virus (HDV). All of these viruses produce acute inflammation of the liver, characterized clinically by fever, nausea, vomiting, and jaundice. The characteristic differences of hepatitis A, B, and non-A, non-B viruses are given in Table 7–1. The delta virus will be considered separately.

Two classic epidemiologic patterns of transmission of viral hepatitis were recognized early and formed the basis for the classification of the disease into two major clinical types. So-called *infectious hepatitis* is the more common variety, which often involves many people and a short incubation period (caused by the type A virus). *Serum hepatitis*, which is caused by the type B virus or the non-A, non-B virus, usually follows blood transfusions or needle wounds and has a longer incubation period.

HEPATITIS A

Hepatitis A (infectious hepatitis) is the type seen in most epidemic outbreaks of hepatitis in the normal population. The disease is transmitted by a fecal-oral route and is therefore more common in countries with low standards of living, where it af-

TABLE 7–1. Characteristics of Hepatitis Viruses

Characteristic	A Virus	B Virus	Non-A, Non-B Virus
Epidemiology	Endemic and epidemic, water-borne and food-borne epidemics	Endemic	Endemic
Transmission	Fecal-oral	Direct inoculation ? venereal	Direct inoculation ? other
Incubation period (weeks)	2–7	4–26	2–8
Disease	Acute	Acute and chronic	Acute and chronic
Size of virus	27 nm	42 nm (27 nm core)	?
Coat protein	No	Yes	?
Nucleic acid	RNA	Circular DNA (mainly double-stranded; molecular weight about 2.1 × 10⁶)	?
DNA polymerase	−	+	?
Cell culture system	+	−	−
Animal infection	Marmosets, chimpanzees	Chimpanzees	Chimpanzees
Chronic carrier	−	+	+
Vaccine	−	+	?
Passive immunity with immunoglobulin	+	+	?+

fects the population at a younger age. Outbreaks also show a seasonal pattern (e.g., when children return to school and interact with one another).

Hepatitis A Virus (HAV)

The virus causing hepatitis A is a nonenveloped, isosahedral, single-stranded RNA particle that be-longs to the family Picornaviridae. It has been isolated from the stool of acutely ill patients by Feinstone *et al.* (1973). Electron microscopic observations with positive staining of the particles showed that many have a dense core that is presumably composed of nucleoprotein (Fig. 7–1). This picornavirus localizes primarily in the cytoplasm of the liver, where it multiplies easily. Unlike

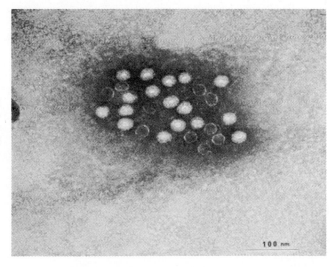

Figure 7–1. Electron micrograph of HAV particles extracted from HAV-infected marmoset liver showing electron-dense cores (× 328,600). (From Braude, A. I.: Medical Microbiology and Infectious Diseases. Philadelphia, W. B. Saunders Company, 1981, p. 628.)

Markers in HAV Infection

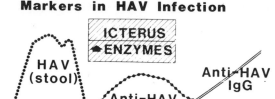

Figure 7–2. Markers in acute HAV infection. (From Pittiglio, D. H. [Ed.]: Modern Blood Banking and Transfusion Practices. Philadelphia, F. A. Davis Co., 1983, p. 388.)

hepatitis B virus, it does not produce a coat protein (see later discussion) and is not detectable in serum. It is stable in ether and to a pH of 3.0. HAV has been classified as an enterovirus (thus becoming enterovirus 72) but continues to be known as hepatitis A virus (Melnick, 1982). Three major polypeptides are associated with the RNA.

Dienhardt *et al.* (1967) attempted to transmit the virus to marmosets (small monkeys found in the tropical forests of the Americas). These studies eventually led to the isolation of strain CR326 of HAV through serial passage in marmosets. HAV has also been purified from human and chimpanzee stool extracts, from infected marmoset and chimpanzee livers, and from bile of infected chimpanzees (Deinstag *et al.*, 1975). In 1987, Provost *et al.* isolated the hepatitis A virus in cell culture directly from human specimens.

Antibodies to HAV (Immunity)

At the onset of clinically apparent hepatitis A, antibodies to HAV appear in the plasma. Initially, the antibody is IgM (anti-HAV IgM), which is subsequently replaced by IgG that persists for years, probably for life (Fig. 7–2). This antibody will aggregate highly purified HAV (Fig. 7–3).

At the present time, there is no vaccine for hepatitis A infection. Passive protection with immune gamma globulin, however, appears to both prevent and ameliorate the disease.

Serologic Tests for HAV

Until quite recently, hepatitis A infection was diagnosed after hepatitis B infection had been ruled

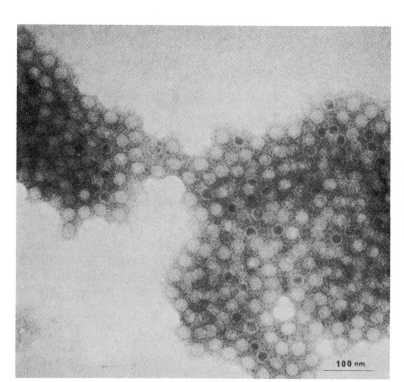

Figure 7–3. Highly purified HAV from preacute phase chimpanzee stool aggregated by anti-HAV (× 256,300). (From Braude, A. I.: Medical Microbiology and Infectious Diseases. Philadelphia, W. B. Saunders Company, 1981, p. 629.)

out by appropriate laboratory tests—therefore by assumption. The recognition that non-A, non-B hepatitis is more common than originally thought, however, has made this assumption less reliable. The HAV antigen (HAAg) has been identified in feces (and occasionally in serum) by rather complex electron microscopic and radioimmunoassay methods—tests that are not readily adapted to the clinical laboratory. Recently, serologic tests have been devised that use antigen extracts from infected marmoset livers or infected human feces. These include a complement fixation test (modified) and an immune adherence hemagglutination assay (IAHA), both of which have been used to demonstrate antibody titer responses to hepatitis A by comparing sera that are obtained two or three weeks apart. The IAHA is based on the principle that human red cells of group O are aggregated in the specific antigen-antibody-complement reaction (Miller, 1975).

Tests for the detection of HAV are not used in the clinical laboratory and are included here only for historical interest. The laboratory diagnosis of hepatitis A is now performed using RIA and ELISA techniques to detect the presence of specific HAV antibodies in the patient's serum (see later discussion).

HEPATITIS B

Formerly known as serum hepatitis and post-transfusion hepatitis, hepatitis B commonly follows parenteral exposure to an infected individual, although other modes of transmission are known to occur (see later discussion). The incubation period is 4 to 26 weeks (i.e., 1 to 6 months). In western Europe and North America, cases of hepatitis B usually appear singly, whereas in Asia, large segments of the population have been found to be infected. In some cases, infection even seems to be acquired. An important advance in the control of the spread of hepatitis B resulted from the discovery, in serum, of an antigen associated with the disease. This antigen was first recognized in the serum of an Australian aborigine and was given the provisional name *Australia antigen*. At first, the antigen appeared to be associated with acute leukemia (Blumberg *et al.*, 1965), yet it was not long before this was realized

not to be, and the association with hepatitis was confirmed (Prince, 1968; Blumberg *et al.*, 1968). Australia antigen is now known to be unassembled viral coat (see later discussion) or "surface" antigen and is termed *HBsAg*.

Hepatitis B Virus (HBV)

HBV is a hepatotropic virus that is microbiologically unrelated to HAV. It is a double-stranded DNA particle that exists in three forms:

1. A spherical (disc) particle, 22 nm in diameter
2. A filamentous form, 22 nm wide by 50 to 200 nm long
3. A Dane particle, 42 nm in diameter, which represents the virion, consisting of a 27-nm nucleocapsid DNA-containing core, surrounded by an outer lipoprotein coat (Figs. 7–4 and 7–5)

The predominant form seen in the blood of patients with hepatitis B is the spherical particle. The filamentous form is slightly less common, and the Dane particle is the least common. It was suggested that the larger particles represented the complete virion and that the other morphological forms were excess coat protein. This suggestion was given experimental foundation when the internal component of the Dane particle was released by treating the particles with 0.5 per cent Tween-80 (polysorbate) in phosphate-buffered saline (Almeida *et al.*, 1971). In addition, the filamentous forms could be converted to the spherical (disc) forms by exposure to mildly acidic buffers.

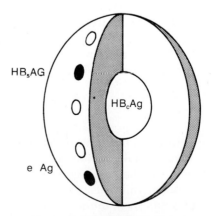

Figure 7–4. The Dane particle.

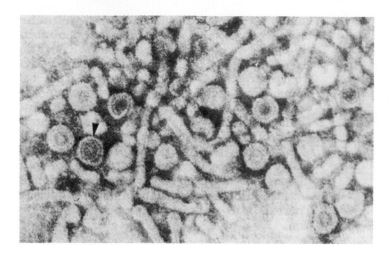

Figure 7–5. Electron micrograph of particulate Australia antigen (HBsAg) showing discs, filaments, and Dane particles (arrow) (× 250,000). (From Braude, A. I.: Medical Microbiology and Infectious Diseases. Philadelphia, W. B. Saunders Company, 1981, p. 630.)

Markers for Hepatitis B Virus

HBsAg. The outer lipoprotein coat (or envelope) of hepatitis B virus is known as *hepatitis B surface antigen (HBsAg)*. It is 22 nm in diameter and is found in the body fluids of patients with hepatitis B viral infection. It is produced in the cytoplasm of infected hepatocytes.

HBcAg. The core of the HBV is known as *hepatitis B core antigen (HBcAg)*. It is 27 nm in diameter and is located in the nuclei of hepatocytes in patients with HBV infection.

HBeAg. The *e antigen (HBeAg)* is also found in some HBsAg-positive sera either bound to immunoglobulins or free in solution. The antigen appears during acute infection and then usually disappears, but it can be carried chronically in patients with chronic hepatitis B antigenemia and chronic hepatitis. The exact nature of the e antigen is unknown. Three antigen subtypes, known as HBe_1Ag, HBe_2Ag, and HBe_3Ag, are recognized. The presence of e antigen appears to be associated with viral replication in the liver. The persistence of the antigen usually indicates chronic hepatitis and may be a marker for infectivity of HBsAg-positive blood.

Subtypes of HBsAg

HBsAg contains a common immunologic determinant, a, and several major subdeterminants that are specified by the viral genome (LeBouvier, 1971). The subdeterminants can be detected by the presence of spurs in immunodiffusion tests with various antisera. Eight distinct categories and two of the mixed subtype have been recognized (Table 7–2). In addition, several minor antigenic subtypes have been described.

The major subtypes consist of various combinations of the subdeterminants d/y and w/r, which appear to constitute two groups, composed of d/y on the one hand and w1, w2, w3, w4, and r on the other. The two mixed subtypes (adwr and adyr) are extremely rare and may be due to phenotypic or genotypic mixing of immunologic markers during simultaneous infection associated with more than one subtype of HBsAg. Of the minor subtypes, g has been found with w2.

Antigenic subtypes ayw2 and ayw3 appear to be more common in Africa and the Middle East, whereas subdeterminant r appears to predominate in the Far East and is very common in Japan. The antigenic subtype adw2 is common in the United States.

TABLE 7–2. Major and Minor Subtypes of Hepatitis B Surface Antigen	
Major Subtypes	**Minor Subtypes**
ayw1	q
ayw2	x
ayw3	f
ayw4	t
ayr	j
adw2	n
adw4	g
adr	
adwy	
adyr	

HBsAg of adw and ayw subtypes appears to differ in both biophysical and biochemical characteristics.

Subtype-specific antibodies are determined by studying inhibition of the antibody reactions with different known HBsAg subtypes in the same passive hemagglutination or radio immunoassay techniques used in anti-HBs detection (see later discussion).

Antibodies to HBAg

Subsequent to infection with HBV, antibodies to HBcAg (anti-HBc) usually appear (often at the same time that enzyme elevations are first seen). Antibody to the surface antigen (anti-HBs) usually appears later, sometimes being delayed by 6 to 12 months after the acute episode and often coinciding with the disappearance of circulating HBsAg.

Both human and animal studies indicate that anti-HBc tends to decrease gradually and may become undetectable after 1 or 2 years, although high titers are found in carriers. During the recovery phase of acute hepatitis B, anti-HBc may be present in the absence of HBsAg and anti-HBs, and donations of blood taken at this time can cause post-transfusion hepatitis (Hoofnagle *et al.*, 1978). Anti-HBs lasts much longer and may persist throughout life. This antibody bestows immunity to further infection with HBV. As mentioned, HBeAg is present during the incubation period of acute hepatitis B, and anti-HBe develops either during recovery or with the onset of overt liver disease. The presence of the antibody is considered to be a good prognostic sign (Fig. 7–6).

Incidence of Hepatitis B

Hepatitis B has now assumed major public health importance in a number of situations, the incidence varying from one geographic area to another. Approximately 200,000 new cases of HBV infection occur annually in the United States. Approximately 150,000 patients remain anicteric, 10,000 require hospitalization, and 12,000 to 20,000 become chronic carriers (Tyrell, 1985). Eight to twelve per cent of adults are antibody-positive. The infection is primarily found among certain "high-risk" groups, such as health care workers (who are repeatedly exposed to blood or blood products), patients (and staff) in hemodialysis units, immunosuppressed patients, institutionalized groups (e.g., prisoners, military recruits), illicit drug users, homosexual males, and individuals from areas in which the virus is endemic (Table 7–3). In addition, 8 to 10 per cent of all cases of post-transfusion hepatitis in the United States in the late 1970s were due to hepatitis B virus (Alter *et al.*, 1978).

HBV infection varies from an unapparent or unrecognized course to a rapidly fatal, fulminant course. Many cases are probably asymptomatic and as such are mistaken for a mild influenza attack. For this reason, many individuals who have no history of hepatitis present with serologic evidence of prior exposure to HBV and HAV (Table 7–4).

Figure 7–6. Markers in acute HBV infection. (From Pittiglio, D. H. [Ed.]: Modern Blood Banking and Transfusion Practices. Philadelphia, F. A. Davis Co., 1983, p. 387.)

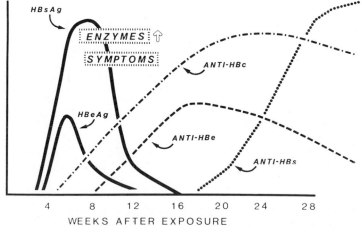

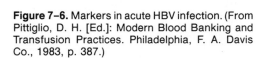

TABLE 7–3. Hepatitis Markers in High-Incidence Groups

Marker	Positive (%)		
	Southeast Asian Immigrants (483)*	Male Homosexuals (1077)*	Renal Dialysis Patients (163)*
Anti-HAV			—
IgG	90.2	35.6	
IgM	1.0	—	
HBsAg	20.3†	4.5	71.7‡
Anti-HBs and Anti-HBc	46.8	50.4	—
Anti-HBs	2.9	—	—
Anti-HBc	1.4	5.1	—
HAV and/or HBV	94.6	67.9	—

*Number tested
†50% HBeAg positive, 50% anti-HBe positive, and 100% anti-HBc positive
‡71.8% HBeAg positive and 100% anti-HBc positive
From Pittiglio, D. H. (Ed.): Modern Blood Banking and Transfusion Practices. Philadelphia, F. A. Davis Co., 1983, p. 389.

Transmission of Hepatitis B

Although parenteral infection is considered to be the most important mode of transmission of hepatitis B, infections can be acquired by casual contact with infected blood or serum, whereby inoculation may occur through often trivial or even unnoticed breaks in the skin or mucous membranes. The minimum infective dose of plasma from a carrier was estimated to be 1×10^{-6} ml (Murray, 1955). Drake *et al.* (1952) found that 4×10^{-5} ml of plasma given by subcutaneous injection could transmit the disease.

Apart from the transfusion of blood or blood products, which still appears to be the most dangerous source of infection, recognized modes of transmission of hepatitis B include the use of common needles and syringes among drug addicts, failure to sterilize dental equipment and tattooing needles, the sharing of razors and toothbrushes, and sexual contact (particularly among male homosexuals). Arthropod spread (mosquitos, bedbugs) is suspected in some tropical areas, although this, like fecal-oral routes, remains uncertain.

Susceptibility to the disease is not confined to any age group; maternal transmission to the fetus or newborn has been reported and often leads to chronic infection of the infant.

The many different modes of transmission of

TABLE 7–4. Viral Hepatitis Markers in Blood Donors With and Without a History of Prior Exposure

	Percentage Positive for One or Several Markers				
	HBsAg	Anti-HBc	Anti-HBc/HBs	Anti-HBc/HBs/HAV	Anti-HAV
Random donors (529)*	0	0.2	4.0	3.5	19.1
Health care personnel (donors) (569)	0	0.002	4.3	0.005	7.7
Donors rejected for hepatitis history (203)	0	0	5.1	1.0	27.6

*Number tested
From Pittiglio, D. H. (Ed.): Modern Blood Banking and Transfusion Practices. Philadelphia, F. A. Davis Co., 1983, p. 390.

hepatitis B are almost certainly due to the fact that almost all body secretions (e.g., saliva, semen, urine, sweat, colostrum) have been shown to contain the viral surface antigen.

Clinical signs and Symptoms of Hepatitis B

Individuals exposed to HBV through accidental needle puncture or transfusion do not usually show the expected initial symptoms (weakness, fatigue, nausea, and jaundice) until about 10 to 16 weeks after exposure. In some individuals, however, pain in the joints and/or rash or urticaria may occur several weeks before the illness is recognized as hepatitis.

The acute phase of the illness is also of variable length but in most cases has a duration of only a few weeks. The vast majority of individuals who develop acute hepatitis recover completely and develop immunity. About 10 per cent, however, do not develop immunity and may become chronic carriers or develop chronic active or chronic persistent hepatitis. The reason that this small minority become carriers is not known, although it may be associated with their immunologic status at the time of exposure. (Note: the clinical signs and symptoms of HAV infection are almost identical to those seen in acute HBV disease.)

Protection Against HBV by Antibody

The administration of immunoglobulin prepared from subjects with relatively potent anti-HBs was found to reduce the risk of hepatitis in individuals accidentally exposed to HBV (Grady and Lee, 1975), whether through inoculation, oral ingestion, or when blood or blood products are splashed onto mucous membranes. In these cases, hepatitis B immunoglobulin with a high titer of anti-HBs should be given in a dose of approximately 5 ml (for adults) as soon as possible after exposure (WHO, 1977).

Standard immunoglobulin is usually of little value in prophylaxis due to a low titer of anti-HBs (Seeff et al., 1977).

HBV Vaccine

The clinical value of a vaccine against HBV infection was demonstrated by Szmuness et al. (1980). The vaccine used was prepared from the plasma of chronic carriers of HBsAg; 20-nm spherical particles were purified from the plasma and then treated with formalin to kill any residual live virus. This material was shown to produce anti-HBs in 96 per cent of vaccinated individuals after two injections given one month apart. In a high-risk population (e.g., male homosexuals), the incidence of both clinical and subclinical HBV infection was significantly less in the vaccinated group (1.4 to 3.4 per cent) than in the control group (18 to 27 per cent). The side effects from the vaccine are minimal, and the vaccine is probably effective in preventing infection even after exposure to HBV. It should be noted that the vaccine is not intended for use in transfusion practice, because most cases of post-transfusion hepatitis are caused by non-A, non-B virus.

The licensing of the HBV vaccine was announced by the U.S. Food and Drug Administration (FDA) in 1981, and the Journal of the American Medical Association (June 1984) stated that the vaccine is safe and recommended for health care personnel worldwide.

Recent work by researchers at Merck, Sharpe and Dohme Research Laboratories, West Point, Pennsylvania (reported in the American Association of Blood Banks News Briefs, July 1984), has resulted in the development of a version of the vaccine made by a recombinant strain of the yeast *Saccharomyces cerevisiae*. This preparation was found to have positive effects on human volunteers. Thirty-seven healthy, low-risk adults were tested, each receiving 10 μg of HBsAg at 0, 1, and 6 months. Antibody to HBsAg was found to be present in 27 to 40 per cent of the vaccinees by 1 month and in 80 to 100 per cent by 3 months. Following the third dose at 6 months, large boosts of titer were noted. The formed antibody was found to be specific for the a determinant of HBsAg. There were no serious reactions to the vaccination—the only common complaint being transient soreness at the site of injection. The researchers pointed out that this may be the first use in humans of a vaccine prepared by recombinant DNA technology.

The three-dose program is believed to offer immunity for about 5 years, when a booster dose would become necessary. The fear of contracting acquired immunodeficiency syndrome (AIDS; see Chapter 13) from these inoculations has been shown to be groundless according to James Maynard, M.D., Ph.D., chief of the Hepatitis Branch of the Centers for Disease Control and director of the World Health Organization Collaborating Center for Reference and Research on Viral Hepatitis.

Many new types of vaccines are currently under investigation, including those made with yeast using a synthetic protein and other recombinant DNA techniques.

NON-A, NON-B HEPATITIS

Until recently, viral hepatitis that could not be associated with hepatitis B, cytomegalovirus, or Epstein-Barr virus infection was presumed to be due to hepatitis A. The development of specific diagnostic methods for all these other agents has shown this to be an erroneous assumption. Because it could be proved that in some cases hepatitis was not caused by HAV or HBV, the rather clumsy term *non-A, non-B hepatitis* was suggested. It is now known that the hepatitis C virus (HCV) is the major cause of NANB hepatitis. The HCV nomenclature refers to blood-borne virus. Water-borne NANBV is referred to as Type E, although the general term NANB has perisisted.

Incidence of Non-A, Non-B Hepatitis

In the United States, between 89 and 100 per cent of cases of post-transfusion hepatitis may be related to NANB hepatitis.

Anicteric cases of post-transfusion hepatitis are more common than icteric cases. For example, Seeff *et al.* (1977) reported a study in the United States in which 2,204 patients were followed and in which post-transfusion hepatitis was diagnosed in 241 patients. The disease was found to be icteric in less than one fifth of these patients. In 14 prospective studies reviewed by Blum and Vyas (1982), the overall frequency of hepatitis in patients receiving blood tested as HBsAg negative (from volunteer donors) varied from 4 to 13 per cent.

The incidence of non-A, non-B hepatitis in patients who have received blood transfusions is di-

rectly related to the level of alanine aminotransferase (ALT) in the relevant blood donors (Aach *et al.*, 1981). Although non-A, non-B hepatitis does develop in some patients who have received blood only from donors with normal ALT levels, it can be deduced that at least 21 per cent of cases of transfusion-associated hepatitis might be prevented by excluding donors with ALT levels above 44 IU (Holland *et al.*, 1981).

Non-A, non-B hepatitis is seen in populations of low socioeconomic status and is associated with a chronic carrier state (Alter, 1980). The minimum carrier rate in volunteer donors in the United States has been estimated to be 1.6 per cent, and, in commercial (paid) donors, it has been estimated to be 5.4 per cent (Blum and Vyas, 1982).

Although non-A, non-B hepatitis is usually associated with transfusion, sporadic cases have also been documented without known exposure to blood or blood products (i.e., due to water-borne [type E] virus).

Transmission of Non-A, Non-B Hepatitis

The mode of transmission of non-A, non-B hepatitis is sometimes similar to that of hepatitis B. Although its association with transfusion is clear, its prevalence among populations of low socioeconomic status suggests transmission by close person-to-person contact.

Experimental transmission of non-A, non-B hepatitis has shown that it can be transmitted from human to human and from human to chimpanzee (Tabor *et al.*, 1978).

Clinical Signs and Symptoms of Non-A, Non-B Hepatitis

The majority of patients with non-A, non-B hepatitis have minimal clinical manifestations, and few patients require hospitalization. The incubation period varies from 6 to 10 weeks, with a peak of about 8 weeks (Alter, 1980). Up to 60 per cent of cases reveal abnormal ALT levels for more than a year; if a liver biopsy is taken, most cases show histologic evidence of a significant chronic liver disease, and about 10 per cent show features of cirrhosis (Alter, 1980). The tendency for serum hepatic enzyme levels to fluctuate markedly over a relatively short period of time is a striking feature of non-A, non-B hepatitis. Although the disease differs in many respects from hepatitis B, there is considerable overlap, and the two forms cannot be differentiated on clinical grounds alone.

Serologic Tests

A variety of test systems have been described with respect to non-A, non-B hepatitis, yet none has been universally accepted as a marker of the infection. The diagnosis of non-A, non-B hepatitis has classically been made by ruling out other known causes of hepatitis by appropriate serologic tests. Surrogate testing for detecting blood-borne NANBV (HCV) in donated blood has been suggested (Anonymous, 1988). This test uses an indirect method of screening for NANBV by measuring first for increased levels of ALT and second for antibody to HBcAg (Anti-HBc). This method, however, will detect only about 50 per cent of NANB-contaminated donor blood. Currently, both radioimmunoassay and enzyme immunoassay are commercially available for the detection of anti-HBc. In each case, the method is based on an inhibition technique in which the solid-phase capture reagent consists of immobilized HBc antigen (prepared by recombinant DNA techniques) and the labeled probe is a standardized anti-HBc. The test sample competes with the labeled probe for antigen sites on the solid-phase reagent; consequently, the presence of anti-HBc in the test sample generates a low signal value, whereas its absence results in a high signal value. The test is open to the possibility of error because it requires careful and consistent attention to pipetting, washing, and other technical procedures. It has also been shown that there is not a clear differentiation between positive and negative donor populations (Kline *et al.*, 1987) and that the test may generate nonreproducible or false-positive results, particularly around the test cutoff (Dodd, 1987).

In 1986, however, blood-collecting agencies decided to implement anti-HBc testing in routine blood donor screening (Zuck *et al.*, 1987). The use of both anti-HBc and ALT tests has been associated with significant decreases in the reported incidence of transfusion-associated NANB hepatitis (Dodd, 1989). At least some of this decrease appears to be attributable to the testing itself; therefore anti-HBc appears to be an independent indicator of infectivity for HBV, albeit of low order (Dodd, 1991).

DELTA HEPATITIS

Delta hepatitis, caused by the hepatitis delta virus (HDV), has been shown to occur worldwide. Populations that are at high risk with respect to HBsAg are also at risk for HDV infections. These include intravenous drug users, recipients of blood products, male homosexuals, and mentally retarded individuals (Bonino *et al.*, 1987; Govindarajan, 1988).

Hepatitis Delta Virus

The hepatitis delta virus (HDV) was first described by Rizzetto *et al.*, (1987). This single-stranded RNA virus (also known as the delta antigen) is spherical in shape with a diameter of 36 nm (Bonino *et al.*, 1987). It is a defective hepatotropic virus in that it requires obligatory helper functions from HBV in order to ensure its replication and infectivity. HBV, for example, provides HDV with a protein coat of HBsAg, which allows it to function as an infectious agent (Govindarajan, 1988).

Antibodies to HDV

The HDV antigen is the first marker to appear in HDV infection, but it is transient in serum (1 to 4 days) and appears prior to symptomatology and elevation of liver enzymes. With the decline of HDV-Ag, IgM antibodies to HDV appear (seroconversion), followed by low levels of IgG antibodies in acute infection. The progression to high levels of IgG anti-HDV in HBsAg-positive individuals indicates the switch to chronic HDV infection.

Transmission of HDV

The transmission of HDV is linked to that of its HBV-helper virus and occurs by parenteral and transmucosal routes. Horizontal transmission occurs in households, and infections increase in non-hygienic, crowded living conditions. In epidemics, mosquitos have been shown to be a vehicle for transmission of HDV (Govindarajan, 1988).

Clinical Signs and Symptoms

HDV infection occurs as either acute or chronic in conjunction with concomitant HBV infection. The acute infection can occur in one of two forms:

1. Coinfection with acute HBV infection. In these cases either both viruses are cleared rapidly or the patient progresses to fulminant hepatitis. There is a higher incidence of fulminant hepatitis and cases of relapse with HDV-HBV coinfection than when HBV is present alone.
2. Superinfection of a chronic HBV infection, in which more than 90 per cent of cases progress to chronic HDV infection.

Chronic HDV infection has a poor prognosis for the patient. Liver necrosis, inflammation, and clinical illness are increased in their severity, and cirrhosis often occurs.

Treatment of Delta Hepatitis

There are no effective antiviral drugs or immunosuppressive agents for treatment of chronic HDV infections. Vaccination against HBV also provides immunity of HDV because HDV is not infectious and cannot replicate without HBV-helper functions.

THE SEROLOGIC DETECTION OF HEPATITIS MARKERS

Serologic Detection of Anti-HAV

The serologic tests that have been described to identify anti-HAV include complement fixation, immune adherence hemagglutination, radioimmunoassay, and ELISA. Of these, only radioimmunoassay is available commercially, and it is the most commonly used technique for this purpose.

The radioimmunoassay test for anti-HAV uses a solid phase (bead) that is coated with an anti-HAV–HAV complex. The bead is incubated with a mixture of the patient's serum and ^{125}I-labeled anti-HAV. The anti-HAV in the patient's serum competes with the known labeled antibody for the available binding sites, resulting in a decrease in counts per minute (cpm). A 50 per cent or greater reduction in the counts when compared with the negative control cpm indicates that the unknown contains anti-HAV.

One of several methods available to identify IgM–anti-HAV involves the use of staphylococcal protein A (Newman DC or Cowen strain) to absorb IgG from diluted serum prior to testing. Other methods, including column chromatography and labeled anti-IgM, have also been used. The radioimmunoassay technique for detecting IgM–anti-HAV involves the incubation of the patient's serum with an anti-IgM–coated solid phase. Purified HAV particles are added to the bound IgM fraction of the patient's serum. These will bind to IgM having anti-HAV specificity. ^{125}I-labeled anti-HAV is added after incubation and washing (to remove unbound protein), and an increase in cpm of the test when compared with the negative control indicates the presence of IgM–anti-HAV in the test sample.

Serologic Detection of HBsAg

The serologic tests used for the detection of HBsAg include:

1. Ouchterlony double diffusion (agar gel diffusion)
2. Counterelectrophoresis
3. Rheophoresis
4. Complement fixation
5. Reversed passive latex agglutination
6. Reversed passive hemagglutination
7. Radioimmunoassay
8. Enzyme-linked immunosorbent assay (ELISA)

These tests may be grouped into first generation, second generation, and third generation, according to sensitivity—third generation being the most sensitive and therefore preferred in most clinical situations. In this connection, Ouchterlony double diffusion (agar gel diffusion) is regarded as a first-generation test; radioimmunoassay, reversed passive hemagglutination, enzyme-linked immunosorbent assay (ELISA), and reversed passive latex agglutination are regarded as third-generation tests; and the remainder, counterelectrophoresis, rheophoresis, and complement fixation, are regarded as second-generation tests (Table 7–5).

TABLE 7–5. Tests Available for HBsAG Detection
Third generation
Radioimmunoassay
Reversed passive hemagglutination
Enzyme-linked immunosorbent assay (ELISA)
Reversed passive latex agglutination
Second generation
Counterelectrophoresis
Rheophoresis
Complement fixation
First generation
Ouchterlony double diffusion (agar gel diffusion)

Sources of antisera for the detection of HBsAg are:

1. Human, including multiply-transfused patients, patients giving an anamnestic response following transfusions of blood and blood products, volunteers stimulated with noninfectious HBsAg-positive material, and sporadic sources (i.e., not associated with blood or blood sources)
2. Animals hyperimmunized with purified HBsAg
3. Laboratory animals (guinea pigs, rabbits, mice, monkeys, chimpanzees)
4. Domestic animals (horses, sheep, goats)

It should be noted that although HBsAg has been found to be present for as long as a year in the serum of carriers, it has also been reported that most patients with clinical or serum enzyme patterns consistent with a diagnosis of serum hepatitis do not retain HBsAg for more than three months after the acute phase of the disease.

PRACTICAL CONSIDERATIONS IN HEPATITIS TESTING

In practice, tests for HBV and HBsAg are performed to:

1. Identify blood donors who are infected with HBV and who might, therefore, transmit the infection to recipients of transfusion.
2. Establish the etiology of clinical cases of hepatitis.

To this end, any method that optimally demonstrates the presence of HBsAg in serum or plasma is satisfactory. Third-generation tests, naturally, are the methods of choice for both of these applications.

In cases of clinical hepatitis in which HBsAg is *not* detected, sensitive methods for the detection of anti-HBs or anti-HBc (see later discussion) are useful, although tests for anti-HBc may be of limited usefulness in many situations (see Serologic Detection of HBcAg and Anti-HBc, later in this chapter). Anti-HBs detection by less sensitive methods is useful in identifying donors whose plasma contains high anti-HBs titer and is therefore suitable for the production of HBIG (hepatitis B immune globulin) and potent antisera for *in vitro* diagnostic methods. When evaluating the safety and effectiveness of passive and active immunization with experimental HBIG preparations and vaccines, however, third-generation methods are preferable.

Suggested Rules for Practical Testing

In testing for hepatitis B surface antigen and antibody (and all other hepatitis-related viruses, antigens, and/or antibodies), extreme caution should be exercised by the technologist to guard against the spread of infection. To this end, the following rules should be followed when handling any biologic specimens known to contain or suspected of containing the viruses.

General Rules

1. Smoking, eating, and drinking should not be permitted in laboratory areas. Food must not be stored in the same refrigerator as blood or blood products.
2. The technologist should avoid all contact between the fingers and the mouth, including the licking of labels, pencils, and so on.
3. Mouth pipetting should be expressly forbidden.
4. Technologists must wash in a hand basin (not a laboratory sink) after handling a specimen. A strong antiseptic solution should be used for this purpose (e.g., povidone-iodine [Betadine Poviodine]).
5. In each laboratory, a safety officer should be appointed to supervise work and to educate staff.

Clothing

1. A plastic apron should be worn in the laboratory, and it should be cleaned with weak hypochlorite and then water after each use.
2. Plastic gloves should be worn, and these should be discarded into a plastic bag and incinerated after use. Gloves should be changed every 2 hours.
3. A clean gown that can be autoclaved after use should be worn.
4. If there is danger of production of an aerosol (e.g., in shaking and gassing of samples), safety spectacles or a visor should be worn.
5. Opening of specimens and all pipetting should be performed in a fume hood.
6. The hands should be washed well with povidone-iodine after gloves are removed.

Work Areas

1. Before and after each use, work benches must be cleaned with strong hypochlorite solution (10,000 ppm available chlorine).
2. A freshly prepared bottle of prepared hypochlorite, a disposal jar with hypochlorite swabs, and a plastic disposable bag should be on hand at all times for wiping up spills.
3. The hypochlorite solution should be checked several times a day with starch iodine paper (paper turns blue if solution is active).
4. All paper work should be done in a separate, clean area.

Specimens

1. Specimens from patients suspected of having serum hepatitis should arrive at the laboratory in a plastic bag with proper identification as "high-risk" specimens attached to the outside of the bag.
2. Any leaking specimen should be discarded unopened.
3. Open the container *carefully* after covering the cork with gauze squares.
4. Pipetting should be done with a rubber teat or other device, and the sample should be expelled *gently* down the wall of the receiving vessel.
5. Pipettes should be completely immersed in hypochlorite immediately after use and then autoclaved before washing.
6. If it is necessary to centrifuge the specimen, do so in a tightly capped tube. If the tube breaks in the centrifuge, any removable contaminated parts should be autoclaved or immersed in 2 per cent activated glutaraldehyde (Cidex), and the rest of the centrifuge should be swabbed with Cidex and left for 1 hour. (Note: hypochlorite corrodes centrifuges.)

Accidents

1. If the eyes or mouth is contaminated, wash the area well with tap water.
2. Pricks or cuts incurred while processing specimens or pre-existing skin lesions that become contaminated with samples for examination should be washed at once with hypochlorite solution, followed by rinsing with water. Any such accidents should be recorded and reported.

SEROLOGIC TEST METHODS

Not all of the test procedures presented here are performed in the modern clinical laboratory. Some are included for historical interest, others for the sake of completeness. The choice of which tests to perform in the routine laboratory is a matter of user preference and choice.

Ouchterlony Double Diffusion (Agar Gel Diffusion)

Ouchterlony double diffusion (or agar gel diffusion) was the first method used in establishing the relationship of HBsAg to type B hepatitis. The technique has the following advantages:

1. It demonstrates specificity by the formation of lines of identity between HBsAg in test samples and in positive control sera.
2. It distinguishes the subtypes of HBsAg by lines of partial identity or spur formation.
3. It is the simplest method available for HBsAg (and anti-HBs) detection in that no special equipment is required.
4. A number of different well configurations and

agar and buffer combinations have given satisfactory results.

The disadvantages of the technique are:

1. It is less sensitive than other techniques.
2. It requires 24 to 72 hours for optimal results.
3. Optimal test conditions are somewhat dependent upon the antiserum used.

Ouchterlony double diffusion can provide a convenient method for the identification of very potent antisera because of its relative insensitivity.

METHOD 1: OUCHTERLONY DOUBLE DIFFUSION (AGAR GEL DIFFUSION)

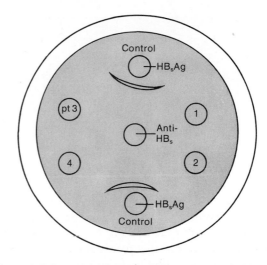

Figure 7–7. Ouchterlony double diffusion (agar gel diffusion).

Materials

1. Buffers—phosphate-buffered saline at pH 7.4. (Good results have also been reported with tris-EDTA or veronal. The pH of the buffer should be between 7.2 and 8.2.)
2. Gels—agarose. Different types of agar (Noble agar, ionagar, and agarose) can be used, but agarose gives the most reproducible results. Agarose concentrations between 0.6 and 2.0 per cent work well; 1.1 per cent is generally most convenient. Dilute in buffer (1).
3. Plates—3¼ × 4¼-inch lantern slides. (Microscope slides or Petri dishes work equally well.) The plates can be prepared and stored provided that they are precoated with a thin film of 2 per cent Noble agar, which is applied when the plates are warm and subsequently dried in a 50°C to 60°C chamber for 30 minutes. Prepunched plates are available from several commercial firms, but they are expensive, and freshness cannot be ensured.

Method

1. Pipette 15 ml of a 1.1 per cent agarose solution onto a lantern slide, giving a gel of about 1.5-mm thickness.
2. After the gel has hardened, punch a 7-hole pattern on the agarose-coated plate with a metal punch. Wells 2 to 3 mm in diameter and from 3 to 4 mm apart give satisfactory results, although

they can be as large as 5 mm in diameter and 6 to 7 mm apart.
3. The wells are filled with a Pasteur (or capillary) pipette; a separate pipette is used for each serum sample. Serum known to contain HBsAg is placed in the upper and lower wells. Anti-HBs is placed in the central well; this allows for the observation of lines of identity or nonidentity between the control precipitins produced by sera under test, which are placed in the four adjacent wells (Fig. 7–7).
4. Incubate the slide in a moist chamber for 24 to 72 hours.

Interpretation

Ideally, plates should be read in a darkened room. The appearance of a white precipitation line (read against a dark background) indicates the presence of HBsAg.

Counterelectrophoresis

The technique of counterelectrophoresis (CEP) is based on the fact that HBsAg and its antibody, anti-HBs, have differing electrophoretic mobilities in an electrical field. Thus, a slide covered with a thin layer of agarose containing a series of punched *opposing* wells, when placed in an electrical field with

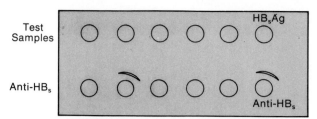

Figure 7–8. Counterelectrophoresis.

antigen and antibody properly oriented in opposite wells, allows the fast migration of antibody and antigen *toward* each other and results in a visible precipitate between the wells where the antigen and antibody meet (Fig. 7–8).

The advantages of this technique in comparison with Ouchterlony double diffusion are twofold:

1. It is possible to obtain a positive reaction in 30 to 90 minutes with CEP, as opposed to 24 to 72 hours with Ouchterlony double diffusion.
2. The reagents are moving in one direction rather than diffusing radially from the wells, so there is a greater degree of sensitivity.

METHOD 2: COUNTERELECTROPHORESIS

Note: A number of CEP reagents and kits are available from commercial sources. For more information, see Alter *et al.,* 1971; Das *et al.,* 1971; Dreesman *et al.,* 1972; and Gocke and Howe, 1970.

Materials

Many variations of this technique exist with respect to reagents, concentrations, and so on. All of the many variations have been reported to give satisfactory results.
1. Buffer—barbital buffer (0.05 M, pH 8.6)
2. Gels—17 ml of agarose (1 per cent concentration) diluted in buffer (1)
3. Plates—3¼ × 4-inch lantern slides

Method

1. Pipette 16 ml of 1 per cent agarose solution onto 3¼ × 4-inch slides to give a gel of uniform thickness.

2. After the agar has cooled and hardened, cut two parallel rows of 15 wells, 3 mm in diameter and 7 mm apart, edge to edge, in the agar with a metal punch.
3. Fill the wells in one row with the sera under test; fill the other set of wells with anti-HBs of adequate potency to form a precipitin reaction in agar gel diffusion (see Fig. 7–8).
4. Connect the slides to the barbital buffer in an electrophoresis cell by wicks of chromatographic paper, with the wells containing anti-HBs proximal to the anode and the wells containing test sera proximal to the cathode.
5. Electrophoresis is carried out for 2 hours at 15 mA constant current per slide.
6. An HBsAg-positive control serum should be included on each slide.

Interpretation

Slides may be examined for immunoprecipitin reaction 1 to 24 hours after completion of electrophoresis. The presence of a white precipitation line (read against a dark background) indicates the presence of HBsAg.

Rheophoresis

The technique known as *rheophoresis* uses the same principle as Ouchterlony double diffusion. In this technique, however, samples containing HBsAg are forced to migrate towards the anti-HBs by evaporation (Fig. 7–9).

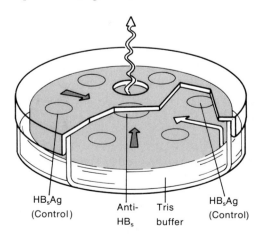

Figure 7–9. Rheophoresis.

Comparison tests with Ouchterlony double diffusion, counterelectrophoresis, and complement fixation performed by Jambazian and Holper (1972) indicate that rheophoresis has sensitivity similar to that of counterelectrophoresis and complement fixation and is more sensitive than the Ouchterlony double-diffusion technique. In addition, rheophoresis was found to be particularly convenient for determining HBsAg subtypes with appropriate subtype-specific antisera.

METHOD 3: RHEOPHORESIS

See Jambazian and Holper, 1972.

Materials

1. Buffer—0.01 M tris buffer, pH 7.6
2. Gel—1.25 ml 0.8 per cent agarose
3. Plate—Ouchterlony double-diffusion dish (a molded plastic cup, 3 cm in diameter and approximately 6 mm deep, will serve the purpose)

Method

1. Fit a gel diffusion dish with a cylindrical Teflon ring (3 cm outside diameter, 2.5 cm inside diameter, and 0.55 cm in length).
2. Pour melted agarose (1.25 ml, 0.8 per cent, pH 7.6) into the dish, and allow it to solidify.
3. Cut a pattern of six peripheral wells (5 mm in diameter) and a central well (3 mm in diameter) in the agar with a center-to-center distance of 7 mm (Fig. 7–9).
4. Carefully remove the Teflon ring, leaving a circular moat around the periphery of the dish.
5. Fill the moat with 0.01 M tris buffer, pH 7.6.
6. Fill two opposing peripheral wells with serum containing HBsAg to serve as a control. Fill the remaining peripheral wells with test samples.
7. Fill the central well with anti-HBs.
8. One minute after adding anti-HBs, cover the central well with a 3-mm plastic cover to prevent evaporation.
9. Place a 3-cm² plastic cover with a central hole (0.8 cm in diameter) over the entire plate with the center of the plastic cover located directly over the antibody well.
10. Incubate the plate at 37°C, and read after 8 to 16 hours' incubation (16 to 24 hours if incubation is at 28°C to 32°C).

Interpretation

The presence of a white precipitate line (read against a dark background) indicates the presence of HBsAg.

Complement Fixation

Complement-fixation techniques are, in general, more sensitive than double diffusion or counterelectrophoresis for measuring HBsAg or anti-HBs but are less sensitive than hemagglutination or radioimmunoassay techniques for measuring anti-HBs. Both quantitative and qualitative complement-fixation tests can be completed within 2 hours; they involve simple, easily obtainable equipment; they are easy to perform with standardized reagents; and they can be automated. The major advantage of this test is that it allows for the detection of antibodies in the patient's serum by their complement-fixing properties.

The test has the following disadvantages:

1. The necessity for standardizing reagents
2. The need to test more than one dilution of serum, especially when testing for HBsAg, to avoid prozoning
3. The possibility of nonspecific anticomplementary reactions in certain sera.

All recognized subtypes of HBsAg can be detected by this technique with high-titer, multi-specific, complement-fixing antibody. It should be noted, however, that there are many examples of "hyperimmune" anti-HBs that do not fix complement, even though they are excellent precipitins.

The most common complement-fixation technique used in HBsAg and anti-HBs detection is the microtiter technique.

METHOD 4: THE MICROTITER COMPLEMENT-FIXATION TECHNIQUE

Note: The microtiter complement-fixation method described here is as described by Barker, *et al.* (1970), which is patterned after the technique originally described by Sever (1962).

Method

1. Heat serum for testing to 56°C for 30 minutes.
2. Prepare a series of twofold dilutions in veronal buffered saline supplemented with calcium and magnesium. Dilutions should start at 1:5, using microtiter plates.
3. Add 0.025 ml of complement, 1.7 to 2 µ, and 0.025 ml of antibody, 2 to 4 µ, to each dilution, and allow to incubate for 16 to 20 hours at 4°C. Note: In practice, overnight fixation at 4°C is commonly used, but short fixation at 37°C for 1 hour allows for completion of the test within 2 hours. Tests by Schmidt and Lennette (1971) revealed that although the shorter test tended to give slightly lower antigen titers, its sensitivity was comparable to that of the overnight test.
4. Add 0.025 ml of 1 per cent suspension of hemolysin-sensitized sheep red blood cells.
5. Incubate for 30 minutes at 35°C, shaking the plates to keep the cells in suspension.
6. Read microscopically.

Interpretation

The endpoint is the highest serum dilution at which 3- to 4-plus fixation of complement occurs.

Reversed Passive Latex Agglutination

The reversed passive latex agglutination test is the most rapid and the most simple first-generation test for HBsAg. The test is, in principle, the agglutination of latex particles coated with anti-HBs by HBsAg in test samples. Because false-positive results are frequently seen, confirmation of this reaction (and all other agglutination reactions) by another method of equal or greater sensitivity is essential.

METHOD 5: REVERSED PASSIVE LATEX AGGLUTINATION

Note: Goat polystyrene-latex particles with a gamma globulin fraction containing rabbit anti-HBs are obtainable from commercial sources. See Fritz and Rivers, 1972; Hirata *et al.,* 1973; Leach and Ruck, 1971; and Malin and Edwards, 1972.

Method

1. Using a small rod, mix one drop of serum under test with one drop of the latex suspension on a black plastic or glass slide.
2. Set up a control in parallel, using serum known to possess HBsAg.
3. Tilt the slide by hand or with an appropriate mechanical shaker for 5 minutes at room temperature.

Interpretation

Agglutination of the particles becomes apparent not later than 5 minutes after mixing when HBsAg is present in the serum under test.

Note: Perform a confirmatory test to guard against false-positives, if necessary.

Reversed Passive Hemagglutination

Agglutination of red cells coated with anti-HBs (reversed passive hemagglutination) provides a rapid, sensitive, and simple method for detecting HBsAg.

The same caution given for reversed passive latex agglutination applies here; because false-positive results are frequently seen, another method is essential before results are finally interpreted.

Reversed passive hemagglutination is based on the principle that antibody globulins are readily bound to the surface of red blood cells that have been treated with tannic acid. Highly purified antibody (from horse serum) is attached to tanned turkey erythrocytes to yield a "sensitized" cell suspension that will agglutinate the presence of HBsAg.

METHOD 6: REVERSED PASSIVE HEMAGGLUTINATION

See Chrystie *et al.*, 1974; Hopkins and Das, 1973; and Juji and Yokochi, 1969.

Materials

1. Test cells—1 per cent suspension of formalinized tanned turkey erythrocytes with purified horse anti-HBs dispersed in phosphate-buffered saline (pH 7.2, 0.15 M containing 5 per cent sucrose, 1.5 per cent normal rabbit serum, and 0.1 per cent sodium azide). This preparation is available from commercial sources.
2. Control cells—formalinized, tanned turkey erythrocytes coated with normal horse globulin.
3. Buffer—sterile 0.15 M phosphate-buffered saline, pH 7.2, containing normal horse serum, normal human serum, and 0.1 per cent sodium azide.

    These reagents can be stored at 4°C. Cells from commercial sources should be reconstituted 15 minutes before use with the manufacturer's recommended volume of sterile distilled water. Once reconstituted, the cells will keep for 1 day at 4°C.
4. Titration plates—U-bottom, disposable.

Method

1. Prepare two dilutions of each test serum by placing three drops of diluent in the first row of wells of a U-bottom, disposable titration plate and one drop in a second row of wells, using a disposable 0.025-ml dropper. Using a 0.025-ml microtiter loop, take up 0.025 ml of the patient's serum and mix with the diluent in the first well, giving a 1:4 dilution. Transfer the diluter to the second well, giving a 1:8 dilution. Rinse the diluter in strong bleach (Javex), and follow with two distilled water rinses. Repeat for each test serum.
2. Set up positive and negative controls using 1 ml of heat-inactivated, diluted HBsAg-positive

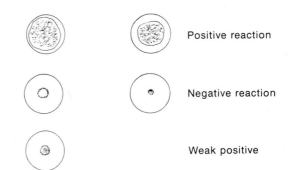

Figure 7–10. Interpretation of passive agglutination results.

human serum as a positive control and 1 ml of normal human serum as a negative control.
3. To each of the 1:8 dilutions, add one drop (0.025-ml dropper) of the test cells.
4. Mix the contents of the wells by gently shaking the plates. Cover with a plastic sealer, and allow to settle at room temperature.
5. Read after 30 to 60 minutes.

Interpretation

Positive Reaction

Cells may be partially or completely agglutinated to form a carpet at the bottom of the well (Fig. 7–10).

Negative Reaction

Cells fall to the base of the U and form a tight ring or button in the center of the well (Fig. 7–10).

Weak Positive Reaction

Incomplete agglutination with a central carpet of agglutinated cells surrounded by a definite ring pattern is seen. The ring is of larger diameter than that of a negative pattern and can usually be distinguished by its slightly crenelated edge (Fig. 7–10).

Note: Perform a confirmatory test to guard against false-positive reactions.

Radioimmunoassay

Radioimmunoassays are the most sensitive methods for the detection of HBsAg and anti-HBs.

The two most widely used techniques are the solid phase radioimmunoassay and the double-antibody or radioimmunoprecipitation (RIP) tests. The solid phase radioimmunoassay system for HBsAg detection uses the "sandwich" principle; test samples are added to plastic tubes or beads coated with anti-HBs. In the radioimmunoprecipitation technique for HBsAg, known quantities of anti-HBs and ^{125}I-labeled HBsAg are incubated with antibody against gamma globulin, and antigen-antibody complexes are precipitated.

Radioimmunoassay methods are more sensitive than hemagglutination methods and are much more sensitive than second-generation methods (e.g., counterelectrophoresis) for the detection of HBsAg and anti-HBs.

METHOD 7: RADIOIMMUNOASSAY

The technique described here is that intended for use with the Austria 11-125 kit provided by Abbott Laboratories, North Chicago, Illinois. See Aach *et al.,* 1971, 1973; Overby *et al.,* 1973.

Materials

The Kit Contains:

1. Beads—coated with HBsAg (guinea pig)
2. Vials (10 ml each) of anti-HBs ^{125}I (human)—approximately 7 μCi per vial; preservative—0.1 per cent sodium azide
3. Vial (5 ml) of negative control (nonreactive for HBsAg); preservative—0.1 per cent sodium azide
4. Vial (3 ml) of positive control (positive for HBsAg); preservative—0.1 per cent sodium azide
5. Four reaction trays—(20 wells each), 8 sealers, and 80 tube identification inserts
6. Counting tubes (8 cartons, 20 tubes each) properly positioned for transfer of beads from reaction trays

Additional Materials Needed (Not Provided with the Kit)

1. Precision pipettes or similar equivalent to deliver 0.2 ml

2. Device for delivery of rinse solution such as Cornwall syringe, Filamatic, or equivalent
3. An aspiration device for washing coated beads, such as a cannula or aspirator tip, and a vacuum source and trap for retaining the aspirate
4. A well-type gamma scintillation detector capable of efficiently counting ^{125}I
5. Gently circulating water bath, capable of maintaining temperature at 45°C ± 1°C
6. Austria confirmatory neutralization test kit (Note: all Austria 11-125 reactive samples must be confirmed with the test procedure provided with this kit)

Collection and Preparation of Samples

1. Only serum and recalcified plasmas can be tested. Collect blood specimens, and separate the serum from the sample. Plasma can be tested only after conversion to serum.
2. If specimens are to be stored, they should be refrigerated at 2°C to 8°C or frozen. If specimens are to be shipped, they should be frozen.

Procedure

Seven negative and three positive controls should be assayed with each run of unknowns. Ensure that reaction trays containing controls and reaction trays of unknowns are subjected to the same process and incubation times. Use a clean pipette or disposable tip for each transfer to avoid cross-contamination.

1. Adjust the temperature of the water bath to 45°C.
2. Remove the cap from the clear plastic tube that contains the antibody-coated beads. Hold the bead dispenser directly over the top of the reaction tray incubation well, and push down with the index finger to release one bead into a well for each sample to be tested.
3. Using precision pipettes, add 0.2 ml of serum and positive and negative controls to the bottom of their respective wells. Ensure that the antibody-coated bead is completely surrounded by serum. Tap the reaction tray to release any air bubbles that may be trapped in the serum sample.
4. Apply a cover sealer to each tray, and incubate the trays in the 45°C water bath for 2 hours.

5. At the end of 2 hours, remove the trays from the water bath. Remove the cover sealer and discard. Using a semiautomated aspiration and rinsing system, aspirate the serum; rinse each well and bead with a total of 5 ml of distilled or deionized water. Repeat this wash procedure one additional time. Note: A manual system of washing the wells and beads may also be used. Using disposable pipettes or cannulas and a Cornwall syringe delivery system, or equivalent, and a vacuum source, rinse each well and bead with extreme care not to overflow the reaction well but ensuring that the bead is totally immersed throughout the wash procedure. Place the pipette or cannula, attached to the vacuum source, into the bottom of the well next to the bead, and simultaneously add slowly, with a Cornwall syringe, 5 ml of distilled or deionized water.

6. With precision pipettes, add 0.2 ml of ^{125}I-labeled anti-HBs (human) to the bottom of each reaction well. Ensure that the antibody-coated bead is surrounded by the labeled antibody solution. Tap the tray to release any air bubbles that may be trapped in the solution.

7. Apply a new cover sealer to each tray, and incubate the trays in the 45°C water bath for 1 hour.

8. At the end of 1 hour, remove the trays from the water bath. Remove the cover sealer, aspirate the antibody solution from each well, and rinse the well and antibody-coated bead it contains with a total of 5 ml of distilled or deionized water, as in step 5.

9. Transfer the beads from the reaction wells to properly identified counting tubes; align the inverted rack of oriented counting tubes over the reaction tray, press the tubes tightly over the wells, and then invert the tray and tubes together so that the beads fall into the properly labeled tubes.

10. Place the counting tubes in a suitable well-type gamma scintillation counter, and determine the count rate. The position of the bead at the bottom of the counting tube is not important. Although it is not critical that the counting be done immediately, it should be performed as soon as practicable. All control samples and unknowns must be counted together.

Interpretation

The presence or absence of HBsAg is determined by relating net counts per minute of the unknown sample to net counts per minute of the negative control mean times the factor 2.1. Unknown samples whose net count rate is higher than the mean cutoff value established with the negative control are to be considered positive with respect to HBsAg.

The mean value for the positive control samples should be at least five times the negative control mean. If not, the technique may be suspect, and the run should be repeated.

Note: For gamma counters that do not automatically subtract machine backgrounds, the gross counts may be used if the cutoff value for the negative control is calculated as described below.

Calculation of the Negative Control Mean

An example of the calculation of the negative control mean is given in Table 7–6.

Elimination of Aberrant Values

Discard those individual values in the negative control samples that fall outside the range of 0.5 to 1.5 times the mean.

Example (from Table 7–6):

$$0.5 \times 386 = 193 \text{ and } 1.5 \times 386 + 579$$

$$\text{Range} = 193 \text{ cpm to } 579 \text{ cpm}$$

TABLE 7–6. An Example of the Calculation of the Negative Control Mean

Negative Control Sample Number	Net Count Rate Per Minute
1	380
2	400
3	410
4	375
5	350
6	390
7	400
	Total 2705

$$\frac{\text{Total net cpm}}{7} = \frac{2705}{7} = \text{net cpm (mean)}$$

Note: In this example, no negative control sample is rejected as aberrant. The negative control mean therefore need not be revised. Typically, all negative control values should fall within the range of 0.5 to 1.5 times the control mean. If more than one value is consistently found to be outside this range, technical problems should be suspected.

Calculation of the Cutoff Value (from Table 7–6)

1. Multiply the net negative control mean, 386 cpm, by the factor 2.1.
2. The calculated cutoff value is then 811 cpm.
3. Unknowns whose net count rate is higher than the cutoff value should be considered positive with respect to HBsAg.

Note: Many gamma counters have no capacity for automatically subtracting background. In this case, as an alternative to subtracting instrument background manually from each sample, uncorrected sample counts per minute can be compared with a cutoff modified as follows:

$$\text{(Negative control mean} - \text{background)} \times 2.1 + \text{background} = \text{cutoff}$$

Example (from Table 7–6):

Gross negative control mean = 436 cpm

Instrument background − 50 cpm

Cutoff = (436 − 50) × 2.1 + 50 = 861

Samples with gross count rates greater than 861 are to be considered reactive with respect to HBsAg.

Calculation of Positive Control to Negative Control Ratio (from Table 7–6)

1. Divide the positive control mean value by the native control mean value after correcting for background.

$$\frac{\text{Net positive control mean}}{\text{Net negative control mean}} = \text{P/N ratio}$$

2. This ratio should be at least 5; otherwise, the technique may be suspect, and the run should be repeated.

Using the figures in Table 7–6:

Net positive control mean value = 5906 cpm

Net negative control mean value = 386 cpm

P/N ratio = 5906 divided by 386 = 15.3

Technique is acceptable, and data may be considered valid.

Limitations of the Procedure

Nonrepeatable Positives

Some positive results may test nonreactive on repeat. This phenomenon is highly dependent upon the technique used in running the test. The most common sources of such nonrepeatable positives are:
1. Inadequate rinsing of the bead.
2. Cross-contamination of nonreactive samples caused by transfer of residual droplets of high-titer, antigen-containing sera on the pipetting device.

Nonspecific False Positives

The nonspecific false positives resulting from cross-reactions with guinea-pig serum are essentially eliminated by using ^{125}I-labeled anti-HBs of human origin; however, all sensitive immune systems have a potential for false positives, and before notifying a patient or donor that he or she may be a carrier of HBsAg, positive results must be confirmed as follows:
1. *Repeatability.* Further testing of the sample in question will verify whether it is repeatedly positive. In making an evaluation of data, consideration should be given to the actual test values obtained. The value 2.1 times the negative control mean is used as the cutoff for single determinations. This value has been selected in order to decrease the total number of nonrepeatable positives.
If repeat testing shows the sample to be less than 2.1 times the negative control mean, the original result may be classified as a nonrepeatable positive. If repeats are above the cutoff value, the sample should be presumed reactive for HBsAg. Such results are contingent on de-

termination of the specificity of the repeatable positive.

2. *Specificity.* Specificity analysis must be performed prior to informing a donor that he or she is an HBsAg carrier. A suitable method must be used for confirmation of screening procedure on all reactive specimens. A repeatable reactive specimen, confirmed by neutralization with human antiserum, must be considered HBsAg-positive.

Enzyme-Linked Immunoassay

The enzyme-linked immunosorbent assay (ELISA) technique is based on the same principle as the radioimmunoassay technique, but an enzyme label rather than a radiolabel is used as an indicator. In this technique, after incubation and washing to remove unbound label, a chromogenic substrate is added. Degradation of the substrate by bound enzyme produces a color change and an optical density increase that is proportional to the HBsAg concentration in the unknown sample.

Serologic Detection of Anti-HBs

Serologic testing for anti-HBs is usually not helpful in diagnosis because the antibody often appears weeks to months after antigenemia has subsided. Testing, however, is useful in determining past infection and possible immunity in individuals who may have been exposed to infection or who are likely to work in situations where exposure risks are high. In these cases, anti-HBs can be easily detected by passive hemagglutination of antigen-sensitized red blood cells or by radioimmunoassay.

Serologic Detection of HBcAg and Anti-HBc

Hepatitis B core antigen and antibody are detectable by several serologic procedures with varying degrees of sensitivity, notably complement fixation, counterelectrophoresis, immune adherence hemagglutination, and radioimmunoassay.

Serologic tests for anti-HBc have proved valuable for seroepidemiologic studies and diagnosis of HBV infection, whereas tests for HBcAg are seldom used in the diagnosis of type B hepatitis. Lack of availability of reagents for both HBcAg and anti-HBc has to some extent limited their use for anti-HBc to research laboratories.

HBcAg has been purified from the following sources:

1. The liver of immunosuppressed chimpanzees experimentally infected with HBV. The HBcAg in these cases is purified by differential centrifugation and isopyknic banding in cesium chloride.
2. Plasma of chronic carriers of HBcAg, which contains large numbers of Dane particles.

In the latter technique, the Dane particles are purified by isopyknic and rate zonal centrifugation procedures. The HBsAg is removed by treatment with a nonionic detergent. The free cores are then purified by isopyknic banding in cesium chloride. Two populations of cores have been detected by such means:

1. "Heavy" cores, with a density of about 1.37 gm per cubic centimeter and a high specific DNA polymerase activity. These cores serve as a source of antigen for radioimmunoprecipitation tests for anti-HBc.
2. "Light" cores, with a density of about 1.30 to 1.32 gm per cubic centimeter and deficient in DNA polymerase activity. These cores have been used successfully as a source of antigen for complement fixation and immune adherence hemagglutination tests for anti-HBc.

Of the tests available, complement fixation is probably the most widely used for anti-HBc detection; although it is insufficiently sensitive to diagnose many unapparent or subclinical infections, almost all patients with chronic infection (clinical or subclinical) have anti-HBc detectable by complement fixation. The source of antigen for complement fixation tests is chimpanzee liver. The test is performed in the same way as complement-fixation tests for anti-HBs (see earlier in this chapter) yet has the disadvantage of requiring a large quantity of antigen compared with other tests for anti-HBc. Counterelectrophoresis is as sensitive as complement fixation for anti-HBc and provides results in 2 hours. Again, relatively large quantities of

HBcAg purified from chimpanzee liver are required. The test procedure is the same as that for HBsAg (see earlier in this chapter).

A more satisfactory test is the immune adherence hemagglutination (IAHA) technique, which, according to Tsuda *et al.* (1975) is about 10 times as sensitive as complement fixation and counterelectrophoresis for detecting anti-HBc. Relatively small quantities of HBcAg are required and therefore can be obtained from Dane particle–rich plasma as well as from liver.

The most sensitive tests for HBcAg and anti-HBc, however, are radioimmunoassays. The antigen source is high-density Dane particle cores purified from HBsAg-positive plasma. The tests are said to be 300 times more sensitive than complement fixation or counterelectrophoresis in anti-HBc detection.

Serologic Detection of HBeAg and Anti-HBe

Tests for HBeAg and anti-HBe are not generally used in a routine setting, because although there may be prognostic implications of such detection, the utilized tests (immunoprecipitation, such as the Ouchterlony double-diffusion method) have not been proved to be sufficiently sensitive in this respect.

Serologic Tests in Delta Hepatitis

Only HBsAg-positive persons need to be tested for HDV infection because of the helper functions from HBV required by HDV. Diagnosis of acute versus chronic HDV infection is based on the detection of IgM anti-HDV and total anti-HDV (IgM and IgG) using commercially available RIA or ELISA kits.

JUST THE FACTS

Introduction: Hepatitis

1. *Hepatitis* is a generic term referring to an inflammation of the liver.
2. In general use, *hepatitis* refers to the clinical, laboratory, and/or histologic effects of liver injury, whether or not inflammation is present.
3. Most cases of hepatitis are the result of damage to hepatocytes.
4. Damage may be caused by viruses, bacteria, fungi, parasites, drugs, toxins, heat, hyperthermia, radiation, or excessive alcohol intake.
5. Some cases are idiopathic.
6. Hepatocytes can be replaced by the regeneration of new cells.
7. When too many hepatocytes are destroyed to maintain basic liver function, the term *fulminant hepatitis* is applied.
8. The morphologic changes that occur in the liver vary with the cause of hepatitis.
9. The term *hepatitis* is qualified with an etiologic modifier dependent on the cause (e.g., viral hepatitis, alcoholic hepatitis, etc.).

The Hepatitis Viruses

1. *Viral hepatitis* and *acute viral hepatitis* are terms used to refer to cases caused by specific hepatotropic viruses (hepatitis A virus, hepatitis B virus, non-A, non-B hepatitis virus, and delta hepatitis virus). (Study Table 7–1.)
2. All of these viruses cause inflammation of the liver with fever, nausea, vomiting, and jaundice.
3. There are two major clinical types of hepatitis:
   a. Infectious hepatitis—caused by type A virus.
   b. Serum hepatitis—caused by type B virus or NANB virus.

Hepatitis A

1. This is the type seen in most epidemic outbreaks in the normal population.
2. Transmission is by the fecal-oral route.
3. It is more common in countries with a low standard of living, where it affects the population at a younger age.
4. Outbreaks show a seasonal pattern.

Hepatitis A virus

1. Hepatitis A virus is a nonenveloped, isosahedral, single-stranded RNA particle that belongs to the family Picornaviridae.
2. It has a dense core that is presumably composed of neucleoprotein.
3. It localizes primarily in the cytoplasm of the liver, where it multiplies easily.

4. It does not produce a coat protein and is not detectable in serum.
5. It is stable in ether and to a pH of 3.0.
6. It is an enterovirus.
7. The virus has been isolated in cell culture directly from human specimens.

Antibodies to HAV (Immunity)

1. Initial antibody is IgM.
2. This is subsequently replaced by IgG that persists for years, probably for life.
3. The antibody will aggregate highly purified HAV.
4. There is no vaccine for hepatitis A infection.
5. Passive protection is provided by immune gamma globulin.

Serologic Tests for HAV

1. Hepatitis A infection was originally diagnosed by assumption (i.e., hepatitis B had been ruled out).
2. Tests are not used in the clinical laboratory, but are sometimes used in research laboratories.
3. Laboratory diagnosis of hepatitis A is performed using tests that detect the presence of antibodies.

Hepatitis B

1. Hepatitis B commonly follows parenteral exposure to an infected individual, although other modes of transmission are known to occur.
2. The incubation period is 4 to 26 weeks.
3. In Western Europe and North America, cases of hepatitis B usually appear singly.
4. In Asia, large segments of the population have been found to be infected. In some cases, infection appears to be acquired.
5. The association antigen was originally called *Australia antigen.*
6. Australia antigen is now known to be unassembled viral coat (surface antigen) and is called HBsAg.

Hepatitis B Virus (HBV)

1. This is a hepatotropic virus.
2. It is a double-stranded DNA particle that exists in three forms:
   a. A spherical (disc) particle (22 nm in diameter)

—the predominant form in the blood of patients with hepatitis B.
   b. A filamentous form (22 nm wide, 50 to 200 nm long)—less common in the blood of patients with hepatitis B.
   c. A Dane particle (42 nm in diameter, containing a 27-nm nucleocapsid DNA-containing core, surrounded by an outer lipoprotein coat)—the least common in the blood of patients with hepatitis B.
3. It is believed that the larger particles represent the complete virion and that the other morphologic forms are excess coat protein.

Markers for Hepatitis B Virus

1. HBsAg is the outer lipoprotein coat—22 nm in diameter—found in body fluids of patients with hepatitis B—produced in the cytoplasm of infected hepatocytes.
2. HBcAg is the core of HBV—27 nm in diameter—located in the nuclei of hepatocytes.
3. HBeAg, also found in some HBsAg-positive sera either bound to immunoglobulins or free in solution, appears during acute infection, then usually disappears (or can be carried chronically); three subtypes are known. The persistence of the antigen usually indicates chronic hepatitis and may be a marker for infectivity of HBsAg-positive blood.

Subtypes of HBsAg

1. HBsAg contains a common immunologic determinant and several major subdeterminants that are specified by the viral genome.
2. The major subtypes consist of various combinations of subdeterminants d/y and w/r, constituting two groups—d/y (1) and w1,w2,w3,w4, and r (2).
3. Mixed subtypes, adwr and adyr, are extremely rare.
4. Subtypes ayw2 and ayw3 appear to be more common in Africa and the Middle East.
5. Subdeterminant r appears to be predominant in the Far East and is common in Japan.
6. Subtype adw2 is common in the United States.
7. HBsAg of adw and ayw appears to differ in both biophysical and biochemical characteristics.
8. Subtype-specific antibodies are determined

using passive hemagglutination or radioimmunoassay techniques (as used in anti-HBs detection).

Antibodies to HBAg

1. Anti-HBc antibodies usually appear subsequent to infection with HBV.
2. Anti-HBs usually appear later (sometimes delayed 6 to 12 months), often coinciding with the disappearance of circulating HBsAg. Anti-HBc decreases and may become undetectable after 1 to 2 years, although high titers are found in carriers.
3. During recovery, anti-HBc may be present in the absence of HBsAg and anti-HBs. (Donations taken at this time can cause post-transfusion hepatitis.)
4. Anti-HBs may persist throughout life, bestowing immunity.
5. The presence of anti-HBe is considered a good prognostic sign.

Incidence of Hepatitis B

1. About 200,000 new cases of HBV infection occur annually in the United States.
2. Eight to twelve per cent of adults are antibody positive.
3. The infection is found primarily in health care workers, patients and staff in hemodialysis units, immunosuppressed patients, institutionalized groups, illicit drug users, homosexual males, and individuals from areas in which the virus is endemic.

Transmission of Hepatitis B

1. The most important mode of transmission is parenteral infection.
2. Casual contact with infected blood can also cause the disease.
3. Recognized modes of transmission include:
   a. Blood transfusion
   b. Common needles and syringes
   c. Unsterilized dental equipment
   d. Tattooing needles
   e. Sharing of razors and toothbrushes
   f. Sexual contact (male homosexuals particularly)

4. Arthropod spread is suspected, although, like fecal-oral routes, it remains uncertain.
5. Susceptibility to the disease is not confined to any age group.
6. The many modes of transmission are almost certainly due to the fact that most body secretions contain viral surface antigen.

Clinical Signs and Symptoms of Hepatitis B

1. Individuals exposed to HBV through accidental needle puncture or transfusion do not show the initial symptoms (weakness, fatigue, nausea, and jaundice) until about 10 to 16 weeks after exposure.
2. Pain in the joints and/or rash or urticaria may occur weeks before the illness is recognized as hepatitis.
3. The acute phase of the illness usually lasts for only a few weeks.
4. Most individuals recover and develop immunity.
5. About 10 per cent do not develop immunity and may become chronic carriers or develop chronic active or chronic persistent hepatitis.

Protection Against HBV by Antibody

1. Immunoglobulin prepared from subjects with relatively potent anti-HBs has been found to reduce the risk of hepatitis in individuals exposed to HBV.
2. Standard immunoglobulin is usually of little value in prophylaxis due to low titer of anti-HBs.

HBV Vaccine

1. Vaccines have been developed that are clinically valuable.
2. Szumness *et al.* developed a vaccine from the plasma of chronic carriers of HBsAg, which is effective in many cases (with the exception of post-transfusion hepatitis).
3. In 1984, a vaccine was developed made by a recombinant strain of the yeast *Saccharomyces cerevisiae*. A three-dose program is believed to offer immunity for about 5 years.
4. Other vaccines are currently under investigation.

Non-A, Non-B Hepatitis

1. Since it was proved that in some cases hepatitis was not caused by HAV or HBV, the term non-A, non-B (NANB) was suggested.
2. Hepatitis C virus (HCV) is the major cause of NANB hepatitis.

Incidence of Non-A, Non-B Hepatitis

1. This type of hepatitis is quite common.
2. Between 89 and 100 per cent of cases of post-transfusion hepatitis in the United States may be related to NANB.
3. Anicteric cases of post-transfusion hepatitis are more common than icteric cases.
4. The incidence of NANB hepatitis in transfusion recipients is directly related to the level of alanine aminotransferase (ALT) in the relevant blood donations.
5. NANB hepatitis is seen in populations of low socioeconomic status and is associated with a chronic carrier state.
6. In volunteer donors, the carrier rate is 1.6 per cent; in paid donors, this rises to 5.4 per cent.
7. Sporadic cases have been documented that are not the result of exposure to blood or blood products.

Transmission of Non-A, Non-B Hepatitis

1. Transmission is by transfusion or (sometimes) by close person-to-person contact.
2. NANB hepatitis can be transmitted from human to human and from human to chimpanzee.

Clinical Signs and Symptoms of Non-A, Non-B Hepatitis

1. Most patients have minimal clinical manifestations and few require hospitalization.
2. The incubation period varies from 6 to 10 weeks, with a peak of about 8 weeks.
3. Up to 60 per cent reveal abnormal ALT levels for more than a year.
4. Liver biopsy reveals histologic evidence of significant chronic liver disease in most cases; about 10 per cent show features of cirrhosis.
5. Serum hepatic enzyme levels fluctuate markedly over a relatively short period of time.

6. NANB and hepatitis B cannot be differentiated on clinical grounds alone.

Serologic Tests

1. No universal test has been accepted as a marker for NANB infection.
2. Surrogate testing that measures increased levels of ALT and then antibody to HBcAg is used but will detect only about 50 per cent of NANB-contaminated donor blood.

Delta Hepatitis

1. This has been shown to occur worldwide.
2. Populations at high risk for HBsAg are also at risk for HDV infections.

Hepatitis Delta Virus

1. HDV is a single-stranded RNA virus (also known as the delta antigen), spherical in shape with a diameter of 36 nm.
2. It is a defective hepatotropic virus that requires helper functions from HBV in order to ensure its replication and infectivity.

Antibodies to HDV

1. HDV is transient in serum (1 to 4 days).
2. As HDV antigen declines, IgM antibodies are formed, followed by low levels of IgG.
3. The progression to high levels of IgG anti-HDV in HBsAg-positive individuals indicates the switch to chronic HDV infection.

Transmission of HDV

1. The transmission of HDV is linked to that of its HBV-helper virus.
2. Transmission occurs by parenteral and transmucosal routes.
3. Horizontal transmission occurs in households.
4. Infections increase in nonhygienic, crowded living conditions.
5. In epidemics, mosquitos have been shown to be a vehicle for transmission.

Clinical Signs and Symptoms of Delta Hepatitis

1. Acute infection can occur as:
   a. Coinfection with acute HBV infection.
   b. Superinfection of a chronic HBV infection.
2. Chronic HDV infection has a poor prognosis for the patient. Liver necrosis, inflammation, and clinical illness are increased in their severity, and cirrhosis often occurs.

Treatment of Delta Hepatitis

1. There are no effective antiviral drugs or immuno-suppressive agents for the treatment of chronic HDV infections.
2. Vaccination against HBV also provides immunity to HDV.

The Serologic Detection of Hepatitis Markers

1. Hepatitis markers can be identified by comple-ment fixation, immune adherence hemagglu-tination, radioimmunoassay, and ELISA.

Practical Considerations in Hepatitis Testing

1. Tests for HBV and HBsAg are performed to identify blood donors who are infected with HBV and to establish the etiology of clinical cases of hepatitis.
2. Third-generation tests are the methods of choice for both of these applications. When HBsAg is not detected, sensitivity methods for the detection of anti-HBs or anti-HBc can be useful.

Suggested Rules for Practical Testing

The student should study this section in the text, which is in point form.

Review Questions

Multiple Choice

Choose the phrase, sentence, or symbol that completes the statement or answers the question. More than one answer may be correct in each case. Answers are given at the end of this book.

1. Hepatitis is the result of damage to hepatocytes, which may be caused by:
   (a) viruses
   (b) drugs
   (c) heat
   (d) excessive alcohol intake
   (Introduction: Hepatitis)

2. Infectious hepatitis:
   (a) is caused by hepatitis A virus
   (b) is caused by hepatitis B virus
   (c) is caused by non-A, non-B hepatitis virus
   (d) usually results from needle punctures or nee-dle wounds
   (The Hepatitis Viruses)

3. Hepatitis A:
   (a) is also known as *serum hepatitis*
   (b) is transmitted by a fecal-oral route
   (c) is more common in countries with low stan-dards of living
   (d) is the type seen in most epidemic outbreaks of hepatitis in the normal population
   (Hepatitis A)

4. The hepatitis A virus:
   (a) produces a coat protein
   (b) is detectable in the serum of patients with hep-atitis A
   (c) is stable in ether
   (d) is stable to a pH of 3.0
   (Hepatitis A Virus [HAV])

5. Anti-HAV:
   (a) appears in the plasma at the onset of clinically apparent hepatitis A
   (b) initially occurs as IgM
   (c) initially occurs as IgG
   (d) persists in the circulation until the symptoms of the disease are no longer apparent
   (Antibodies to HAV [Immunity])

6. Hepatitis B:
   (a) is also known as *post-transfusion hepatitis*
   (b) commonly follows parenteral exposure to HBV

(c) has an incubation period of 2 to 4 weeks
(d) has an incubation period of 1 to 6 months
(Hepatitis B)

7. The hepatitis B virus:
   (a) exists in three forms
   (b) is microbiologically related to hepatitis A virus
   (c) is a double-stranded DNA particle
   (d) is none of the above
   (Hepatitis B Virus [HBV])

8. The outer lipoprotein coat (or envelope) of hepatitis B virus is known as:
   (a) HBsAg
   (b) HBcAg
   (c) HBeAg
   (d) HDV
   (Markers for Hepatitis B Virus)

9. The number of antigenic subtypes that have been recognized for HBeAg is:
   (a) one
   (b) two
   (c) three
   (d) none
   (Markers for Hepatitis B Virus)

10. The two mixed subtypes of HBeAg, adwr and adyr, are:
    (a) extremely common in Japan
    (b) extremely rare
    (c) possibly due to phenotypic mixing of immunologic markers during simultaneous infection associated with more than one subtype of HBsAg
    (d) none of the above
    (Subtypes of HBsAg)

11. Antibodies to HBsAg:
    (a) occur at the onset of clinically apparent hepatitis B
    (b) often appear in coincidence with the disappearance of circulating HBsAg
    (c) bestow immunity to further infection with hepatitis B virus
    (d) may persist throughout life
    (Antibodies to HBAg)

12. Which of the following individuals may be considered "high-risk" groups with respect to hepatitis B infection?
    (a) patients in hemodialysis units
    (b) homosexual males
    (c) immunosuppressed patients
    (d) illicit drug users
    (Incidence of Hepatitis B)

13. Hepatitis B may be transmitted through:
    (a) transfusion of blood or blood products
    (b) unsterilized dental equipment
    (c) sexual contact
    (d) all of the above
    (Transmission of Hepatitis B)

14. Viral surface antigen has been found in:
    (a) saliva
    (b) semen
    (c) sweat
    (d) colostrum
    (Transmission of Hepatitis B)

15. An HBV vaccine made by a recombinant strain of the yeast *Saccharomyces cerevisiae:*
    (a) has been found to have positive effects on human volunteers
    (b) causes the production of antibody in recipients after a three-dose program
    (c) produces an antibody in recipients that is specific for the a determinant of HBsAg
    (d) has several serious side effects
    (HBV Vaccine)

16. The transmission of non-A, non-B hepatitis is:
    (a) associated with transfusion of blood or blood products
    (b) similar to that of hepatitis B
    (c) believed to be through close person-to-person contact
    (d) not possible between humans and chimpanzees
    (Transmission of Non-A, Non-B Hepatitis)

17. The hepatitis delta virus:
    (a) is a single-stranded RNA virus
    (b) has a diameter of 36 nm
    (c) is a defective hepatotropic virus
    (d) requires obligatory helper functions from HBV in order to ensure its replication and infectivity
    (Hepatitis Delta Virus)

18. Sources of antisera for the detection of HBsAg include:
    (a) horses
    (b) mice
    (c) multiply-transfused human patients
    (d) goats
    (Serologic Detection of HBsAg)

19. In practical testing of HBsAg:
    (a) mouth pipetting is acceptable under certain circumstances
    (b) pipetting should be performed in a fume hood
    (c) leaking specimens should be carefully cleaned before use
    (d) specimens should be centrifuged in a tightly capped tube
    (Practical Considerations)

20. HBcAg has been purified from:
    (a) latex particles
    (b) the liver of immunosuppressed chimpanzees experimentally infected with HBV
    (c) cesium chloride
    (d) the plasma of chickens
    (Serologic Detection of HBcAg and Anti-HBc)

Answer "True" or "False"

1. The term hepatitis refers to inflammation of the liver.
   (Introduction: Hepatitis)

2. Serum hepatitis is caused by type B virus or the NANB virus.
   (The Hepatitis Viruses)

3. Hepatitis A is not transmitted by a fecal-oral route.
   (Hepatitis A)

4. The hepatitis A virus belongs to the family Picornaviridae.
   (Hepatitis A Virus [HAV])

5. An effective vaccine exists for hepatitis A infection.
   (Antibodies to HAV [Immunity])

6. HBcAg was originally known as Australia antigen.
   (Hepatitis B)

7. The Dane particle is the most common form of HBV seen in patients with hepatitis B.
   (Hepatitis B Virus [HBV])

8. Three subtypes of HBsAg have been recognized.
   (Subtypes of HBsAg)

9. Populations that are of high risk with respect to HBsAg are also at risk for HDV infections.
   (Delta Hepatitis)

10. Post-transfusion hepatitis is usually related to the NANB virus.
    (Incidence of Non-A, Non-B Hepatitis)

GENERAL REFERENCES

Baron, E.J., and Finegold, S.M.: Bailey and Scott's Diagnostic Microbiology, 8th ed. St Louis, C. V. Mosby Company, 1990.

Freeman, B.A.: Burrows Textbook of Microbiology, 27th ed. Philadelphia, W. B. Saunders Company, 1985.

Henry, J.B.: Clinical Diagnosis and Management by Laboratory Methods. Philadelphia, W. B. Saunders Company, 1991.

Sheehan, C.: Clinical Immunology: Principles and Laboratory Diagnosis. Philadelphia, J. B. Lippincott, 1990.

8

C-Reactive Protein (CRP) and Other Plasma Proteins

OBJECTIVES

The student shall know, understand, and be prepared to explain:
1. The characteristics of C-reactive protein
2. The properties of C-reactive protein
3. Current and potential uses of C-reactive protein determination in:
    a. Bacterial and viral infections
    b. Rheumatic diseases
    c. Myocardial infarction
    d. Burn injuries
    e. Renal transplantation
4. The laboratory tests for C-reactive protein
5. The properties and characteristics of other plasma proteins, particularly:
    a. Haptoglobin
    b. Fibrinogen
    c. Alpha$_1$-antitrypsin
    d. Ceruloplasmin
    e. Alpha$_2$-macroglobulin

C-REACTIVE PROTEIN

C-reactive protein (CRP) is a trace constituent of serum that was originally defined by its calcium-dependent precipitation with the C-polysaccharide of *Pneumococcus* (Tillet and Francis, 1930). The protein was originally thought to be an antibody to C-polysaccharide and specific for patients with pneumococcal infections, but later studies dis-pelled this contention, and the relative *nonspecificity* of CRP is now well recognized.

The outstanding characteristic of CRP is that it appears in the sera of individuals in response to a variety of inflammatory conditions and tissue necrosis and disappears when the inflammatory condition has subsided. It is consistently found in cases of bacterial infection (particularly the colon-typhoid group) (Dawson, 1957), active rheumatic

173

fever (Anderson and McCarthy, 1950), and many malignant diseases, and it is commonly found in cases of active rheumatoid arthritis, viral infection, and tuberculosis. In addition, CRP has been detected in the sera of patients following surgical operations (Crockson *et al.*, 1966) and blood transfusions, as well as in bullous fluid aspirated from patients with thermal burns, pemphigus vulgaris, and other bullous lesions. The protein usually appears rapidly after the onset of disease (14 to 26 hours) and may increase in concentration by as much as 1,000 times its normal amount; thus, it is a useful clinical indicator of disease states (Hayashi and LoGrippo, 1972; Table 8–1).

During the 1940s and 1950s, laboratory testing for CRP was widely used as an aid to diagnosis of a variety of inflammatory conditions; however, certain problems with the test subsequently came to be realized, namely:

1. The nonspecificity of the test, which was considered to be a major problem in clinical interpretation.
2. The quantitative nature of the original assay procedure, which made it impossible to establish any correlation between the positivity of the test and the severity of a clinical disease.

In addition to these problems, new tests were being developed for monitoring acute-phase reactions, the most popular of which was the erythrocyte sedimentation rate (ESR).

For these reasons, the CRP test gradually lost its popularity and by the mid-1970s was being performed by very few laboratories.

The potential role of CRP in the clinical laboratory as a mediator or modulator of the immune response has recently restimulated interest in the protein due to studies on the purification of the CRP molecule, the preparation of an antiserum specific for it, and the development of sensitive, specific, rapid, and quantitative techniques for its measurement in serum. This resurgence of interest is also stimulated by the fact that a molecule that is produced in such large amounts during the acute infammatory response must have biologic significance, even if such significance is as yet unrealized.

Properties of C-Reactive Protein

Human CRP is a homogeneous molecule (molecular weight 120,000) with a sedimentation coefficient of 6.5 and an electrophoretic mobility in the gamma region (Volanakis *et al.*, 1978) that consists of five probably identical, noncovalently bound subunits of approximately 21,500 to 23,500 d each, linked in the form of a cyclic pentamer. It is made up of 100 per cent peptide and has an amino acid composition similar to that of immunoglobulin (IgG). In addition, CRP shares with immunoglobulin the ability to initiate certain functions of potential significance to host defense and inflammation, including precipitation (Tillet and Francis, 1930; Abernathy and Francis, 1937), agglutination (Gal and Miltenyi, 1955), opsonization (Kindermark, 1971), capsular swelling (Lofstrom, 1944), and complement activation (Kaplan and Volanakis, 1974; Siegel *et al.*, 1974). C-reactive protein also combines with T lymphocytes and inhibits certain of their functions (Mortensen *et al.*, 1975), and it inhibits the aggregation of platelets induced by aggregated human gamma globulin and thrombin (Fiedel and Gewurz, 1975). CRP differs from immunoglobulin in antigeneity (MacLeod and Avery, 1941), tertiary structure, homogeneity (Gotschlich and Edelman, 1965), stimuli required for formation and release, and binding specificities (for which CRP, in certain reactivities, requires calcium) (Gotschlich and Edelman, 1967), and in that it is produced entirely by hepatocytes or liver parenchymal cells (Kushner and Feldmann, 1978).

In a physical sense, CRP is thermolabile, being destroyed by heating at 70°C for 30 minutes, and does not cross the human placenta.

The elevation of CRP in a patient above the normal (i.e., 0.5 mg/dl) indicates tissue damage or inflammation or both, with great reliability. If these

TABLE 8–1. Presence of C-Reactive Protein in Disease

Normally Present	Occasionally Present	Absent
Active rheumatic fever	Pericarditis	Skin diseases
Acute myocardial infarction	Rheumatoid arthritis	URI (upper respiratory infections)
Carcinoma	Pyelitis	Renal disease
Streptococcal infections	Nephritis	Localized infections
Pneumonia	Tuberculosis	

evaluations are monitored sequentially, they can provide an excellent means of assessing disease activity and guiding therapy.

Current and Potential Uses of CRP Determination

The serum levels of alpha$_1$-antitrypsin, haptoglobin, ceruloplasmin, alpha$_1$-acid glycoprotein, and CRP increase during active inflammation or tissue injury. Serum CRP levels, however, increase within 4 to 6 hours after an acute tissue injury, whereas the serum levels of all the other acute-phase reactants increase from 12 to 24 hours after the injury. CRP, therefore, is an earlier and more reliable indicator of clinical disease and its severity than the other reactants.

Studies by Fisher et al. (1976) have shown that the CRP test can also be useful as a means of evaluating the postoperative clinical course of a patient as opposed to the traditional parameters used for this purpose (e.g., body temperature, white blood count, erythrocyte sedimentation rate), which are often unreliable. In general, serum CRP levels in uncomplicated surgical cases increase within 4 to 6 hours, reach peak value (usually 25 to 35 mg/dl) between 48 and 72 hours postoperatively, then begin to decrease after the third postoperative day, and reach normal values between the fifth and twelfth postoperative days. In using CRP levels in this regard, it is important to run tests in series rather than at single, isolated points in the clinical course; it is also important that the preoperative CRP levels be determined. Further, the CRP levels must be determined quantitatively in order to be clinically meaningful and useful.

CRP determinations have also been found to be useful in evaluating the clinical course of bacterial and viral infections, rheumatic diseases, myocardial infarction, burn injuries, and renal transplantation.

Bacterial and Viral Infections. In the differential diagnosis of infectious diseases, CRP was reported by McCarthy et al. (1978) to be useful in distinguishing bacterial from viral infections. Studies of sequential determinations of CRP in acute childhood pyelonephritis (Jodal and Hanson, 1976) showed that levels of the protein decreased promptly following successful treatment yet continued to rise or remained unaffected when drug therapy was ineffective. Pepys et al. (1977), in studying inflammatory bowel disease, reported that CRP was useful in distinguishing Crohn's disease or transmural colitis from chronic ulcerative colitis—a distinction that is not always possible on clinical and histopathologic grounds.

Rheumatic Diseases. CRP measurements can reflect the activity of various rheumatic diseases. In cases of rheumatoid arthritis, for example, CRP has been shown to be a more reliable indicator of disease activity than the ESR, because the ESR reflects certain blood changes that are not necessarily altered in inflammation (e.g., immunoglobulin and cholesterol concentrations, anemia, the size and shape of erythrocytes), whereas CRP does not (Walsh et al. 1979).

Myocardial Infarction. A sharp increase in the serum CRP level accompanies myocardial infarction (especially in the acute phase), and this increase usually parallels the size of the infarct (Smith et al., 1977). CRP quantitation, therefore, can be useful in differentiating acute infarction from angina. Serious complications are indicated by continued increase (or subsequent increase) of the CRP level.

Burn Injuries. Daniels et al. (1974), in studying the serum protein profiles in thermal burns, showed that an increase in CRP levels correlated with the severity of the burn.

Renal Transplantation. Sandoval (1981) observed a sudden increase in the serum CRP level that correlated with the onset of homograft rejection, thereby suggesting the potential of using CRP testing in monitoring patients with kidney transplants.

CRP testing has also proved useful in cases of systemic lupus erythematosus.

Discussion

Although little is known about the precise function of CRP, it is possible that the interactions of this protein with various lymphocyte and monocyte subpopulations may constitute the function of "paving the way" for subsequent, more specific immune response. The finding that CRP has a particularly strong affinity for monocytes bearing Fc receptors may be significant in this respect, although the true nature of this interaction remains yet to be elucidated.

LABORATORY TESTS FOR CRP

CRP protein determination is now considered to be of greater practical significance than all other indices of inflammation in assessing inflammatory diseases. For example, CRP is present at all times when the ESR is abnormally elevated, and whereas ESR determinations may provide "borderline" results and may, in some cases, remain elevated in the absence of inflammation (e.g., in anemia due to a decrease in number of erythrocytes, in pregnancy due to an increase in fibrinogen, and in nephrosis due to loss of albumin and relative increase in globulin), CRP does not have a variable range between normal and abnormal and is not influenced by anemia or serum protein alteration.

Serologic tests for CRP use the patient's serum and either purified pneumococcal C-polysaccharide or anti-CRP serum obtained from rabbits immunized with purified CRP, the latter being preferred.

The tests that have been devised for CRP can be divided into different categories, depending upon the type of procedure involved:

1. *Agglutination.* Agglutination tests for CRP are performed using latex particles coated with antibodies to human CRP, which interact with the patient's serum either on a microscope slide or in a test tube. This test, known as the latex-fixation test, is by far the most popular of the CRP tests and is claimed to be the most sensitive (Fishel, 1967). (The technique is described later in this chapter.)
2. *Complement fixation.* Complement fixation tests for CRP are not generally suitable for use in the routine clinical laboratory and, therefore, are considered to be of historic and academic interest only.
3. *Fluorescent antibody.* Fluorescent antibody tests are useful in studying the binding of CRP to lymphocytes and their subpopulations and are used primarily as research tools for localizing CRP in tissues.
4. *Precipitation.* Precipitation tests for CRP can be done either in the fluid phase (by a capillary or a tube method) or in the solid gel phase (by the Ouchterlony, Oudin, or Mancini methods). In addition, CRP gel tests involving electrophoresis or electroimmunodiffusion have been described.

In 1976, Deaton and Maxwell described the use of laser nephelometry in the measurement of CRP (and other serum proteins). This technique is sensitive, rapid, and reproducible and makes it possible reliably to perform CRP determinations on a large number of samples. In brief, the procedure involves the measurement of light (from a laser-light source) that is scattered by insoluble immune complexes in a liquid medium containing polyethylene glycol. The patient's serum sample and standards are incubated for 2 hours at room temperature with a specific anti-CRP antiserum diluted in polyethylene glycol containing a buffer (pH 7.4). With the use of a nephelometer, the laser beam is passed from the source through the sample and control solutions, which contain the insoluble CRP immune complexes. The forward-scatter light is measured within the range of the standard sera, with a photomultiplier tube. The concentration of CRP is proportional to the amount of forward-scatter light displayed by the instrument. Note: In order to attract nonspecific background-scatter light, which is related to the patient's serum or the reagents or both, it is necessary to run appropriate blank samples in parallel with the test. In some cases (e.g., when using specimens that have been frozen and thawed), levels of background-scatter light can be extremely high: this represents the only inconvenience of this technique.

5. *Radioimmunoassay.* An extremely sensitive radioimmunoassay has been described that is capable of detecting levels of CRP in the nanogram range. For most routine studies of CRP, however, this degree of sensitivity is unnecessary.

METHOD 1: C-REACTIVE PROTEIN RAPID LATEX AGGLUTINATION TEST

The C-reactive protein (CRP) agglutination test is based on the reaction between patient serum and the CRP antibody coated to the treated surface of latex particles.

The test procedure given here is adapted from the C-reactive protein test (latex) product insert provided in a kit from ICL Scientific, Fountain Valley, California.

Materials

The kit contains:

1. CRP latex reagent with dropper assembly
2. One per cent suspension of stabilized polystyrene latex particles coated with specific antihuman CRP produced in goats or sheep. Note: Store at 2°C to 8°C—DO NOT FREEZE. Properly stored reagent is stable until expiration date indicated on the label. Reagent that does not produce appropriate quality-control results should be discarded after verification by repeat testing.
3. Glycine-saline buffer (pH 8.2 ± 0.1. Note: Store at 2°C to 8°C. Properly stored reagent is stable until expiration date indicated on the label. Reagent that does not produce appropriate quality-control results should be discarded after verification by repeat testing. Discard if contaminated, i.e., evidence of cloudiness or particulate material in solution.
4. Capillary pipettes
5. Applicator sticks
6. Glass slide
7. Positive control serum (human) prediluted. Store at 2°C to 8°C.
8. Negative control serum (human) prediluted. Store at 2°C to 8°C.

Additional Material Required:

1. Stopwatch or timer
2. 12 × 75 mm test tubes
3. Serologic pipettes (1 ml graduated) and safety pipetter
4. Calibrated pipetter (optional)

Procedure (Quantitative)

Note: All reagents and specimens must be at room temperature before testing. A positive and negative control must be tested with each unknown patient specimen. (CAUTION: Since the control sera is derived from human sources, it should be handled in the same manner as clinical serum specimens.) When using the positive control, failure to obtain a positive reaction indicates deterioration of the latex reagent and/or the control itself. When using the negative control, a smooth or slightly granular reaction must be observed. If agglutination is exhibited with this control, the test should be repeated. If the repeat yields the same result, the reagents must be replaced, and test results considered invalid.

1. Fill one of the capillary pipettes provided with undiluted serum to approximately two-thirds of the pipette length. While holding the capillary pipette perpendicular to the slide, deliver one free-falling drop to the center of one of the oval divisions of the slide.
2. Fill a capillary pipette with undiluted serum to approximately two-thirds of the pipette length. While holding the capillary pipette perpendicular to the slide (to ensure correct delivery of consistent amounts of test serum), deliver one free-falling drop to the center of one of the oval divisions of the slide. Note: Do not reuse capillary pipettes or applicator sticks. If a calibrated pipetter is used instead of a capillary pipette, adjust the pipetter to deliver 0.05ml (50 μl) of the specimen.
3. Using the squeeze dropper vials provided, add one drop of the prediluted positive control and one drop of the prediluted negative control to separate labeled divisions of the slide.
4. Resuspend the CRP latex reagent by gently mixing until the suspension is homogeneous. Using the dropper provided, add one drop of the CRP latex reagent to each serum specimen and to each control.
5. Using separate applicator sticks, mix each specimen and each control thoroughly. The contents of the mixtures should be spread evenly over the entire area of their respective divisions on the slide.
6. Tilt the slide back and forth gently for 2 minutes. Place the slide on a flat surface and observe immediately for macroscopic agglutination using a direct light source.

Note: The latex reagent, controls, and buffer contain 0.1 per cent sodium azide as a preservative. Since this may react with lead and copper plumbing to form highly explosive metal azides, they should be flushed with a large volume of water upon disposal, to avoid azide buildup.

The Semiquantitative Slide Test

If a patient's serum gives a positive reaction, the serum may be serially diluted with glycine-saline buffer to determine a semiquantitative estimate of the CRP level. After mixing each dilution, 0.05 ml is placed on a separate division of the glass slide and tested as in steps 4 through 6 above. The titer of CRP is the last dilution that exhibits a positive reaction.

When performing this test, a dilution control should be run simultaneously, using one drop of latex reagent and one drop of glycine-saline buffer. Agglutination in this control invalidates the test.

Interpretation of Results

Agglutination of the latex suspension indicates a level of CRP equal to or greater than 1.0 ± 0.2 mg/dl. A positive reaction is reported when either the undiluted or 1:5 dilution specimen (or both) demonstrates agglutination (Table 8–2). Agglutination in the 1:5 dilution is indicative of a CRP level greater than 5 mg/dl.

Positive reactions are reported as follows:

1+   Very small clumping with an opaque fluid background

2+   Small clumping with slightly opaque fluid in the background

3+   Moderate clumping with slightly opaque fluid in the background

4+   Moderate clumping with clear fluid background

Sources of Error and Limitations

False-positive results may be observed with this technique if serum specimens are lipemic, hemolyzed, or heavily contaminated with bacteria. If the reaction time is longer than 2 minutes, a false-positive result may also be produced as a result of drying. False-negative results may be observed in undiluted serum specimens because of high levels of CRP (antigen excess). A 1:5 dilution of serum is tested for this reason.

This test is not ideal in cases where quantitative determination is indicated because the strength of reaction is not always indicative of CRP concentration. In such cases it is preferable to use nephelometry. Also, this test, which has an assessed

TABLE 8–2. Interpretation of Tests for C-Reactive Protein

Undiluted Serum	Diluted Serum	Interpretation
0 to 2+	2+ to 4+	Strongly positive
3+ to 4+		Positive
1+ to 2+	0 to 2+	Weakly positive
	Negative	
Negative	Negative	Negative

sensitivity of 93 per cent, will detect levels of CRP of ±1 mg/dl and, therefore, patients with values lower than 1 mg/dl may be undetected.

OTHER PLASMA PROTEINS

Haptoglobin

Haptoglobin is a 100,000-d plasma glycoprotein with α electrophoretic mobility. Its principal function is to irreversibly bind to free hemoglobin released by intravascular hemolysis, forming a complex that is rapidly cleared by hepatocytes in the liver, thus preventing the loss of free hemoglobin in the liver (Javid, 1978). Haptoglobin levels increase twofold to fourfold attendant to injury, and haptoglobin is frequently found in inflammatory exudates. The rise in plasma haptoglobin in response to inflammation is due to the *de novo* synthesis of the protein by the liver and does not involve the release of previously formed haptoglobin from other sites.

Haptoglobin levels are decreased due to intravascular hemolysis or (in some cases) due to decreased synthesis as a result of liver disease. Since relatively minor hemolytic events have the potential of markedly depleting the haptoglobin level in the absence of an inflammatory response, no quantitative correlation between the plasma haptoglobin content and the severity of hemolysis can be made. Conversely, infection or inflammation can lead to a twofold to tenfold increase in haptoglobin. In such situations, a normal haptoglobin level does not rule out the diagnosis of intravascular hemolysis. The levels of other acute-phase protein (e.g.,

CRP) should be taken into account when interpreting the haptoglobin levels.

Haptoglobin has two major genetic variants, designated Hp1 and Hp2.

Fibrinogen

After a surgical incision, fibrinogen accumulates at the site of injury for 1 to 2 weeks. Fibrin is then formed in the presence of enzymes, which are released from PMNs and platelets (Powanda and Moyer, 1981). This fibrin increases the tensile strength of the wound and stimulates fibroblast proliferation and growth. Fibrinogen or fibrin degradation products (FDP) can indirectly stimulate fibrinogen synthesis by hepatocytes (through the production of IL-1 by peripheral blood monocytes or Kupffer cells), which suggests an amplification loop (Fuller and Ritchie, 1982).

Alpha$_1$-Antitrypsin

Alpha$_1$-antitrypsin is one of a family of serine protease inhibitors in human plasma. The physiologic targets are the proteases released from leukocytes rather than trypsin; therefore, the name antitrypsin is not quite accurate yet is still applied (Carrell, 1986).

The activity of these proteases released during digestion of microorganisms and other debris causes lung tissue damage in pulmonary inflammation. Once bound to alpha$_1$-antitrypsin, the activity of these proteases are completely inhibited, being later removed and catabolized. Alpha$_1$-antitrypsin is synthesized by the liver, which can increase synthesis fourfold when stimulated by an inflammatory process. The alpha$_1$-antitrypsin–protease complexes are not taken up by macrophages (as is the case with alpha$_2$-macroglobulin–protease complexes) (Powanda and Moyer, 1981), although there is experimental evidence that proteases can be transferred between alpha$_1$-antitrypsin and alpha$_2$-macroglobulin.

Homozygous alpha$_1$-antitrypsin deficiency can result in:

Premature emphysema, particularly in a patient who also smokes, where onset can occur as early as 30 years of age, with death by age 50. These patients are also affected by air pollution and respiratory infections.

Liver disease. Infants may develop neonatal cholestasis, which can progress to cirrhosis in children. Adults invariably show histologic evidence of liver damage, with about one-fifth developing cirrhosis.

Individuals who have heterozygous alpha$_1$-antitrypsin deficiency are at elevated risk of developing liver disease, connective tissue disease (e.g., rheumatoid arthritis), inflammatory eye disease, and glomerulonephritis (Breit *et al.*, 1985). Alpha$_1$-antitrypsin has a role in several mediator pathways in the inflammatory response. The absence of this protein, therefore, allows the proteases to attack the tissue surrounding the inflammatory process and cause damage that may lead to chronic inflammation.

Ceruloplasmin

The glycoprotein known as ceruloplasmin is the principal copper-transporting protein in human plasma. Eighty to 95 per cent of circulating copper is bound to ceruloplasmin, the remainder being bound more loosely to albumin and amino acids. Ceruloplasmin appears to be the primary copper transport protein for transferring copper to cytochrome C oxidase (vital to aerobic energy production), which, along with glycolysis, increases during wound healing (Goldstein *et al.*, 1982). Ceruloplasmin, along with the copper it carries, has two major functions:

1. It is essential to collagen formation and the extracellular cross-linking and maturation of collagen and elastin (Powanda and Moyer, 1981).
2. It may serve to protect the matrix of healing tissue against superoxide ions, generated by phagocytes in the course of clearing tissue debris and microorganisms.

Ceruloplasmin depletion or absence is associated with Wilson's disease, a degenerative, autosomal recessive-trait disease that is relatively rare (Foley, 1974). In this disease, there is a gastrointestinal absorption defect that allows copper to be taken up in excessive amounts. Copper is massively increased in the tissues and there are massive renal tubular reabsorption defects that result in excessive urinary excretion of proteins, glucose, and other elements.

Alpha₂-Macroglobulin

Alpha$_2$-macroglobulin, like alpha$_1$-antitrypsin, is a protease inhibitor in human plasma. The inhibitor binds to proteolytic enzymes released from damaged tissues as well as from phagocytic cells, thus partially inhibiting their activity. These alpha$_2$-macroglobulin-protease complexes are rapidly phagocytosed by macrophages and fibroblasts (Van Leuven *et al.*, 1978). Alpha$_2$-macroglobulin appears to be a scavenger protease inhibitor that binds excess molecules that cannot be handled by the intended inhibitor. In that role, it functions in hemostasis, coagulation, fibrinolysis, and complement pathways (Roberts, 1985). No diseases have been associated with a deficiency of alpha$_2$-macroglobulin. This may indicate that death results from a deficiency of the protein.

JUST THE FACTS

C-Reactive Protein

1. C-reactive protein (CRP) is a nonspecific trace constituent of serum.
2. CRP appears in the sera of individuals in response to a variety of inflammatory conditions and tissue necrosis and disappears when the inflammatory condition has subsided.
3. CRP is consistently found in bacterial infection, active rheumatic fever, and many malignant diseases.
4. CRP is commonly found in active rheumatoid arthritis, viral infection, and tuberculosis.
5. CRP has been detected in patients following surgical operations and blood transfusions.
6. Bullous fluid aspirated from patients with thermal burns, pemphigus vulgaris, and other bullous lesions has been found to contain CRP.
7. CRP appears after the onset of disease (14 to 26 hours).
8. It may increase in concentration by as much as 1,000 times its normal amount and is, therefore, a useful clinical indicator of disease states.
9. Testing for CRP is complicated by nonspecificity and by the lack of correlation between positivity of the test and the severity of the disease.
10. The biologic significance of CRP is not clear.

Properties of C-Reactive Protein

1. Human CRP is a homogeneous molecule (molecular weight 120,000).
2. It has a sedimentation coefficient of 6.5.
3. Its electrophoretic mobility is in the gamma region.
4. It consists of five probably identical non-covalently bound subunits of approximately 21,500 to 23,500 d each, linked in the form of a cyclic pentamer.
5. It is made up of 100 per cent peptide.
6. It has an amino acid composition similar to that of IgG.
7. It shares with immunoglobulin the ability to initiate precipitation, agglutination, opsonization, capsular swelling, and complement activation.
8. It binds with and inhibits certain T-lymphocyte functions.
9. It inhibits the aggregation of platelets induced by aggregated human gamma globulin and thrombin.
10. It differs from immunoglobulin in antigeneity, tertiary structure, homogeneity, required stimuli for formation, and release and binding specificities, and in that it is produced entirely by hepatocytes or liver parenchymal cells.
11. CRP is thermolabile—it is destroyed by heating to 70°C for 30 minutes.
12. CRP does not cross the human placenta.
13. CRP elevation above the normal (0.5 mg/dl) indicates tissue damage or inflammation or both. Sequential monitoring aids in assessing disease activity and the guiding of therapy.

Current and Potential Uses of CRP Determination

1. CRP is an early, reliable indicator of clinical disease compared to other plasma proteins.
2. CRP tests can be useful as a means of evaluating the postoperative clinical course of a patient.
3. CRP tests are useful in evaluating the clinical course of bacterial and viral infections, rheumatic diseases, myocardial infarction, burn injuries, and renal transplantation.

Laboratory Tests for CRP

1. Tests for CRP can be divided into different categories, depending on the type of procedure in-

volved. These include agglutination tests (using latex particles coated with antibodies to human CRP), complement-fixation tests (not generally used in the routine laboratory), fluorescent antibody tests (primarily a research test), precipitation, and radioimmunoassay (which provides an unnecessary degree of sensitivity).
2. The most frequently used test for CRP is the rapid latex agglutination test.

Other Plasma Proteins

Haptoglobin

1. Haptoglobin is 100,000-d plasma glycoprotein with α electrophoretic mobility.
2. Its principal function is to irreversibly bind to free hemoglobin released by intravascular hemolysis, forming a complex that is rapidly cleared by hepatocytes in the liver, thus preventing the loss of free hemoglobin in the liver.
3. Haptoglobin levels increase two- to fourfold attendant to injury.
4. It is frequently found in inflammatory exudates.
5. There is no quantitative correlation between plasma haptoglobin content and the severity of hemolysis.
6. "Normal" haptoglobin levels do not necessarily rule out a diagnosis of intravascular hemolysis.
7. Haptoglobin has two major genetic variants, Hp1 and Hp2.

Fibrinogen

1. After a surgical incision, fibrinogen accumulates at the site of injury for 1 to 2 weeks.
2. Fibrin is formed, which increases the tensile strength of the wound and stimulates fibroblast proliferation and growth.
3. Fibrinogen or fibrin degradation products can indirectly stimulate fibrinogen synthesis by hepatocytes, which suggests an amplification loop.

Alpha$_1$-Antitrypsin

1. This is one of a family of serine protease inhibitors in human plasma.
2. The physiologic targets are the proteases released from leukocytes rather than trypsin.
3. These proteases cause lung tissue damage and

pulmonary inflammation. Once bound to alpha$_1$-antitrypsin, their activity is completely inhibited, being later removed and catabolized.
4. The protein is synthesized in the liver.
5. Synthesis can increase fourfold when stimulated by inflammation.
6. The alpha$_1$-antitrypsin–protease complexes are not taken up by macrophages, although proteases can be transferred between alpha$_1$-antitrypsin and alpha$_2$-macroglobulin.
7. Homozygous deficiency of the protein can result in premature emphysema and liver disease.
8. Heterozygous deficiency of the protein results in an elevated risk of liver disease, connective tissue disease, inflammatory eye disease, and glomerulonephritis.
9. The protein has a role in several mediator pathways in the inflammatory response. Absence of the protein allows proteases to attack the tissue surrounding the inflammatory process and cause damage that may lead to chronic inflammation.

Ceruloplasmin

1. This is the principal copper-transporting protein in human plasma.
2. Ceruloplasmin and the copper it carries are essential to collagen formation and the extracellular cross-linking and maturation of collagen and elastin and may serve to protect the matrix of healing tissue against superoxide ions, generated by phagocytes in the course of clearing tissue debris and microorganisms.
3. Ceruloplasmin depletion or absence is associated with Wilson's disease.

Alpha$_2$-Macroglobulin

1. This is also a protease inhibitor in human plasma.
2. It binds to proteolytic enzymes released from damaged tissues as well as from phagocytic cells, thus partially inhibiting their activity.
3. The complexes formed are rapidly phagocytosed by macrophages and fibroblasts.
4. Alpha$_2$-macroglobulin appears to be a scavenger protease inhibitor that binds excess molecules that cannot be handled by the intended inhibitor.

5. The protein functions in hemostasis, coagulation, fibrinolysis, and complement pathways.

6. No diseases are associated with deficiency of this protein, suggesting that it may be essential for life.

Review Questions

Multiple Choice

Choose the phrase, sentence, or symbol that completes the statement or answers the question. More than one answer may be correct in each case. Answers are given at the end of this book.

1. C-reactive protein:
   (a) is a trace constituent of serum
   (b) was originally defined by its potassium-dependent precipitation with the C-polysaccharide of *Pneumococcus*
   (c) was originally thought to be an antibody to C-polysaccharide
   (d) is a nonspecific protein
   (C-Reactive Protein)

2. CRP is consistently found in cases of:
   (a) bacterial infection
   (b) active rheumatic fever
   (c) active rheumatoid arthritis
   (d) viral infection
   (C-Reactive Protein)

3. After the onset of disease, CRP usually appears in the serum within:
   (a) 1 to 3 hours
   (b) 14 to 26 hours
   (c) 3 to 5 weeks
   (d) 1 to 6 months
   (C-Reactive Protein)

4. Human CRP:
   (a) is a β globulin
   (b) is made up of 100 per cent peptide
   (c) has an amino acid composition similar to that of IgG
   (d) is not involved in the initiation of complement activation
   (Properties of CRP)

5. CRP has the ability to initiate:
   (a) precipitation
   (b) agglutination
   (c) opsonization
   (d) capsular swelling
   (Properties of CRP)

6. CRP:
   (a) crosses the human placenta
   (b) does not cross the human placenta
   (c) is thermostable
   (d) is thermolabile
   (Properties of CRP)

7. The elevation of CRP above the normal indicates:
   (a) the termination of the disease process
   (b) tissue damage
   (c) inflammation
   (d) none of the above
   (Properties of CRP)

8. CRP:
   (a) is present at all times when the ESR is elevated
   (b) is absent when the ESR is normal
   (c) has a variable range between normal and abnormal
   (d) is influenced by anemia or serum protein alteration
   (Laboratory Tests for CRP)

9. Tests for CRP include:
   (a) precipitation tests
   (b) the latex-fixation test
   (c) the slide agglutination test
   (d) all of the above
   (Laboratory Tests for CRP)

10. The molecular weight of CRP is:
    (a) 120,000 to 140,000
    (b) 250,000 to 300,000
    (c) 500,000 to 800,000
    (d) 60,000 to 80,000
    (Properties of CRP)

11. Haptoglobin:
    (a) is a 100,000-d plasma glycoprotein
    (b) binds to free hemoglobin released by intravascular hemolysis
    (c) increases as a result of intravascular hemolysis
    (d) all of the above
    (Haptoglobin)

12. Fibrinogen accumulates at the site of surgical incision for:
    (a) 6 to 7 hours
    (b) 1 to 2 weeks
    (c) 1 to 2 months
    (d) 1 to 2 minutes
    (Fibrinogen)

13. Alpha₁-antitrypsin:
    (a) is a serine protease inhibitor
    (b) is synthesized by the liver
    (c) increases when stimulated by an inflammatory process
    (d) targets the proteases released from trypsin
    (Alpha₁-Antitrypsin)

14. Ceruloplasmin:
    (a) appears to be the primary copper-transport protein for transferring copper to cytochrome C oxidase
    (b) is a glycoprotein
    (c) when absent is associated with Wilson's disease
    (d) all of the above
    (Ceruloplasmin)

15. Alpha₂-macroglobulin:
    (a) is a protease inhibitor in human plasma
    (b) is the principal copper-transporting protein in human plasma
    (c) appears to be a scavenger protease inhibitor that binds excess molecules that cannot be handled by the intended inhibitor
    (d) functions in hemostasis, coagulation, fibrinolysis, and complement pathways
    (Alpha₂-Macroglobulin)

Answer "True" or "False"

1. CRP is retained at high levels for many years after conditions of inflammation have subsided.
   (C-Reactive Protein)

2. CRP has been detected in the sera of patients following surgical operations.
   (C-Reactive Protein)

3. After the onset of disease, CRP may increase in concentration by as much as 5000 times its normal amount.
   (C-Reactive Protein)

4. The monitoring of CRP elevations in sequence is of no value in assessing disease activity.
   (Properties of CRP)

5. The latex-fixation test for CRP is considered to be more sensitive than other techniques.
   (Laboratory Tests for CRP)

6. There is a quantitative correlation between the plasma haptoglobin content and the severity of hemolysis.
   (Haptoglobin)

7. Fibrinogen or fibrin degradation products can indirectly stimulate fibrinogen synthesis by hepatocytes.
   (Fibrinogen)

8. Homozygous alpha₁-antitrypsin deficiency can result in premature emphysema.
   (Alpha₁-Antitrypsin)

9. Ceruloplasmin is the principal copper-transporting protein in human plasma.
   (Ceruloplasmin)

10. Several disease states are associated with alpha₂-macroglobulin deficiency.
    (Alpha₂-Macroglobulin)

GENERAL REFERENCES

Baron, E.J., and Finegold, S.M.: Bailey and Scott's Diagnostic Microbiology, 8th ed. St Louis, C. V. Mosby Company, 1990.

Bennington, J.L.: Saunders Dictionary and Encyclopedia of Laboratory Medicine and Technology. Philadelphia, W. B. Saunders Company, 1984.

Freeman, B.A.: Burrows Textbook of Microbiology, 27th ed. Philadelphia, W. B. Saunders Company, 1985.

Henry, J.B.: Clinical Diagnosis and Management by Laboratory Methods. Philadelphia, W. B. Saunders Company, 1991.

Sheehan, C.: Clinical Immunology: Principles and Laboratory Diagnosis. Philadelphia, J. B. Lippincott, 1990.

9

Streptococcus pyogenes

OBJECTIVES

The student shall know, understand, and be prepared to explain:

1. The etiology and morphologic characteristics of *Streptococcus pyogenes*
2. The epidemiology and manifestations (signs and symptoms) of *S. pyogenes* infections
3. The extracellular products of *S. pyogenes,* specifically to include:
   a. The characteristics of streptolysin O
   b. The properties of streptolysin O
   c. The significance of the antistreptolysin O reaction
   d. A comparison of streptolysin O and streptolysin S
   e. The serologic tests for antistreptolysin O
   f. The method of antistreptolysin O titration
   g. The rapid latex agglutination ASO procedure

Introduction

Streptococcus pyogenes (S. pyogenes) are cell wall antigens of Lancefield group A contained by most streptococci. They are gram-positive cocci that are β-hemolytic and are divided into serogroups A through O on the basis of the immunologic action of the cell wall carbohydrate. So-called *fimbriae,* which contain important surface components of the streptococcus, arise near the plasma membrane and project through the cell wall and capsule. The fimbriae contain lipotechoic acid, which is important in the adherence of the organism to human epithelium and the initiation of infection. Also on the fimbriae are the M and R antigens, which are structurally similar but immunologically distinct. R antigen has no known biologic role.

The major virulence factor of *S. pyogenes* is the M protein, a cell protein found in association with the hyaluronic capsule. This M protein is the basis for the subclassification of group A streptococci into over 60 M serotypes. Strains of *S. pyogenes* that lack M protein cannot cause infection. M protein inhibits phagocytosis, and antibody synthesized against M protein provides type-specific immunity to group A streptococci.

S. PYOGENES INFECTIONS

A number of infections are the result of *S. pyogenes.* These infections or conditions can lead to subsequent development of complications that are more important in terms of human morbidity and mortality.

Manifestations of *S. pyogenes* Infection

The manifestations of *S. pyogenes* include:

Upper Respiratory Infection. The manifestations of upper respiratory infection depend on the age of the subject. Infants and young children show an insidious onset of rhinorrhea (which is sometimes purulent), coughing, fever, vomiting, and anorexia. Cervical adenopathy may also be present. The syndrome is known as *streptococcosis*. Streptococcal pharyngitis is seen in children over 3 years of age. Most cases result in a fever, mild sore throat, and pharyngeal erythema without exudate (similar to viral pharyngeal erythema, which is not easily differentiated on clinical signs and symptoms alone). In some cases, however, pharyngeal erythema with purulent tonsillar exudate and petechiae may be observed on the palate, posterior pharynx, and tonsils, with younger children experiencing abdominal pain, nausea, and vomiting.

Scarlet Fever. This is the result of pharyngeal infection with a strain of group A streptococcus that produces erythrogenic toxin and is responsible for the characteristic rash, which usually develops on the second day of illness and results in hyperkeratosis with subsequent peeling. The signs and symptoms of scarlet fever are the same as those of streptococcal pharyngitis with the addition of a rash.

Skin Infections. These include impetigo, which begins as a lesion that itches and eventually crusts over and heals; cellulitis, caused by subcutaneous infection with group A streptococci and characterized by a warm, red, tender area that may be mildly swollen; and erysipelas, a distinct cellulitis syndrome that usually involves the face and may be associated with pharyngitis. Erysipelas is characterized by toxicity and a high fever and can be fatal if untreated.

Complications of *S. pyogenes* Infection

The attendant complications of *S. pyogenes* infection include:

Acute Rheumatic Fever. All M serotypes that infect the throat appear to be capable of causing rheumatic fever. A few serotypes have been identified that cause a much lower proportion of cases than would be expected from their frequency as a cause of pharyngitis. The incidence of rheumatic fever is directly proportional to the strength of the antibody response for streptolysin O. Prognosis is good when carditis is absent during the initial infection.

Glomerulonephritis. This may occur after pharyngitis or skin infections (pyoderma) with one of a limited number of nephritogenic M serotypes. The reason that these serotypes cause glomerulonephritis is unknown.

The Extracellular Products of *S. pyogenes*

Streptolysin O (SLO) is a bacterial toxin produced by virtually all strains of *S. pyogenes*. It is one of two extracellular hemolysins (or cytolysins), the other being *streptolysin S* (SLS). SLO is released during infection as indicated by antibody production to it. The toxin is a protein with a molecular weight of approximately 70,000, which, in its reduced state, brings about the lysis of red and white blood cells.

PROPERTIES OF STREPTOLYSIN O

Streptolysin O is so called because of its oxygen lability, and it is quite distinct from SLS (see later discussion). It is hemolytically inactive in the oxidized form and is characteristic of a group of cytolytic toxins known as the *oxygen-labile toxins* (Bernheimer, 1970), which are produced by several different gram-positive bacteria and possess a number of common properties—they are activated by sulfhydryl (SH) compounds, they appear to be antigenically related, and their biologic activity is completely inhibited by low concentrations (1.0 μg/ml) of cholesterol and certain related sterols.

Hemolysis of erythrocytes occurs within minutes after the addition of SLO, and toxic effects of SLO have been demonstrated on several types of mammalian cells in culture (Cinader, 1973). SLO is also cardiotoxic. It may cause interstitial myocarditis in experimental animals and systolic arrest of perfused mammalian hearts. Its cardiotoxicity is probably caused by inducing the release from atria of acetylcholine, which poisons ventricles. The first, the f site, contains two cystine residues and is responsible for the attachment of the molecule to the red blood cells; the second site, the t site, is concerned with the final hemolytic event.

It is evident that membrane cholesterol is the binding site of SLO, because only those cells that contain cholesterol in their membranes are susceptible to the toxin. In addition, SLO is inactivated only by the membrane lipid fraction that contains cholesterol; the addition of exogenous cholesterol to SLO inhibits toxic action, and treatment of erythrocyte membranes with alfalfa saponin or filipin inhibits the absorption of SLO (Shany *et al.*, 1974). These agents are known to bind to cholesterol in the membrane. The actual *mechanism* that results in cell lysis remains to be explained, however.

SIGNIFICANCE OF THE ANTISTREPTOLYSIN O REACTION

Streptolysin O is antigenic, eliciting the formation of antibodies that effectively neutralize its hemolytic action. A high proportion of patients with streptococcal infections show an antibody response during convalescence; therefore, the measurement of serum antistreptolysin O (ASO) has become a valuable and reliable indicator of streptococcal infection (particularly in cases of rheumatic fever and glomerulonephritis).

COMPARISON OF STREPTOLYSIN O WITH STREPTOLYSIN S

Unlike SLO, SLS is an oxygen-stable nonantigenic peptide with a molecular weight of about 2,800. Whereas SLO is synthesized only by growing streptococci, SLS is synthesized by both growing and resting cells and is found on the surface of washed streptococcal cells as a cell-bound hemolysin. The peptide, however, is loosely bound and can be released into the surrounding medium by a variety of carrier molecules (e.g., serum albumin, α-lipoproteins, yeast RNA, and nonionic detergents such as tweens and tritons). Upon release by the carriers, the hemolysin becomes recognized as SLS. Extracellular SLS, therefore, is a complex between a nonspecific carrier molecule and the specific hemolytic peptide. The peptide can be transferred among the various carriers and finally to the surface of mammalian cells. After the interaction with membrane phospholipids, the hemolytic peptide is inactivated. SLS is inhibited by lecithin and β-lipoproteins, but, unlike SLO, it is not inhibited by cholesterol. Further, red cells treated with SLO show distinct lesions similar to those caused by complement, yet red cells similarly treated with SLS show no such lesions. SLS, when injected intravenously, causes necrosis of the liver and kidney tubules and massive intracellular hemolysis. When injected intra-articularly, it can induce a chronic arthritis.

TESTS FOR ANTISTREPTOLYSIN O

The most widely used test for SLO is the neutralization test used to detect ASO in serum. This test is based on the fact that ASO can be specifically fixed to SLO *in vitro*, where it will neutralize its hemolytic activity. The test, therefore, by doubling dilution, estimates the amount of antibody that, in the presence of a constant dose of SLO, can completely inhibit hemolysis of a given number of red cells.

In the interpretation of ASO titers, many variables, including age, the severity of the infection, previous exposure to streptococcal infection, and the individual's ability to respond immunologically to the toxin, must be taken into account, because no set "normal" titer has been established. Most healthy adults (99 per cent) have ASO titers of 125 Todd units (or less). (The original ASO test procedure was developed by Todd, whose name is still used to express the levels of antibody titer. One Todd unit is that amount of antibody that completely neutralizes two and one-half minimal hemolytic doses of SLO.) Children, however, show fluctuating ASO titers from 5 to 125 Todd units. The usual titer normally decreases after 50 years of age, probably owing to a weakened immunologic response.

A rise in ASO titer of at least 30 per cent over the previous level is usually regarded as significant. In cases of rheumatic fever and glomerulonephritis, a marked increase in ASO titer is often seen during the symptom-free period preceding an attack of the illness. ASO titers in acute cases of rheumatic fever are usually between 300 and 1,500 Todd units and are usually maintained at high levels for a period of 6 months from the onset of disease. Drugs commonly used in the treatment of patients with rheumatic fever (e.g., sodium salicylate, aureum salts, and aminophenazone with phenylbutazone [Irgapyrin]) do not affect the production of SLO *in vivo*, but antibiotics (e.g. penicillin, Aureomycin), hormones, and cortisone inhibit the production of the toxin.

Increased ASO titers have been found in a large number of diseases (e.g., scarlet fever, cholera minor, tuberculous diseases, pneumococcal pneumonia, gonorrhea), although they are rarely above 500 Todd units unless the patient has had a recent streptococcal infection. Very low titers are observed in all states of the nephrotic syndrome, possibly as a result of a defect in formation, increased destruction of antibody protein, or loss of antibody protein in the urine.

A single high ASO titer is of little value to the clinician because a small number of healthy individuals have high titers. Significance should only be attached to changes in ASO titers determined by serial titration.

In addition to the ASO titration, a particle agglutination test has been described, which is generally less frequently used. This test involves coated particles (e.g., latex, treated erythrocytes, or certain bacteria) that are then mixed with diluted test serum on a slide. If the particles agglutinate, ASO can be regarded as present. It is possible to use erythrocytes as particles, because the SLO is in the oxidized state and, therefore, is nonhemolytic. The main advantage of this test when compared with the ASO titration is that lipoproteins, oxidized SLO, or bacterial growth products do not give false-positive results.

The streptozyme test is a particle agglutination test in which erythrocytes are coated with a crude mixture of streptococcal antigens. It is good for screening but has limited value as a quantitative test.

METHOD 1: ANTISTREPTOLYSIN O TITRATION

Antistreptolysin O titration allows the quantitative analysis of the antibody, based on an internationally recognized unit system (Todd, 1932). The system defines a minimal hemolytic dose of SLO as that amount of toxin that will completely hemolyze 0.5 ml of a 5 per cent suspension of rabbit red blood cells, measured in Todd units.

Materials

1. Saline—0.85 per cent
2. Streptolysin O buffer—this is commercially available from a number of supply houses. It is prepared as follows:
   7.4 gm sodium chloride
   3.17 gm potassium phosphate
   1,081 gm sodium phosphate
   Add to 1,000 ml of distilled water. The final pH should be between 6.5 and 6.7. The buffer may be stored at 4°C for up to 1 week.
3. Streptolysin O—this is available in dehydrated form from commercial supply houses and should be rehydrated just prior to use. Once rehydrated, the solution should not be subjected to vigorous shaking, and it must be used within 1 hour or discarded, because the active reagent is subject to inactivation by oxidation.
4. Red blood cells—a 5 per cent suspension of fresh (not more than 1 week old) human red blood cells (group O) is most commonly used in this test, although rabbit red blood cells are equally sensitive to SLO. The cells must be washed three times in diluent, and the buffy coat (white blood cells) must be removed. The final centrifugation should be at 1,500 rpm for 10 minutes, following which the packed red cells may be measured to achieve a 5 per cent suspension. Prepare the final suspension in SLO buffer.
5. Test tubes—12 × 100 mm are commonly used (round bottom).

Procedure

1. Prepare dilutions of fresh or inactivated serum as follows, using SLO buffer as a diluent:
   1:10 —0.5 ml of serum + 4.5 ml of buffer
   1:100—1.0 ml of 1:10 serum dilution + 9.0 ml of buffer
   1:500—2.0 ml of 1:100 serum dilution + 8.0 ml of buffer
   The first two serum dilutions are usually sufficient for preliminary titrations.
2. Set up the test according to the protocol given in Table 9–1.

TABLE 9–1. Protocol for Antistreptolysin O Titration

Serum Dilutions	1:10		1:100					1:500					Red Cell Control	SLO Control
Tube	1	2	3	4	5	6	7	8	9	10	11	12	13	14
Add serum dilution, ml	0.8	0.2	1.0	0.8	0.6	0.4	0.3	1.0	0.8	0.6	0.4	0.2	0	0
Add buffer solution, ml Shake gently to mix	0.2	0.8	0	0.2	0.4	0.6	0.7	0	0.2	0.4	0.6	0.8	1.5	1.0
Add streptolysin O, ml Shake gently to mix. Incubate at 37°C for 15 minutes	0.5	0.5	0.5	0.5	0.5	0.5	0.5	0.5	0.5	0.5	0.5	0.5	0	0.5
Add 5 per cent red cell suspension, ml	0.5	0.5	0.5	0.5	0.5	0.5	0.5	0.5	0.5	0.5	0.5	0.5	0.5	0.5
Shake gently to mix. Incubate at 37°C for 45 minutes, shaking tubes after first 15 minutes. Following incubation, centrifuge tubes for 1 minute at 1,500 rpm														
Todd unit value	12	50	100	125	166	250	333	500	625	833	1250	2500		

Interpretation

The ASO titer expressed in Todd units is the reciprocal of the serum dilution that completely neutralizes the SLO. For example, a serum showing no hemolysis in tubes 1 through 4, a trace of hemolysis in tube 5, and marked to complete hemolysis in the remaining tubes is reported as containing 125 Todd units.

Before reporting results, always ensure that the controls give the expected results.

METHOD 2: RAPID LATEX AGGLUTINATION ANTISTREPTOLYSIN O PROCEDURE

The rapid latex agglutination antistreptolysin O (ASO) procedure is based on the principle that, if polystyrene latex particles are coated with streptolysin O antigen, visible agglutination will be exhibited in the presence of the corresponding antistreptolysin O antibody.

Materials

Stanbio Laboratory Inc., San Antonio, Texas, provides the ASO Quicktest Kit for this test.

The kit contains:

1. ASO latex reagent coated with streptolysin O. Store at 2° to 8°C. Mix well before use.
2. 0.9 per cent NaCl solution. This is a saline solution containing sodium azide as a preservative.

3. Positive control serum. A prediluted serum containing at least 200 U/ml of ASO. This control should exhibit visible agglutination at the end of the 3-minute test period.
4. Negative control serum. A prediluted serum containing less than 100 U/ml of ASO. This control should exhibit a smooth or slightly granular appearance at the end of the 3-minute test period.
5. Glass slides with 6 wells. Use only the glass slide provided. The slide should be rinsed in distilled water and thoroughly dried with a soft cloth or tissue after each use.

Additional materials required but not provided in the kit:

1. Applicator sticks
2. Timer
3. 12 × 75 mm test tubes
4. Pasteur pipettes and rubber bulb
5. Serologic pipettes and safety bulb
6. 50 µl disposable pipettes and safety bulb
7. High-intensity direct light

Procedure (Screening Test)

Note: All reagents and specimens should be at room temperature before testing.

1. Label a 12 × 75 mm test tube for each patient to be tested.
2. Pipette 1 ml of saline into each test tube.
3. Add 1 drop of patient serum to each of the appropriately labeled test tubes using a Pasteur pi-

pette. Cover the tube and mix the dilution thoroughly by inverting the tube several times.

4. Label 1 division of the 6-cell slide for the positive control, negative control, and the respective patient sera to be tested.
5. Pipette 50 µl of the controls and patient sera onto the appropriately labeled cells. Use a fresh pipette for each specimen.
6. Add 1 drop of latex reagent to each cell.
7. Mix each specimen with a separate applicator stick. Spread the mixture evenly over the cell.
8. Rotate the slide for exactly 3 minutes.
9. Examine immediately with a bright source of direct light.

Interpretation

Agglutination indicates a positive result and no agglutination indicates a negative result, provided that the controls have given the expected results.

Agglutination demonstrates 200 U/ml or more of ASO. Positive result should be retested quantitatively. In semiquantitative testing, the U/ml of the highest dilution of serum to produce visible agglutination is the reported value.

The patient's serum should be prepared as follows:

Dilution	U/ml
1:30	300
1:40	400
1:60	600
1:80	800
1:100	1,000

Discussion

False-positive reactions can result from bacterial contamination of the specimen or if the reaction is observed after 3 minutes. Markedly lipemic serum or plasma may produce nonspecific reactions.

Most individuals will have a detectable ASO titer that varies with age and geographical location. A titer of 200 U/ml or greater may be associated with rheumatic fever or glomerulonephritis. A patient with an elevated titer should be retested over a period of 4 to 6 weeks to plot the course of the titer.

JUST THE FACTS

S. pyogenes Infections

1. *S. pyogenes* infections include upper respiratory infections, scarlet fever, and skin infections.
2. The attendant complications that can result from *S. pyogenes* infection include acute rheumatic fever and glomerulonephritis.

The Extracellular Products of *S. pyogenes*

1. Streptolysin O (SLO) is a bacterial toxin produced by virtually all strains of *S. pyogenes.*
2. The other extracellular hemolysin (cytolysin) is streptolysin S (SLS).
3. SLO (molecular weight 70,000) is released during infection as indicated by antibody production to it.
4. In its reduced state, SLO brings about the lysis of red and white blood cells.

Properties of Streptolysin O

1. SLO is so called because of its oxygen lability.
2. In the oxidized form, it is hemolytically inactive.
3. It is produced by several different gram-positive bacteria.
4. Like other oxygen-labile toxins, SLO is activated by SH compounds and is antigenically related, and its biologic activity is completely inhibited by low concentrations of cholesterol and certain related sterols.
5. SLO hemolyzes erythrocytes.
6. SLO is cardiotoxic.
7. Only cells that contain membrane cholesterol are susceptible to the toxin; therefore, membrane cholesterol is the binding site of SLO.
8. SLO is inactivated by the membrane lipid fraction that contains cholesterol.
9. The mechanism that results in cell lysis is unknown.

Significance of the Antistreptolysin O (ASO) Reaction

1. A high proportion of patients with streptococcal infections show an antibody response to SLO during convalescence.

2. The measurement of serum ASO is a valuable and reliable indicator of streptococcal infection.

Comparison of Streptolysin O with Streptolysin S

1. SLS is oxygen stable and non-antigenic (molecular weight 2,800).
2. SLS is synthesized by both growing and resting cells.
3. SLS is found on the surface of washed streptococcal cells as a cell-bound hemolysin.
4. The peptide is loosely bound and can be released into the surrounding medium by, for example, serum albumin, α-lipoproteins, yeast RNA, tweens, and tritons.
5. Extracellular SLS is a complex between a nonspecific carrier molecule and a specific hemolytic peptide.
6. SLS can be transferred among the various carriers and finally to the surface of mammalian cells.
7. After the interaction with membrane phospholipids, the hemolytic peptide is inactivated.
8. SLS is inhibited by lecithin and β-lipoproteins, but not by cholesterol.
9. SLS does not cause lesions on red cells (as does SLO).
10. Intravenous injection of SLS causes necrosis of the liver and kidney tubules and massive intracellular hemolysis.
11. When injected intra-articularly, it can induce a chronic arthritis.

Tests for Antistreptolysin O

1. The most widely used test for SLO is the neutralization test used to detect ASO in serum.

2. ASO titers must be interpreted, taking into account the variables caused by age, infection severity, previous exposure to streptococcal infection, and the individual's ability to respond immunologically to the toxin.
3. There is no set "normal" titer for ASO.
4. Most healthy adults have ASO titers of 125 Todd units (or less).
5. Children show fluctuating ASO titers from 5 to 125 Todd units.
6. The usual titer decreases after age 50.
7. A rise in ASO titer of 30 per cent over a previous level is regarded as significant.
8. In cases of rheumatic fever and glomerulonephritis, a marked increase in ASO titer is often seen during the symptom-free period preceding an attack of the illness.
9. In cases of rheumatic fever, ASO titers are usually between 300 and 1,500 Todd units. They are maintained at these high levels for about 6 months from the onset of disease. Drugs used in treatment do not affect the production of SLO, but antibiotics, hormones, and cortisone inhibit its production.
10. Increased ASO titers, although rarely above 500 Todd units unless the patient has had a recent streptococcal infection, are seen in scarlet fever, cholera minor, tuberculous diseases, pneumococcal pneumonia, and gonorrhea.
11. Low ASO titers are seen in all stages of nephrotic syndrome.
12. A single high ASO titer is of little value because a number of healthy individuals have high titers.
13. Other tests for ASO include a particle agglutination test, which does not give false-positive results with oxidized SLO or bacterial growth products, and the streptozyme test, which is good for screening but has little value as a quantitative test.

Review Questions

Multiple Choice

Choose the phrase, sentence, or symbol that completes the statement or answers the question. More than one answer may be correct in each case. Answers are given at the end of this book.

1. *Streptococcus pyogenes:*
   (a) are cell wall antigens of Lancefield group A
   (b) are contained by most streptococci
   (c) are gram-negative cocci
   (d) are gram-positive cocci
   (Introduction)

2. The attendant complications of *S. pyogenes* infection include:
   (a) acute rheumatic fever
   (b) systemic lupus erythematosus
   (c) glomerulonephritis
   (d) all of the above
   (S. pyogenes Infection)

3. Streptolysin O:
   (a) is a bacterial toxin produced by virtually all strains of *S. pyogenes*
   (b) is a viral toxin
   (c) is released during infection
   (d) is not antigenic
   (The Extracellular Products of S. pyogenes)

4. Streptolysin O:
   (a) in a reduced state brings about the lysis of red and white blood cells
   (b) in a reduced state brings about the lysis of red cells only
   (c) is so called because of its oxygen lability
   (d) is the same as streptolysin S
   (Properties of Streptolysin O)

5. The molecular weight of streptolysin O is:
   (a) about 5,000
   (b) about 70,000
   (c) about 250,000
   (d) about 300,000
   (The Extracellular Products of S. pyogenes)

6. The oxygen-labile toxins:
   (a) are activated by sulfhydryl compounds
   (b) are not related antigenically to one another
   (c) are inactivated by sulfhydryl compounds
   (d) are inhibited in their biologic activity by low concentrations of cholesterol
   (Properties of Streptolysin O)

7. Streptolysin O possesses:
   (a) two active sites
   (b) three active sites
   (c) four active sites

   (d) six active sites
   (Properties of Streptolysin O)

8. Streptolysin S:
   (a) is an oxygen-labile toxin
   (b) is nonantigenic
   (c) has a molecular weight similar to that of streptolysin O
   (d) is synthesized only by growing streptococci
   (Comparison of Streptolysin O with Streptolysin S)

9. In the interpretation of ASO titers, which of the following must be taken into account:
   (a) the age of the patient
   (b) previous exposure to streptococcal infection
   (c) the individual's ability to respond immunologically to the toxin
   (d) all of the above
   (Tests for Antistreptolysin O)

10. The ASO titer in children is:
    (a) usually high
    (b) usually below 5 Todd units
    (c) usually between 5 and 125 Todd units
    (d) usually between 300 and 500 Todd units
    (Tests for Antistreptolysin O)

11. The production of streptolysin O *in vivo* is inhibited by:
    (a) sodium salicylate
    (b) penicillin
    (c) aureum salts
    (d) cortisone
    (Tests for Antistreptolysin O)

12. The particle agglutination test for streptolysin O:
    (a) is more frequently used than the antistreptolysin O titration
    (b) involves particles coated with latex, treated erythrocytes, or certain bacteria
    (c) is unreliable because of the probability of false-positive results
    (d) is a useful quantitative test
    (Tests for Antistreptolysin O)

Answer "True" or "False"

1. Strains of *S. pyogenes* that lack M protein cannot cause infection.
   (Introduction)

2. Impetigo is not one of the manifestations of *S. pyogenes* infection.
   (S. pyogenes Infections)

3. Streptolysin O is quite distinct from streptolysin S.
   (Properties of Streptolysin O)

4. Streptolysin O is cardiotoxic.
   (Properties of Streptolysin O)

5. Streptolysin O is inactivated by the membrane lipid fraction of cells that lack cholesterol.
   (Properties of Streptolysin O)

6. Red cells treated with streptolysin O show distinct lesions similar to those caused by complement.
   (Comparison of Streptolysin O with Streptolysin S)

7. Increased ASO titers have been found in cases of scarlet fever, where the level is usually more than 1,000 Todd units.
   (Tests for Antistreptolysin O)

GENERAL REFERENCES

Baron, E.J., and Finegold, S.M.: Bailey and Scott's Diagnostic Microbiology, 8th ed. St Louis, The C. V. Mosby Company, 1990.

Bennington, J.L.: Saunders Dictionary and Encyclopedia of Laboratory Medicine and Technology. Philadelphia, W. B. Saunders Company, 1984.

Dorland's Illustrated Medical Dictionary, 27th ed. Philadelphia, W. B. Saunders Company, 1988.

Freeman, B.A.: Burrows Textbook of Microbiology, 27th ed. Philadelphia, W. B. Saunders Company, 1985.

Henry, J.B.: Clinical Diagnosis and Management by Laboratory Methods. Philadelphia, W. B. Saunders Company, 1991.

Sheehan, C.: Clinical Immunology; Principles and Laboratory Diagnosis. Philadelphia, J. B. Lippincott, 1990.

10

Cold Agglutinins;
Streptococcus MG

OBJECTIVES

The student shall know, understand, and be prepared to explain:
1. The characteristics of cold agglutinins
2. Cold agglutinin syndrome
3. Cold agglutinins in *Mycoplasma pneumoniae* infection and infectious mononucleosis
4. Cold agglutinins in other disease states
5. Tests for cold agglutinins, specifically:
   a. Rapid screen for cold agglutinins
   b. Titration of cold agglutinins
6. The characteristics of streptococcus MG
7. The tests for streptococcus MG, specifically the streptococcus Mg agglutination test

COLD AGGLUTININS

Introduction

Cold agglutinins were initially demonstrated by Landsteiner (1903) through the observation that agglutination would occur when the serum of an animal was mixed with its own red cells at a temperature near 0°C. It was later shown that this phenomenon also applied to most human subjects (Landsteiner and Levine, 1926). The significance of these cold agglutinins with respect to human disease, however, was not fully appreciated until many years later.

At a shallow but convenient level, cold agglutinins can be divided into two groups: those that are "harmless," having anti-I or anti-H or (rarely) anti-Pr specificity and present in all normal sera; and those that are "harmful," the so-called pathologic cold autoagglutinins, which have anti-I, anti-i, and (rarely) other specificities and are found in cases of chronic cold agglutinin syndrome and transiently following mycoplasmal infection.

A detailed study of cold agglutinins is unnecessary for the serologist although the interested reader is referred to the excellent texts by Mollison, *et al.* (1987) and Petz and Garratty (1980) for more detailed information (see General References at the end of this chapter). This discussion will be confined to those areas that involve the serology laboratory. Cold agglutinins with respect to autoimmune hemolytic anemia are discussed in Chapter 14.

Characteristics

By definition, cold agglutinins are antibodies that react best with red blood cells at temperatures *below* 37°C. The reaction strength is often greatest at temperatures of 0° to 4°C. At temperatures of 25° to 30°C, these reactions are generally not manifest, although the thermal maximum is dependent upon the concentration and binding affinity of the cold agglutinin. Those cold agglutinins that are active only to a temperature of 10° to 15°C are regarded as harmless, whereas those that are active *in vitro* up to a temperature of 30°C or more are generally associated with such harmful effects as blocking of small vessels on exposure to cold due to red cell agglutination, and with the production of hemolytic anemia. Between these two extremes are many examples of cold agglutinins that are active up to a temperature of 25°C and are found in association with disease.

The agglutination observed with cold agglutinins can be eliminated by warming and may be reversed to the original agglutinated state by recooling the specimen. The antibody agglutinates all adult human red blood cells, regardless of group, although some variation in reaction strength is often observed. In addition, the agglutinating serum reacts with the erythrocytes of many unrelated species. They may be absorbed to exhaustion by erythrocytes in the cold but are unaffected by absorption at 37°C. They may be stored in the cold with only a slight diminution of potency.

Cold Agglutinin Syndrome

Cold agglutinin syndrome is a condition in which there is a high titer of cold agglutinins causing intravascular agglutination when the blood is cooled in peripheral parts of the body exposed to the cold, which may cause mild hemolytic anemia as a result of complement fixation. The condition is reversible by rewarming the exposed parts of the body.

The syndrome occurs in two distinct clinical settings:

1. In the elderly, chronic cold agglutinin syndrome usually has a gradual onset and chronic course. The agglutinins usually contain monoclonal κ light chains. This condition may also be due to the presence of a lymphoma in some individuals.

2. Postinfectious cold agglutinin syndrome, which commonly follows infection with *Mycoplasma pneumoniae* or infectious mononucleosis.

Those affected with cold agglutinin syndrome, in addition to a high titer of cold agglutinins, are also found to have large amounts of C3d, resulting in a positive direct antiglobulin test.

Cold Agglutinins in *Mycoplasma pneumoniae* Infection and Infectious Mononucleosis

Cold agglutinins are found in approximately 55 per cent of patients with *M. pneumoniae* pneumonia. In such cases, subclinical hemolysis is common and in a few patients there is an episode of hemolytic anemia (Tanowitz *et al.*, 1978).

Generally, cold agglutinin syndrome in *M. pneumoniae* infections occurs in the second or third week after the onset of the disease. The onset of hemolysis is usually rapid, and abnormal IgM cold agglutinins, which characteristically have anti-I specificity, increase in titer, reaching a peak at day 12 to day 15 and then rapidly decreasing after day 20. In some cases, the patient may already have recovered from the respiratory infection, then become ill again. Increasing pallor and jaundice occur, and splenomegaly is generally present. In a few cases, acrocyanosis and hemoglobinuria are seen (Pirofsky, 1969), and, in rare cases, gangrene may result from exposure to the cold. The hemolytic anemia, if this occurs, proceeds at an alarming rate and may be fatal (Dacie, 1962; Tanowitz *et al.*, 1978). The disorder may be more pronounced in cases of glucose-6-phosphate dehydrogenase (G-6-PD) deficiency and sickle-cell disease (Tanowitz *et al.*, 1978).

The involvement of cold agglutinins in *M. pneumoniae* infections has been the subject of several investigations. The fact that the antibody has anti-I specificity suggests the possibility of the presence of I-like antigen in the *M. pneumoniae* organism and a cross-reactive response (Janney *et al.*, 1978). This is supported by the fact that, whereas intact *M. pneumoniae* organisms do not inhibit anti-I, lipopolysaccharide prepared from them does. Furthermore, the cold agglutinins produced in rabbits following an injection of *M. pneumoniae* will inhibit these organisms (Costea *et al.*, 1972).

In *M. pneumoniae* pneumonia, there is a positive correlation between the frequency of cold agglutinins and the severity of the disease, the extent of pulmonary involvement, and the duration of the illness. Extremely high titers are sometimes found in cases of hemolytic anemia. A fourfold rise in titer is significant of acute involvement. Antibiotic therapy may interfere with the development of cold agglutinins.

In infectious mononucleosis, cold agglutinins of anti-I specificity are frequently present as a transient phenomenon (Jenkins *et al.*, 1965; Rosenfield *et al.*, 1965). Worlledge and Dacie (1969), in reviewing published cases, concluded that anti-i is present in about 50 per cent of patients with the disease. Fourteen of 30 sera from afflicted individuals agglutinated cord red cells (which possess the highest concentration of the i antigen) to a titer of 16 or more, whereas normal sera agglutinated the same cells only to a titer of 4 at 4°C. The antibody in patients with infectious mononucleosis is normally detectable *in vitro* up to a temperature of about 24°C, although in patients who developed a hemolytic syndrome (less than 1 per cent), the antibody was found to be active *in vitro* up to a temperature of at least 28°C.

Goldberg and Barnett (1967), in investigating a case of hemolytic anemia complicating infectious mononucleosis, found that the agglutinin involved was an IgG-IgM complex. The autoantibody (presumably anti-i) was found to be IgG, and the IgM was an anti-IgG antibody. Both antibodies reacted more strongly at 4°C, and the separated IgG was found *not* to be an agglutinin, although it sensitized red cells to agglutination by anti-IgG. Capra *et al.* (1969) suggested that these findings represented the rule in infectious mononucleosis with hemolytic anemia, although subsequent investigations have cast doubt on this conclusion (Chaplin, 1980). Many examples of IgM anti-i infectious mononucleosis have been reported (e.g., Troxel *et al.*, 1966; Wolheim and Williams, 1966).

Infectious mononucleosis is further discussed in Chapter 12.

Cold Agglutinins in Other Disease States

In the early literature on cold agglutinin syndrome an association with several pathogenic states was reported, although the significance of the relationship, in most cases, is questionable. Included in this group are trypanosomiasis, relapsing fever, cirrhosis, malaria, septicemia, pernicious anemia, and various forms of carcinoma (Pirofsky, 1969). The production of high-titer cold agglutinins has also been found (by the same author) to occur during influenza virus infection, occasionally involving an episode of hemolytic anemia.

Tests for Cold Agglutinins

In the serology laboratory, tests for cold agglutinins are most commonly requested in cases of suspected primary atypical pneumonia, where rapid screening tests have proved useful. If strongly positive reactions or reactions that increase in strength as the temperature decreases are observed, titration of the antibody is recommended. Tests should be performed regularly, because an increase in titer through the duration of the illness is of greater significance than a positive result on a single specimen.

The fact that cold agglutinins are absorbed by erythrocytes under cold conditions is of major importance in the determination of cold agglutinins. If specimens are stored and/or transported in the cold, most cold agglutinins of significance will attach themselves to the red blood cells and will therefore be absent from the serum when testing is performed. For this reason, specimens should be collected at 37°C and transported to the laboratory submerged in water at 37°C. If this is not possible, specimens should be warmed to 37°C for 30 minutes before the serum is separated from the cells. Centrifugation is not recommended, but if it is unavoidable, refrigerated centrifuges must not be used.

METHOD 1: RAPID SCREEN FOR COLD AGGLUTININS

Method

1. Place the specimen in a water bath at 37°C as soon as it arrives in the laboratory.
2. Separate the serum from the clot when the clot has retracted completely.

3. Using a Pasteur pipette, transfer the serum into a labeled tube and centrifuge at 400 rpm for 2 minutes.
4. Prepare a 5 per cent suspension of the patient's cells.
5. Set up 2 test tubes in a test tube rack.
6. Place 2 drops of the patient's serum in each tube. To each tube add consecutively:
   a. One drop of patient's red cells.
   b. One drop of group O cord red cells.
7. Incubate the serum-cell mixture at 20°C for 1 hour.
8. Read and record results.
9. Incubate the same tubes in a water bath at 15°C for 1 hour.
10. Read and record results.

Interpretation

If agglutination is observed at 15°C and 20°C, proceed with the titration technique as described in Method 2.

If agglutination is observed at 15°C but disappears as the tube is warmed to 20°C or higher, record the result as negative.

METHOD 2: TITRATION OF COLD AGGLUTININS

Method

1. Set out 10 tubes in a test tube rack.
2. Place 1.5 ml of diluent (physiologic saline) in tube 1 and 1.0 ml of diluent (physiologic saline) in tubes 2 through 10.
3. Add 0.5 ml of the patient's serum to tube 1, mix and transfer 1.0 ml to tube 2, mix and transfer 1.0 ml to tube 3, and so on, through tube 9. Tube 10 will serve as a cell control. By this method, dilutions will be 1:4 to 1:1,024.
4. Add 0.1 ml of the patient's own red cells (2 per cent suspension) to each tube.
5. Mix the contents by vigorous shaking of the test tube rack, and place racks at 4°C overnight.
6. Remove the tubes from the refrigerator and read immediately.

Interpretation

The titer of cold agglutinins is read as the reciprocal of the highest dilution exhibiting any agglutination (1+ agglutination is usually taken as the weakest when read macroscopically). After reading, place the tubes at 37°C for 2 hours and reread. If the titer was due to cold agglutinins, the erythrocytes will be dispersed and no agglutination will be seen.

Note: As for the rapid screen, specimens for titration of cold agglutinins must be kept at 37°C at all times until the serum and cells are separated.

STREPTOCOCCUS MG

Streptococcus MG is a nonhemolytic, gram-positive coccus that is isolated from the throats of patients with primary atypical pneumonia. During convalescence, patients with this disease often develop antibodies to streptococcus MG, which are specific and react with the capsular polysaccharide of the organism.

Forty-four per cent of patients with primary atypical pneumonia demonstrate positive streptococcus MG reactions. Agglutinins occur in more than 75 per cent of patients with severe attacks of the disease of long duration; only 20 per cent of patients with mild attacks of short duration develop agglutinins.

Streptococcus MG agglutinins occur in normal serum at low titers (1:10). A titer of 400 or greater in a single specimen is considered to be suggestive of primary atypical pneumonia, but a fourfold rise in titer of antibodies to streptococcus MG during convalescence is of greater diagnostic significance than a single positive result. These agglutinins are usually detectable approximately 2 to 3 weeks after the onset of the disease.

Antibodies to streptococcus MG are distinct from cold agglutinins, many individuals showing one but not the other reaction. The agglutinins to streptococcus MG are found in only about 4 per cent of patients with other diseases where they have no value as a diagnostic aid, the titers varying considerably yet never being extremely high.

Tests for Streptococcus MG

The most common test for the detection of streptococcus MG is the streptococcus MG agglutination test. Specimens for this test may be allowed to clot in the refrigerator, because antibodies to streptococcus MG are not absorbed by red blood cells as are cold agglutinins. The serum should be separated from the red cells and stored at 4°C. Excellent commercial antigens for streptococcus MG are available from Difco Laboratories, Detroit, MI, and from Baltimore Biological Laboratories, Cockeysville, MD.

It should be noted that, although the streptococcus MG agglutination test is helpful in the diagnosis of primary atypical pneumonia, the coccus itself is not the etiologic agent of the disease.

METHOD 3: THE STREPTOCOCCUS MG AGGLUTINATION TEST

Method

1. Set up 10 tubes in a test tube rack.
2. Add 0.2 ml of diluent (physiologic saline) to each tube.
3. Add 0.2 ml of the patient's serum to tube 1. Mix and transfer 0.2 ml to tube 2. Continue mixing and transferring, and discard 0.2 ml from tube 9. Tube 10 will then serve as an antigen control.
4. Add 0.2 ml of antigen suspension to each tube. The final dilutions are 1:4 through 1:1,024.
5. Shake the rack, and incubate at room temperature or 37°C for 18 hours.
6. Read and record results.

Interpretation

The highest dilution showing definite agglutination (1+) is taken as the endpoint. The titer is expressed as the reciprocal of this dilution (e.g., if the agglutination endpoint occurs at 1:1:28, the titer is 128). Note that low titers (i.e., less than 20) are not considered significant.

JUST THE FACTS

Cold Agglutinins

Introduction

1. *Cold agglutinins* refers to the reaction of serum and cells at a temperature near 0°C.
2. Cold agglutinins can be divided into two groups:
   a. Harmless—having anti-I, anti-H, or (rarely) anti-Pr specificity and present in all normal sera.
   b. Harmful—having anti-I, anti-i, and (rarely) other specificity, found in cases of chronic cold agglutinin syndrome and transiently following mycoplasmal infection.

Characteristics

1. Cold agglutinins are antibodies that react best with red blood cells at temperatures below 37°.
2. The reaction strength is often greatest at 0° to 4°C.
3. Reactions are generally not seen at 25° to 30°C.
4. Harmless cold agglutinins are reactive only to a temperature of 10° to 15°C.
5. Those cold agglutinins that react up to a temperature of 30°C are usually associated with harmful effects (the blocking of small vessels on exposure to the cold due to red cell agglutination, and the production of hemolytic anemia).
6. Between these extremes of temperature are many examples of cold agglutinins that are active up to 25°C and that are found in association with disease.
7. Agglutination with cold agglutinins can be eliminated by warming and reversed by recooling the specimen.
8. The antibody agglutinates all adult human red blood cells regardless of group, although some variation in reaction strength is often observed.
9. The agglutinating serum reacts with the erythrocytes of many unrelated species.
10. They may be absorbed to exhaustion by erythrocytes in the cold but are unaffected by absorption at 37°C.
11. Specimens may be stored in the cold with only slight diminution of antibody potency.

Cold Agglutinin Syndrome

1. This is a condition in which there is a high titer of cold agglutinins causing intravascular agglutination when the blood is cooled in peripheral parts of the body exposed to the cold, which may cause mild hemolytic anemia as a result of complement fixation.
2. The syndrome occurs in the elderly (sometimes due to the presence of a lymphoma) and occurs at all ages following *Mycoplasma pneumoniae* infection or infectious mononucleosis.
3. Patients with cold agglutinin syndrome also have large amounts of C3d resulting in a positive direct antiglobulin test.

Cold Agglutinins in Mycoplasma pneumoniae *Infection and Infectious Mononucleosis*

1. Cold agglutinins are found in approximately 55 per cent of patients with *M. pneumoniae* pneumonia.
2. Cold agglutinins occur in the second or third week after the onset of disease.
3. The IgM cold agglutinins characteristically have anti-I specificity.
4. The titer of these cold agglutinins reaches a peak at days 12 to 15, then rapidly decreases after day 20.
5. It is believed that there is an I-like antigen in the *M. pneumoniae* organism.
6. There is a positive correlation between the frequency of cold agglutinins and the severity of *M. pneumoniae* pneumonia.
7. A fourfold rise in titer is significant of acute involvement.
8. Antibiotic therapy may interfere with the development of cold agglutinins.
9. In infectious mononucleosis:
   a. Cold agglutinins of anti-I specificity are frequently present as a transient phenomenon.
   b. About 50 per cent of patients have cold agglutinins with anti-i specificity.
   c. The antibody is normally detectable *in vitro* up to a temperature of 24°C.
   d. In patients who develop a hemolytic syndrome (less than 1 per cent), the antibody could be active at 28°C.

e. The agglutinin appears to be an IgG-IgM complex. The autoantibody (presumably anti-i) is IgG and the IgM is anti-IgG.

Cold Agglutinins in Other Disease States

1. Cold agglutinin syndrome has been reported to be associated with several pathogenic states (e.g., trypanosomiasis, relapsing fever, cirrhosis, malaria, septicemia, pernicious anemia, and various forms of carcinoma). The significance of the relationship in most cases is questionable.

Tests for Cold Agglutinins

1. Tests for cold agglutinins are commonly requested in cases of suspected atypical pneumonia.
2. Titration is useful because an increase in titer through the duration of the illness is of greater significance than a positive result on a single specimen.
3. Specimens for cold agglutinin tests must be kept at 37°C.

Streptococcus MG

1. This is a nonhemolytic, gram-positive coccus that is isolated from the throats of about 44 per cent of patients with primary atypical pneumonia.
2. During convalescence, patients often develop antibodies to streptococcus MG.
3. Streptococcus MG agglutinins occur in normal serum at low titers.
4. A titer of 400 or greater in a single specimen is suggestive of primary atypical pneumonia, but a fourfold rise in titer of antibodies to streptococcus MG during convalescence is of greater diagnostic significance.
5. Antibodies are usually detectable 2 to 3 weeks after the onset of disease. The antibodies are distinct from cold agglutinins, many individuals showing one but not the other reaction.
6. Antibodies to streptococcus MG are found in only 4 per cent of patients with other disease, where they have no value as a diagnostic aid.

Tests for Streptococcus MG

1. The common test is the streptococcus MG agglutination test.

2. The test is helpful in diagnosis, but the coccus is not the etiologic agent of the disease.

Review Questions

Multiple Choice

Choose the phrase, sentence, or symbol that completes the statement or answers the question. More than one answer may be correct in each case. Answers are given at the end of this book.

1. The term "cold agglutinins":
   (a) refers to antibodies that react best with red blood cells at temperatures below 37°C
   (b) refers to antibodies that react best with red blood cells at temperatures above 37°C
   (c) refers to antibodies that have a thermal range between 25° and 30°C
   (d) refers to antibodies that most often react best at 0° to 4°C
   (Characteristics)

2. The thermal maximum of cold agglutinins is:
   (a) 0°C
   (b) 4°C
   (c) 10°C
   (d) dependent upon the concentration and binding affinity of the cold agglutinin
   (Characteristics)

3. The agglutination observed with cold agglutinins:
   (a) can be eliminated by warming the specimen
   (b) is reversible with changes in temperature
   (c) cannot be eliminated by warming the specimen
   (d) can be eliminated by cooling the specimen below 0°C
   (Characteristics)

4. Cold agglutinins:
   (a) agglutinate all adult human red blood cells regardless of group
   (b) agglutinate red blood cells of group O only
   (c) exhibit varying reaction strength from one sample to another
   (d) can be absorbed to exhaustion by erythrocytes at 37°C
   (Characteristics)

5. Chronic cold agglutinin syndrome in the elderly:
   (a) usually has a gradual onset and a chronic course
   (b) produces agglutinins in the patient that usually contain polyclonal κ light chains
   (c) may be due to the presence of a lymphoma in some individuals
   (d) produces agglutinins in the patient that usually contain monoclonal λ chains
   (Cold Agglutinin Syndrome)

6. Those individuals affected with cold agglutinin syndrome:
   (a) have a high titer of cold agglutinins
   (b) have large amounts of C3d on their cells
   (c) have a positive direct antiglobulin test
   (d) usually have a negative direct antiglobulin test
   (Cold Agglutinin Syndrome)

7. In *Mycoplasma pneumoniae* infection:
   (a) all patients have high titers of cold agglutinins
   (b) about 55 per cent of patients have abnormal cold agglutinins that have anti-I specificity
   (c) hemolytic anemia is the result in the vast majority of patients
   (d) there is a positive correlation between the frequency of cold agglutinins and the severity of the disease
   (Cold Agglutinins in Mycoplasma pneumoniae *Infection and Infectious Mononucleosis)*

8. In infectious mononucleosis:
   (a) cold agglutinins of anti-I specificity are frequently present
   (b) cold agglutinins of anti-i specificity are frequently present and thereafter persist throughout life
   (c) a hemolytic syndrome may develop in fewer than 1 per cent of cases
   (d) the cold agglutinins formed will react with cord red blood cells to a temperature of about 24°C
   (Cold Agglutinins in Mycoplasma pneumoniae *Infection and Infectious Mononucleosis)*

9. Streptococcus MG:
   (a) is a nonhemolytic, gram-positive coccus
   (b) is a nonhemolytic, gram-negative coccus
   (c) is isolated from the throats of patients with primary atypical pneumonia
   (d) often stimulates the production of antibodies in patients with primary atypical pneumonia
   (Streptococcus MG)

10. Agglutinins to streptococcus MG:
    (a) are found in 44 per cent of patients with primary atypical pneumonia
    (b) occur in normal serum at high titers (1:40 or greater)
    (c) are the same as cold agglutinins
    (d) are found in high titers in patients with a number of diseases
    (Streptococcus MG)

Answer "True" or "False"

1. Cold agglutinins that are active only to a temperature of 10° to 15°C are regarded as harmless.
   (Characteristics)

2. Cold agglutinins will react with the erythrocytes of many unrelated species.
   (Characteristics)

3. Cold agglutinins are found in approximately 90 per cent of patients with *Mycoplasma pneumoniae* infection.
   (Cold Agglutinins in Mycoplasma pneumoniae Infection and Infectious Mononucleosis)

4. Antibiotic therapy has no effect on the development of cold agglutinins.
   (Cold Agglutinins in Mycoplasma pneumoniae Infection and Infectious Mononucleosis)

5. Anti-i is present in all normal sera to a titer of 16.
   (Cold Agglutinins in Mycoplasma pneumoniae Infection and Infectious Mononucleosis)

6. Specimens for cold agglutinin testing should be collected at 37°C and, if possible, transported to the laboratory submerged in water at 37°C.
   (Tests for Cold Agglutinins)

7. Streptococcus MG is the etiologic agent of primary atypical pneumonia.
   (Tests for Streptococcus MG)

8. Antistreptococcus MG antibodies react with the capsular polysaccharide of streptococcus MG.
   (Streptococcus MG)

GENERAL REFERENCES

Baron, E.J., and Finegold, S.M.: Bailey and Scott's Diagnostic Microbiology, 8th ed. St Louis, The C. V. Mosby Company, 1990.

Bennington, J.L.: Saunders Dictionary and Encyclopedia of Laboratory Medicine and Technology. Philadelphia, W. B. Saunders Company, 1984.

Dorland's Illustrated Medical Dictionary, 27th ed. Philadelphia, W. B. Saunders Company, 1988.

Freeman, B.A.: Burrows Textbook of Microbiology, 27th ed. Philadelphia, W. B. Saunders Company, 1985.

Henry, J.B.: Clinical Diagnosis and Management by Laboratory Methods. Philadelphia, W. B. Saunders Company, 1991.

Mollison, P.L., Englefriet, C.P., and Contreras, M.: Blood Transfusion in Clinical Medicine, 8th ed. Oxford, Blackwell Scientific Publications, 1987.

Petz, L.D., and Garrity, G.: Acquired Immune Hemolytic Anemias. New York, Churchill Livingstone, 1980.

Pittiglio, D.H.: Modern Blood Banking and Transfusion Practices. Philadelphia, F. A. Davis Company, 1983.

Sheehan, C.: Clinical Immunology: Principles and Laboratory Diagnosis. Philadelphia, J. B. Lippincott, 1990.

11

Herpes Viruses

OBJECTIVES

The student shall know, understand, and be prepared to explain:

1. The general characteristics of herpes viruses
2. The general characteristics of the herpes simplex virus (HSV)
3. The transmission and clinical manifestations of herpes simplex virus type 1 (HSV-1)
4. The transmission and clinical manifestations of herpes simplex virus type 2 (HSV-2)
5. A comparison of HSV-1 transmission and HSV-2 transmission
6. The laboratory diagnosis of HSV
7. Cytomegalovirus (CMV) with respect to:
   a. General characteristics
   b. Epidemiology
   c. Congenital infection
   d. Acquired infection
   e. Latent infection
8. The effects of CMV on the immune system
9. Antigens and antibodies in CMV infection
10. Laboratory tests for CMV
11. Serologic tests for CMV, including:
    a. Passive latex agglutination
    b. The cytomegalovirus IgM assay
12. The varicella-zoster (V-Z) virus with respect to:
    a. General characteristics
    b. Epidemiology
    c. Laboratory diagnosis
13. The characteristics and incidence of human herpesvirus-6 (HHV-6)
14. The laboratory diagnosis of HHV-6
    Note: The Epstein-Barr virus is discussed in Chapter 12.

Introduction

There are currently six recognized human herpes viruses, known as herpes simplex type 1, herpes simple type 2, cytomegalovirus, Epstein-Barr virus, varicella-zoster virus, and human herpesvirus-6. All are fairly large, enveloped DNA viruses that undergo a replicative cycle involving DNA expression and nucleocapsid assembly within the nucleus. The viral structure gains an envelope when the virus buds through the nuclear membrane that is altered to contain specific viral proteins.

The viruses of the herpes family produce a number of clinical diseases, although they share the basic characteristic of being cell-associated, which may in part account for their ability to produce subclinical infections that can be reactivated under appropriate stimuli.

HERPES SIMPLEX VIRUS (HSV)

The most usual manifestation of HSV infection is the common cold sore or fever blister (herpes labialis). Although this manifestation has been described since ancient times, it was only in 1919 that the virus was isolated by inoculation of herpes labialis vesicle fluid into a rabbit cornea. The transmissibility of HSV was demonstrated by reinoculation from the infected rabbit cornea into the cornea of a blind man. The virus was shown to be etiologically related to a wide variety of clinical syndromes after its successful growth in cell culture. It was also shown to be related to subclinical infection, occurring with either primary or recurrent disease. Recurrent HSV disease usually occurs as a result of reactivation of latent virus residing in paraspinal or cranial nerve ganglia innervating the site of primary infection, but other distant sites may be involved. The activated virus presumably travels down the axon to the skin (or other site) and induces disease. In some cases, however, exogenous reinfection also occurs. Recurrence with cell-to-cell spread of virus occurs in the presence of serum-neutralizing antibodies.

HSV is widespread, and humans are the only natural hosts or known reservoir of infection for the human herpes viruses, although herpes viruses of other vertebrates do occur. The incubation period is 2 to 12 days, and there is no apparent sexual or seasonal predilection for infection. It has been reported that the incidence of seropositivity rises to nearly 100 per cent in some populations by age 45, with approximately 70 to 80 per cent of individuals having contact with the virus by age 25. Antibody prevalence in adults varies greatly with socioeconomic class (30 to 50 per cent of upper socioeconomic class adults have detectable antibody to HSV as compared to 80 to 100 per cent of adults in lower socioeconomic groups). HSV can be cultured from the oropharynx in about 1 per cent of healthy adults and from the genital tract of slightly less than 1 per cent of asymptomatic adult women who are not pregnant.

Malnutrition, concurrent debilitating disease, a variety of acute childhood illnesses, and prematurity all predispose to disseminated primary infections in infants and young children. Neonatal HSV infections may be acquired in the antenatal or perinatal period. The majority are acquired perinatally as a result of exposure to an infected birth canal during delivery. Acquired HSV infection in the mother's genital tract late in pregnancy with active lesions present at the time of birth presents the greatest risk to the fetus, although more than half of clinically infected infants are born to asymptomatic mothers. The spectrum of disease occurring in an infected neonate varies from subclinical to severe. Symptoms and signs reflect the organ of involvement. In cases of overwhelming generalized infection, encephalitis and respiratory and/or hepatic failure with increasing jaundice and adrenal insufficiency may occur. Infants that survive infection are often, but not always, left with some degree of neurologic damage and may manifest recurrent vesicular skin lesions for many years.

Two cross-reacting antigenic types of HSV have been identified, known as herpes simplex type 1 (HSV-1) and herpes simplex type 2 (HSV-2).

Herpes Simplex Type 1 (HSV-1)

HSV-1 is generally found in and around the oral cavity and in skin lesions that occur above the waist. The transmission of the virus is usually nonvenereal but probably requires close contact (e.g., hand-to-mouth and kissing). Young children and preadolescents (i.e., beyond the neonatal period) are infected almost exclusively with HSV-1.

The most common clinical manifestation of primary HSV-1 infection is acute gingivostomatitis, which occurs most frequently in children between the ages of 1 and 4 years. Other manifestations of primary HSV infections include rhinitis, keratoconjunctivitis, meningoencephalitis, eczema herpeticum (Kaposi's varicelliform eruption), and traumatic herpes (e.g., herpetic whitlow and generalized infection). In young adults, primary HSV-1 infection may frequently produce an acute upper respiratory illness with pharyngitis and tonsillitis (Glezen et al., 1975).

Follicular conjunctivitis with chemosis, edema, and corneal ulcers is also caused by primary HSV-1 infection. The ulcers may progress from small dendritic ulcers to large "geographic" ulcers. Secondary bacterial infection may then lead to opacification of the lens. Herpes labialis and dendritic corneal ulcers are the most common manifestation of symptomatic, recurrent HSV-1 infection. A predilection for esophageal ulceration and interstitial pneumonitis (as well as disseminated disease) is seen in immunosuppressed patients with primary or recurrent disease. HSV-1 will also (occasionally) cause a severe necrotizing encephalitis, usually affecting the temporal or frontal lobes. About 15 per cent of patients with HSV encephalitis (which has no age, sex, or socioeconomic predilection) have a history of recurrent herpes labialis, which is similar to the frequency observed in the general population. About 33 per cent of patients with encephalitis will manifest herpes labialis during the course of encephalitis.

Herpes Simplex Type 2 (HSV-2)

Herpes simplex type 2 (HSV-2) is isolated primarily from the genital tract and skin lesions *below* the waist, commonly from genital lesions in persons in the 15- to 30-year age group. The most common form of HSV-2 primary and recurrent disease has been recognized for about 200 years, but interest was reactivated because of the discovery of widespread venereal transmission and neonatal infection.

HSV-2 is the most common cause of genital vesicular lesions in humans. Primary HSV-2 genital infection in adults is occasionally accompanied by a benign aseptic meningitis, either from neurologic ascent or via hematogenous spread. Transient myelitis or myeloradiculitis can also occur concurrent with the infection.

Discussion

Although HSV-1 and HSV-2 have different modes of transmission and associated clinical disease, some overlap does occur. HSV-2 infection, for example, can occur in the oral cavity, and HSV-1 can infect the genital tract. When HSV-1 genital disease occurs in pregnant women, it may cause neonatal disease as well. Cutaneous vesicular eruptions, which are indistinguishable from varicella-zoster, can be caused by both types of viruses, and erythema multiforme, which is probably a result of an immune reaction to HSV, has been associated with both HSV-1 and HSV-2.

Laboratory Diagnosis

Several methods for the laboratory diagnosis of HSV are available, including isolation of the virus and the direct detection of antigen in tissues or cytologic preparation, using immunofluorescence or immunoenzyme methods (Cleveland, 1987). In addition, the detection of the virus in body fluids (using monoclonal antibodies) can be performed using immunoassays or immunoblots (Lakeman, 1987).

The cytology and histology laboratories can be supportive in diagnosis in the proper clinical setting, but the tests performed are not as sensitive as viral culture.

The serology laboratory plays a supporting role in the determination of the prevalence of exposure to HSV and for diagnosing primary infection when a fourfold or greater rise in titer is demonstrated. Titers may rise significantly in early recurrent infections but usually become stabilized (at moderately high levels) following multiple recurrences. The immunoglobulin class of the antibody produced in response to the virus may be determined using indirect immunofluorescence and enzyme immunoassay methods.

CYTOMEGALOVIRUS (CMV)

Cytomegalovirus (CMV) is a ubiquitous human viral pathogen that is indistinguishable in negative-

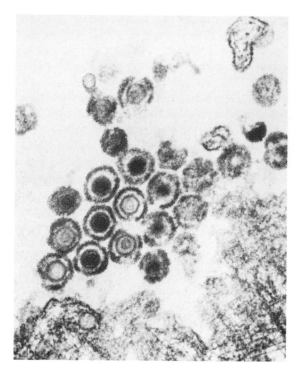

Figure 11–1. A group of negatively stained CMV particles. Note the "owl's eye" appearance. (From Krugman, S. *et al.*: Infectious Diseases of Children, 8th ed. St Louis, The C. V. Mosby Co., 1985, p. 9. Courtesy of Janet P. Smith, Ph.D.)

staining microscopy from herpes simplex and varicella. The characteristic changes now associated with CMV infection (i.e., striking epithelial cell cytomegaly with a single, large, red intranuclear inclusion surrounded by a halo, which gives the cell the appearance of an owl's eye [Fig. 11–1]) were first described in 1904, but it was not until 1956 and 1957 that the CMV was isolated in the laboratory. In 1966, the actual isolation of the virus following transfusion was reported, as was the observation of elevated antibody titers.

CMV infections have a long incubation period (from weeks to months), which parallels a slow replicative cycle in tissue culture. The infections may be local or systemic and can be either active or latent.

Epidemiology

CMV infection is endemic worldwide. It is most prevalent among very young children, particularly those living in crowded conditions, and may be transmitted by oral, respiratory, or venereal routes. It may also be transmitted through organ transplant or in fresh transfused blood. The most likely mode of transmission is venereal as a result of contact with the virus in body secretions. Transmission appears to require direct and intimate contact with secretions or excretions (urine, tears, respiratory secretions, genital secretions, feces, blood, and breast milk). Occasionally, the transfusion of blood from a healthy, asymptomatic donor is followed by active CMV infection in the recipient. It would appear that blood leukocytes and transplanted tissues are the sources of CMV.

The prevalence of viral excretion in the urine, which denotes active infection, varies from 0.5 to 2 per cent at birth to 10 to 56 per cent at 6 months of age, depending on the socioeconomic status and living conditions of the population studied. By 1 year of age, the prevalence of viral excretion usually plateaus or declines to a point where only about 1 per cent of healthy adults excrete virus in the urine (except in pregnancy, where about 4 to 13 per cent of women excrete the virus in urine). Seropositivity, which also reflects exposure to CMV, increases slowly during childhood and rises significantly during adolescence. By age 35, between 35 and 100 per cent of adults have detectable antibodies (again, depending on the socioeconomic status of the population under study).

Congenital Infection

CMV is believed to be the most common cause of congenital infection in humans, affecting 0.5 to 2.4 per cent of live births. The mode of natural transmission of virus from mother to fetus is ill defined because generally the transmission is asymptomatic. About 1 per cent of newborns manifest damage caused by CMV, some becoming seriously ill, with death occurring in some premature infants. Maternal CMV infections are subject to recurrence (like herpes simplex virus infections), especially in the genital tract. The role of recurrent infection in intrauterine transmission, however, is poorly understood.

Symptomatic congenital CMV infections are characterized by a high incidence of neurologic symptoms as well as neuromuscular disorders, splenomegaly, mild hepatomegaly with moderately abnormal liver functions, and jaundice. Newborns are more prone to develop severe cytomegalic inclusion disease (CID), which can be fatal or can cause mental retardation, deafness, vision defects, microcephaly, and motor dysfunction. In some causes, asymptomatic newborns develop hearing and neurologic impairment in later life. Infants sometimes excrete extremely high titers of CMV in the urine for as long as a year or more after birth and could therefore function as a source of acquired infection for others (see below).

Acquired Infection

Primary CMV infection can be acquired via oral or venereal routes, or parenterally by organ transplantation or blood transfusion. This type of infection is a major cause of morbidity and often mortality in patients with acquired immunodeficiency syndrome (AIDS). In general, CMV infection is asymptomatic and can persist in the host as a chronic or latent infection. Occasionally, a self-limiting, heterophil-negative, mononucleosis-like syndrome results with symptoms that include sore throat, fever, chills, profound malaise, and myalgia, with lymphadenopathy and splenomegaly in some cases. The virus may be excreted in the urine during both primary and recurrent acquired CMV infection and can persist sporadically for years. Later reinfection with the same or different strains of CMV or reactivation of a latent infection causes titers of virus in the urine and/or saliva to rise as high as 10^6 infective units/ml, and these levels can be sustained for weeks or months. Seroconversion usually results from infections occurring in immunocompetent individuals

CMV infection in normal adults and children usually does not produce complications. Infrequently, however, CMV infection can produce interstitial pneumonitis, hepatitis, Guillain-Barré syndrome, meningoencephalitis, myocarditis, thrombocytopenia, and hemolytic anemia.

Organ Transplantation. Seronegative patients who receive an allograft transplant from seropositive tissue are at risk of infection, the great majority of infections being transmitted by the donor kidney or arising from the reactivation of the recipient's latent virus. In immunosuppressed patients, only those who are seronegative appear to be at risk of developing CMV infection. Symptoms in these cases include fever, arthralgia, pneumonitis, leukopenia, and hepatitis. Other diseases in posttransplant patients include retinitis and glial-nodule encephalitis. Some of these conditions can be life threatening. For example, interstitial pneumonitis is a major cause of death following allogenic bone marrow transplantation.

Blood Transfusion. Studies of the acquisition rate of CMV infection following the transfusion of blood or blood components containing white cells suggest a 5 to 12 per cent donor CMV carrier rate. Neonates of low birth weight are also at high risk of transfusion-acquired CMV infection as a result of blood or blood component transfusion (estimated at 12.5 per cent). These infected infants can become severely ill with symptoms including pneumonia and hepatitis (Yeager, 1981).

Latent Infection

Latent infections, which are characterized by periods of reactivation of a virus, have not been clearly demonstrated with respect to CMV, the evidence being indirect and circumstantial. Cytomegalovirus has been recovered from the peripheral blood leukocytes of patients with active CMV infection, but attempts to recover the virus from the leukocytes of healthy donors have remained unsuccessful with the exception of one report.

Effects of CMV on the Immune System

Infection with CMV diminishes the immune response in both normal and immunocompromised individuals, which results in a decreased proliferative response to the CMV antigens. Alterations in the number of T-lymphocyte subsets, which persist for months, occur in patients with CMV mononucleosis-like syndrome, which increases the number of OKT8 lymphocytes (suppressor) and decreases the number of OKT4 lymphocytes (helper).

There is circumstantial evidence linking CMV to human malignancies (especially Kaposi's sarcoma), but so far no cause-and-effect relationship has been found.

Antigens and Antibodies in CMV Infection

Several antigens appear at varying times in cells infected with CMV.

Immediate Early Antigens. These appear within 1 hour of cellular infection before replication of viral DNA takes place.

Early Antigens. These appear within 24 hours of cellular infection before replication of viral DNA takes place.

Late Antigens. These are demonstrated in the nucleus and cytoplasm of infected cells at about 72 hours after infection, or at the end of the viral replication cycle.

The antibody response associated with infection differs in incidence and significance. In primary infection, a transient virus-specific IgM antibody is produced with eventual seroconversion and the production of IgG antibodies. The reactivation of latent infection in seropositive individuals is usually accompanied by a significant rise in IgG titer (no IgM antibodies are produced). When reinfection occurs due to a strain of CMV that is different from the original infecting virus, a significant IgG response occurs. Whether IgM is produced at this stage remains to be elucidated.

Laboratory Tests for CMV

The method of choice for confirming CMV infection is viral culture, which is routinely performed by direct immunofluorescent antibody (DFA) examination. It is also possible to demonstrate CMV in bronchoalveolar lavage specimens by DFA examination.

Hematologic examination of the blood usually reveals a characteristic lymphocytosis, with over 20 per cent variant lymphocytes being a common finding. Abnormal liver function tests may also be observed. The demonstration of inclusion bodies in leukocytes in urinary sediment offers another assessment of the presence of infection.

The isolation of CMV from urine or blood samples or the demonstration of CMV-specific IgM or increasing CMV-specific IgG antibody titers offers a definitive diagnosis. Several methods are available for the detection of CMV antibodies (see Table 11–1).

Electron microscopy can be used to detect virus

TABLE 11–1. Test Methods for Cytomegalovirus

Test Specific for	Method
Antibody	Complement fixation Latex particle agglutination
IgG antibody	Anticomplement immuno-fluorescence
IgM antibody	Indirect fluorescent antibody
IgG and IgM antibody	Enzyme immunoassay
Antigen	Direct electron microscopy Enzyme immunoassay
Cytomegalovirus mRNA	Nucleic acid probe
cDNA probe	*In situ* hybridization

in urine, and this method is reliable if a positive result is obtained. A negative result, however, does not rule out CMV infection.

The detection of IgM virus antibodies can aid in the diagnosis of primary infection or rare reactivation of infection. Contaminating antibodies (e.g., rheumatoid factor, antinuclear antibody, and nonspecific cold agglutinins) can cause false-positive results, however. Tests for heterophil, Epstein-Barr virus, and *Toxoplasma* antibodies are generally negative. The presence of large amounts of virus-specific IgG antibodies can hamper efforts to demonstrate IgM. In addition, an IgM response is not seen in about 50 to 90 per cent of congenital infections (depending on the method used) even in the presence of virus excretion in the urine.

Significant increases in CMV-specific IgG antibody demonstrated by complement fixation, anticomplement immunofluorescence (ACIF), and enzyme immunoassay (EIA) suggest recent infection or reactivation of latent infection but offer no proof of this. The EIA method for IgM and IgG antibodies to CMV has replaced CF, ACIF, and IFA methods. Useful screening tests to obtain seronegative blood donors include latex particle agglutination and indirect hemagglutination.

Recently, newer methods for the detection of CMV have been examined. These include EIA and cDNA tests for CMV detection in urine and *in situ* hybridization (ISH) with cDNA of CMV, which allows for the detection of RNA transcript of CMV DNA in peripheral blood mononuclear cells. The ISH technique could become a new early detection method for CMV expression, since it is more sensitive than dot-blot hybridization (Northern blot).

Serologic Tests for Cytomegalovirus

Passive Latex Agglutination

The passive latex agglutination method for the detection of antibodies to CMV involves the mixing of latex particles (which have been previously CMV-sensitized) with the patient's serum. If antibody is present in the patient's serum, the agglutinated particles will be visible macroscopically. If antibody is not present, or in the event of low antibody concentration, the latex particles will appear smooth and evenly dispersed. The presence of CMV antibodies suggests that the patient has been exposed to the virus.

METHOD 1: PASSIVE LATEX AGGLUTINATION FOR THE DETECTION OF ANTIBODIES TO CYTOMEGALOVIRUS IN HUMAN SERUM

The technique described here is intended for use with the CMV Scan Kit provided by Becton Dickinson Microbiology Systems, Cockeysville, MD.

Materials

The kit contains:
1. CMV antigen-coated latex particles prepared from disrupted CMV that has been judged to be inactivated by bioassay procedures. The preparation contains 0.02 per cent gentamicin and 0.02 per cent sodium azide. Store at 2° to 8°C and return to refrigerator when not in use. Do not freeze.
2. Phosphate-buffered saline, pH 7.4, containing bovine serum albumin with 0.02 per cent sodium azide. Store at 2° to 8°C and return to refrigerator when not in use. Do not freeze.
3. Test cards, which must be flat for proper reactions. Care should be taken not to finger-mark the test areas, since this may result in an oily deposit and improper test results. Use each card once and discard. Store cards (in original packaging) in a dry area at room temperature.
4. Plastic stirrers

5. Dispensing needle, 21-gauge, green hub. At the end of each test day, remove the needle from the dispensing bottle and recap. Rinse the needle in distilled water. Do not wipe the needle because it is silicone coated and wiping could remove the silicone.
6. High-reactive control serum (human) with 0.1 per cent sodium azide
7. Low-reactive control serum (human) with 0.1 per cent sodium azide
8. Nonreactive control serum (human) with 0.1 per cent sodium azide

Additional material needed (not provided with the kit):
1. Centrifuge
2. Rotator with humidifying cover. Rotation should be between 95 and 110 rpm, with 100 rpm being the ideal. The rotator should circumscribe a circle approximately 2 cm in diameter in the horizontal plane. A moistened humidifier cover must be used to prevent drying of the test specimens during rotation.
3. High-intensity incandescent lamp
4. Micropipettors, 25 µl delivery
5. Vortex mixer

Specimen Requirements

A minimum of 2 ml of clotted blood or anticoagulated blood is required. The specimen should be centrifuged promptly and an aliquot of serum or plasma removed. Plasma specimens containing EDTA or heparin as an anticoagulant can be used for qualitative or quantitative testing using the same technique as for serum samples. Plasma specimens containing citrate phosphate dextrose adenine (CPDA-1) as an anticoagulant must be brought to a 1 per cent dilution in buffer before testing.

Specimens may be stored for up to 1 week in the refrigerator. If longer storage is required, store frozen at −18°C or lower. Serum specimens that show obvious microbial contamination should not be used for testing. The presence of mild lipimea or hemolysis, however, will not affect the test.

Note: Successful testing has been performed on plasma specimens in CPDA-1 from platelet units stored at 22°C for 5 days and from red cell units prepared for transfusion and stored at 2° to 6°C for 14 days.

Procedure (Qualitative)

Before beginning the procedure, allow the reagents to reach room temperature. Do not mix reagents from different kit lot numbers and avoid microbial contamination of reagents. The latex reagent should be mixed for 5 to 10 seconds (using the highest speed setting for variable speed mixers). Vortexing is necessary at the beginning of each batch of specimens even if more than one batch is tested per day. Remove the cap from the latex reagent and attach the green hub needle to the tapered fitting. Label each circle of the card with the appropriate identification of patient sera and controls.

1. Using a micropipettor, place 25 μl of each specimen (patient, high-reactive control, and negative-reactive control) on the appropriately labeled, separate circles, using a new tip each time.
2. Using a new plastic stirrer for each circle, spread the serum to fill the entire circle.
3. Hold the bottle cap over the tip of the needle and gently invert the latex reagent dispensing bottle several times. While holding the bottle in an inverted, vertical position, dispense several drops of the latex reagent into the bottle cap until a drop of uniform size has been formed. This pre-dropped reagent may be recovered after testing by aspirating it back into the bottle.
4. Dispense 1 free-falling drop (approximately 15 μl) of latex reagent onto each circle containing serum. (Note: To ensure proper drop delivery, the dispensing bottle *must* be held vertically.)
5. Hand rotate the card back and forth 3 or 4 times to distribute the latex antigen throughout the circle. Avoid cross-contamination with adjacent circles.
6. Place the card on a rotator and mix for 8 minutes under a moistened humidifying cover.
7. Immediately after rotation, read the card macroscopically in the wet state. To help differentiate weak agglutination from no agglutination, a brief hand rotation of the card (3 or 4 back-and-forth motions) can be made following mechanical rotation. Tests should be read under a high-intensity incandescent lamp. Fluorescent light is generally insufficient to distinguish minimally reactive results.

Note: For quantitative determination, perform serial dilutions of each specimen (25 μl) on the card, using a separate row for each specimen. Controls should also be run with the quantitative procedure.

Interpretation

Any agglutination of the latex reagent is regarded as positive. If the suspension remains evenly dispersed with no agglutination, report as negative. In the quantitative method, report reactivity in terms of the highest dilution showing any agglutination of the latex reagent. If the controls do not react as expected, the test must be considered invalid.

Discussion

A negative test result suggests that the patient has not been previously exposed to CMV; however, in the early stages of primary infection, antibodies may not be detectable. The presence of CMV antibodies in qualitative testing on a single acute-phase or convalescent-phase specimen is an indication of previous exposure to the virus but does not indicate immunity to subsequent reinfection.

In the quantitative test, a fourfold or greater rise in antibody titer on specimens collected 2 weeks apart may suggest recent infection, although absence of a fourfold titer rise does not definitely rule out the possibility of exposure and infection. Conversion from seronegativity to positivity or a change in antibody titer between specimens collected apart from one another may occasionally be caused by influenza A or *Mycoplasma pneumoniae* infections, suggesting stress reactivation of CMV antibody.

The following should be noted with respect to this procedure and in all procedures that involve CMV antibody detection:

1. Patients with acute infection may not have detectable antibody.
2. Seroconversion may indicate recent infection, but an increase in antibody titer by this method does not differentiate between a primary and a secondary antibody response.
3. The timing of antibody response during a primary infection may differ slightly. The pattern of antibody response during a primary CMV infection has not been demonstrated.
4. Test results from neonates should be interpreted with caution since the CMV antibody detected may be maternal in origin.
5. Although the CMV latex procedure will detect

IgM and IgG antibodies, detection of IgA and IgE has not yet been demonstrated.

6. A negative CMV test may be useful in excluding possible infection, but the diagnosis of CMV should be confirmed by demonstrating the presence of the virus directly or by viral culture.

The Cytomegalovirus IgM Assay

This test, which is an indirect enzyme-labeled immunosorbent assay, detects IgM antibodies to cytomegalovirus, using antigen-coated microwells as a solid phase. The test is useful as a clinical aid in the diagnosis of primary CMV infection. It should be noted, however, that specific IgM antibody has been reported in reactivations and reinfections, and that IgM antibody may persist for as long as 9 months in immunocompetent individuals and for even longer periods in immunosuppressed patients.

IgM responses vary between different individuals. For example, 10 to 30 per cent of infants congenitally infected with CMV fail to develop IgM antibody, and 27 per cent of adults with primary infection likewise do not demonstrate IgM antibody. In pregnant women, the presence or absence of CMV IgG or IgM response is of limited value in predicting congenital CMV infection. The presence of CMV-specific IgM antibody in the circulation of the newborn, however, is indicative of infection.

METHOD 2: CYTOMEGALOVIRUS IgM ASSAY (QUANTITATIVE)

The technique described here is intended for use with the kit provided by Sigma Chemical Co, St Louis, MO.

Materials

The kit contains:
1. Microplate wells coated with CMV antigen (strain AD 169). Store at 2° to 6°C with desiccant in the reusable plastic bag and reseal after opening.
2. Holder for wells.
3. Sample diluent, a buffered protein solution containing surfactant and blue dye, pH 7.5. It contains absorbent (heat-aggregated human IgG) and 0.1 per cent sodium azide. Store at 2° to 6°C.
4. Calibrator. This is human serum containing IgM antibodies to CMV at 100 arbitrary units (AU/ml). It contains 0.1 per cent sodium azide as a preservative and should be stored at 2° to 6°C.
5. Conjugate. This contains goat antibodies to human IgM labeled with calf alkaline phosphatase. It contains pink dye and 0.02 per cent sodium azide. Store at 2° to 6°C.
6. Substrate. This contains p-nitrophenyl phosphate, disodium, and hexahydrate 1 mg/ml, pH 9.6. This solution may develop a slightly yellow color on storage. Do not use if the absorbance of the undiluted substrate is greater than 0.4 at 405 nm when measured against water using a microplate reader or a spectrophotometer with a 1 cm lightpath.
7. Wash concentrate. This is a buffer solution concentrate with surfactant. It is prepared by adding the contents of the bottle to 1 liter of deionized water. Mix well. The wash concentrate contains 0.1 per cent sodium azide as a preservative and should be stored at 2° to 6°C.
8. Stop solution, an alkaline solution, pH 12.0. Store at room temperature. Note: This solution causes irritation. Contact with eyes, skin, and clothing should be avoided, as should breathing the vapor. Wash thoroughly after handling.
9. Positive control. This is human serum containing IgM antibodies to CMV and 0.1 per cent sodium azide as a preservative. The content (expected range) is stated as a percentage of calibrator on the label.
10. Negative control. This is human serum containing no detectable antibodies to CMV and 0.1 per cent sodium azide as a preservative. The negative control should be less than 30 per cent of the calibrator.

Note: Reagents from different lots should not be interchanged.

Additional material required (not provided with kit):
1. Spectrophotometer that accommodates a 1 ml volume, or microplate reader capable of accurately measuring absorbance at 405 nm.
2. Pipettes (10 μl, 100 μl, and 200 μl) and pipettor
3. Timer

4. 1 liter measuring cylinder
5. Squeeze bottle for dispensing wash solution
6. Dilution plates or tubes
7. Test tubes or cuvettes, 1.0 ml

Specimen Requirements

A minimum of 2 ml of clotted blood or anticoagulated blood is required. The specimen should be centrifuged promptly and an aliquot of the serum (plasma) removed. The specimen is unsuitable for testing if lipemia, hemolysis, or bacterial contamination is observed. If the specimen contains visible particulate matter, it should be clarified by centrifugation before testing. The specimens should *not* be heat-inactivated, as this will cause false-positive results.

If the test cannot be performed immediately, the specimen should be refrigerated or frozen. Frozen serum should be thawed rapidly at 37°C.

Procedure

1. Dilute calibrator, positive and negative controls, and test samples by combining 10 µl of each with 200 µl of sample diluent in labeled tubes or dilution plates.
2. Place the desired number of antigen wells in the holder.
3. Using a pipette tip, mix the samples and diluent by drawing up and expelling two or three times. Transfer 100 µl of each diluted specimen to the appropriate antigen well.
4. Include one well that contains only 100 µl sample diluent. This serves as a reagent blank and is used to zero the photometer.
5. Allow the plate to stand at room temperature for 30 (± 2) minutes.
6. Shake out or aspirate the contents of the wells. Wash the wells by filling them with wash solution from a squeeze bottle and shaking out or aspirating. Wash three times. Drain the wells on a paper towel to remove excess fluid. (Note: This washing procedure must be performed thoroughly to achieve accurate results. Bubbles should be avoided.)
7. Place 2 drops (or 100 µl) conjugate in each well, including the reagent blank well.
8. Allow to stand at room temperature for 30 (± 2) minutes.
9. Wash wells by repeating step 6.
10. Place 2 drops (or 100 µl) substrate into each well, including the reagent blank well.
11. Allow to stand at room temperature for 30 (± 2) minutes.
12. Place 2 drops (or 100 µl) stop solution into each well.
13. Read and record absorbance of each test at 405 nm within 2 hours after the reaction has been stopped.

Calculation of Results

Microplate Reader

Set absorbance at 405 nm to 0 with water as reference. Read and record absorbance of reagent blank. Then set absorbance to 0 with the reagent blank as a reference. Read and record absorbance of samples and calibrator. The CMV IgM antibody concentration is then expressed as a percentage by dividing the absorbance value of the calibrator into the absorbance value of the sample and multiplying by 100.

Spectrophotometer

Completely remove the contents of each well and transfer to cuvette or test tube. Add 800 µl of deionized water to each sample and mix. Set absorbance at 405 nm to 0 with water as a reference. Read and record the absorbance of each sample including the reagent blank. Subtract the absorbance of the reagent blank from the absorbance of each sample. Express the antibody concentration as a percentage by dividing the absorbance value of the calibrator (minus the absorbance of the reagent blank) into the absorbance value of the sample (minus the absorbance of the reagent blank) and multiplying by 100.

Interpretation

± 30 per cent of calibrator = positive for IgM antibodies to CMV

Less than 30 per cent of calibrator = negative for IgM antibodies to CMV

Note: Specimens giving absorbance values above

that of the calibrator should be diluted and re-assayed. The value obtained should be multiplied by the dilution factor. If cord blood is tested, there is a possibility of contamination with maternal blood. A follow-up specimen taken directly from the newborn should be tested to confirm positive results.

Discussion

In this procedure, false-negative results can be due to a low level of specific IgM antibodies (due to the specimen being obtained too early in the development of infection) or interference by competitive antigen-specific CMV-specific IgG (especially in congenitally infected newborns because of the presence of maternal IgG).

False-positive results can be due to interference by IgM rheumatoid factor (if present at very high levels) or interference by specific IgG. Serum containing very high levels of antibody to DNA (greater than 2,000 IU/ml), as can occur in systemic lupus erythematosus patients, may yield false-positive results.

Viral infections have also been reported to elicit heterotypic CMV IgM responses. About 30 per cent of sera from patients with heterophil (antibody-positive) mononucleosis show heterotypic CMV IgM responses. In addition, varicella-zoster virus (see later in this chapter) has been reported to cause heterotypic CMV IgM responses.

This test is of limited value in determining the timing of primary infection. It should be noted that the test is an *aid* to diagnosis and is not diagnostic in itself.

VARICELLA-ZOSTER VIRUS

The name of this virus reflects two associated diseases—varicella (chickenpox) and zoster (shingles). Primary infection with the virus results in the clinical manifestations of chickenpox. Following this, the virus enters a latent phase, presumably within nuclei of neutrons in dorsal root ganglia. The reactivation of the virus results in the clinical manifestations characteristic of zoster. Humans are the only natural hosts of the varicella-zoster (V-Z) virus.

Epidemiology

Varicella (chickenpox) primarily affects children in the 2- to 5-year age group, although susceptible individuals of any age can become infected. The disease is endemic, with superimposed epidemics every 2 to 5 years. The disease is highly contagious, although immunity is lifelong, with an 80 to 90 per cent clinical attack rate. It is presumed that the mode of transmission is via the respiratory tract, although the virus has only very occasionally been isolated from this site.

Zoster, which is less communicable than varicella, is a sporadic disease that occurs most frequently in middle-aged individuals (45 years and older). There is no sex, racial, geographic, or seasonal predilection for infection. Humoral immunity to varicella does not protect against reactivation and/or clinical zoster. The reactivation of V-Z virus is associated with a depressed host immune response. Manipulation of the spinal cord, local radiation therapy, and underlying diseases or therapy that suppress cellular immunity have all been associated with triggering the onset of zoster.

Characteristics

Varicella has a usual incubation period of 14 to 17 days, after which there may be a 1- to 3-day prodromal period of fever, headache, and malaise before the eruption of the characteristic red macular rash, which progresses to papules, vesicles, and pustules that crust over and shed without scarring. The rash usually involves the trunk more than the extremities, and for 2 to 6 days, successive crops of lesions continue to appear so that lesions in various stages of development are seen at one time.

There are a number of possible complications associated with varicella infection. For example, adults sometimes develop an interstitial nodular pneumonitis, which occurs concomitantly with the typical skin rash and follows a course of variable severity depending on the host's immune competence. Primary infection may also be complicated by several rare hemorrhagic varicella syndromes. Febrile purpura, which can occur a few days after the onset of the rash, is seen in both children and adults and is characterized by thrombocytopenia and hemorrhage into the vesicles. Another complication is postinfection purpura, which begins 1 or 2 weeks after appearance of the rash and is characterized by thrombocytopenia with gastrointestinal, genitourinary, cutaneous, and mucous membrane hemorrhage. More severe hemorrhagic complications include malignant varicella with purpura and purpura fulminants.

Encephalitic complications of varicella include cerebral involvement and acute cerebellar ataxia. Other complications include nephritis, nephrosis, hepatitis, myocarditis, arthritis, and Reye syndrome. Susceptible individuals who are immunosuppressed have a greater risk of complications following V-Z virus exposure.

Neonatal varicella may be acquired *in utero* or in the perinatal period. This can result in congenital abnormalities in the infant. It appears that if the mother's illness occurs 4 days or less prior to delivery, the infant is at greatest risk (Meyers, 1974).

Zoster infection is characterized by neuralgia for a few days to weeks, followed by the characteristic eruption typically confined to one or two adjacent dermatomes, although the distribution occasionally involves multiple dermatomes and may cross the midline. Persistent neuralgia is seen in older patients and can be severe, lasting several months to 1 year. The thoracic dermatomes are usually involved in zoster infection, followed in frequency by lumbar, cervical, and trigeminal nerve distribution. Encephalomyelitis may develop when cranial nerve roots are involved, and pleural inflammation may accompany a thoracic eruption.

Laboratory Diagnosis

The serologic methods most commonly used in clinical diagnosis of varicella infection are indirect immunofluorescence, an immunofluorescence method to detect antibodies to specific membrane antigens (FAMA), or enzyme immunoassay (Shehab, 1983). Complement fixation is also useful in confirming recent infection, but it is relatively insensitive.

The best way to confirm infection, however, is to recover the virus in human diploid fibroblast cell cultures. Rapid diagnosis can also be made by direct immunofluorescence to detect viral antigens in vesicular lesions (Drew, 1980).

Other methods for presumptively diagnosing V-Z virus infection include scraping the base of a vesicular lesion and histologically observing multinucleated giant cells containing intranuclear inclusions, or observing herpesvirus particles by electron microscopy. It should be noted, however, that these methods will not differentiate between V-Z and herpes simplex virus infections.

EPSTEIN-BARR VIRUS

The Epstein-Barr virus is discussed in Chapter 12.

HUMAN HERPESVIRUS-6

A "new" virus, classified as a herpesvirus because of its shape, size, and *in vitro* behavior, was isolated from peripheral blood leukocytes of six patients during studies of lymphoproliferative disorders (Salahuddin, 1986). Genomic analysis showed the virus to be molecularly unrelated to other human herpesviruses (Josephs, 1986). Initially, the virus was called B-lymphotropic virus, but subsequent studies (Lopez, 1988) indicated that T cells are the primary target of infection. The agent is currently classified as human herpesvirus-6 (HHV-6). Niederman (1988) reported patients with mild, nonspecific symptoms and cervical lymphadenopathy associated with serologic evidence of acute HHV-6 infection. Ueda (1989) and Asano (1989) implicated the same agent as the cause of roseola infantum (exanthem subitum).

Up to 75 per cent of infants develop antibody to HHV-6 by 10 to 11 months of age (Ueda, 1989), which suggests a high rate of seropositivity in the general population.

Laboratory Diagnosis of HHV-6

Culture methods include cocultivation of a patient's peripheral blood cells with cord blood mononuclear cells and examination of cultures after 5 to 10 days by electron microscopy and anticomplement immunofluorescence. Anticomplement immunofluorescence of infected cell cultures has also been used for antibody detection and titration (Lopez, 1988).

JUST THE FACTS

Introduction

1. There are six recognized human herpes viruses.
2. All are fairly large, enveloped DNA viruses.
3. All undergo a replicative cycle involving DNA expression and nucleocapsid assembly within the nucleus.
4. The viral structure gains an envelope when the virus buds through the nuclear membrane that is altered to contain specific viral proteins.
5. The herpes viruses produce a number of clinical diseases.
6. The herpes viruses are all cell-associated, which may in part account for their ability of produce subclinical infections that can be reactivated under appropriate stimuli.

Herpes Simplex Virus (HSV)

1. The most usual manifestation of HSV infection is the common cold sore or fever blister (herpes labialis).
2. The virus was isolated in 1919 by inoculation of herpes labialis vesicle fluid into rabbit cornea.
3. The transmissibility of HSV was demonstrated by reinoculation from the infected rabbit cornea into the cornea of a blind man.
4. The virus is related to a wide variety of clinical syndromes.
5. The virus is also related to subclinical infection, occurring with either primary or recurrent disease.
6. Recurrent HSV disease usually occurs as a result of reactivation of latent virus residing in paraspinal or cranial nerve ganglia innervating the site of primary infection, but other distant sites may be involved.
7. The activated virus presumably travels down the axon to the skin or other site and induces disease.
8. Recurrence with cell-to-cell spread of virus occurs in the presence of serum-neutralizing antibodies.
9. Humans are the only natural hosts or known reservoirs of infection for the human herpesvirus (herpes viruses of other vertebrates do occur).

10. The incubation period for the virus is 2 to 12 days.
11. There is no apparent sexual or seasonal predilection for infection.
12. Seropositivity rises to nearly 100 per cent in some populations by age 45 years.
13. Seventy to 80 per cent of individuals have contact with the virus by age 25.
14. Thirty to 50 per cent of adults in the upper socioeconomic class have detectable antibody, compared to 80 to 100 per cent of adults in the lower socioeconomic class.
15. HSV can be cultured from the oropharynx in about 1 per cent of healthy adults.
16. HSV can be cultured from the genital tract of slightly less than 1 per cent of asymptomatic adult women who are not pregnant.
17. Predisposition to primary infection in infants and young children can be caused by malnutrition, concurrent debilitating disease, and a variety of childhood illnesses.
18. Neonatal HSV infection may be acquired in the perinatal (most) or antenatal period.
19. The spectrum of disease occurring in an infected neonate varies from subclinical to severe, with symptoms and signs reflecting the organ of involvement.

Herpes Simplex Type 1 (HSV-1)

1. HSV-1 is generally found in and around the oral cavity and in skin lesions that occur *above* the waist.
2. The transmission of the virus is usually nonvenereal but probably requires close contact.
3. Young children and preadolescents are infected almost exclusively with HSV-1.
4. The most common clinical manifestation of primary HSV-1 infection is acute gingivostomatitis, which occurs most frequently in children aged 1 to 4 years.
5. Other manifestations include rhinitis, keratoconjunctivitis, meningoencephalitis, eczema herpeticum, traumatic herpes, and follicular conjunctivitis with chemosis, edema, and corneal ulcers.
6. Upper respiratory illness with pharyngitis and tonsillitis is frequently seen in young adults.
7. Herpes labialis and dendritic corneal ulcers are the most common manifestations of symptomatic, recurrent HSV-1 infection.

8. HSV-1 will also occasionally cause a severe necrotizing encephalitis, which has no age, sex, or socioeconomic predilection.

Herpes Simplex Type 2 (HSV-2)

1. HSV-2 is primarily isolated from the genital tract and skin lesions *below* the waist.
2. HSV-2 is most commonly isolated from genital lesions in the 15- to 30-year age group.
3. The most common form of HSV-2 primary and recurrent disease has been recognized for about 200 years, but interest was reactivated because of the discovery of widespread venereal transmission and neonatal infection.
4. HSV-2 is the most common cause of genital vesicular lesions in humans.
5. Primary HSV-2 genital infection in adults is occasionally accompanied by a benign aseptic meningitis, either from neuronal ascent or via hematogenous spread. Transient myelitis or myeloradiculitis can also occur.

Discussion

1. HSV-1 and HSV-2 have different modes of transmission and associated clinical disease, but overlap does occur.
2. HSV-2 infection can occur in the oral cavity, and HSV-1 can infect the genital tract.
3. When HSV-1 genital disease occurs in pregnant women, it may cause neonatal disease as well.
4. Both types of virus may cause cutaneous vesicular eruptions that are indistinguishable from varicella-zoster.
5. Erythema multiforme (probably as a result of an immune reaction to HSV) has been associated with both HSV-1 and HSV-2.

Laboratory Diagnosis

1. Several methods of laboratory diagnosis of HSV are available, including isolation of the virus and the direct detection of antigen in tissues or cytologic preparation, using immunofluorescence or immunoenzyme methods.
2. The detection of the virus in body fluids (using monoclonal antibodies) can be performed using immunoassays or immunoblots.
3. Cytology and histology can be supportive in di-

agnosis in the proper clinical setting, but the tests used are not as sensitive as viral culture.
4. The role of the serology laboratory lies in the determination of prevalence of exposure to HSV and for diagnosing primary infection when a fourfold or greater rise in antibody titer is demonstrated.
5. Early recurrent infections may significantly boost antibody titers, but following multiple recurrences, titers often become stabilized at moderately high levels.
6. The immunoglobulin class of antibody response can be determined using indirect immunofluorescence and enzyme immunoassay methods.

Cytomegalovirus

1. Cytomegalovirus is indistinguishable from herpes simplex and varicella in negative-staining electron microscopy.
2. CMV has a long incubation period (from weeks to months).
3. Infections may be local or systemic and can be either active or latent.

Epidemiology

1. CMV is endemic worldwide.
2. It is most prevalent among very young children, particularly those living in crowded conditions.
3. It may be transmitted by oral, respiratory, or venereal (most likely) routes, by organ transplant, or in fresh transfused blood.
4. Transmission appears to require direct contact with secretions or excretions.
5. Occasionally, the transfusion of blood from a healthy, asymptomatic donor is followed by active CMV infection in the recipient.
6. Blood leukocytes and transplanted tissues appear to be the sources of CMV.
7. One-half to 2 per cent of newborns show viral excretion in the urine (active infection).
8. These figures rise to 10 to 56 per cent at 6 months of age.
9. By age 1 year the percentage plateaus or declines.
10. One per cent of healthy adults excrete virus in the urine (except in pregnancy, where it rises to 4 to 13 per cent).

11. Seropositivity increases slowly during childhood and rises significantly during adolescence.
12. By age 35 years, 35 to 100 per cent of adults have detectable antibodies.
13. These percentages vary with the socioeconomic status of the population under study.

Congenital Infection

1. CMV affects 0.5 to 2.4 per cent of live births.
2. Transmission is generally asymptomatic.
3. About 1 per cent of newborns manifest damage caused by CMV; some become seriously ill, and death can occur in premature infants.
4. Congenital CMV infections are characterized by neurologic as well as neuromuscular disorders, splenomegaly, and mild hepatomegaly with moderately abnormal liver functions and jaundice.
5. Newborns are prone to develop severe cytomegalic inclusion disease, which can be fatal or cause mental retardation, deafness, vision defects, microcephaly, and motor dysfunction.
6. In some cases, asymptomatic newborns develop hearing and neurologic impairment in later life.
7. Infants sometimes excrete extremely high titers of CMV in the urine for as long as 1 year or more after birth and could therefore function as a source of acquired infection for others.

Acquired Infection

1. Primary CMV infection can be acquired via oral or venereal routes or parenterally by organ transplantation or blood transfusion.
2. This type of infection is a major cause of morbidity and often mortality in patients with AIDS.
3. Acquired CMV infection is generally asymptomatic and can persist in the host as a chronic or latent infection.
4. The virus may be excreted in the urine during both primary and recurrent acquired CMV infection and can persist sporadically for years.
5. Later reinfection with the same or different strains of CMV, or reactivation of a latent infection can cause titers of virus in urine and/or saliva to rise to as high as 10^6 infective units/ml.
6. CMV infection in normal adults and children usually does not produce complications.
7. Infrequently, it can produce interstitial pneumonitis, hepatitis, Guillain-Barré syndrome, meningoencephalitis, myocarditis, thrombocytopenia, and hemolytic anemia.
8. Seronegative patients who receive an allograft transplant from seropositive tissue are at risk of infection with CMV.
9. Five to 12 per cent of donor blood carries CMV, which is transmitted during transfusion.

Latent Infection

1. Latent infection is suspected but has not been clearly demonstrated with respect to CMV.

Effects of CMV on the Immune System

1. Infection with CMV diminishes the immune response in both normal and immunocompromised individuals, which results in a decreased proliferative response to the CMV antigens.
2. Suppressor T lymphocytes are increased; helper T lymphocytes are decreased.
3. The evidence linking CMV to human malignancies is circumstantial.

Antigens and Antibodies in CMV Infection

1. The antigens that appear at varying times in cells infected with CMV include immediate early antigens (within 1 hour), early antigens (within 24 hours), and late antigens (within 72 hours).
2. In primary infection IgM antibody is produced, with eventual seroconversion and the production of IgG.
3. The reactivation of latent infection in seropositive individuals is usually accompanied by a significant rise in IgG (no IgM is produced).
4. When reinfection occurs due to a strain of CMV that is different from the original infecting virus, IgG is produced (it is not known if IgM is produced).

Laboratory Tests for CMV

1. Viral culture is the method of choice for confirming CMV infection.
2. Characteristic lymphocytes (20 per cent) are seen in hematologic examination.
3. Abnormal liver function tests may be observed.

4. Inclusion bodies in leukocytes in urine sediment also suggests infection.
5. Definitive diagnosis of infection can be made through the isolation of CMV from urine or blood samples or by the demonstration of CMV-specific IgM or increasing CMV-specific IgG antibody titers.
6. Electron microscopy can detect the virus in urine. Absence of the virus does not rule out CMV infection.
7. The detection of IgM virus antibodies suggests primary infection or rare reactivation of infection. Contaminating antibodies can give false-positive results.
8. The presence of large amounts of virus-specific IgG antibodies can hamper efforts to demonstrate IgM.
9. IgM response is not seen in 50 to 90 per cent of congenital infections.
10. Significant increases in IgG suggest, but do not prove, recent infection or reactivation of latent infection.
11. EIA methods for detecting IgM and IgG antibodies have replaced CF, ACIF, and IFA methods.
12. Latex particle agglutination and indirect hemagglutination are useful screening tests for donors.
13. Newer methods include EIA and cDNA tests for CMV detection in urine and *in situ* hybridization (ISH) with cDNA of CMV.

Serologic Tests for Cytomegalovirus

1. The tests used in the serology laboratory for detection of CMV antibody are passive latex agglutination and quantitative determination of IgM antibodies to CMV in human serum.

Varicella-Zoster Virus

1. The name of this virus reflects two diseases, varicella (chickenpox) and zoster (shingles).
2. Primary infection results in chickenpox; reactivation results in shingles.
3. Between primary infection and reactivation, the virus enters a latent phase.
4. Humans are the only known natural hosts of the V-Z virus.

Epidemiology

1. Varicella primarily affects children in the 2- to 5-year age group.
2. The disease is endemic—epidemic outbreaks occur every 2 to 5 years.
3. The disease is highly contagious—immunity is lifelong.
4. The mode of transmission is assumed to be via the respiratory tract.
5. Zoster is less communicable than varicella.
6. Zoster is a sporadic disease that occurs most frequently in individuals 45 years of age and older.
7. There is no sex, racial, geographic, or seasonal predilection for zoster infection.
8. Humoral immunity to varicella does not protect against reactivation of clinical zoster.
9. The reactivation of V-Z virus is associated with a depressed host immune response.
10. Manipulation of the spinal cord, local radiation therapy, and underlying diseases or therapy that suppress cellular immunity have all been associated with triggering the onset of zoster.

Characteristics

1. Varicella has an incubation period of 14 to 17 days.
2. The characteristic rash appears after a possible 1- to 3-day period during which there is fever, headache, and malaise.
3. The rash progresses to papules, vesicles, and pustules that crust over and shed without scarring.
4. The rash involves the trunk rather than the extremities.
5. There are a number of complications associated with varicella infection.
6. Neonatal varicella may be acquired *in utero* or in the perinatal period.
7. If the mother's illness occurs 4 days or less prior to delivery, the infant is at greatest risk and can demonstrate congenital abnormalities.
8. Zoster is characterized by neuralgia for a few days and weeks, followed by the characteristic eruption, typically confined to one or two adjacent dermatomes (sometimes multiple dermatomes are involved).
9. Persistent neuralgia is seen in older patients

and can be severe, lasting several months to 1 year.

10. The thoracic dermatomes are usually involved in zoster infection.
11. When cranial nerve roots are involved, encephalomyelitis may develop.
12. Pleural inflammation may accompany a thoracic eruption.

Laboratory Diagnosis

1. Serologic methods include indirect immunofluorescence or enzyme immunoassay or complement fixation.

Epstein-Barr Virus

See Chapter 12.

Human Herpesvirus-6

1. This "new" virus is classified as a herpesvirus because of its size, shape, and *in vitro* behavior.
2. T cells are the primary target of infection.
3. Up to 75 per cent of infants develop antibody to HHV-6 by 10 to 11 months of age.

Laboratory Diagnosis of HHV-6

1. Culture methods include cocultivation of the patient's peripheral blood cells with cord blood mononuclear cells and examination of the cultures after 50 to 10 days by electron microscopy and anticomplement immunofluorescence.
2. Anticomplement immunofluorescence of infected cell cultures has also been used for antibody detection and titration.

Review Questions

Multiple Choice

Choose the phrase, sentence, or symbol that completes the statement or answers the question. More than one answer may be correct in each case. Answers are given at the end of this book.

1. Which of the following are currently recognized human herpesviruses?
   (a) cytomegalovirus
   (b) varicella-zoster virus
   (c) Epstein-Barr virus
   (d) HIV-1
   (Introduction)

2. The incubation period for HSV is:
   (a) 2 to 12 days
   (b) 2 to 12 months
   (c) 30 to 40 days
   (d) none of the above
   (Herpes Simplex Virus [HSV])

3. HSV-1:
   (a) is generally found in and around the oral cavity
   (b) can produce upper respiratory illness in young adults
   (c) is transmitted by the venereal route
   (d) can be transmitted by kissing
   (Herpes Simplex Type 1 [HSV-1])

4. HSV-2:
   (a) is isolated primarily from the genital tract
   (b) is isolated from skin lesions above the waist
   (c) is isolated from skin lesions below the waist
   (d) is the most common cause of genital vesicular lesions in humans
   (Herpes Simplex Type 2 [HSV-2])

5. Erythema multiforme:
   (a) has been associated with HSV-1 only
   (b) has been associated with HSV-2 only
   (c) has been associated with both HSV-1 and HSV-2
   (d) is probably a result of an immune reaction to HSV
   (Discussion)

6. Cytomegalovirus:
   (a) is a ubiquitous human viral pathogen
   (b) is indistinguishable in negative-staining electron microscopy from herpes simplex and varicella
   (c) causes an infection that has a long incubation period
   (d) all of the above
   (Cytomegalovirus)

7. CMV infection:
   (a) is endemic worldwide
   (b) may be transmitted through oral routes

(c) can follow the transfusion of blood from a healthy asymptomatic donor
(d) none of the above
(Epidemiology)

8. Congenital CMV infection:
   (a) affects 50 to 60 per cent of live births
   (b) affects 2 to 4 per cent of live births
   (c) is generally asymptomatic
   (d) causes symptoms in about 1 per cent of newborns
   (Congenital Infection)

9. Acquired CMV Infection:
   (a) can result from blood transfusion
   (b) can result from organ transplant
   (c) is the major cause of morbidity and often mortality in AIDS patients
   (d) is generally asymptomatic
   (Acquired Infection)

10. Infection with CMV:
    (a) diminishes the immune response
    (b) enhances the immune response
    (c) causes an increase in the number of OKT8 lymphocytes in patients with CMV mononucleosis-like syndrome
    (d) causes an increase in the number of OKT4 lymphocytes in patients with CMV mononucleosis-like syndrome
    (Effects of CMV on the Immune System)

11. The antigens that occur in cells infected with CMV include:
    (a) early antigens
    (b) immediate early antigens
    (c) late antigens
    (d) all of the above
    (Antigens and Antibodies in CMV infection)

12. The method of choice for the confirmation of CMV infection is:
    (a) complement fixation
    (b) electron microscopy
    (c) viral culture
    (d) heterophil antibody tests
    (Laboratory Tests for CMV)

13. Varicella:
    (a) affects children in the 2- to 5-year age group
    (b) is highly contagious
    (c) is less contagious than zoster
    (d) is always isolated from the respiratory tract of infected individuals
    (Epidemiology)

14. The usual incubation period for varicella is:
    (a) 1 to 3 days
    (b) 14 to 17 hours
    (c) 14 to 17 days
    (d) 2 to 3 months
    (Characteristics)

15. The serologic methods used in the clinical diagnosis of varicella infection are:
    (a) indirect immunofluorescence
    (b) enzyme immunoassay
    (c) complement fixation
    (d) passive hemagglutination
    (Laboratory Diagnosis)

16. The primary targets of infection of human herpesvirus-6 are:
    (a) T cells
    (b) B cells
    (c) both B and T cells equally
    (d) platelets
    (Human Herpesvirus-6)

Answer "True" or "False"

1. The viruses of the herpes family are capable of causing subclinical infections.
   (Introduction)

2. Neonatal HSV infections are most commonly acquired during the antenatal period.
   (Herpes Simplex Virus [HSV])

3. Young children and preadolescents are infected almost exclusively by HSV-2.
   (Herpes Simplex Type 1 [HSV-1])

4. HSV-2 infection can occur in the oral cavity.
   (Discussion)

5. About 1 per cent of healthy adults excrete CMV in the urine.
   (Epidemiology)

6. In immunosuppressed patients, only those who are seropositive appear to be at risk of developing CMV infection.
   (Acquired Infection)

7. CMV has been recovered from the peripheral blood leukocytes of patients with active CMV infection.
   (Latent Infection)

8. CMV may be linked to human malignancies, although this has not been proved.
   (Effects of CMV on the Immune System)

9. Early antigens appear in cells infected with CMV after replication of viral DNA has taken place.
   (Antigens and Antibodies in CMV Infection)

10. Significant increases in CMV-specific IgG antibody demonstrated by complement fixation offer proof of recent infection or reactivation of latent infection.
    (Laboratory Tests for CMV)

11. Zoster occurs most frequently in children in the 2- to 5-year age group.
    (Epidemiology)

12. Neonatal varicella may be acquired *in utero* or in the perinatal period.
    (Characteristics)

13. Complement fixation is useful in confirming varicella infection, but it is relatively insensitive.
    (Laboratory Diagnosis)

14. Human herpesvirus-6 is molecularly unrelated to other human herpes viruses.
    (Human Herpesvirus-6)

GENERAL REFERENCES

Baron, E.J., and Finegold, S.M.: Bailey and Scott's Diagnostic Microbiology, 8th ed. St Louis, The C. V. Mosby Company, 1990.

Bennington, J.L.: Saunders Dictionary and Encyclopedia of Laboratory Medicine and Technology. Philadelphia, W. B. Saunders Company, 1984.

Dorland's Illustrated Medical Dictionary, 27th ed. Philadelphia, W. B. Saunders Company, 1988.

Freeman, B.A.: Burrows Textbook of Microbiology, 27th ed. Philadelphia, W. B. Saunders Company, 1985.

Henry, J.B.: Clinical Diagnosis and Management by Laboratory Methods. Philadelphia, W. B. Saunders Company, 1991.

Turgeon, M. L.: Immunology and Serology in Laboratory Medicine. St. Louis, C. V. Mosby Company, 1990.

12

Infectious Mononucleosis

OBJECTIVES

The student shall know, understand, and be prepared to explain:

1. The Epstein-Barr virus (EBV)
2. The characteristics of infectious mononucleosis
3. A general outline of heterophil antibodies
4. The role of heterophil antibodies in infectious mononucleosis
5. Other antigens expressed by EBV-infected B lymphocytes, specifically:
   a. Viral capsid antigen (VCA) and antibody
   b. Early antigen (EA) including early antigen-diffuse (EA-D) and early antigen-restricted (EA-R), and their antibodies
   c. Epstein-Barr nuclear antigen (EBNA) and antibody
5. The serologic tests for infectious mononucleosis, including:
   a. The Paul-Bunnell test
   b. The Davidsohn differential test
   c. Rapid differential slide tests (spot tests)

Introduction

Infectious mononucleosis is a self-limiting disease caused by the Epstein-Barr virus (EBV). The disease may be confused with similar but more serious diseases such as diphtheria, pharyngitis, Vincent's angina, lymphadenitis with scarlet fever, hepatitis, or pertussis (whooping cough). Currently, the most effective method of diagnosis is serologic.

THE EPSTEIN-BARR VIRUS

The Epstein-Barr virus is an enveloped, human herpes double-stranded DNA virus that belongs to the family Herpetoviridae. It is ubiquitous and may be transmitted through saliva, blood transfusions, transplacental routes, and possibly by mosquitos, although under normal circumstances transmission of the virus through transfusion or transplacental routes is unlikely. Infectious mononucleosis results from primary infection with EBV, after which neutralizing antibodies develop and lifelong immunity protects against further exogenous reinfections. The virus infects B lymphocytes, but the variant lymphocytes produced in response to infection and seen in microscopic examination of the peripheral blood have T-cell characteristics. Once infected, an individual remains a lifelong carrier of the virus. EBV has been known to survive in peripheral blood lymphocytes and in epithelial cells of the oropharynx for years without producing disease.

EBV is present worldwide, and infection during childhood appears to be quite frequent, especially in less affluent socioeconomic groups, where 80 per cent of 5-year-old children are seropositive as compared to 40 to 50 per cent of 5-year-old children from higher socioeconomic groups.

In Western society, primary exposure to EBV occurs in two waves: approximately half the population is exposed to the virus before age 5 with the second wave of seroconversion occurring during late adolescence. Eighty to 90 per cent of healthy adults have antibody to EBV.

Individuals who lack antibodies to the virus are at risk of contracting infectious mononucleosis. EBV represents a minor problem for immunocompetent individuals, but immunologically compromised patients are at major risk. Blood transfusion from an immune donor to a nonimmune recipient may result in a primary infection in the recipient, known as IM postperfusion syndrome.

A minor percentage of patients experience symptomatic reactivation. This reactivation of latent infection has been implicated in a persistent illness referred to as the EBV-associated fatigue syndrome, but this phenomenon is not universally accepted.

The frequency of clinically apparent IM has been estimated to be 45:100,000 in adolescents. In immunosuppressed patients, the incidence of EBV infection ranges from 35 to 47 per cent. There is a carrier state after primary infection, as occurs with other herpes viruses.

Several different diseases are associated with EBV, notably Burkitt's lymphoma and nasopharyngeal carcinoma.

EBV has several different antigens that may be used to relate different diseases to EBV infections. The viral capsid antigens (VAC) are found in all persons affected by acute phase infectious mononucleosis. The antibody to VAC achieves maximum strength during the second week of the disease, then gradually decreases in strength, remaining at a low level throughout life. The so-called early antigens (EA) are also found in cases of infectious mononucleosis, but they disappear early after recovery. Both of these antigens can be detected by immunofluorescence techniques (see later discussion).

CHARACTERISTICS

Infectious mononucleosis is an acute infectious disease of the mononuclear-phagocyte system. It is typically seen in young adults and often occurs without significant signs and symptoms, especially in children under 5 years of age. Clinically, the disease presents as fever, malaise, lethargy, sore throat with exudate, enlarged lymph nodes in the neck, mild hepatitis, enlarged spleen, and sometimes blotchy skin rash. The disease has an incubation period of from 10 to 50 days, and once fully developed usually lasts about 1 to 4 weeks, although convalescence may take months. Characteristic of infectious mononucleosis are enlarged lymphocytes with atypical nuclei (so-called Downey cells), which present after a short period of time. They usually follow the presence of heterophil antibodies, persisting after the disappearance of these antibodies.

HETEROPHIL ANTIBODIES: DESCRIPTION

Experimental work by Forssman (1911) revealed that emulsions of guinea pig organs injected into rabbits provoked the formation of antibodies that lysed sheep erythrocytes in the presence of complement. Subsequently, the name "Forssman antigen" was used for any substance that stimulated the formation of sheep hemolysin. The sheep antibody produced in this way is an example of a "heterophil" antibody, heterophil being the name given to several groups of antigens that occur in cells or fluids of apparently unrelated animals and microorganisms; yet they are so closely related that they cross-react with antibodies against any one member of the particular heterophil group. The Forssman antigen is found in the red cells of many species (horse, sheep, dog, cat, mouse, fowl) as well as in some bacteria such as pneumococci, certain strains of dysentery and paratyphoid bacilli, *Clostridium welchii*, and *Neisseria catarrhalis*. It is absent in humans, monkeys, rabbits, rats, ducks, and cows.

Although the Forssman antigen was the first example of a heterophil antigen, it is important to recognize that there are many heterophil systems, of which the Forssman is only one. Among some investigators, the terms *Forssman antigen* and *hetero-*

phil antigen are used synonymously; yet the Forssman antigen is the antigen that was discovered in guinea pig tissues, whereas the term *heterophil antigen* refers to a broad group of antigens in various plants and animals whose characteristics are similar to those of the Forssman antigen.

Apart from their intrinsic interest, heterophil systems are of some practical importance in that they can be put to (albeit limited) diagnostic use in some cases of typhus, primary atypical pneumonia, serum sickness, and infectious mononucleosis.

HETEROPHIL ANTIBODIES IN INFECTIOUS MONONUCLEOSIS

Paul and Bunnell (1932) observed that heterophil antibodies developed in patients suffering from infectious mononucleosis. The antibodies were found to react with a heat-stable antigen on sheep erythrocytes that is shared by ox (beef) erythrocytes but not by guinea pig kidney (i.e., they were non-Forssman in nature).

The reasons for the development of heterophil antibodies in infectious mononucleosis are not clear, although it has been suggested that because the disease induces the formation in lymph nodes of lymphocytes and monocytes in increased numbers and abnormal forms, and because lymphocytes may participate in the formation of globulin, this may be contributory. IgM agglutinins are usually observed within 2 weeks after the development of symptoms, lasting from 4 to 8 weeks and reaching maximal titers during the second and third weeks. The titer does not, in fact, correlate with the severity of the disease, and, because heterophil agglutinins appear in 50 to 80 per cent of cases of infectious mononucleosis, negative tests do not rule out the possibility of infection (see below).

OTHER ANTIGENS

EBV-infected B lymphocytes express a variety of other antigens encoded by the virus, namely viral capsid antigen (VCA), early antigen (EA), and nuclear antigen (NA). These antigens produce specific antibody responses, for which assays are available.

Testing for these specific antibodies can be helpful in determining the immune status, and the time of their appearance may be indicative of the stage of the disease.

Viral Capsid Antigen. This antigen is produced by infected B cells and is found in the cytoplasm. The corresponding IgM antibody is detectable early in the course of the infection, but it disappears within 2 to 4 months and is normally present in low concentration. An IgG anti-VCA is usually detected within 4 to 7 days after the onset of clinical signs and symptoms. This antibody persists for a long period of time and can be present for life.

Early Antigen. This antigen is a complex of two components, each of which produces corresponding antibodies.

Early Antigen-Diffuse (EA-D) and Anti-EA-D. The antigen EA-D is found in both the nucleus and the cytoplasm of B cells. Anti-EA-D occurring as IgG strongly indicates active infection but is not detectable in 10 to 20 per cent of infected individuals. The antibody usually disappears in about 3 months. A rise in titer is demonstrated during reactivation of a latent EBV infection. In general, the antibody is not a consistent indicator of the disease stage.

Early Antigen-Restricted (EA-R) and Anti-EA-R. The antigen is usually found as a mass in the cytoplasm only. Anti-EA-R (IgG) is sometimes demonstrated in the serum of very young children but usually not in the serum of young adults during the acute phase. The antibody appears transiently in the later convalescent stage. Like anti-EA-D, anti-EA-R is generally not an indicator of the disease stage.

Epstein-Barr Nuclear Antigen (EBNA) and Antibody. EBNA is found in the nucleus of all EBV-infected cells. The antigen is synthesized before EA synthesis during the infection of B cells but does not stimulate antibody until after the incubation period of IM, at which time the EBV genome-carrying B cells are destroyed by T lymphocytes. The IgG anti-EBNA does not appear until the convalescent stage but is almost always present in sera containing IgG antibodies to VCA unless the patient is in the early acute stage. The antibody titer rises slowly to reach a plateau at about 3 to 12 months after infection. Because of the persistent viral carrier state that follows primary EBV infection, the antibody remains at detectable levels (titers ranging from 1:10 to 1:160) indefinitely. The levels of antibody in patients with EBV-associated malignancies vary from very high in cases of nasopharyngeal carcinoma to barely detectable in some cases of Burkitt's lymphoma (although patients with Burkitt's lymphoma can also possess high levels of antibody).

A diagnosis of IM should be made taking into account the patient's symptoms, clinical history, and antibody response patterns to EBV-VCA and EA. Note: Patients with severe immunologic defects or immunosuppressive diseases may not produce anti-EBNA, even when anti-VCA is present.

SEROLOGIC TESTS FOR INFECTIOUS MONONUCLEOSIS

The Paul-Bunnell Test

Sheep erythrocytes carry an antigen associated with infectious mononucleosis, an antigen associated with serum sickness, and the Forssman antigen. The Paul-Bunnell test uses simple dilutions of a patient's serum to which small amounts of sheep erythrocytes are added. Agglutination of the sheep cells is of limited value, however, because it reveals that one (or more) of the three types of antibodies mentioned is present in the test serum. The Paul-Bunnell test, therefore, is incapable of determining specificity and is only indicative of the presence or absence of heterophil antibodies. As a screening test, however, the test is useful because it is simple and inexpensive and, when negative results are obtained, the need for further testing is eliminated.

METHOD 1: THE PAUL-BUNNELL TEST FOR INFECTIOUS MONONUCLEOSIS: PRESUMPTIVE TEST (UNABSORBED)

Specimen Requirements

An amount of 2 ml of clotted blood is required. The presence of hemolysis renders the specimen unsuitable for testing.

Reagents, Supplies, and Equipment

1. 2 per cent suspension of washed sheep cells in normal saline (prepared using 0.2 ml of packed erythrocytes in 9.8 ml of saline). Note: cells should be no more than 1 week old.
2. 0.9 per cent saline
3. 12 × 75 mm test tubes
4. Graduated serologic pipettes
5. Centrifuge
6. Incubator (37°C) (optional)

Note: As a control, a known positive should be run in parallel with the test procedure.

Method

1. Inactivate the patient's serum for 30 minutes at 56°C.
2. To a row of 10 test tubes (12 × 75 mm), add 0.4 ml of normal saline solution to the first tube and 0.25 ml of normal saline to each of the remaining 9 tubes. (Note: A second set of 10 tubes should be set up as the control.)
3. Add 0.1 ml of the patient's inactivated serum to tube 1, mix and transfer 0.25 ml to tube 2, mix and transfer 0.25 ml to tube 3, repeating the transfer until the last tube is reached, and discard 0.25 ml.
4. Add 0.1 ml of 2 per cent sheep cell suspension to each tube. Shake the tubes thoroughly. Incubate tubes for 1 hour at 37°C or at room temperature overnight.
5. Centrifuge for 1 minute at 1,500 rpm.
6. Read macroscopically after gently shaking the tubes to resuspend the red cell sediment. Viewing with a low-power objective of the microscope is permissible.

Interpretation

A titer of 1:56 is considered to be a positive presumptive test in the presence of clinical and/or cytologic findings suggestive of infectious mononucleosis.

The Davidsohn Differential Test

Davidsohn (1937) designed a classic differential test to distinguish between heterophil sheep cell agglutinins in human serum due to Forssman antigen, serum sickness, and infectious mononucleosis. The principle of the test is based on the fact that some of the antigens that cause agglutination of sheep erythrocytes are carried on ox (beef) erythrocytes but not on the kidney cells of the guinea pig: therefore, exposure of the test serum to both guinea pig kidney cells and ox (beef) erythrocytes causes absorption of either one or both of these antibodies. The absorbed agglutinins can be removed by centrifugation and aspiration of the resultant fluid, which is then tested with sheep erythrocytes. The actions of the two antigens in their absorption patterns are shown in Table 12–1.

METHOD 2: THE DAVIDSOHN DIFFERENTIAL TEST

Beef cells and guinea pig cells for this test are available from Baltimore Biologicals, Cockeysville, MD, and from Difco Laboratories, Detroit, MI.

Materials

1. Test serum—inactivated at 56°C for 30 minutes
2. Diluent—0.85 per cent normal saline
3. Red cells—2 per cent suspension of sheep erythrocytes in saline. Cells should be between 24 hours and 1 week old.
4. Beef cells—20 per cent beef erythrocytes
5. Guinea pig cells—20 per cent suspension of guinea pig kidney cells
6. Test tubes—10 × 75 mm (round bottomed)
7. Positive and negative controls

TABLE 12–1. Absorption Patterns in Davidsohn Differential Test

Type of Heterophil Antibody	Absorbed by Guinea Pig Kidney Cells	Absorbed by Beef Erythrocytes
Forssman	yes	no
Infectious mononucleosis	no	yes
Serum sickness	yes	yes

Method

1. Place 1.0 ml of beef cells into a test tube and 1.0 ml of guinea pig cells into a second test tube.
2. Add 0.25 ml of test serum to each tube and shake.
3. Place at room temperature for 5 minutes, shaking periodically to bring the cells back into suspension.
4. Centrifuge at 1,500 rpm for 10 minutes.
5. Carefully remove 0.25 ml of clear supernatant from each tube, and place into separate tubes (marked 1 and 2, respectively).
6. Place tube 1 and tube 2 in row 1 and row 2, respectively, of a test tube rack.
7. Place 7 additional tubes in each row.
8. Add 0.25 ml of diluent to each tube.
9. With a clean pipette, mix the contents of tube 1 and transfer 0.25 ml to tube 2 of row 1. Mix and transfer 0.25 ml from tube 2 to tube 3. Continue this process to tube 8, and discard 0.25 ml of the final dilution in tube 8. Repeat this step for row 2.
10. Add 0.1 ml of sheep erythrocytes to each tube.
11. Shake and leave at room temperature for 2 hours.
12. Read and record results.

Interpretation

The titer is recorded as the reciprocal of the highest dilution showing agglutination. Interpret the results of the tests as follows:

Infectious Mononucleosis

1. The titer of the Paul-Bunnell test is 1:56 or higher.
2. The titer in row 1 is reduced more than eightfold.
3. The titer in row 2 is reduced more than fourfold.

Serum Sickness

1. The titer of the Paul-Bunnell test is 1:56 or higher.
2. The titer in row 1 is reduced more than eightfold.
3. The titer in row 2 is reduced more than eightfold.

Forssman Antigen

1. The titer of the Paul-Bunnell test is 1:56 or higher.
2. The titer in row 1 is not reduced.
3. The titer in row 2 is reduced more than eightfold.

Note: Positive and negative infectious mononucleosis serum controls should give the appropriate reactions when tested in parallel with the test. Results should not be considered valid unless controls give the expected results (see Table 12–1).

Rapid Differential Slide Tests (Spot Tests)

A number of rapid slide tests have been developed for which many commercial houses provide kits. These procedures can be divided into two main categories: those using papain-treated sheep erythrocytes, and those using horse erythrocytes.

The procedure using papain-treated sheep erythrocytes is based on Wallner's discovery that when papain is added to sheep erythrocytes, the receptors for the antibodies of infectious mononucleosis are specifically inactivated. The diagnosis of infectious mononucleosis is achieved in this test by testing the suspect serum with native as well as papain-treated sheep erythrocytes. Interpretation is as shown in Table 12–2.

Horse erythrocytes are used as an indicator in a rapid specific test for infectious mononucleosis. The test involves two stages: absorption of sera with guinea pig kidney and with ox cells. The ox

TABLE 12–2. Interpretation of Rapid Differential Slide Tests Using Native and Papain-treated Sheep Erythrocytes

Serum	Native Sheep Cells	Papain-Treated Sheep Cells
Normal serum (greater than 1:64) Infectious mononucleosis serum	Agglutination	No agglutination (occasional weak or late clumping
Serum sickness or other heterophil antibodies	Agglutination	Agglutination (clump before N-cells)

cells contain heterophil antigen to infectious mononucleosis but do not contain the Forssman antigen. Agglutination with the horse erythrocytes and the serum absorbed with guinea pig kidney, therefore, indicates a positive reaction. The test is marketed under the name Monospot (Ortho Diagnostic, Raritan, NJ) (see Method 3, below). It is considered convenient because it is all performed on a glass slide and the agglutination occurs within minutes. It should be noted, however, that false-positive results with the Monospot test have been reported in patients with pancreatic carcinoma, rubella, and rheumatoid arthritis. The test can also be used to distinguish serum sickness from infectious mononucleosis.

METHOD 3: MONOSPOT

The Monospot test uses the principle of agglutination of horse erythrocytes by heterophil antibody present in infectious mononucleosis. Because horse red cells exhibit antigens directed against both Forssman and infectious mononucleosis antibodies, a differential absorption of the patient's serum is necessary to distinguish the specific heterophil antibody from those of the Forssman type. Serum or plasma from the patient are absorbed with both guinea pig kidney and beef erythrocyte stroma. Guinea pig kidney contains only the Forssman antigen, and beef erythrocytes contain only the antigen associated with infectious mononucleosis. Guinea pig kidney will absorb only heterophil antibodies of the Forssman type, and beef erythrocytes will absorb only the heterophil antibody of infectious mononucleosis. Agglutination of horse red blood cells by the absorbed patient specimen is indicative of a positive reaction for heterophil antibody.

Specimen Requirements

If blood is obtained from the patient by venipuncture, at least 2 ml is required. This may be collected into a dry tube (to obtain serum) or into a tube containing EDTA, sodium oxalate, potassium oxalate, sodium citrate, ACD solution, or heparin as anticoagulants (to obtain plasma).

As an alternative, capillary specimens may be used. In this case, four heparinized or nonheparinized capillary pipettes (75 mm length, 1.1 mm to 1.2 mm inside diameter, 85 μl volume) should be collected by finger puncture. The required 0.05 ml of serum or plasma can be obtained from four such capillary tubes if the patient's hematocrit is less than 50 per cent. If the hematocrit is greater than 50 per cent, additional tubes will be required. The tubes should be sealed at the dry end and centrifuged for 5 minutes in a microhematocrit centrifuge. The tubes are then broken at the interface between the plasma or serum and the cells.

The Kit contains:

1. Guinea pig antigen—a suspension of guinea pig kidney antigen preserved with 1 per cent sodium azide
2. Beef erythrocyte stroma—a suspension of beef erythrocyte stroma antigen preserved with 1 per cent sodium azide
3. Horse erythrocytes—a suspension of stabilized horse red blood cells preserved with 1:3,000 chloramphenicol and 1:10,000 neomycin sulfate. Note: These three reagents should be stored at 2° to 8°C. Improper storage may invalidate the expiration date.
4. Glass slide
5. Microcapillary pipettes (20 λ) for indicator cells
6. Rubber bulbs
7. Plastic pipettes for delivery of serum or plasma samples
8. Wooden applicator sticks
   Note: A stopwatch or laboratory timer (not included with the kit) is also required.
9. Positive control serum—human serum containing the heterophil antibody of IM, preserved with 0.1 per cent sodium azide
10. Negative control serum—human serum lacking the heterophil antibody of IM, preserved with 0.1 per cent sodium azide
    Note: The control sera should be checked when the kit is received and periodically during the dating period.

Procedure (Qualitative Method)

1. Place the slide on a flat surface under a direct light source.
2. Invert the vial of horse (indicator) erythrocytes to resuspend the cells. Using a clean micro-

capillary tube, place 10 λ of cells on one corner of both squares on the slide.

To use the microcapillary tube, insert the end of the pipette marked with a heavy black line ¼-inch into the neck of the rubber tube. Hold the rubber bulb between the thumb and the third finger. Tilt the vial of cells and insert the pipette. Allow the pipette to fill to the top (20 λ) mark by capillary action. Do not draw the cells into the bulb.

To deliver 10 λ of cells to the slide, place the index finger over the hole in the top of the bulb and squeeze gently until the level of cells in the pipette reaches the first mark. Touch the pipette top to a corner of square 1 to release the cells. Repeat the process to deliver the remaining 10 λ of cells to the corner of square 2.

3. Put 1 drop of thoroughly mixed guinea pig antigen (reagent 1) in square 1.
4. Put 1 drop of thoroughly mixed guinea pig antigen (reagent 2) in square 2.
5. Using a disposable plastic pipette, add 1 drop of the patient's serum or plasma to the center of each square on the slide.
6. Mix the serum/plasma and the guinea pig antigen in square 1 at least 10 times with a clean wooden applicator stick. *Avoid the horse erythrocytes.*
7. Mix the serum/plasma and the beef erythrocyte stroma in square 2 at least 10 times with a clean wooden applicator stick. *Avoid the horse erythrocytes.*
8. Blend the horse (indicator) erythrocytes over the entire surface of each square. Use a clean wooden applicator for each side, and use no more than 10 stirring motions to blend.
9. Start a timer upon completion of the final mixing. Do not move or pick up the slide during the reaction period.
10. Observe for agglutination for no longer than 1 minute after the final mixing.

Interpretation

1. If the agglutination pattern is stronger on the left side (square 1) the test is positive.
2. If the agglutination pattern is stronger on the right side (square 2) the test is negative.
3. If no agglutination appears on either side (1 or 2) of the slide or if agglutination is equal on both squares of the slide the test is negative.

Procedure (Semiquantitative Method)

If a positive qualitative result is obtained, a titration may be performed to provide a semiquantitative indication of the level of heterophil antibody.

1. Prepare serial dilutions of serum by pipetting 0.5 ml of 0.85 per cent saline into each of the desired number of tubes. Pipette 0.5 ml of the patient's serum into the first tube, mix and transfer 0.5 ml of the diluted serum to the second tube. Repeat this process until the final tube is reached. Discard 0.5 ml of the diluted serum from the last tube.
2. Place a titration slide on a flat surface under a direct light source. Treat each of the dilutions as if they were individual sera and follow the steps for the qualitative procedure for each of the appropriately labeled squares. *(Omit the use of beef stroma, and use only the guinea pig antigen.)*
3. The highest dilution in which visible agglutination occurs is the endpoint. If agglutination is present in all of the dilutions, extend the serial dilutions.
4. Record results as the reciprocal of the highest dilution that showed agglutination.

Note: The titer of Monospot cannot be compared with titration values obtained with other slide or tube test procedures because of variations in sensitivity of the erythrocytes used. The titer is not indicative of the severity of the disease but may be a useful indicator when sequential examinations are made.

JUST THE FACTS

Introduction

1. Infectious mononucleosis is a self-limiting disease caused by the Epstein-Barr virus.
2. The disease may be confused with diphtheria, pharyngitis, Vincent's angina, lymphadenitis with scarlet fever, hepatitis, or pertussis.

The Epstein-Barr Virus (EBV)

1. EBV is an enveloped, double-stranded DNA, human herpes virus that belongs to the family Herpetoviridae.
2. The virus is ubiquitous.

3. It is transmitted through saliva, blood transfusions, transplacental routes, and possibly by mosquitos.
4. Transmission through transfusion or transplacental routes is unlikely under normal circumstances.
5. Primary infection with EBV results in infectious mononucleosis, after which neutralizing antibodies provide lifelong immunity.
6. EBV infects B lymphocytes. The variant lymphocytes produced in response to infection have T-cell characteristics.
7. Once infected, the individual remains a lifelong carrier of the virus.
8. EBV may survive in peripheral blood lymphocytes and in epithelial cells of the oropharynx for years without producing disease.
9. EBV is present worldwide.
10. Infection during childhood appears to be quite frequent, especially in less affluent socioeconomic groups (80 per cent of 5-year-olds being seropositive) than in higher socioeconomic groups (40 to 50 per cent of 5-year-olds being seropositive).
11. In Western society, about half the population is exposed to the virus before age 5. A second "wave" of seroconversion occurs during late adolescence.
12. From 80 to 90 per cent of healthy adults have antibody to EBV.
13. Individuals who lack antibodies are at risk of contracting IM.
14. EBV represents a minor problem for immunocompetent individuals.
15. Immunologically compromised patients are at major risk.
16. Infection resulting from blood transfusion is known as IM postperfusion syndrome.
17. A minor percentage of patients experience symptomatic reactivation.
18. The frequency of clinically apparent IM has been estimated to be 45:100,000 in adolescence.
19. The incidence in immunosuppressed patients ranges from 35 to 47 per cent.
20. There is a carrier state after primary infection.
21. Several diseases are associated with EBV (Burkitt's lymphoma, nasopharyngeal carcinoma).

Characteristics

1. IM is an acute infectious disease of the mono-nuclear-phagocyte system.
2. It is typically seen in young adults.
3. It often occurs without significant signs and symptoms, especially in children under age 5.
4. It presents as fever, malaise, lethargy, sore throat with exudate, enlarged lymph nodes in the neck, mild hepatitis, enlarged spleen, and sometimes blotchy skin rash.
5. The incubation period is from 10 to 50 days.
6. The disease lasts about 1 to 4 weeks, although convalescence may take months.
7. Enlarged lymphocytes with atypical nuclei (Downey cells) are characteristic. They are present for a short period of time and usually follow the presence of heterophil antibodies, persisting after the disappearance of these antibodies.

Heterophil Antibodies: Description

1. The antibody to the "Forssman" antigen was the first example of a "heterophil" antibody.
2. Heterophil is the name given to several groups of antigens that occur in the cells or fluids of apparently unrelated animals and microorganisms, yet are so closely related that they will cross-react with antibodies against any one member of the particular heterophil group.
3. The Forssman antigen is found in the red cells of many species (horse, sheep, dog, cat, mouse, fowl) as well as in some bacteria.
4. The Forssman antigen is absent in humans, monkeys, rabbits, rats, ducks, and cows.
5. There are many heterophil systems of which Forssman is only one.
6. Heterophil systems are of some practical importance in that they can be put to limited diagnostic use in some cases of typhus, primary atypical pneumonia, serum sickness, and infectious mononucleosis.

Heterophil Antibodies in Infectious Mononucleosis

1. Heterophil antibodies develop in patients suffering from IM.
2. The antibodies react with heat-stable antigen on sheep erythrocytes that is shared by ox (beef) erythrocytes but not by guinea pig kidney (i.e., not Forssman).
3. Because the disease induces the formation of lymphocytes and monocytes in the lymph nodes in increased numbers and abnormal forms, and because lymphocytes may participate in the formation of globulin, this may contribute to the reason why heterophil antibodies are formed.
4. IgM agglutinins are usually observed within 2 weeks after the development of symptoms.
5. These IgM antibodies last for 4 to 8 weeks, reaching maximal titers during the second and third weeks.
6. The titer does not correlate with the severity of the disease.
7. Heterophil agglutinins appear in 50 to 80 per cent of cases of IM; therefore negative tests do not rule out the possibility of infection.

Other Antigens

1. EBV-infected B lymphocytes produce a variety of other antigens encoded by the virus.
2. Testing for the corresponding antibody can be helpful in determining immune status.
3. The time of appearance of these antibodies may be indicative of the stage of the disease.
4. Viral capsid antigen (VCA) is found in the cytoplasm. IgM anti-VCA (normally present in low concentration) is detectable early in the course of infection but disappears after 2 to 4 months. IgG anti-VCA is usually detected within 4 to 7 days after onset of signs and symptoms and persists for a long period of time and can be present for life.
5. Early antigen (EA) is made up of early antigen-diffuse (EA-D) and early antigen-restricted (EA-R).
6. EA-D is found both in the nucleus and in the cytoplasm of B cells.
7. Anti-EA-D occurring as IgG strongly indicates active infection but is not detected in 10 to 20 per cent of infected individuals. The antibody usually disappears after 3 months. A rise in titer is demonstrated during reactivation of a latent EBV infection. The antibody is not a consistent indicator of the disease stage.
8. EA-R is found as a mass in the cytoplasm only.
9. Anti-EA-R (IgG) is sometimes demonstrated in

the serum of very young children but not in young adults during the acute stage.
10. The antibody appears transiently in the later convalescent stage.
11. The antibody is not an indicator of the disease stage.
12. Epstein-Barr nuclear antigen (EBNA) is found in the nucleus of all EBV-infected cells.
13. The antigen is synthesized before EA synthesis during the infection of B cells.
14. EBNA does not stimulate antibody until after the incubation period of IM, at which time the EBV genome-carrying B cells are destroyed by T lymphocytes.
15. IgG anti-EBNA does not appear until the convalescent stage but is almost always present in sera containing IgG antibodies to VCA unless the patient is in the early acute stage (except in patients with severe immunologic defects or immunosuppressive diseases).
16. IgG anti-EBNA titer rises slowly to reach a plateau at about 3 to 12 months after infection.
17. IgG anti-EBNA remains at detectable levels indefinitely.

18. The levels of antibody in patients with EBV-associated malignancies are very high in nasopharyngeal carcinoma and vary from high to barely detectable in some cases of Burkitt's lymphoma.
19. IM diagnosis should be made taking into account the patient's symptoms, clinical history, and antibody response patterns to EBV-VCA and EA.

Serologic Tests for Infectious Mononucleosis

1. The Paul-Bunnell test, which is a useful screening test but cannot determine specificity.
2. The Davidsohn differential test, which differentiates the heterophil types of antibody associated with IM, serum sickness, or Forssman antigen.
3. Spot tests, which are also differential but require absorption of the patient's serum to distinguish the specific heterophil antibody from the Forssman type.

Review Questions

Multiple Choice

Choose the phrase, sentence, or symbol that completes the statement or answers the question. More than one answer may be correct in each case. Answers are given at the end of this book.

1. Infectious mononucleosis may be confused with:
   (a) diphtheria
   (b) Vincent's angina
   (c) pertussis
   (d) all of the above
   (Introduction)

2. The Epstein-Barr virus:
   (a) belongs to the family Herpetoviridae
   (b) may be transmitted through saliva
   (c) is usually transmitted by transfusion
   (d) rarely causes infection in children
   (The Epstein-Barr Virus)

3. The frequency of clinically apparent infectious mononucleosis in adolescents has been estimated to be:
   (a) 1:100,000
   (b) 45:100,000

   (c) 90:100,000
   (d) 128:100,000
   (The Epstein-Barr Virus)

4. The incubation period for infectious mononucleosis is:
   (a) 1 to 10 days
   (b) 10 to 50 days
   (c) 5 to 10 weeks
   (d) 4 to 6 hours
   (Characteristics)

5. The Forssman antigen is found on the red cells of:
   (a) sheep
   (b) rats
   (c) humans
   (d) fowl
   (Heterophil Antibodies: Description)

6. The heterophil antibodies associated with infectious mononucleosis react with heat-stable antigen on the erythrocytes of:
   (a) sheep

(b) ox (beef)
(c) guinea pig kidney
(d) all of the above
(Heterophil Antibodies in Infectious Mononucleosis)

7. The Viral capsid antigen (VCA):
   (a) is produced by infected B cells
   (b) is found in the nucleus of B cells
   (c) is found in the cytoplasm of B cells
   (d) is found in the nucleus of T cells
   (Other Antigens)

8. The Epstein-Barr nuclear antigen:
   (a) is found in the nucleus of all EBV-infected cells
   (b) is found in the cytoplasm of all EBV-infected cells
   (c) is found both in the nucleus and the cytoplasm of all EBV-infected cells
   (d) is synthesized before EA synthesis during the infection of B cells
   (Other Antigens)

Answer "True" or "False"

1. Infectious mononucleosis is caused by the Epstein-Barr virus.
   (Introduction)

2. EBV presents a major problem for immunocompetent individuals.
   (The Epstein-Barr Virus)

3. Infectious mononucleosis often occurs without significant signs and symptoms, especially in children under the age of 5.
   (Characteristics)

4. Forssman is one of many heterophil systems.
   (Heterophil Antibodies: Description)

5. Heterophil antibodies appear in *all* cases of infectious mononucleosis.
   (Heterophil Antibodies in Infectious Mononucleosis)

6. Early antigen-diffuse (EA-D) is found in both the nucleus and the cytoplasm of B cells.
   (Other Antigens)

7. Patients with severe immunologic defects always produce anti-EBNA when anti-VCA is present.
   (Other Antigens)

8. The Paul-Bunnell test can be used to determine the specificity of the heterophil antibody present in a given serum.
   (Serologic Tests for Infectious Mononucleosis)

GENERAL REFERENCES

Baron, E.J., and Finegold, S.M.: Bailey and Scott's Diagnostic Microbiology, 8th ed. St Louis, The C. V. Mosby Company, 1990.

Bennington, J.L.: Saunders Dictionary and Encyclopedia of Laboratory Medicine and Technology. Philadelphia, W. B. Saunders Company, 1984.

Dorland's Illustrated Medical Dictionary, 27th ed. Philadelphia, W. B. Saunders Company, 1988.

Freeman, B.A.: Burrows Textbook of Microbiology, 27th ed. Philadelphia, W. B. Saunders Company, 1985.

Henry, J.B.: Clinical Diagnosis and Management by Laboratory Methods. Philadelphia, W. B. Saunders Company, 1991.

Turgeon, M. L.: Immunology and Serology in Laboratory Medicine. St. Louis, C. V. Mosby Company, 1990.

13

Acquired Immunodeficiency Syndrome (AIDS)

OBJECTIVES

The student shall know, understand, and be prepared to explain:
1. A brief history of AIDS
2. A description of the human immunodeficiency virus (HIV)
3. The structure of the human immunodeficiency virus
4. The HIV genome
5. The life cycle of HIV
6. The incidence of AIDS
7. The modes of transmission of HIV
8. The clinical manifestations of AIDS to include:
   a. The primary stage
   b. The intermediate stage (AIDS-related complex)
   c. The final stage
9. Factors influencing the progression of AIDS
10. The effects of HIV on the immune system
11. AIDS treatment
12. The development of vaccines
13. The prevention of HIV infection
14. The prevention of HIV infection in health care workers
15. Antibody development in AIDS
16. The laboratory diagnosis of AIDS
17. The tests used to detect HIV antibody, specifically:
    a. Enzyme-linked immunosorbent assay (ELISA)
    b. Western blot (WB) assay
    c. Indirect immunofluorescent assay (IFA)
    d. Slide agglutination tests
    e. Radioimmunoassay
    f. Radioimmunoprecipitation assay
18. The tests used to detect HIV antigen, specifically:
    a. HIV isolation
    b. Enzyme-linked immunosorbent assay (ELISA)
    c. Indirect immunofluorescent assay (IFA)

d. Slide agglutination tests
19. The tests used for detecting HIV genes, specifically:
    a. *In situ* hybridization
    b. Filter hybridization
    c. Southern blot hybridization
    d. DNA amplification

Introduction: History

During 1981 several reports appeared in the literature regarding the development of *Pneumocystis carinii* pneumonia, other opportunistic infections, and a disseminated form of Kaposi's sarcoma in apparently previously healthy, young homosexual men in New York City and San Francisco (Gottlieb *et al.*, 1981; Friedman-Kien *et al.*, 1981; Gottlieb *et al.*, 1981; Masur *et al.*, 1981; Siegal *et al.*, 1981). The constellation of infections seen in these men had essentially never occurred before in people with a normal immune function, and therefore it was suspected that they were suffering a severe immune defect. Kaposi's sarcoma, prior to this time, was rarely seen in North America, and this unprecedented occurrence in clusters of young men raised suspicion of a new illness and not merely a newly recognized one.

Subsequent to the initial reports of these diseases in homosexual men, a task force was formed by the Centers for Disease Control to study the epidemic systematically. For reasons of surveillance and reporting, patients were defined as having the syndrome if (1) they had a reliably diagnosed disease (e.g., *P. carinii* pneumonia or Kaposi's sarcoma and were less than 60 years of age) that suggested an underlying cellular immune defect, and (2) the disease occurred in the absence of a cellular immune deficiency that could be ascribed to another factor (e.g., the use of immunosuppressive drugs or the presence of a lymphoreticular malignancy) (CDC Task Force, 1982). Although this definition is obviously restrictive, it still technically defines AIDS.

The task force formed by the Centers for Disease Control discovered that no patients fitting the case definition had been found prior to 1978 and that all but one patient of the 159 initially reported had been men, and, when sexual preference was known, 92 per cent of these men were either bisexual or homosexual. It is important to note, however, that there is no gender-determined resistance to AIDS (Masur *et al.*, 1982; Harris *et al.*, 1983), and in fact it has been suggested that the syndrome can be transmitted by a single vaginal intercourse (Cabane *et al.*, 1984).

It was also discovered that AIDS could develop in heterosexual intravenous drug abusers and heterosexual (non–drug abusing) classic hemophilia patients (Masur *et al.*, 1981; Ehrenkranz *et al.*, 1982), which suggested that the etiologic agent was transmissible by blood or blood products. In addition, it was discovered that transmission can occur between mother and fetus *in utero* (Jensen *et al.*, 1984; Rawlinson *et al.*, 1984; Rubinstein *et al.*, 1983; Scott *et al.*, 1984).

Several theories have been offered about the origins of AIDS, though all must be considered speculation. It is unlikely that the syndrome originated in North America. One theory that appears to have gained tentative acceptance is that the causative retrovirus existed in exceedingly remote pockets of Africa (possibly as an agent with a nonhuman primate reservoir) and that recent population shifts could have introduced the agent into certain urban centers of Central Africa, which, in effect, could have simultaneously conveyed the virus to North America (DeVita, Hellman, and Rosenberg, 1985). This theory is supported by the fact that the etiologic agent of AIDS, human immunodeficiency virus (see below) has been shown through studies of cross-reactions of viral proteins to be closely related to simian T-cell lymphotropic virus type III (STLV-III), which causes a form of AIDS in African green monkeys.

HUMAN IMMUNODEFICIENTY VIRUS (HIV)

The etiologic agent of AIDS is a human retrovirus known as human immunodeficiency virus (HIV). Retroviruses are defined as viruses that contain a single positive-stranded RNA, which contain the virus's genetic information, and a special enzyme known as "reverse transcriptase" in their core. This enzyme enables the virus to convert viral RNA to DNA in contrast to the normal process of transcription where DNA is converted to RNA.

Two types of HIV have been classified:

1. HIV-1, the causative agent of AIDS in the United States and Europe
2. HIV-2, associated with immunodeficiency and a clinical syndrome similar to AIDS in West Africa (Clavel *et al.*, 1987)

HIV was formerly known as lymphadenopathy-associated virus (LAV) (Barré-Sinoussi *et al.*, 1983), human T-cell lymphotropic virus Type III (HTLV-III) (Popovic *et al.*, 1984), or AIDS-related virus (ARV) (Levy *et al.*, 1984). It is believed to be a member of a group of nontransforming, cytopathic retroviruses called lentiviruses (based on genomic sequence homologies, morphology, and life cycle), which cause chronic neurodegenerative and wasting diseases in animals similar to the wasting disease and neurologic disorders produced by HIV in humans.

The Structure of the Human Immunodeficiency Virus

The HIV virus particle (virion) is about 100 nm in diameter and consists of three parts—an outer envelope derived from the host cell membrane, a core shell of protein, and a cone-shaped inner core that contains two identical strands of RNA (the viral genome—see below) with associated reverse transcriptase and core polypeptides (Fig. 13–1). Embedded in the lipid bilayer are virally encoded membrane proteins (p18 and p24). A large glycoprotein traverses the lipid bilayer membrane at regular intervals and protrudes above the surface in a knoblike structure. This glycoprotein has two components—gp41, which transverses the membrane, and gp120, which extends beyond the surface as a knob. Note: The names of these proteins are derived

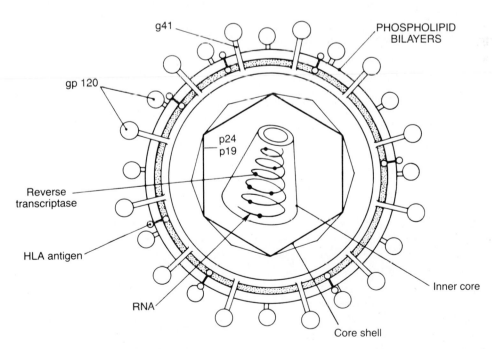

Figure 13–1. Structure of the HIV virion. (Modified from Sheehan, C.: Clinical Immunology: Principles and Laboratory Diagnosis. Philadelphia, J. B. Lippincott Company, 1990, p. 242.)

from their molecular weight (gp41 = a glycoprotein of molecular weight 41,000 d). The gp120 component provokes an immune response.

Also on the outer envelope are human leukocyte antigens (HLA), which are derived from human cell membranes when new HIV virions bud from human cells during the process of virus particle formation.

The HIV Genome

Ratner *et al.*, (1985) and Wain-Hobson *et al.*, (1985) have determined the complete nucleotide sequences of the HIV genome, making it possible to identify viral genes and some of the relationships between viral gene products and the clinical course of AIDS. The HIV genome shares the basic structure of all known retroviruses, yet is unique in its complexity. In addition to the usual structural genes (*gag, pol,* and *env*) it has at least five other regulatory genes (*tat, art/trs, sor, 3'orf,* and *R*) whose products regulate viral reproduction in various ways, as described below (Table 13–1).

1. The *gag* (*g*roup *a*ntigen) gene codes for core structural proteins, which are cleaved from a large polyprotein (55kd) found in high levels of infected cells. The cleavage products form the three core proteins p18, p24, and p15.
2. The *pol* (*pol*ymerase) gene codes for:
   a. *Reverse transcriptase,* which transcribes single-stranded RNA into double-stranded DNA. It is an immunogenic protein designated p66/51.
   b. *RNase,* which is an enzyme that digests the RNA in RNA-DNA hybrids that form as intermediates in the creation of viral DNA.
   c. *Protease (p31),* which cleaves itself from an initial polyprotein and cleaves other enzymes and structural proteins from their polyproteins.
   d. *Integrase,* which is responsible for inserting the viral DNA into the host DNA.
3. The *env* (*env*elope) gene codes for the glycoprotein gp160, which is found in infected cells. It is cleaved to form gp120 and gp41.

TABLE 13–1. Genes of the Human Immunodeficiency Virus		
Gene	**Viral Gene Products**	**Function**
gag	p55 precursor, p17, p24m, p15 Mature proteins	Codes for core proteins
pol	Reverse transcriptase	Transcribes single-stranded RNA into double-stranded DNA
	RNase	An enzyme that digests RNA in RNA-DNA hybrids that form as intermediates in the creation of viral DNA
	Protease (p31)	Cleaves itself and other enzymes and structural proteins from their polyproteins
	Integrase	Inserts the viral DNA into the host DNA
env	gp160, precursor gp120, gp41	gp120 binds CD4 for infection gp41 is required for viral fusion with cell
sor	p23	Related to viral infectivity
tat	p14	Accelerates viral protein production Required for viral replication
R	p15	Unknown
art/trs	p20	Regulates the translation of the viral genome
3'orf	p27	Latency of the virus

4. The *tat* (*trans-activation translation*) gene, which produces p14, speeds up the production of viral protein and is required for viral replication. When *tat* is not present, no virus particles are formed and only minimal RNA is produced (Fisher *et al.*, 1986).

5. The *art/trs* (*anti-repression transactivator*) gene regulates the translation of the viral genome (Muesing *et al.*, 1987). It produces p20, an anti-repression transactivator protein that regulates the expression of the components of the viral gene.

6. The *sor* (*short open reading frame*) gene is related to viral infectivity. It produces p23, which is present in the filtrate of virus-infected cultures and against which antibodies form in the serum of HIV-infected individuals (Aiya and Gallo, 1986).

7. The *3'orf* (*3' open reading frame*) gene slows down viral reproduction tenfold in CD4 cells and is considered responsible for the latency of the virus. It produces p27 against which antibodies have been found in infected individuals (Luciw *et al.*, 1987).

8. The R (*reading frame*) gene codes for an immunogenic product, (p15), whose function is unknown (Wong-Staal *et al.*, 1987).

The viral genome has identical ends known as LTR (*long terminal ends*), which contain a terminator, an enhancer, and a promoter for the process of transcription (Fig. 13–2).

The Life Cycle of HIV

The life cycle of the human immunodeficiency virus begins when the gp120 protein on the viral envelope binds to the CD4 protein receptor on the surface of the target cell. The primary target cell is the helper-inducer subset of T lymphocytes, although macrophages, about 40 per cent of the peripheral blood monocytes, cells in the skin, lymph nodes, and other organs, as well as about 5 per cent of the B lymphocytes, express CD4 and can be infected by HIV. Although CD4 receptors have also been identified on some glial cells, and neuroleukin receptors have been identified on neurons that are capable of binding gp120, their clinical importance remains uncertain. In addition, cells of the gastrointestinal system, which do not produce appreciable amounts of CD4, do sometimes appear to be infected by HIV *in vivo*. This suggests that gastrointestinal infection may be what leads to the AIDS-associated weight loss and emaciation known in Africa as "slim disease."

After HIV binds to the CD4-containing cell, it penetrates the host cells and loses its outer layer (i.e., it injects its core into the cell). This core, as mentioned, contains two strands of RNA, which are then exposed. The viral RNA is transcribed into DNA by the enzyme DNA-polymerase, which initially makes a single-stranded DNA copy of the viral RNA. Ribonuclease, an associated enzyme, destroys the original RNA and the polymerase makes a second complementary copy of DNA, using the first DNA strand as a template. The viral genetic information is now in the form of double-stranded DNA, which is the same form in which the cell carries its own genetic makeup. From here, the DNA migrates into the cell nucleus where a third enzyme, integrase, is believed to "splice" the HIV genome into the host cell's DNA, which means that the provirus will be duplicated

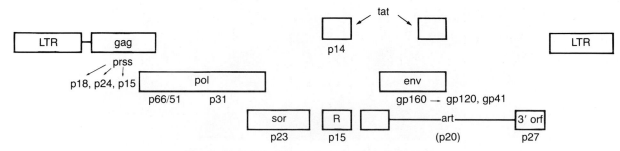

Figure 13–2. The HIV genome showing viral genes.

together with the cell's own genes every time the cell divides.

From this stage, the production of new virus particles takes place, although this replication is sporadic and involves only some of the infected cells. This phase begins when nucleotide sequences in the LTR's direct enzyme belonging to the host cell to copy the DNA of the integrated virus into RNA. Some of the RNA will provide the genetic material for a new generation of virus. Others will serve as the messenger RNA that guides the synthesis of structural proteins and enzymes of the new virus. Once the viral proteins are formed, they are assembled into a complete virus particle, which buds from the cell membrane (Fig. 13–3). Once these viruses are released into the circulation, they have the ability to infect new target cells.

When HIV replication occurs, the CD4 cell is killed. This results in a severe depletion of helper-inducer T lymphocytes. This depletion correlates to the progressive severity of AIDS and to the increased susceptibility to opportunistic disease and malignancies seen in its clinical course.

DISEASE CHARACTERISTICS

Incidence

The ultimate dimensions of AIDS are difficult to assess with any accuracy. Many leading authorities have predicted the number of cases that can be expected over the next few years, yet these predictions are speculative at best. As of July 4, 1988, there had been 66,464 reported cases of AIDS in the United States. By March 31, 1989, this number had grown to 89,501, and by July 31, 1991, it had reached 182,834 (Centers for Disease Control, Atlanta, Georgia, personal communication, 1991). Of adult AIDS patients, approximately 63 per cent are homosexual or bisexual men, 19 per cent are heterosexual intravenous drug abusers, 7 per cent are homosexual or bisexual IV drug abusers, 4 per cent are heterosexual men and women, 3 per cent are recipients of blood or blood-product transfusions (usually prior to 1985), 1 per cent are patients with hemophilia or other coagulation disorders, and 3 per cent have unknown risk factors (Heyward and Curran, 1988). Of the 1,054 pediat-

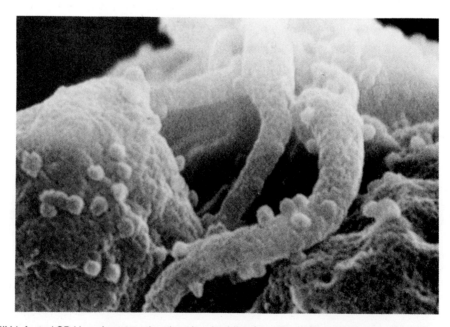

Figure 13–3. HIV-infected CD4 lymphocytes showing virus budding from the plasma membrane. (Courtesy of CDC Archives.)

ric AIDS cases reported in 1988, 78 per cent of the infections occurred perinatally and most could be traced to IV drug abuse by the child's parent (or parents) and 19 per cent had resulted from blood transfusions or treatment for hemophilia or were traced to parents who either had AIDS or had practiced high-risk behavior. The majority of adult AIDS patients in the United States are white (59 per cent); blacks account for 26 per cent, and the remaining 14 per cent are hispanic (Heyward and Curran, 1988).

In addition, there have been a small number of cases of AIDS in health care workers with occupational exposure to HIV but without other known risk factors. Of the 13 cases reported by Carlson (1988), five involved accidental needle puncture, six involved exposure to blood or body fluid with ungloved hands or skin lesions, one involved a lacerated finger while working, and one involved unknown exposure.

Modes of Transmission

The primary mode of transmission of HIV is through the exchange of body fluids (semen and vaginal secretions) during sexual contact (heterosexual, homosexual, or bisexual). The virus can also be transmitted through intimate contact with blood from an infected individual (through blood or blood products or by sharing blood-contaminated drug paraphernalia), transplacental routes, and possibly breast milk (Redfield, 1987).

Only these four body fluids (semen, vaginal secretions, blood, and possibly breast milk) have been implicated in transmission of HIV to date, in spite of the fact that HIV has also been isolated in saliva, tears, cerebrospinal fluid (CSF), amniotic fluid, and urine.

There have been no cases of AIDS being transmitted by food, water, insects, or casual contact with an AIDS patient, although it is believed that viral transmission can occur from contact with inanimate objects that have been recently contaminated with infected blood or certain body fluids and are transferred to broken skin or mucous membranes.

CLINICAL MANIFESTATIONS

Primary Stage

Patients in the early stages of HIV infection are either completely asymptomatic or may show a mild, chronic lymphadenopathy. This stage may last from many months to many years after initial infection. The virus often replicates abundantly after first entering the body, and free virus is found in the CSF surrounding the brain and spinal cord and in circulating blood. After a few weeks, this viral concentration drops suddenly and the initial symptoms disappear.

Certain infected individuals experience a brief, mononucleosis-like illness that has the appearance of influenza (fever malaise and possibly skin rash). These symptoms occur at or about the same time as the first wave of HIV replications. At about the same time, antibodies to HIV can be detected for the first time (usually about 2 weeks to 3 months after infection, rarely later).

Following these initial mild symptoms, the individual may remain asymptomatic for years.

Intermediate Stage

After the primary stage, the disease progresses to an intermediate stage of symptomatic infection with persistent lymphadenopathy and quantitative T-cell deficiencies, especially a decreased CD4-positive cell count and an inverted CD4/CD8 ratio, but without the opportunistic infections and cancers seen in AIDS. This state is known as AIDS-related complex (ARC).

Patients with ARC usually present with prolonged constitutional symptoms of fatigue, night sweats, fever, diarrhea, and weight loss (HIV wasting syndrome). A diagnosis is made according to Centers for Disease Control criteria if *two* of the following clinical manifestations plus *two* laboratory abnormalities are found in a patient without explainable etiology (Redfield, 1987):

Clinical Manifestations

1. Lymphadenopathy of more than 3 months' duration
2. Fever of over 100°F of more than 3 months' duration

3. More than 10 per cent weight loss
4. Persistent diarrhea
5. Fatigue
6. Night sweats

Laboratory Abnormalities

1. CD4 cells less than 400/mm²
2. CD4/CD8 ratio less than 1.0
3. Leukopenia
4. Thrombocytopenia
5. Anemia
6. Elevated serum globulins
7. Anergy to skin tests
8. Reduced blastogenesis
9. Positive HIV antibody test

Final Stage

From 2 to 10 years after initial infection, replication of the virus begins again and the disease progresses to a syndrome of severe CD4 depletion, resulting in opportunistic infections and cancers suggestive of severe cell-mediated immunity defects (Table 13–2). This final stage is called AIDS. Clinical features include extreme weight loss, fever, and multiple secondary infections.

Of the opportunistic infections seen during this phase, lethal *P. carinii* pneumonia and candidi-asis are extremely common; other infections may exist concurrently. The most frequent malignancy observed is an aggressive, invasive variant of Kaposi's sarcoma, which produces tumors in the skin and linings of internal organs, lymphomas, and cancers of the rectum and tongue (Fig. 13–4).

Discussion

Certain factors can influence the progression of AIDS. For example, patients who are weakened by a pre-existing medical condition before infection may progress toward AIDS more quickly than would usually be seen. Disease progression can also be hastened by stimulation of the immune system in response to later infections.

Other pathogenic microorganisms such as human herpesvirus-6 (HHV-6) (see Chapter 11) can interact with HIV in a way that may increase the severity of the HIV infection. Although HHV-6 is normally controlled by the immune system, the presence of HIV and its weakening effect on the immune system may allow HHV-6 to replicate more freely. HHV-6 usually invades the B cells but can also invade T4 cells. If T cells are also infected with HIV, HHV-6 can stimulate the virus, thereby further impairing the immune system and hastening the course of the disease.

AIDS can sometimes be controlled by experimental treatments but cannot currently be cured. In developed countries, half of the patients infected with HIV die within 18 months of diagnosis, and 80 percent die within 36 months.

Effects of HIV on the Immune System

Inducer-helper T lymphocytes play a central role in the induction of most immune responses. HIV infection can lead to the lysis of CD4+ T lymphocytes or functional inactivation of these cells without cytolysis. This diminished inducer-helper T cell activity results in the impairment of all types of immune responses.

The fact that CD4+ T cells are lysed by HIV is reflected in the marked reduction of these cells in AIDS patients. In normal individuals, the ratio of CD4+ T cells to CD8+ T cells is approximately 2:1, whereas in AIDS patients this ratio is often reduced to as low as 0.5:1 (i.e., the ratio is reversed). This

TABLE 13–2. Opportunistic Infections and Neoplasms Associated with AIDS

Opportunistic Infections	Neoplasms
Cytomegalovirus	Kaposi's sarcoma
Epstein-Barr virus	Burkitt-like lymphoma
Adenovirus	Undifferentiated non-Hodgkin's lymphoma
Herpes simplex	
Herpes zoster	Hodgkin's disease
Mycobacterium avium-intracellulare	
Mycobacterium kansasii	*Pneumocystis carinii*
Mycobacterium tuberculosis	*Toxoplasma gondii*
Streptococcus pneumoniae	*Cryptosporidium* species
Haemophilus influenzae	*Isospora belli*
Salmonella species	*Candida albicans*
Syphilis	*Coccidioides*
	Histoplasma capsulatum
	Cryptococcus neoformans
	Aspergillis species

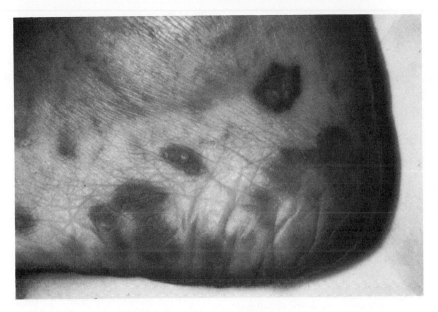

Figure 13–4. Typical lesions in Kaposi's sarcoma. (Courtesy of CDC Archives.)

dramatic reduction in CD4+ T cells occurs in spite of the fact that probably less than 1 per cent of these cells are *directly* infected with HIV, with more than 99 per cent being latently infected without detectable viral RNA transcripts. Furthermore, HIV-infected individuals have various immunologic abnormalities even before their CD4+ T cells are reduced in numbers. The answer as to why the number of CD4+ T cells destroyed is far greater than the number infected is not known.

In addition to the depletion of CD4+ T cells, which becomes most significant in the late stages of the disease, HIV also causes functional impairment of these cells in ways not directly related to cytotoxic effects or T cell depletion. Uninfected T cells, for example, have a decreased expression of IL-2 receptors and diminished secretion of IL-2 in response to soluble antigens both *in vivo* and *in vitro*. Humoral responses to soluble antigens and CTL responses to certain viruses are also impaired, probably as a result of the failure of the CD4+ T cells to secrete adequate amounts of the appropriate cytokines required for functional differentiation of B cells and CTLs.

The immunosuppressive effects of HIV may also be partly related to effects the virus has on cells other than CD4+ T cells. Abnormalities in B-lymphocyte activation are frequently observed in HIV-

infected individuals. This may be due to diminished T-cell help, as well as refractoriness of the B cells themselves.

Macrophages can also be infected by HIV, although these cells are relatively resistant to the cytolytic effects of the virus, possibly because high levels of CD4 expression may be required not only for viral entry into cells but also for virus-induced cytotoxicity. Macrophage functions, however, are impaired, characterized by decreased chemotaxis, IL-1 production, and oxygen metabolite-dependent killing of microbes. In addition, the antigen-presenting capabilities of monocytes and macrophages are reduced, possibly due to the down-regulation of class I MHC expression that is reported to occur in HIV-infected macrophages.

Functional impairment is also reported to affect NK cells, and this may be the reason for inadequate antiviral immunity in these individuals.

Treatment

The treatment of AIDS usually involves the treatment of the opportunistic infections and cancers that are its complications. To date, no effective intervention has been developed, although increasing knowledge of the structure and replicative cycle of HIV has allowed for the development of drugs that will inhibit viral replication or reduce the budding of the virus from the cell membranes. The most important of these is 3'azido-3'deoxy-thymidine, called zidovudine (formerly known as azidothymidine or AZT). This drug is an inhibitor of reverse transcriptase and is also a DNA chain terminator. Clinical trials conducted by Fischi *et al.*, (1987) showed that the drug reduced mortality, morbidity, and the number of opportunistic infections in AIDS patients. The drug is taken orally and crosses the blood-brain barrier. The problems with the use of the drug are the many side effects, which include megaloblastic anemia, neutropenia, nausea, insomnia, and myalgia (Weller, 1987). It is also highly toxic to bone marrow. These problems were to some extent overcome by work performed by Dr. Nigel Philips at the Montreal General Hospital, who used liposomes (tiny, spherical sacs of water derived from body cells) as a transport mechanism to carry zidovudine to target cells. Liposomes do not travel to bone marrow, so when they are used to carry the drug to other destinations, the drug's toxic effects are greatly reduced or eliminated (Medical Research Council of Canada communique, February, 1991). Unfortunately, zidovudine does not eliminate latent virus and ultimately fails to stem the progression of immunodeficiency since, over a period of time, HIV develops resistance to the drug.

Other promising drugs that inhibit reverse transcriptase and/or cause DNA chain termination include dideoxycytidine (non FDA approved), phosphonoformate, and rifabutin. In another treatment strategy, AIDS patients have been treated with soluble CD4 molecules in an attempt to interfere with the spread of the virus. The approach has had limited success. Further, α-interferon, which reduces viral budding from infected cell surfaces, has been undergoing clinical trials and has been shown to be of use in the treatment of Kaposi's sarcoma.

Finally, it has been proposed by Dr. Paul Jolicoeur of Montreal that anticancer drugs may be useful in treating AIDS. The treatment is admitted to be paradoxical because the cancer drug proposed for use is immunosuppressive. Despite this, the treatment is reported to have eliminated an AIDS-like disease in mice and could have a similar effect on human AIDS (Medical Research Council of Canada communique, February, 1991).

The Development of Vaccines

The development of an effective vaccine for immunoprophylaxis has become a priority for medical research institutions worldwide. The task has been complicated by the genetic potential of the virus for great antigenic variability and the lack of good animal models for vaccine trials. In spite of these complications, several vaccines have been developed, which fall into three groups (types): genetically engineered HIV subunit vaccines (combined with adjuvant or in a virus vector), anti-idiotype vaccines (antibodies against CD4), and killed-virus vaccine. These vaccines will require lengthy clinical trials, yet the initial findings are promising and it is not unrealistic to assume that an effective vaccine will be developed in the not too distant future. (See New Hopes for AIDS Vaccines, Communique of the Medical Research Council of Canada, February, 1991).

Prevention of HIV Infection

HIV transmission can be curtailed through the practice of safe sex. Several recommendations have been made in this respect, including the use of condoms and the avoidance of fluid interchange between sexual partners (except in the case of uninfected partners in monogamous relationships).

In recent years, the screening of blood donors and donors of organs, tissue, and semen as well as blood products for HIV has reduced the risk of transmission to minimal levels. In addition, heat treatment and techniques such as monoclonal absorption have eliminated the risk of blood-borne HIV transmission to hemophiliacs.

In the case of drug abusers, it would perhaps be naive to recommend discontinuance of the practice (although this would obviously be the wisest choice), but the use of sterile equipment and the avoidance of shared needles would eliminate this mode of transmission.

Prevention of HIV Infection in Health Care Workers

The Centers for Disease Control offer the following recommendations for health care workers who deal with AIDS patients and blood specimens:

1. Contamination of the outside of containers

upon specimen collection should be carefully avoided. Ensure that the lid is on tight.

2. Gloves should be worn when processing patient specimens. Masks and protective eyewear should be used if splashing or aerosolization is anticipated. Gloves should be changed at the end of processing, and hands should be washed carefully and thoroughly.

3. Biological safety cabinets should be used when blending, sonicating, and mixing specimens.

4. Mouth pipetting should be expressly forbidden in the laboratory.

5. Precautions should be taken when handling needles. Bending, breaking, recapping, and removing needles from disposable syringes should be avoided. Needles should always be placed in puncture-resistant containers.

6. Work surfaces should be decontaminated with a chemical germicide after spills and when work is completed.

7. Contaminated materials should be disposed of in bags and in accordance with institutional policies for the disposal of infective waste.

8. Equipment should be decontaminated before repair or shipping.

9. Hands should be washed before leaving the laboratory.

10. Protective clothing should be removed before leaving the laboratory.

Antibody Development in AIDS (Fig. 13–5)

All of the protein and glycoprotein gene products (p and gp) may induce an antibody response in the infected individual. Groopman *et al.*, (1986) found that the first antibody to be observed is directed against the p24 core protein, followed by a mixture of antibodies usually including antibodies to the gp41 envelope glycoprotein. These antibodies are seen in both symptomatic and asymptomatic HIV-

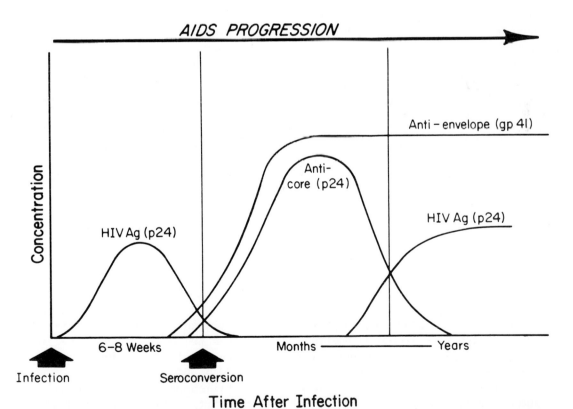

Figure 13–5. The antigen and antibody response in AIDS. (From McNamara, A.M.: Acquired immunodeficiency syndrome. In Sheehan, C.: Clinical Immunology: Principles and Laboratory Diagnosis. Philadelphia, J. B. Lippincott Company, 1990, p. 245.)

seropositive individuals and act as markers for HIV infection. In the late stages of AIDS, when patients deteriorate clinically, the titer of gp24 declines (see Fig. 13–5). Antibodies to the envelope gene products (gp160, gp120, and gp41) can be detected in almost all HIV-positive individuals, and antibodies to p31, p51, and p66 (the polymerase gene products) are also commonly detected (Jackson and Balfour, 1988). There does not appear to be any consistency in the development of other antibodies.

LABORATORY DIAGNOSIS

A wide range of test methods have been devised to isolate HIV, detect HIV antibodies, and detect HIV antigen in a patient's blood and body fluids. The isolation of HIV and methods used to detect HIV antigens are mainly used to detect early HIV infection before antibodies develop. They are also used to detect the progression from asymptomatic to symptomatic AIDS infection by monitoring an increase in p24 antigen.

It should be noted that while the detection of HIV antigen indicates *active* HIV infection, the detection of antibody to HIV denotes prior exposure to HIV (Jackson and Balfour, 1988).

HIV antibody tests are of two major classes: screening tests and supplementary tests.

It is currently possible to detect HIV-2 antibodies, proteins, and genes through the modification of test methods for HIV-1. It should be noted that HIV-2 positive sera may cross-react with HIV-1 core proteins but probably not with HIV-1 envelope proteins. The test methods discussed in this text refer to HIV-1 detection.

TESTS TO DETECT HIV ANTIBODY

Enzyme-Linked Immunosorbent Assay

The most widely used screening test for HIV antibodies is the enzyme-linked immunosorbent assay (ELISA) procedure, mainly because it is simple to perform, can be used to screen large numbers of specimens in a short period of time (less than 4 hours), and is relatively inexpensive.

In this test, HIV antigens, which are derived from disrupted virus particles (first-generation assays),

recombinant antigens, or chemically synthesized peptides (second-generation assays), are immobilized onto microtiter wells or plastic or metal beads. The patient's serum is then incubated with the fixed antigen and washed. Anti-IgG antibody, conjugated either to horseradish peroxidase, glucose oxidase, or alkaline phosphatase, is added and allowed to incubate. After washing, the appropriate chromogenic enzymatic substrate is added and a color change occurs that is proportional to the amount of human IgG present.

The results are interpreted with the use of a spectrophotometer by comparing the values obtained from positive and negative controls to those of the test specimen. This results in an absorbance cutoff value above which the test is considered reactive. If the test is modified to include a mixture of heavy- and light-chain antibodies to human immunoglobulin, it can also be used to detect IgM antibodies.

Antibody can also be detected in the ELISA test if the method is modified to a competitive assay format. In this procedure, patient serum or plasma specimens are incubated with enzyme-labeled HIV antibodies in microtiter wells coated with HIV antigens. Patient and enzyme-labeled HIV antibodies then compete for the binding sites on the immobilized HIV antigens. The more unbound patient HIV antibody that binds to the antigen, the less labeled HIV antibody binds and the less color development occurs when the substrate is added. Color development is therefore inversely proportional to the amount of HIV antibodies present in the patient's specimen.

The sources of error in this technique are as follows:

False-Positive Results

1. Technical error
2. The patient is suffering from:
   a. An autoimmune disease. The false-positive result is due to shared membrane antigens between the HIV virion and the human host cell, i.e., T-cell antigens, HLA antigens, nuclear and cellular antigens.
   b. Alcoholism
   c. Lymphoproliferative diseases
   d. Adult T-cell leukemia-lymphoma
   e. Syphilis
   f. No known risk

False-Negative Results

1. AIDS is in the incubation stage (between the time of infection and the development of detectable antibody).
2. AIDS is in the late stage (when antibody titers typically decrease).
3. Envelope glycoproteins (i.e., gp41 and gp120) are lost (due to overstringent purification methods).
4. There is insufficient p24 in antigen mixtures as a result of glycoprotein enrichment procedures.

When a reactive test is encountered, the test is repeated in duplicate to rule out technical error. If the specimen is reactive in at least two of three tests, it is referred to as "repeatedly reactive." In this case, a supplementary test is performed to confirm the result.

The Predictive Value Positive (PVP)

The PVP is an important concept in ELISA testing, giving the probability of a positive test being a true positive. The PVP is dependent on the prevalence of a disease in a given population. A reactive ELISA test in a high-risk person or population is most likely indicative of true infection, whereas a reactive test result in a low-risk individual or population may indicate a false-positive.

The sensitivity and specificity of ELISA antibody tests are better than 98 per cent when compared with Western blot assays.

ELISA tests have also been modified to detect HIV antigen (see discussion later in this chapter).

Western Blot Assay

In the Western blot (WB) assay, HIV virus is disrupted and HIV proteins are separated by molecular weight into discrete bands by electrophoresis onto polyacrylamide gels (Lombardo, 1987). The viral proteins are then transferred onto nitrocellulose sheets and cut into strips. Individual strips are incubated overnight with patient serum, washed, and incubated with anti-human immunoglobulin conjugated with enzymes or biotin. After the addition of the appropriate substrate, color develops to show discrete bands where antigen-antibody reactions have occurred.

Interpretation of the results of the tests is gener-

ally governed by Centers for Disease Control guidelines and individual laboratory experiences. The Centers for Disease Control recommends that tests be considered positive when the gp41 band appears alone or when an envelope antibody (gp41, gp120, or gp160) appears in combination with another HIV characteristic band (p15, p18, p24, gp41, p51, p55, p66, gp120, or gp160). In some cases, kits supplied by commercial companies will have special interpretive instructions, and these should obviously be followed when using the particular kit. The test is considered negative when no bands appear. If there is isolated reactivity to a single HIV protein or a pattern of reactivity to multiple proteins from the same viral gene product (i.e., polymerase gene products: p31, p51/66 only), the test result is considered doubtful (or indeterminate). In this case, a follow-up specimen from the patient should be collected in 6 months and the test repeated in case the patient is in the early stages of HIV infection.

False-positive WB reactions may occur in healthy individuals, in HTLV-1 or HIV-2 infections, in bilirubinemia, in connective tissue disease, in polyclonal gammopathies, and in patients with HLA antibodies (Jackson and Balfour, 1988).

Western blot is the most widely used supplementary test for confirming reactive HIV ELISA antibody tests, although the test has certain disadvantages—it is cumbersome to perform, it requires overnight incubation, and interpretation is often difficult.

Indirect Immunofluorescent Assay

The indirect immunofluorescent assay (IFA) is another test currently in use as a supplemental test for confirming reactive ELISA tests. The source of antigen is HIV-infected H9 or HUT 78 cells (i.e., malignant T-cell lines) dried and fixed with acetone to wells of a fluorescent slide (Lennette et al., 1987). Serum or plasma from the patient is then added and the mixture is washed with an Evans blue counterstain. The results are interpreted using a fluorescent microscope by noting the degree of fluorescence intensity, the percentage of fluorescent cells, and the localization of the fluorescence to cell surfaces. (Note: It is the gp160 and gp120 envelope proteins that are reacting in this test.)

IFA is more sensitive and specific than WB; the

test is simple and results are obtained generally in less than 2 hours (Jackson and Balfour, 1988; Khan and Hunter, 1988). The procedure has the disadvantage of nonspecific staining. There is also a certain amount of difficulty associated with interpretation. In addition, the fluorescence fades quickly so that slides cannot be stored. A further disadvantage is the expense of the required equipment, in particular the fluorescent microscope.

Slide Agglutination Tests

Rapid slide agglutination tests are widely used in field work in Africa to detect HIV antibodies in blood products and patients. The advantages of these screening tests over ELISA antibody tests are that they are simple and fast (requiring only 5 minutes to 2 hours), the results are not affected by heat inactivation, all materials are portable, and results can be read macroscopically (Yoshida *et al.*, 1987; Riggin *et al.*, 1987). An additional advantage is that slide agglutination tests simultaneously detect both IgG and IgM HIV antibodies.

In principle, the test is that of an antigen-antibody reaction made visible on a slide by linking the detector antigens to polystyrene or polyvinyl beads or to gelatin carriers. Addition of the patient's serum or plasma results in visible agglutination.

Other Tests for Antibody Detection

Other tests used in the detection of HIV antibody include radioimmunoassay and radioimmunoprecipitation assay. Both of these are usually used as research techniques (rarely used in the diagnostic laboratory) because they are expensive and time consuming and require the use of radioactive materials for the labeling of antibodies.

The principles of these tests are as follows:

Radioimmunoassay. Radioactive labeled (usually ^{125}I) anti-HIV antibodies compete with unlabeled patient serum (unlabeled antibody) for binding sites of solid-phase, fixed HIV antigen. The radioactivity of bound antibodies is measured in a gamma counter. The amount of HIV antibody is inversely proportional to the number of counts detected (Janda, 1985).

Radioimmunoprecipitation Assay. HIV-infected cells are exposed to a radioactive isotope, lysed, and centrifuged in an ultracentrifuge to ob-

tain a cell lysate containing radiolabeled viral proteins. The patient's serum is preabsorbed with protein A-Sepharose beads, then mixed with the cell lysate. Immunoprecipitates are formed by boiling in buffer, and the immunoprecipitate is separated by electrophoresis on sodium dodecyl sulfate-polyacrylamide gels. Banding patterns similar to those of WB are formed and interpreted.

TESTS TO DETECT HIV ANTIGEN

HIV Isolation

The technique of HIV isolation is used to detect HIV antigen in early infection (before antibodies develop) and to monitor antiviral drug therapy (viral isolation will decrease if therapy is successful).

The technique involves the collection of monocytes from peripheral blood samples by Ficoll-Hypaque gradients. Monocytes from HIV-negative donors are also collected, and these are stimulated with phytohemagglutinin for 2 to 4 days before mixing with patient monocytes and interleukin-2. The cell mixture is cocultivated in tissue culture flasks with added cell culture medium for up to 1 month (Janda, 1985). Culture fluid is removed weekly and tested for the presence of HIV by reverse transcriptase assays, antigen indirect immunofluorescence assay, or antigen ELISA testing.

In general this technique is not used in routine laboratories because it is costly and time consuming and has the risk of exposing personnel to high virus concentrations (Jackson and Balfour, 1988; Khan and Hunter, 1988).

Enzyme-Linked Immunosorbent Assay

Modification of the ELISA test allows for the detection of HIV antigen in serum, plasma, culture fluids, and cerebrospinal fluid. The test is that of an antibody sandwich in which monoclonal or polyclonal anti-HIV antibody is coated to the microwell or bead. The patient's specimen is added, incubated, and washed, and rabbit or goat anti-HIV antibody is added. If the patient's sample contains HIV antigen, an antibody-antigen-antibody complex is formed. Enzyme-conjugated antibody to rabbit or goat immunoglobulin is then added, followed by the appropriate substrate. The kits available for this test primarily detect free p24 HIV antigens.

If the ELISA antigen test is repeatedly reactive, an antibody neutralization assay should be performed on the specimen. In this assay, the patient's specimen is incubated with human antibody to HIV before performing the ELISA antigen test. If HIV antigen is present in the specimen, it will be neutralized by the human antibody and attachment to the ELISA antibody coated microwell or bead will not occur. This results in a reduction in absorbance when compared with a concomitant nonabsorbed patient specimen.

Indirect Immunofluorescent Assay (IFA)

The indirect immunofluorescent assay can be modified to detect HIV antigen by treating HIV-infected cells with polyclonal or monoclonal antibody raised against HIV proteins p18 or p24. The test procedure is then the same as for the IFA antibody assay.

Slide Agglutination Tests

Slide agglutination tests can be used for HIV antigen detection by substituting detector antibodies for the detector antigens and mixing with the patient's serum or plasma on a slide (see Slide Agglutination Tests, above).

TESTS FOR DETECTING HIV GENES

Recent techniques have been developed that detect the presence of the viral genes rather than the products of these genes. These techniques are most appropriate for use when the production of virus is low or when the virus may exist in a latent condition.

In Situ Hybridization

In situ hybridization uses a ^{35}S-labeled RNA probe, which binds with viral nucleic acids and is specific for viral RNA. The test procedure involves the fixation of infected cells on a slide, acetylation,

and application of hybridization mixture containing radioactive probe (nonradioactive probes can also be used in modifications of this technique) on the slide, and autoradiograph. The slides are dipped in photographic emulsion, dried, and kept in the dark for 2 days at 4°C, during which time the probe emits radioactive particles and creates a latent image. After 2 days, the slides are developed, dried, stained with Wright stain, and analyzed by light microscopy. The location of HIV-1 is represented by microscopic black dots, with 20 to 100 being observed per infected cell. One to three copies are represented by each dot, which are located over the nucleus and cytoplasm.

This test detects the presence of HIV-1 in lymphocytes in primary lymph nodes and in peripheral blood.

Filter Hybridization

Filter hybridization involves the isolation and denaturation of cytoplasmic RNA from infected cells, transfer of the denatured material to a nylon filter, incubation of the filter with a radioactive probe, and autoradiography. Prehybridization and hybridization are performed using ^{32}P-labeled DNA. The cloned fragment represents the entire HIV-1 genome, excluding the leftmost 224 nucleotides.

Filter hybridization is able to detect one infected cell in 100 peripheral blood leukocytes. It is a relatively rapid procedure, simple and inexpensive, and can be used to monitor viral growth in cell culture.

Southern Blot Hybridization

Southern blot can be used to detect HIV-1 sequence in peripheral blood cells and tissues (lymph nodes, liver, and kidney). It is extremely useful for detecting a specific sequence that may be present in integrated or unintegrated form in infected cells.

The procedure involves the digestion of DNA isolated from HIV-1-infected cells or primary tissues with a panel of restriction enzymes and the separation of DNA fragments according to size using agarose gel electrophoresis. The DNA fragments are then transferred (blotted) onto a membrane, and the membrane is incubated with a cloned HIV-1 probe.

It is possible with this technique to achieve hybridization of 18 viral DNA isolates to the full length of the cloned probe. Complications due to the presence of unintegrated linear and circular DNA, as well as integrated proviral DNA within the infected cells, are avoided by this method.

DNA Amplification

This is an ultrasensitive polymerase chain reaction technique that allows for the direct detection of HIV-1 through the amplification of minute amounts of viral nucleic acid in lymphocyte DNA, after which isotope or nonisotope methods are used to detect the amplified product.

The test can be modified to specifically amplify RNA, which, when performed in addition to DNA amplification, could prove to be a better indicator of biologically active virus than DNA detection alone.

Alternatively, sandwich hybridization can be used, which requires two adjacent, nonoverlapping probes (an immobilized capture probe and a labeled detection probe).

DNA amplification is currently revolutionizing HIV-1 detection. It can be used as confirmatory testing or to monitor the inactivation of HIV-1 by drugs. In time, this technique will provide more accurate and predictive HIV-1 testing and better testing for other latent viruses.

JUST THE FACTS

Introduction: History

1. During 1981 several reports appeared regarding the development of *P. carinii* pneumonia, other opportunistic infections, and a disseminated form of Kaposi's sarcoma in apparently previously healthy, young, homosexual men in New York City and San Francisco.
2. It was suspected that these men were suffering a severe immune defect.
3. Since Kaposi's sarcoma had rarely been seen in North America prior to that time, it was suspected that the illness was new and not merely a newly recognized one.
4. A task force was formed by the Centers for Disease Control to study the epidemic.
5. The task force discovered that no patients fit-

ting the case definition had been found prior to 1978, and that 92 per cent of infected men were either bisexual or homosexual.
6. There is no gender-determined resistance to AIDS.
7. AIDS can develop in intravenous drug abusers and heterosexual (non–drug abusing) classic hemophilia patients (i.e., the etiologic agent is transmissible by blood or blood products).
8. Transmission can also occur between mother and fetus *in utero.*
9. It is unlikely that AIDS originated in North America.
10. It is possible that the causative retrovirus existed in exceedingly remote pockets of Africa (possibly as an agent with a nonhuman primate reservoir) and that recent population shifts could have introduced the agent into certain urban centers of Central Africa, which, in effect, could have simultaneously conveyed the virus to North America. This theory is supported by the fact that HIV is closely related to simian T-cell lymphotropic virus type III, which causes a form of AIDS in African green monkeys.

Human Immunodeficiency Virus (HIV)

1. HIV is a human retrovirus that is the etiologic agent of AIDS.
2. There are two types of HIV.
3. HIV-1 is the causative agent of AIDS in the United States and Europe.
4. HIV-2 is associated with immunodeficiency and a clinical syndrome similar to AIDS in West Africa.
5. HIV was formerly known as lymphadenopathy-associated virus (LAV), human T-cell lymphotropic virus type III, or AIDS-related virus (ARV).
6. HIV is considered to be a member of the lentivirus subfamily.

The Structure of the Human Immunodeficiency Virus

1. The HIV virus particle (virion) is about 100 nm in diameter.
2. It consists of an outer envelope, a core shell of protein, and a cone-shaped inner core that con-

tains two identical strands of RNA with associated reverse transcriptase and core polypeptides.

3. Virally encoded membrane proteins, p18 and p24, are embedded in the lipid bilayer.
4. A large glycoprotein traverses the lipid bilayer membrane, which has two components—gp41 traverses the membrane and gp120 extends beyond the surface as a knob.
5. The gp120 component provokes an immune response.
6. HLA antigens are also on the outer envelope, derived from human cell membranes when the HIV virions bud from human cells during the process of virus particle formation.

The HIV Genome

1. The complete nucleotide sequences of the HIV genome have been determined, making it possible to identify viral genes and some of the relationships between viral gene products and the clinical course of AIDS.
2. The HIV genome shares the basic structure of all known retroviruses but has six additional genes (*tat, art/trs, sor, 3'orf,* and *R*) in addition to the usual three structural genes (*gag, pol,* and *env*).
3. The *gag* (*g*roup *a*nti*g*en) codes for core structural proteins, which are cleaved from a 55kd polyprotein found in high levels of infected cells. The cleavage products form the three core proteins p18, p24, and p15.
4. The *pol* (*pol*ymerase) gene codes for reverse transcriptase, RNase, protease, and integrase.
5. The *env* (*env*elope) gene codes for the glycoprotein gp160, found in infected cells. It is cleaved to form gp120 and gp41.
6. The *tat* (*t*rans-*a*ctivation *t*ranslation) gene speeds up viral protein production and is required for viral replication.
7. The *art/trs* (*a*nti-*r*epression *t*ransactivator) gene regulates the translation of the viral genome. It produces p20.
8. The *sor* (*s*hort *o*pen *r*eading frame) gene is related to viral infectivity. It produces p23.
9. The *3'orf* (3' *o*pen *r*eading *f*rame) gene slows down viral replication tenfold in CD4 cells and is considered responsible for the latency of the virus. It produces p27.
10. The *R* (*r*eading frame) gene codes for an immunogenic product, p15, whose function is unknown.
11. The viral genome has identical ends known as LTRs (*l*ong *t*erminal *e*nds) which contain a terminator, an enhancer, and a promoter for the process of transcription.

The Life Cycle of HIV

1. The life cycle of HIV begins when the gp120 protein on the viral envelope binds to the CD4 protein receptor on the surface of the target cell.
2. The primary target cell is the helper-inducer subset of T lymphocytes.
3. Other target cells include macrophages, about 40 per cent of peripheral blood monocytes, cells in the skin, lymph nodes, and other organs, and about 5 per cent of B lymphocytes.
4. After HIV binds to the CD4-containing cell, it penetrates the host cells and loses its outer layer, injecting its core into the cell.
5. The RNA in the core is transcribed into DNA by DNA-polymerase.
6. The original RNA is destroyed by ribonuclease, and a second complementary copy of DNA is made by polymerase, using the first DNA strand as a template.
7. DNA migrates into the cell nucleus where it is "spliced" to the host cells' DNA.
8. New virus particles are produced in the nucleotide sequences in the LTRs, which direct enzyme belonging to the host cell to copy the DNA of the integrated virus into RNA.
9. When HIV replication occurs, the CD4 cell is killed, which results in a depletion of helper-inducer T lymphocytes.

Disease Characteristics

Incidence

1. As of July 4, 1988, there had been 66,464 reported cases of AIDS in the United States.
2. By March 31, 1989, this number had grown to 89,501.
3. On July 31, 1991, the reported number was 182,834.
4. The majority of AIDs patients are homosexual or bisexual men (63 per cent). Other high-risk individuals are heterosexual IV drug abusers (19 per

cent), homosexual or bisexual IV drug abusers (7 per cent), heterosexual men and women (4 per cent), recipients of blood or blood product transfusion (usually before 1985) (3 per cent), hemophiliacs or patients with other coagulation disorders (1 per cent), and unknown (3 per cent).

5. Of pediatric AIDS cases, 78 per cent could be traced to IV drug abuse by the child's parent (or parents). The other 19 per cent had resulted from blood transfusions or treatment for hemophilia or were traced to parents who either had AIDS or had practiced high-risk behavior.

6. In the United States, 59 per cent of AIDS patients are white, 26 per cent are black, 19 per cent are Hispanic.

7. A small number of health care workers have become infected through accidental needle puncture, ungloved hands, or skin lesions.

Modes of Transmission

1. HIV can be transmitted by sexual contact (with the exchange of body fluids), intimate contact with blood from an infected individual (blood transfusion or the sharing of blood-contaminated drug paraphernalia), and transplacental routes.

2. Only semen, vaginal secretions, blood, and possibly breast milk have been implicated in the transmission of HIV to date.

3. AIDS is not known to be transmitted by food, water, insects, or casual contact.

4. Transmission is believed to be possible through contact with inanimate objects that have been recently contaminated with infected blood or certain body fluids if transferred to broken skin or mucous membranes.

Clinical Manifestations

Primary Stage

1. Patients in the early stages of HIV infection are either completely asymptomatic or may show a mild, chronic lymphadenopathy.

2. This stage may last from many months to many years after infection.

3. Initially, the virus replicates abundantly—free virus is found in the cerebrospinal fluid surrounding the brain and spinal cord and in the circulating blood.

4. This viral concentration drops suddenly after a few weeks, and the initial symptoms disappear.

5. A brief mononucleosis-like illness occurs in certain infected individuals.

6. This illness parallels the first wave of HIV replications.

7. At the same time, antibodies to HIV are detected for the first time (2 weeks to 3 months after infection, rarely later).

8. Following these initial mild symptoms, the individual may remain asymptomatic for years.

Intermediate Stage

1. This is characterized by persistent lymphadenopathy and quantitative T-cell deficiencies (especially decreased CD4-positive cell count and an inverted CD4/CD8 ratio) but without opportunistic infections and cancers seen in AIDS.

2. This state is known as AIDS-related complex (ARC).

3. Patients present with fatigue, night sweats, fever, diarrhea, and weight loss.

4. Diagnosis is made on the basis of Centers for Disease Control criteria if two clinical manifestations and two laboratory abnormalities are found in a patient without explainable etiology.

Clinical Manifestations:
a. Lymphadenopathy of more than 3 months' duration
b. Fever of over 100°F for more than 3 months
c. More than 10 per cent weight loss
d. Persistent diarrhea
e. Fatigue
f. Night sweats

Laboratory Abnormalities:
a. CD4 cells fewer that 400/mm²
b. CD4/CD8 ratio less than 1.0
c. Leukopenia
d. Thrombocytopenia
e. Anemia
f. Elevated serum globulins
g. Anergy to skin tests
h. Reduced blastogenesis
i. Positive HIV antibody test

Final Stage

1. From 2 to 10 years after initial infection, the disease progresses to AIDS.
2. In this stage there is severe CD4 depletion resulting in opportunistic infections and cancers.
3. The clinical features include extreme weight loss, fever, and multiple secondary infections.
5. *Pneumocystis carinii* pneumonia is a common opportunistic infection.
6. The most frequent malignancy is a variant of Kaposi's sarcoma, which produces tumors in the skin and linings of the internal organs, lymphomas, and cancers of the rectum and tongue.

Effects of HIV on the Immune System

1. Inducer-helper T lymphocytes play a central role in the induction of most immune responses.
2. HIV infection can lead to the lysis of CD4+ T lymphocytes or functional inactivation of these cells without cytolysis.
3. CD4+ T cells are reduced in AIDS patients.
4. The CD4 to CD8 ratio is reduced from 2:1 to 0.5:1 (reversed).
5. Less than 1 per cent of CD4+ T cells are *directly* infected with HIV.
6. More than 99 per cent of CD4+ T cells are latently infected without detectable viral RNA transcripts.
7. Individuals have various immunologic abnormalities even before their CD4+ T cells are reduced in numbers. The reason for this is unknown.
8. HIV infection also causes impairment of function of CD4+ T cells, including:
   a. Decreased expression of IL-2
   b. Diminished secretion of IL-2
   c. Humoral responses to soluble antigens
   d. CTL responses to certain viruses
9. Abnormalities in B-lymphocyte activation are frequently observed.
10. Macrophages can also become infected by HIV, although they are fairly resistant to the cytolytic effects of the virus.
11. Macrophage functions are impaired, including:
    a. Decreased chemotaxis
    b. Decreased IL-1 production
    c. Decreased oxygen metabolite-dependent killing of microbes
12. The antigen-presenting capabilities of monocytes and macrophages are reduced.
13. Functional impairment is also reported to affect NK cells, and this may be the reason for inadequate antiviral immunity in these individuals.

Treatment

1. The treatment of AIDS usually involves the treatment of the opportunistic infections and cancers that are its complications.
2. The most promising drug for treatment is zidovudine (formerly known as azidothymidine or AZT).
3. The drug is reasonably effective but has many side effects, and HIV eventually becomes immune to it.
4. Other promising drugs include dideoxycytidine, phosphonoformate, and rifabutin.
5. Soluble CD4 molecules have been used in an attempt to interfere with the spread of the virus.
6. α-Interferon has been shown to be useful in the treatment of Kaposi's sarcoma.
7. It has been proposed that anticancer drugs may be useful in treating AIDS.

Prevention of HIV Infection

1. HIV transmission can be curtailed through the practice of safe sex.
2. Screening of blood donors and donors of organs, tissue, and semen, as well as blood products, has reduced the risk of transmission to minimal levels.
3. Heat treatment techniques have eliminated the risk of blood-borne transmission to hemophiliacs.
4. Drug abusers should use sterile equipment and avoid sharing needles (discontinuance of drug abuse would be preferable).

Prevention of HIV Infection in Health Care Workers

The recommendations of the CDC are:
1. Contamination of the outside of containers upon specimen collection should be carefully avoided. Ensure that the lid is tight.
2. Gloves should be worn when processing pa-

tient specimens. Masks and protective eyewear should be used if splashing or aerosolization is anticipated. Gloves should be changed at the end of processing, and hands should be washed carefully and thoroughly.

3. Biological safety cabinets should be used when blending, sonicating, and mixing specimens.
4. Mouth pipetting should be expressly forbidden in the laboratory.
5. Precautions should be taken when handling needles. Bending, breaking, recapping, and the removal of needles from disposable syringes should be avoided. Needles should always be placed in puncture-resistant containers.
6. Work surfaces should be decontaminated with a chemical germicide after spills and when work is completed.
7. Contaminated materials should be disposed of in bags and in accordance with institutional policies for the disposal of infective waste.
8. Equipment should be decontaminated before repair or shipping.
9. Hands should be washed before a person who has handled infected material leaves the laboratory.
10. Protective clothing should be removed before leaving the laboratory.

The Development of Vaccines

1. The development of an effective AIDS virus is complicated by the genetic potential of the virus for great antigenic variability and the lack of good animal models for vaccine trials.
2. Several vaccines have been developed that are:
   a. Genetically engineered HIV subunit vaccines
   b. Anti-idiotype vaccines
   c. Killed-virus vaccine
3. These vaccines will require lengthy clinical trials, but the initial finds are promising.

Antibody Development in AIDS

1. The first antibody to be observed in HIV-infected individuals is directed against the p24 core protein, followed by a mixture of antibodies usually including antibodies to gp41.
2. These antibodies are seen in symptomatic and asymptomatic HIV-seropositive individuals and act as markers for HIV infection.

3. Antibodies to gp24 decline in the late stages of AIDS.
4. Antibodies to the envelope gene products (gp160, gp120, gp41) can be detected in most HIV-positive individuals.
5. Antibodies to polymerase gene products (p31, p51, and p66) are also commonly detected.
6. The development of other antibodies does not appear to show consistency.

Laboratory Diagnosis

1. Tests have been developed to isolate HIV and to detect HIV antibodies and antigens in blood and body fluids.
2. Isolation of HIV and detection of HIV antigens are mainly used to detect early HIV infection before antibodies develop or to detect the progression from asymptomatic to symptomatic AIDS infection by monitoring an increase in p24 antigen.
3. Detection of HIV antigen indicates active HIV infection.
4. Detection of HIV antibodies denotes prior exposure to HIV.
5. HIV-2 antibodies, proteins, and genes can be detected through the modification of test methods for HIV-1.
6. HIV-2-positive sera may cross-react with HIV-1 core proteins but probably not with HIV-1 envelope proteins.

Tests to Detect HIV Antibody

1. The tests used to detect HIV antibody are:
   a. Enzyme-linked immunosorbent assay (ELISA)
   b. Western blot (WB) assay
   c. Indirect immunofluorescent assay (IFA)
   d. Slide agglutination tests
   e. Radioimmunoassay
   f. Radioimmunoprecipitation assay
2. The tests used to detect HIV antigen are:
   a. HIV isolation
   b. Enzyme-linked immunosorbent assay (ELISA)
   c. Indirect immunofluorescent assay (IFA)
   d. Slide agglutination tests
3. The tests used to detect HIV genes are:
   a. In situ hybridization
   b. Filter hybridization
   c. Southern blot hybridization
   d. DNA amplification

Review Questions

Multiple Choice

Choose the phrase, sentence, or symbol that completes the statement or answers the question. More than one answer may be correct in each case. Answers are given at the end of this book.

1. The human immunodeficiency virus:
   (a) is a human retrovirus
   (b) occurs in three types: HIV-1, HIV-2, and HIV-3
   (c) was formerly known as lymphadenopathy-associated virus (LAV)
   (d) all of the above
   (Human Immunodeficiency Virus)

2. The two components of the large glycoprotein that traverses the lipid bilayer membrane of the human immunodeficiency virus are:
   (a) gp41 and gp120
   (b) gp18 and gp181
   (c) gp18 and gp24
   (d) p41 and p24
   (The Structure of the Human Immunodeficiency Virus)

3. The *pol* genes code for:
   (a) structural proteins
   (b) reverse transcriptase
   (c) RNase
   (d) gp160
   (The HIV Genome)

4. The primary target cells of the human immunodeficiency virus are:
   (a) B lymphocytes
   (b) peripheral blood monocytes
   (c) helper-inducer subset of T lymphocytes
   (d) glial cells
   (The Life Cycle of HIV)

5. The majority of adult AIDS patients are:
   (a) white
   (b) IV drug abusers
   (c) homosexual IV drug abusers
   (d) homosexual or bisexual men
   (Incidence)

6. Which of the following body fluids have been implicated in the transmission of HIV:
   (a) semen
   (b) tears
   (c) cerebrospinal fluid
   (d) vaginal secretions
   (Modes of Transmission)

7. After infection with HIV, antibodies can usually be detected within:
   (a) 6 months
   (b) 6 days to 2 months
   (c) 2 weeks to 3 months
   (d) 1 year
   (Clinical Manifestations: Primary Stage)

8. Patients with ARC usually present with:
   (a) fatigue
   (b) night sweats
   (c) fever
   (d) weight loss
   (Intermediate Stage)

9. The most frequent malignancy observed in the final phase of HIV infection is:
   (a) *Pneumocystis carinii* pneumonia
   (b) Kaposi's sarcoma
   (c) Burkitt-like lymphoma
   (d) none of the above
   (Final Stage)

10. In normal individuals, the ratio of CD4+ T cells to CD8+ T cells is approximately:
    (a) 4:1
    (b) 10:1
    (c) 2:1
    (d) 0.5:1
    (Effects of HIV on the Immune System)

11. The side effects associated with the use of zidovudine in AIDS treatment include:
    (a) megaloblastic anemia
    (b) neutropenia
    (c) myalgia
    (d) nausea
    (Treatment)

12. Mouth pipetting:
    (a) is acceptable in certain laboratories
    (b) should only be used when the specimen is known not to contain HIV
    (c) should be forbidden at all times
    (d) is acceptable when the specimen is kept sterile
    (Prevention of HIV Infection in Health Care Workers)

13. The first antibody to be observed in an HIV-infected individual is directed against:
    (a) the p24 core protein
    (b) the gp41 envelope protein
    (c) the gp160 envelope protein
    (d) the p31 gene product
    (Antibody Development in AIDS)

14. A false-positive result can occur in ELISA testing if the patient is suffering from:
    (a) an autoimmune disease
    (b) syphilis

(c) a lymphoproliferative disease
(d) all of the above
(Tests to Detect HIV Antibody: ELISA)

15. Slide agglutination tests:
    (a) detect IgG HIV antibodies only
    (b) detect IgM HIV antibodies only
    (c) simultaneously detect IgG and IgM HIV antibodies
    (d) must be read microscopically
    (Slide Agglutination Tests [Antibody])

Answer "True" or "False"

1. There is no gender-determined resistance to AIDS.
   (Introduction: History)

2. Reverse transcriptase enables a retrovirus to convert viral DNA to RNA.
   (Human Immunodeficiency Virus)

3. The outer envelope of HIV contains HLA antigens.
   (The Structure of the Human Immunodeficiency Virus)

4. The *sor* gene is related to viral infectivity and produces p23.
   (The HIV Genome)

5. When HIV replication occurs the CD4 cell is killed.
   (The Life Cycle of HIV)

6. The majority of pediatric AIDS cases can be traced to IV drug abuse by the child's parent (or parents).
   (Disease Characteristics: Incidence)

7. There have been cases of HIV being transmitted by food.
   (Modes of Transmission)

8. Patients in the early stages of HIV infection are either completely asymptomatic or may show a mild, chronic lymphadenopathy.
   (Clinical Manifestations: Primary Stage)

9. T cells that are unaffected by HIV have a decreased expression of IL-2.
   (Effects of HIV on the Immune System)

10. Zidovudine is highly toxic to bone marrow.
    (Treatment)

11. Needles should be removed from disposable syringes after use as a precaution against AIDS transmission.
    (Prevention of HIV Infection in Health Care Workers)

12. Antibodies to gp160, gp120, and gp41 are rarely detected in HIV-positive individuals.
    (Antibody Development in AIDS)

13. The detection of HIV antigen indicates active HIV infection.
    (Laboratory Diagnosis)

14. The most widely used screening test for HIV antibodies is the enzyme-linked immunosorbent assay.
    (Tests to Detect HIV Antibody: ELISA)

15. Tests for the detection of HIV genes are most appropriate for use when the production of virus is at its greatest.
    (Tests for Detecting HIV Genes)

GENERAL REFERENCES

Baron, E.J., and Finegold, S.M.: Bailey and Scott's Diagnostic Microbiology, 8th ed. St Louis, C. V. Mosby Company, 1990.

Bennington, J.L.: Saunders Dictionary and Encyclopedia of Laboratory Medicine and Technology. Philadelphia, W. B. Saunders Company, 1984.

DeVita, V.T., Hellman, S., and Rosenberg, S.A. (Eds.): AIDS. Philadelphia, J. B. Lippincott Company, 1985.

Dorland's Illustrated Medical Dictionary, 27th ed. Philadelphia, W. B. Saunders Company, 1988.

Henry, J.B.: Clinical Diagnosis and Management by Laboratory Methods. Philadelphia, W. B. Saunders Company, 1991.

McNamara, A.M.: Acquired immunodeficiency syndrome. *In* Sheehan, C.: Clinical Immunology: Principles and Laboratory Diagnosis. Philadelphia, J. B. Lippincott Company, 1990.

Turgeon, M.L.: Immunology and Serology in Laboratory Medicine. St. Louis, C. V. Mosby Company, 1990.

14

Autoimmune Diseases

OBJECTIVES

The student shall know, understand, and be prepared to explain:
1. The classification and characteristics of autoimmune diseases
2. The possible mechanisms in the initiation of autoimmune diseases
3. The criteria for autoimmune diseases
4. Genetic control of autoimmune diseases
5. The systemic autoimmune diseases, including:
   a. Systemic lupus erythematosus, with respect to:
      i. Characteristics
      ii. Laboratory observations
      iii. Etiology
      iv. Serologic tests
   b. Rheumatoid arthritis, with respect to:
      i. Characteristics of the disease
      ii. Characteristics of rheumatoid factors
      iii. Serologic tests
   c. Ankylosing spondylitis
   d. Necrotizing angiitis (vasculitis)
   e. Polymyositis and dermatomyositis
   f. Progressive systemic sclerosis (scleroderma)
   g. Mixed connective tissue disease
   h. Sjögren's syndrome
6. The organ-specific autoimmune diseases, including:
   a. Autoimmune diseases of the blood, including:
      i. Autoimmune hemolytic anemias:
         (a) Warm type
         (b) Cold type
         (c) Paroxysmal cold hemaglobinuria
         (d) Drug-induced hemolysis
      ii. Autoimmune thrombocytopenic purpura
      iii. Neutropenia
      iv. Lymphocytopenia
      v. Autoimmune aplastic anemia
   b. Autoimmune diseases of the kidney (Types I, II, III, IV, and other forms)
   c. Autoimmune diseases of the endocrine organs, including:
      i. Autoimmune thyroiditis (Hashimoto's thyroiditis)
      ii. Myxedema
      iii. Thyrotoxicosis (Graves' disease)

d. Autoimmune diseases of the pancreas
e. Autoimmune diseases of the adrenals
f. Autoimmune diseases of the parathyroids
g. Autoimmune diseases of the ovary and testis
h. Autoimmune diseases of the nervous system, including:
  i. Disseminated encephalomyelitis
  ii. Idiopathic polyneuritis
  iii. Landry's paralysis
  iv. Multiple sclerosis
j. Autoimmune diseases of the stomach and intestines, including:
  i. Pernicious anemia
  ii. Gastric atrophy
  iii. Regional ileitis (Crohn's disease)
  iv. Ulcerative colitis
  v. Gluten-sensitive enteropathy (Celiac disease)
k. Autoimmune diseases of the liver, including:
  i. Hepatitis
  ii. Drug-induced liver diseases
  iii. Primary biliary cirrhosis
  iv. Portal cirrhosis
l. Autoimmune diseases of the muscle
m. Autoimmune diseases of the eye
n. Autoimmune diseases of the skin, including:
  i. Pemphigus vulgaris
  ii. Bullous pemphigoid
  iii. Cicatricial pemphigoid
  iv. Dermatitis herpetiformis
  v. Systemic lupus erythematosus
o. Autoimmune diseases affecting the heart

Introduction

In most individuals, there exists a tolerance and "self-recognition" of all body components; that is, normal individuals generally do not produce destructive responses to their own tissue antigens. In a minority of the population, however, disorders occur in which tissue injury is primarily caused by an apparent immunologic reaction of the host to his own tissues: these disorders are known as *autoimmune diseases*.

It should be noted that the terms *autoimmune disease* and *autoimmune response*, often used synonymously, do not refer to the same thing. In *autoimmune response*, an autoantibody directed against a "self" antigen can be demonstrated with respect to either erythrocytes or lymphocytes. The autoimmune response, although usually considered to be abnormal, often does not result in disease and frequently occurs in otherwise healthy individuals (e.g., T-agglutinin, anti-I cold autoantibody, and antibodies to smooth muscle). Although it is thought that autoimmune diseases result from tissue injury caused by autoimmune responses, it is not known whether the autoimmune phenomena are a cause, a result, or an accompanying finding in autoimmune disease. It is common, for example, to see autoimmune phenomena in association with infectious diseases (e.g., cold hemagglutinins in infection with *Mycoplasma pneumoniae*), yet there is no evidence that this response results in self-perpetuating protracted autoimmune disease.

Recent evidence suggests that some autoimmunity is necessary and beneficial to the host. For example, to initiate an immune response, an MHC (major histocompatibility locus) molecule must accompany an antigen. MHC class II molecules and antibodies must be coexpressed on an antigen-presenting cell to activate helper T cells, and MHC class I molecules and antigen are needed to activate cytotoxic T cells. In addition, regulation of an immune response occurs by an idiotype–anti-idiotype interaction. An idiotype network based on the ability of B lymphocytes to recognize the idiotype of an antibody molecule and to produce an anti-idiotype antibody was proposed by Jerne (1974). This anti-idiotype antibody then modulates the activity of B cells and T cells.

POSSIBLE MECHANISMS IN THE INITIATION OF AUTOIMMUNE DISEASES

The precise mechanisms that initiate autoimmune diseases are not known, but several theories have been proposed:

Forbidden Clone Theory. The forbidden clone theory postulates a clone (i.e., the progeny of a single cell) of changed or altered lymphocytes arising through cell mutation. Mutant cells carrying a foreign surface antigen would be destroyed by normal lymphocytes, but mutant cells lacking foreign surface antigen would *not* be destroyed by normal lymphocytes. With the proliferation of these antigen-deficient mutants (so-called forbidden clones), these cells, because of genetic dissimilarity, would be capable of reacting with target tissues. The mutations responsible could occur at the level of the macrophage, T or B lymphocytes, or their progenitor cells.

Altered Antigen Theory. In addition to mutation (described previously), altered surface antigens (neoantigens) can be created by chemical, physical, or biologic means, possibly resulting in an autoimmune disease when a portion of the immune response is directed against the altered antigen. Altered antigens can be formed by autocoupling haptens, through physical forces (e.g.,

visible and ultraviolet light, pressure, and cold), which cause the molecule to expose or create a new antigenic determinant, or through photosensitization.

Sequestered Antigen Theory. The sequestered antigen theory proposes that certain antigens are "hidden" (sequestered) in the circulation under conditions of normal health. The antigens often grouped as sequestered include lens proteins of the eye, milk casein antigens of the reproductive system (especially of the male), thyroglobulin, and so on. Exposure of the sequestered antigen to the lymphoreticular system in later life through trauma or infection results in autoimmune disease.

Immunologic Deficiency Theory. The concept of immunologic deficiency is based on the loss or deficiency of immunoregulation. The fact that T-helper and T-suppressor cells have pronounced effects on B cells and certain T-cell subsets is now well recognized. This would suggest that a total or partial functional loss of these cells would result in diminished suppressor cell activities, reflected in heightened immunoglobulin levels or T-cell responses. Normal individuals who develop autoimmune disease therefore have an underlying immune deficiency that renders them susceptible to autoimmune states.

Loss of immunoregulation can be compared with loss of "tolerance." During embryonic life, antigens exposed to the lymphoreticular system (i.e., prior to the time of immunologic maturation) are recognized as "self," whereas antigens not exposed to the lymphoreticular system during that time are regarded as "nonself." The body is "tolerant" of self antigens (i.e., does not react immunologically to them) and "intolerant" of nonself antigens. The continued presence of self antigens ensures continued tolerance; however, mutation or the loss of immunoregulatory powers results in the condition in which self antigens behave as foreign antigens; this results in autoimmune disease.

The Cross-Reactive Antigen Theory. The cross-reactive antigen theory proposes that, because of the size of antigenic determinants, it is possible that complex foreign structures could possess structural parts that are similar or identical to self-structures, resulting in immunologic cross-reactivity. This cross-reactivity may, in certain circumstances, be sufficient to initiate autoimmune disease.

CRITERIA FOR AUTOIMMUNE DISEASES

Many different diseases are associated with autoimmune phenomena. These diseases can be *systemic* (involving more than one organ) or *organspecific* (in which the major effect involves a single organ).

With respect to these diseases, it is not always easy to determine whether the involved autoantibodies are merely associated with the disease or whether they play a central role in the cause. Certain criteria were devised by Koch (known as Koch's postulates) and by Witebsky to aid in this determination.

1. The autoimmune response must be regularly associated with the disease.
2. It must be possible to induce a replica of the disease in laboratory animals.
3. The immunopathologic changes observed in the natural and experimental diseases should parallel each other.
4. It should be possible to transfer the autoimmune illness from the diseased individual to a normal recipient through the transfer of serum or lymphoid cells.

In applying these criteria, it becomes clear that in certain of these diseases, the autoantibodies seem not to have any role in the origin or continuation of the disease and serve as a convenient diagnostic support. In other diseases, any conclusion regarding the relationship of the immunologic phenomenon to the disease etiology is not possible with certainty, and therefore it can only be stated that autoantibodies are often associated with the disease.

GENETIC CONTROL OF AUTOIMMUNE DISEASES

Any hypothesis seeking to explain the development of the autoimmune state must recognize the genetic control of the immune system. It is well documented that certain immune disorders are characterized by predominance in the female and in families. The immune response gene is closely linked to the MHC on chromosome number 6.

There are two approaches to determine whether an autoimmune disease is a genetic trait: family studies and population studies. A link between the disease and HLA is suggested when family members with a presumed autoimmune disease are found to share common HLA haplotypes. In cases in which family studies are not possible (due to death or where the family is small), population studies must be used. In this latter approach, antigen frequencies among large groups of patients with a specific illness are compared with those of a healthy group.

The autoimmune disease with the highest relative risk (the criteria for HLA-disease relationship) is ankylosing spondylitis. In this disease, the HLA-B27 antigen yields a relative risk of approximately 90 per cent. Other diseases showing varying levels of risk are given in Table 14–1.

SYSTEMIC AUTOIMMUNE DISEASES

Systemic Lupus Erythematosus

The autoimmune disease for which the most information is available is systemic lupus erythematosus (SLE), a disease of the connective tissue occurring primarily in women and having a strong hereditary tendency. The clinical differences between SLE and rheumatoid arthritis (discussed later in this chapter) are few, and the dividing line between the two would be difficult to draw.

Characteristics

Systemic lupus erythematosus (SLE) is a generalized disorder of unknown cause that expresses itself as a vasculitis (i.e., inflammation of a vessel), usually involving many organ systems. The disease affects females four times more frequently than males and occurs primarily in young adults between the ages of 20 and 40 years, although diagnosis has been made in patients of all ages (Peacock and Tomar, 1980). There is a higher incidence of SLE in blacks than in whites (Rodnan and Schumacher, 1983).

SLE is an immune complex disease (i.e., tissue injury is caused by immune complexes that, when deposited in tissue, can initiate an inflammatory response). These immune complexes are believed to be the result of depressed suppressor T-cell func-

			Control	
		Patients	Subjects	
	Associated	Possessing	Possessing	Relative
Disease	HLA Antigen	Antigen (%)	Antigen (%)	Risk

TABLE 14–1. Relationship of HLA and Autoimmune Diseases

Disease	Associated HLA Antigen	Patients Possessing Antigen (%)	Control Subjects Possessing Antigen (%)	Relative Risk
Ankylosing spondylitis	B27	79–100	4–13	90
Addison's disease	B8	20–69	18–24	1–7
Reiter's syndrome	B27	65–100	4–14	36
Graves' disease	B8	25–47	16–27	1.8–2.4
Yersinia arthritis	B27	58–78	9–14	18
Salmonella arthritis	B27	60–69	8–10	18
Sjögren's syndrome	Dw3	68–69	10–24	8–16
Adult rheumatoid arthritis	Dw4	38–65	18–31	4.4
Autoimmune thyroiditis	Bw35	63–73	9–14	16.8
Anterior uveitis	B27	37–58	7–10	9.4
Myasthenia gravis (MG)	B8	38–65	13–18	4.4
Multiple sclerosis (MS)	B7	12–46	14–30	1.7

Modified from Barrett, J. T.: Textbook of Immunology, 4th ed. St. Louis, C. V. Mosby Co., 1983.

tion, which allows for the overproduction or inappropriate production of autoantibodies, which combine with autoantigens to form immune complexes (Miller and Schwartz, 1982). The most important of these is the production of DNA-anti-DNA complexes.

There is evidence that the expression of the autoimmune reaction seen in SLE comes under genetic influence. In first-degree relatives, the incidence of SLE is more than 200 times greater than in the general population (Rodnan and Schumacher, 1983). An association exists between SLE and HLA-DRw3 (Theofilopoulos, 1987), HLA-B8, and HLA-DRw2. First-degree relatives of patients with SLE have also been found to have impaired suppressor T-cell function (Miller and Schwartz, 1979).

There is no common clinical pattern for SLE and the severity of the disease varies from one individual to another. The general clinical manifestations include fever, weight loss, malaise, and weakness. Arthritis is the most common manifestation and may precede multisystem involvement. Joint involvement in SLE is symmetrical, is rarely deforming, and can involve almost any joint.

The disease also commonly manifests itself by skin lesions (usually in the form of a red rash across the nose and upper cheeks, from which the disease gets the name *lupus erythematosus,* the red wolf) or photosensitivity. More serious internal lesions involve the kidney, blood vessels, blood cells, and heart. In addition, there may be joint pain affecting several joints bilaterally. At least 50 per cent of

patients have central nervous system involvement, arising from direct inflammation of the cerebral vessels or from the hypertension often found in these individuals. Widespread infarction of cerebral tissue may also be found, and SLE may present clinically as a seizure disorder or a psychiatric disturbance. Renal involvement occurs in the majority of cases, and the resultant decrease in kidney function is the primary cause of death in severe SLE. According to the World Health Organization's Classification of Lupus Nephropathy (based on histopathologic criteria), five classes of glomerulonephritis are associated with SLE (class I through class V), with class II being characterized by mesangial deposits of immunoglobulin and the C3 components of complement and class V being the most severe form of involvement (Table 14–2).

There is no cure for SLE, but steroids and immunosuppressive drugs are often helpful in controlling its course.

Laboratory Observations

Several immunologic phenomena are associated with SLE. The most striking feature of the disease from a laboratory standpoint is the appearance in the serum of numerous globulins with the properties of antibodies that are directed against various cell nuclei (antinuclear antibodies [ANA]). These are usually IgG, but they may be IgM or IgA. Because of these antinuclear factors, patients with SLE may have a false-positive serologic test for

Histologic type	Class I Normal	Class II Mesangial	Class III Focal Proliferative	Class IV Diffuse Proliferative	Class V Membranous
Frequency (%)	>5	15	20	50	15
Proteinuria		68	100	100	100
Nephrotic syndrome		0	15	87	88
Death (%)		18	30	58	38
Uremic death (%)		0	11	36	6

TABLE 14–2. Classification System for Renal Involvement in Systemic Lupus Erythematosus*

*Classification of the World Health Organization

syphilis (Wassermann reaction and Kahn flocculation test), hemolytic anemia with a positive antiglobulin test for antibody to red cell antigen, leukopenia, and thrombocytopenia.

The most relevant laboratory observation in SLE, however, is the lupus erythematosus (LE) cell phenomenon. This was first described in 1948 by Hargreaves, who detected unusual cells in the serum of SLE patients. The LE cell is a polymorphonuclear leukocyte found in the bone marrow and peripheral blood of patients with SLE. The LE cell is characterized by the presence of a homogeneous, cytoplasmic mass that often fills the cytoplasm of the phagocyte (Fig. 14–1). This mass

(known as the LE body) is not always engulfed by the phagocyte and occasionally can be seen free in stained blood films (shown in Fig. 14–1). Often, free LE bodies that are not engulfed are surrounded by viable neutrophils, producing a rosette formation (see Fig. 14–1). These viable phagocytes are apparently in competition with one another for phagocytosis of the deranged LE nucleus.

The development of these structures has been revealed by mixing the serum from an SLE patient with normal whole blood and then observing the changes using microcinematography. In these experiments, the nuclei of certain white blood cells lyse first, becoming homogeneous, and then swell

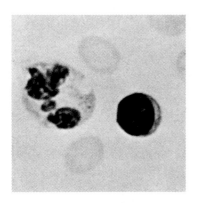
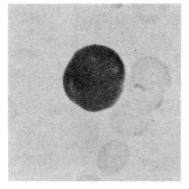
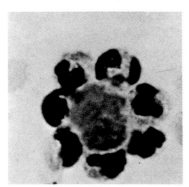
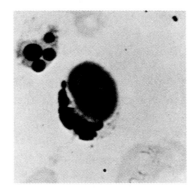

Figure 14–1. The LE cell phenomenon. *Upper left,* a normal neutrophil and lymphocyte; *upper right,* a free LE body; *lower left,* a rosette; and *lower right,* a single LE cell. (From Anderson, J. R., Buchanan, W. W., and Goudie, R. B.: Autoimmunity, 1967. Courtesy of Charles C Thomas, Publisher, Springfield, Illinois.)

to as much as three or four times their normal size. The cells lose their dark staining quality and become paler and spherical. Those phagocytes that are unaffected approach the LE body (producing the rosette formation), strip away its cytoplasm, and engulf it. This final cell, the polymorphonuclear leukocyte with the lysed nucleus as an inclusion body, is an LE cell.

The LE *factor* (which is responsible for these changes) is a 7S IgG antibody, which reacts with deoxyribonucleoprotein (i.e., anti-DNP) and complement, attaching to the nuclei from any source in agreement with the known nonspecificity of anti-DNA antibody. The LE factor is found in more than 95 per cent of SLE patients and in less than 4 per cent of normal individuals. It should be noted, however, that the LE factor is not specific as an indicator of SLE; it is also present (as are LE cells) in the serum of patients suffering from certain other autoimmune diseases (e.g., rheumatoid arthritis, scleroderma, and polydermatomyositis).

Several different specificities of ANA have been found in patients suffering from SLE, mostly revealed through the use of fluorescent ANA techniques, which include antibodies to DNA (almost 60 to 70 per cent), DNA-histone, RNA, and ENA (extractable nuclear antigen). ENA is known to be a mixture of several acidic antigens, few of which have been characterized chemically other than for the presence of dsDNA, dsRNA, ssDNA (or ssRNA), and protein. Certain ENAs (notably Sm and MA antigens) have a high degree of specificity for SLE. Sm antibodies are found in 25 per cent of patients with SLE.

Other antibodies found in SLE patients react with nRNP (nuclear ribonucleoprotein); PCNA (proliferating cell nuclear antigen); Sjögren's syndrome antigens, SS-A and SS-B; the histone antigens, H1, H3, and H4; and others.

These autoantibodies do not cause tissue damage *directly*; tissue damage is triggered by the *depositing* of antigen-antibody *complexes* in the capillaries of affected organs. The removal of these complexes in the kidney accounts for the glomerulonephritis characteristic of the disease. The deposition of these complexes activates complement, leading to tissue destruction. As a result of this complement activation, about 75 per cent of SLE patients develop hypocomplementemia. The excessive antibody production results in hypergammaglobuli-nemia (an excess of gamma globulin), which is characteristic of many autoimmune diseases.

Etiology

In general, SLE arises spontaneously, caused by the formation of antibodies against the body's own tissues, probably due to a genetic depletion of suppressor T cells. This theory is supported by the success of immunosuppressive treatment. In some cases, SLE may be induced by certain drugs (e.g., hydralazine, penicillin, oral contraceptives, and procainamide). Although this form of the disease may appear within a few weeks after the initiation of therapy, a prodromal period of several months is more common. The condition is usually reversible by discontinuance of the drug.

The fact that a disproportionate number of females between puberty and menopause (i.e., childbearing age) suffer from SLE, and that the disease worsens during pregnancy, raises the possibility that estrogens may play a potentially harmful role in disease development and progression.

A variety of environmental factors and bacterial and viral infections are capable of inducing or exacerbating the signs and symptoms of SLE. Ultraviolet light, for example, may cause DNA to form dimers, which significantly alter the antigenicity of DNA and could result in anti-DNA formation.

In individuals who are genetically predisposed to the disease, viral infections are thought to be an important etiologic factor.

Serologic Tests

The laboratory tests for SLE involve two main procedures: the demonstration of the LE cell and the detection of ANA. Although both procedures are discussed here, it should be noted that the LE test is no longer widely used because, although LE cell formation is a useful diagnostic aid when *positive*, many patients produce negative tests because of the difficulty in performing and interpreting these tests. For this reason, fluorescent antinuclear antibody (FANA) and other ANA tests have supplemented LE cell procedures.

FANA in the sera of SLE patients is identified by the indirect fluorescent antibody procedure. It should be noted, however, that the LE cell factor is only one of the *variety* of ANA that are directed against many nuclear antigens. These antibodies may be detected in 3 to 7 per cent of normal adults (as well as about 40 per cent of elderly persons) and also as a result of inflammatory conditions, in 15 per cent of patients with rheumatoid arthritis, and (although usually at low titers) in some patients with chronic hepatitis, periarteritis nodosa, scleroderma, acute drug sensitivity, tuberculosis, lymphoma, and others. The detection of ANA, therefore, is not *diagnostic* of SLE; however, because these antibodies are so frequently found in patients with this disease, their absence can be used as a means of ruling out the disease.

There are several other methods that can be applied to the diagnosis of SLE, including methods for detecting antibodies to DNA and nucleoprotein, which include radioimmunoassay (RIA) and hemagglutination assays.

METHOD 1: INDIRECT FLUORESCENT ANTIBODY TEST FOR THE DETECTION OF ANTINUCLEAR ANTIBODIES (ANA) IN HUMAN SERUM

An ANA test kit for qualitative and semiquantitative detection of ANA by the technique of indirect immunofluorescence is available from Meloy Laboratories, Inc., Toronto, Canada. A similar test kit is available from Electro-Nucleonics, Inc., Bethesda, MD. The following is a description of the use of the Meloy Test Kit.

Principle

Immunofluorescent techniques are used extensively to detect the presence of ANA activity in sera from patients with SLE and other connective tissue diseases. The indirect immunofluorescent assay is based on the use of fluorescein-conjugated antiglobulin. In the Meloy assay, a serum specimen or control is delivered into a well on a microscope slide containing a mouse liver substrate. If present, ANA will bind to nuclear antigens present in the nuclei of the liver sections. After a specific time, under controlled incubation conditions, the slide is carefully washed to remove nonspecific protein and the antigen-antibody complexes are subsequently stained with fluorescein-conjugated anti-human globulins. A lattice or "sandwich" complex of nuclear anti-

human ANA and fluorescein-labeled anti-human globulins is thus formed. Several characteristic patterns of fluorescent staining emerge singly or in any combination. The most commonly encountered fluorescent staining patterns are homogeneous, peripheral, speckled, and nucleolar.

Reagents

1. ANA mouse liver substrate slides: These should be stored in a foil pouch at −20°C until ready for use. At the time of use, remove the required number of slides from the freezer (each slide contains 8 wells) and allow them to equilibrate to room temperature for 7 to 10 minutes. Carefully remove the slides by cutting the foil with scissors and lifting the foil away gently. The slides should not slide out of the foil pouch; this may cause the tissue to be dislodged.

2. ANA control sera—positive and negative: These should be stored at −20°C until first use, and thereafter at 2° to 5°C. They should not be refrozen. The prediluted control is ready for use when thawed.

3. FITC conjugate: This should be stored at −20°C until first use and thereafter at 2° to 5°C. Do not refreeze. The primary activity of FITC (fluorescein isothiocyanate-conjugated goat anti-human globulin) is its reaction to human IgG. The reagent is prediluted and is ready for use when thawed.

4. PBS salts: These should be stored either at −20°C or at 2° to 5°C before reconstitution. Store at 2° to 5°C after reconstitution. One vial of PBS salts results in 1,000 ml of reconstituted buffer (ph 7.0 ± 0.2). To reconstitute, place the PBS salts in a volumetric flask and bring to 1,000 ml with distilled water. Mix thoroughly until salts are dissolved.

5. Buffered glycerol: This should be stored at −20°C until first use and thereafter at 2° to 5°C. Do not refreeze. The kit contains 2 × 6.0 ml vials of buffered glycerol (pH 8.0). One per cent sodium azide is included as a preservative. The reagent is ready for use after thawing.

Precautions

1. All human components have been tested by radioimmunoassay for hepatitis B surface anti-

gen (HBsAg) and have been found to be negative. It should be noted, however, that this does not ensure the absence of HBsAg.

2. The sodium azide (0.1 per cent w/v) included in the reactive and nonreactive ingredients is toxic if ingested. It should be noted that sodium azide may react with lead and copper plumbing to form highly explosive metal azides. If disposing of the agent through plumbing fixtures, flush with a large volume of water to prevent azide build-up.

3. Readings should be taken in the center of the substrate wells; avoid readings at the edge of the well.

4. Care should be taken that the wells are not subject to any abrasion.

5. Individual components in the kit are tested together to ensure compatibility; they should not be interchanged with components of kits that bear different lot numbers.

Specimen Collection and Handling

The blood specimens for the test should be collected aseptically. Serum should be separated from the clot promptly to avoid hemolysis and should be stored at 2° to 5°C for analysis within 24 hours. If not tested within this time period, the sample should be stored frozen. Repeated freezing and thawing of the specimen should be avoided. Plasma may also be used and should be similarly stored.

Materials

The kit contains:
1. 10 ANA substrate slides
2. Positive ANA control serum
3. Negative ANA control serum
4. FITC anti-human globulin conjugate
5. Buffered glycerol
6. Phosphate-buffered saline (PBS) salts

Additional equipment required:

1. Fluorescent microscope with 250× or greater capability
2. Magnetic stirring unit with bars
3. Coverslips—No. 1 glass coverslips
4. Staining dishes
5. Pasteur and serologic pipettes
6. Squeeze bottle
7. Small test tubes with caps
8. 1,000-ml volumetric flask
9. Distilled water

Method

1. Slide preparation: Remove the required number of slides from the freezer. Allow the slides to equilibrate to room temperature for at least 7 to 10 minutes. Remove from foil pouch by cutting with scissors.

2. Sample application:
   Screening Test: Dilute each patient's serum 1:20 with PBS. Save the undiluted sera for possible use in subsequent titration tests if positive screening test results are obtained.
   Titration Test: Sera found to be positive in the screening test should be titrated to endpoint. Prepare a fresh 1:20 dilution of each positive serum, then prepare serial twofold dilutions from this 1:20 dilution. Typically, sera strongly positive in the screening test should be assayed at serial dilutions ranging from 1:20 to 1:5120 in the titration test. Sera weakly positive in the screening test may be tested over the range of 1:20 to 1:640 dilutions.

3. Apply 1 drop (approximately 50 µl) of diluted patient sera to the wells, taking care not to overfill them. Include positive and negative control sera on each slide. Positive and negative control sera provided with the test kit are prediluted and should be applied without further dilution.

4. Incubate in a moist, covered chamber at room temperature for 30 minutes.

5. Hold the slide in a horizontal position, and tilt slightly toward you. Squirt the slide with PBS from a squeeze bottle back and forth between the wells to rinse sera off the bottom row of wells. Tilt the slide away from you, and repeat as above to wash off the top row of wells. Note: Do not aim directly at the wells. Wash in PBS for 5 minutes. Repeat the 5-minute wash with fresh PBS. (Note: Washing may be facilitated by placing the slides [up

to 4] upright against the slides of a staining dish containing 250 ml of PBS, adding a magnetic stirring bar, and agitating on a magnetic stirrer. Thorough washing is essential to remove nonspecifically bound immunoglobulin, which may subsequently bind fluorescein-conjugated antiglobulin to give a false-positive reaction).

6. Shake off the excess PBS, and apply prediluted conjugate to each well.
7. Incubate in a moist, covered chamber at room temperature for 30 minutes.
8. Squirt a light stream of PBS from a squeeze bottle above the wells as in step 5. Wash in PBS for 5 minutes. Repeat the 5-minute wash with fresh PBS.
9. Shake off excess PBS, and immediately apply 1 drop of buffered glycerol to each well.
10. Place a 24- × 50-mm coverslip over the glycerol saturated slide. Use only No. 1 glass coverslips for this purpose.
11. Examine for fluorescent nuclear reaction at a magnification of 250× or greater. Slides should be read by fluorescent microscopy as soon as possible; however, they can be stored in the dark at 4°C for up to 48 hours prior to reading.
12. Sera positive in the screening test should be subsequently titrated to endpoint.

Interpretation

Note: Before reading, ensure that the positive and negative control results conform to the following specifications:

Negative Control: No green-gold fluorescence of greater than ± intensity.

Positive Control: Strong green-gold fluorescence of 3+ or greater intensity.

Negative Readings: In negative sera, the liver section nuclei contain no green-gold fluorescence.

Positive Readings: Results from the screening test should be recorded as positive or negative. The degree of fluorescence may be semiquantitated on a scale of 1+ to 4+. When titrating the serum, the end point should be considered as the highest dilution at which a definite fluorescent pattern may be distinguished. Positive samples show homogenous, peripheral, speckled, or nucleolar fluorescence, or anti-centromere antibody pattern.

1. *Homogenous (solid, diffuse):* The whole nucleus fluoresces evenly green-gold, although nonfluorescent vacuoles are sometimes seen. This pattern characterizes anti-deoxyribonucleic acid-nucleoprotein antibodies, i.e., antibodies to nDNA, dsDNA, ssDNA, DNP, or histones. Antibodies to DNP have been shown to have the same specificity as the LE factor. This pattern is typically seen in rheumatoid disorders. High titers of homogenous ANA are suggestive of SLE; low titers may be found in SLE, rheumatoid arthritis, Sjögren's syndrome, and mixed connective tissue disease (MCTD).

2. *Peripheral (ring, membranous, shaggy, or thready):* This pattern is characterized by sharp green-gold fluorescence of the outer edge of the nucleus (nuclear membrane), with a gradually darkening inner border blending with a dark nuclear center. The pattern results from antibodies to DNA (i.e., nDNA, dsDNA, or DNP) and is associated with SLE in the active stage of the disease and in Sjögren's syndrome

3. *Speckled (mottled):* This pattern is characterized by numerous round speckles of green-gold nuclear fluorescence of various sizes against a dark background (giving the appearance of "pepper dots"). This pattern occurs in the presence of antibody to any extractable nuclear antigen devoid of DNA or histone. The antibody is detected against the saline extractable nuclear antigens: anti-RNP and anti-Smith (anti-Sm). These anti-Sm antibodies have been shown to be highly specific for patients with SLE and appear to be a "marker" antibody. Anti-RNP has been found in patients with a wide variety of rheumatic diseases including SLE, rheumatoid arthritis, Sjögren's syndrome, progressive systemic sclerosis, mixed connective tissue disease, and dermatomyositis.

4. *Nucleolar:* This pattern is characterized by multiple round, smooth, green-gold fluorescing nucleoli of various sizes. It reflects an antibody to nucleolar RNA. It is present in about 50 per cent of patients with scleroderma (progressive systemic sclerosis), Sjögren's syndrome, and in SLE. This pattern can also be observed in

undiagnosed illnesses manifesting Raynaud's phenomenon.

5. *Anti-centromere antibody (ACA):* This pattern is discrete and speckled. The antibody reacts with centromeric chromatin of metaphase and interphase cells and appears to be highly selective for the CREST variant of progressive systemic sclerosis. The antibody is found infrequently in the serum of patients with SLE, mixed connective tissue disease (MCTD), and systemic sclerosis.

Note: Each laboratory should use its own judgment concerning the degree of fluorescence required for a positive test result. It is recommended that a panel of normal and abnormal sera be evaluated to determine a minimum fluorescent endpoint. If a maximum of 1+ reaction on a scale of 1+ to 4+ is considered positive, sera from apparently healthy individuals demonstrate negative results.

Limitations and Expected Values

The test system described should be interpreted keeping in mind the following:

1. ANA is a substance that has been shown to be present in several disease states and in some apparently normal individuals. The appearance of a positive ANA result, therefore, does not necessarily indicate a disease process. Further, data generated by this test should be reviewed in the framework of all available medical evidence.
2. Some positive reactions have been reported in patients suffering from a connective tissue disease or in relatives of patients who may develop such a disease at a later stage. Various therapeutic agents have been shown to induce ANA in the serum of patients receiving these drugs.
3. Procainamide hydrochloride has been the most frequent and most accepted of the "SLE inducers" since 1965. After procainamide therapy, up to 50 per cent of patients develop ANA; however, most patients have remissions when the drug is discontinued. The following drugs have also been implicated as activators of SLE: aminosalicylic acid, phenytoin, griseofulvin, hydralazine, isoniazid, mephenytoin, methylthiouracil, penicillin, phenylbutazone, propylthiouracil,

streptomycin sulfate, sulfadimethoxine, sulfamethoxypyridazine, tetracycline, trimethadione, methyldopa, and ethosuximide.

4. In some patients, the ANA may not be detected if it is present as a complex with circulating antigen. Some evidence indicates its detection may occasionally be facilitated by treating the serum with the enzyme deoxyribonuclease (DNase).
5. Sera shown to be positive at 1:20 should be titrated to endpoint. A homogenous staining pattern may mask other fluorescent patterns. Upon titration of such sera, these other patterns may be observed.

Expected values with this kit as prescribed with a 1:20 dilution of patient's serum are as follows:

1. The normal individual can be expected to give a negative reaction.
2. The patient population with SLE, progressive systemic sclerosis (PSS), and rheumatoid arthritis (RA) will give a positive test in approximately the same percentage as shown in the clinical survey in Table 14–3.

Note: Laboratory personnel are cautioned to consult and follow all manufacturer's recommended procedures for microscope and light source maintenance. It is further recommended that the laboratory maintain a log on lamp usage and change the bulb(s) after the elapsed usage time recommended by the manufacturer.

TABLE 14–3. Positive Reactions Using Recommended Procedure for ANA in Systemic Lupus Erythematosus (SLE), Progressive Systemic Sclerosis (PSS), and Rheumatoid Arthritis (RA)

Titer	Normal Population	SLE	PSS	RA
Negative Tests				
1:10 (or lower)	96	1	4	15
Positive Tests				
1:20	0	0	2	0
1:49–1:80	0	2	4	4
1:160–1:320	0	4	3	1
1:640–1:1280	0	7	4	0
1:2560 (or higher)	0	6	0	0
Per cent positive	0	95	76	25

METHOD 2: ANTINUCLEAR ANTIBODY (ANA) VISIBLE METHOD

Principle

The antinuclear antibody visible method is an indirect immunoenzyme method that uses tissue culture cells (human epithelial cells) as a substrate for the detection and titration of circulating antinuclear antibodies in human serum. Patient serum samples are diluted in buffer and added to microscope slide wells with HEp-2 (human epithelial) cells cultured in them. HEp-2 cells are characterized by extremely large nuclei and the presence of mitotic figures to aid in detection. If specific antibodies are present, stable antigen-antibody complexes are formed that bind anti-human gamma globulin labeled with horseradish peroxidase (HRP). The presence of HRP is indicated by a reaction with 3,3'-diaminobenzidine stain. The resulting dark brown to black staining patterns of the nuclei can be seen with a light microscope. The presence of one or more types of circulating autoantibodies is the hallmark of systemic rheumatic diseases.

Specimen Collection and Preparation

The patient should be in a fasting state prior to specimen collection. A minimum of 5 to 8 ml of clotted blood is required. The blood should be allowed to clot at room temperature. The specimen should be centrifuged promptly and the serum should be separated from the red cells *immediately.* Serum specimens may be stored at 2° to 8°C if they are to be tested within 24 to 48 hours. If testing is not to take place within this period of time, the specimen should be stored frozen (−20°C or below). Do not freeze and thaw sera more than once. Allow the serum specimens to reach room temperature before testing. Avoid the use of sera exhibiting a high degree of lipemia, hemolysis, or microbial growth, since these characteristics may result in increased background staining, a decrease in titers, and/or unclear staining patterns

Reagents, Supplies, and Equipment

A test kit for this procedure is available from ISOLAB, Akron, OH.

The kit contains:

1. Substrate slides. Each HEp-2 slide well contains HEp-2 cells grown and fixed on the slide. The slides are stable until the labeled expiration date when stored at −20°C. The foil envelope should be handled at the edges to protect the cells. Care should be taken to avoid handling the flat surface of the slide.
2. HRP lyophilized conjugate. This is stable before reconstitution (within the labeled expiration date) when stored at 2° to 8°C. The reconstituted conjugate is stable to 90 days when similarly stored.
3. HRP stain reagent. Each vial contains 0.4 per cent diaminobenzidine-HCl and phosphate buffer. Thimerosal is added as a preservative. Reconstitute the stain reagent with deionized water as directed on the label. Add the contents of 1 vial of 0.3 per cent H_2O_2 immediately before use. The unreconstituted stain reagent is stable (within the expiration date) when stored at 2° to 8°C. *It should be noted that Diaminobenzidine-HCl is a possible carcinogen. Ingestion and skin contact should be avoided.*
4. Hydrogen peroxide, 0.3 per cent, ready for use, and stable (within the expiration date) when stored at 2° to 8°C.
5. Phosphate-buffered saline (PBS). Each unit contains dry powder phosphate-buffered saline blend. Dissolve contents in distilled or deionized water as directed on the label and store at 2° to 8°C.
6. Mounting medium. Ready for use. Contains phosphate-buffered glycerol. Thimerosal is added as a preservative.
7. Positive control serum. ANA (homogenous positive control serum [human]), ready for use in a dropper vial containing antinuclear antibodies demonstrating a strong homogenous staining reaction (1:40 dilution). Sodium azide (0.1 per cent w/v) is added as a preservative. Store at 2° to 8°C. The ANA positive control should demonstrate homogenous staining in the nuclei of the HEp-2 cells.
8. Negative control serum. Ready to use in a dropper vial containing no detectable autoantibodies (1:40 dilution). Sodium azide (0.1 per cent w/v) is added as a preservative. Store at 2° to 8°C. The

ANA negative control serum should demonstrate little or no nuclear staining.

Additional equipment required:

1. 12 × 75 mm test tubes and rack
2. Pasteur and calibrated pipettes
3. Staining dish or Coplin jar
4. Moist chamber for incubation
5. Volumetric flask for PBS
6. Distilled or deionized water: CAP Type 1 or equivalent, pH 6.0–7.0
7. Forceps
8. Coverslips
9. Squeeze bottle
10. Blotting or bibulous paper
11. Light microscope.

Procedure

Note: Allow serum specimens to reach room temperature before testing. Do not interchange components from other sources.

1. Prepare sample by diluting each serum 1:40 in PBS. If a serum has previously tested positive, it should be titered to its endpoint.
2. Allow slides to equilibrate to room temperature for 15 to 30 minutes before use, then remove them from the envelope and label. (Note: Handle the envelope and slide by the edges only.)
3. Apply the samples and controls. Use 1 drop of the screening dilution or titration dilution per well. Apply 1 drop of the positive control and 1 drop of the negative control to the appropriate wells on at least 1 slide of each test run. (Note: From this step on, the slides must remain wet.)
4. Incubate the slides in a covered moist chamber at room temperature for 30 minutes.
5. Remove the slides from the chamber and rinse briefly with a gentle stream of PBS. Direct the stream away from the wells.
6. Place the slides in a Coplin or staining jar filled with PBS for 5 minutes to wash. Agitate the slide initially, at midpoint, and prior to removal. Repeat the wash process with fresh PBS.
7. Remove the slides one at a time from the wash solution and drain the excess PBS. If blotting is preferred, blot gently around slide periphery only, with the end of the blotting or bibulous paper. Do not blot directly over the wells. Return to moist chamber.
8. Apply conjugate by dispensing 1 drop (approximately 20 to 30 μl) of conjugate to each well on each slide used.
9. Incubate the slides in a moist chamber at room temperature for 30 minutes. Protect the slides from excess light.
10. Remove the slides from the moist chamber and rinse briefly with a gentle stream of PBS. Direct the stream away from the wells.
11. Place the slides in a Coplin or staining jar filled with PBS to wash. Leave the slides in the PBS for 5 minutes with occasional agitation (initially, at midpoint, and before removing the slides from the wash). Repeat this washing procedure once with fresh PBS.
12. Reconstitute with 10 ml of distilled water. Add the contents of 1 vial of 0.3 per cent H_2O_2 immediately before use. Mix well by gentle inversion or agitation.
13. Remove the slides from the wash buffer, drain the excess PBS, and return to the moist chamber. Flood the wells with the stain reagent. Do not allow the wells to dry. Discard any unused reconstituted stain.
14. Incubate the slides for 15 minutes in a covered moist chamber at room temperature. Again, protect the slides from light.
15. Remove the slides from the moist chamber and rinse with a gentle stream of PBS. Place the slides in a Coplin or staining jar filled with PBS for 10 minutes. Agitate at entry, midpoint, and prior to removal.
16. Remove the slides (one at a time) from the wash buffer and drain excess PBS by gently tapping the horizontal edge of the slide. If blotting is preferred, see directions in step 7.
17. Apply 1 small drop of mounting media in each specimen well. Gently apply coverslip without pressure.
18. Examine the slides with a light microscope using high (4×) magnification

Interpretation

Note: Before reading, ensure that the positive and negative controls have given the expected results. If not, the run should be repeated.

Negative: No cytoplasmic or nuclear specific stain is observed. The cells may be slightly colored due to some nonspecific reaction of the peroxidase stain reagent.

Positive: A serum is considered to be positive if the nuclei of the cells stain more intensely than the negative control well and there is a clearly discernible pattern of colorations. Positive specimens should be confirmed by repeating the test with two-fold dilutions of serum. All positive ANA patterns should be titered to endpoint dilution to detect possible mixed antinuclear reactions that may not be apparent when interpreting a single screening dilution. The endpoint titer is the last serial dilution in which a 1+ coloration with a clearly discernible pattern is detected.

Limitations and Expected Values

The HRP technique has the advantage of resulting in a permanent slide and requires only a conventional light microscope with no special equipment. It is also comparable in sensitivity and patterns of reactivity to fluorescent methods.

False-negative results can occur if the ANA happens to be specific for an antigen other than the one used in the procedure. They can also occur if the substrate is fixed in acetone and is inadequately washed. Without fixation, however, some soluble nuclear antigen may be lost. False-negative results may also be related to the binding of antinuclear factor to circulating immune complexes and to low antibody titer.

False-positive results may occur because of non-specific staining, which may resemble a speckled pattern of reactivity. These staining reactions occur whenever the conjugate or the serum contains antibodies to other tissue antigens, and can be minimized by careful rinsing and removal of excess fluoresceinated conjugate.

The test must be interpreted with caution in the evaluation of patients with connective tissue disease. Under normal testing conditions, the test generally rules out SLE. A negative test, however, can result from autoimmune disease in remission or nuclear autoantibodies not detectable with indirect immunofluorescent or peroxidase immunoenzyme procedures.

The significance of a positive ANA depends on the titer and (although to a lesser extent) on the observed patterns (see previous discussion under "Interpretation" in Method 1). Many apparently normal individuals may show some degree of staining at the 1:40 screening dilution. ANA titers at dilutions of 1:10 to 1:80 usually have little significance but may be seen in patients with rheumatoid arthritis or scleroderma. Antinuclear antibodies are also known to be sex and age dependent, and a positive reaction may be "normal" for certain individuals. In general, the higher the titer, the more likely is the diagnosis of connective tissue disorder. Changes in antibody titer can also be used to observe disease activity.

In the case of a positive ANA test, additional immunologic evaluations are necessary to determine the specificity of the reaction, including double immunodiffusion, counter immunoelectrophoresis, passive hemagglutination, radioimmunoassays, and identification of nuclear antigens by immunoprecipitation or immunoblotting. Such evaluations may demonstrate that more than one ANA specificity is present in a serum. An LE cell preparation is not considered useful, since it would only be positive in 75 per cent of patients with confirmed SLE.

In this, as in all laboratory tests, clinical findings should be correlated with laboratory findings before a definitive diagnosis is made.

METHOD 3: RAPID SLIDE TEST (QUALITATIVE) FOR ANTINUCLEOPROTEIN FACTORS ASSOCIATED WITH SYSTEMIC LUPUS ERYTHEMATOSUS

Principle

Systemic lupus erythematosus (SLE) reagent contains stabilized animal erythrocytes coated with a preparation of deoxyribonucleoprotein (DNP) from calf thymus, the antigen for detection of antinucleoprotein. When the reagent is mixed with serum containing nucleoprotein antibodies, macroscopic agglutination occurs. The procedure is positive in SLE and systemic rheumatic diseases such as rheumatoid arthritis, scleroderma, Sjögren's syndrome, mixed connective tissue disease, and drug-induced lupus erythematosus.

Specimen Collection and Handling

No special preparation of the patient is required prior to specimen collection. A minimum of 2 ml of clotted blood is required. The specimen should be centrifuged immediately and an aliquot of serum removed. The test should be performed immediately, using fresh serum. If this is not possible, the serum should be stored at 2° to 8°C for no longer than 48 hours. If more than 48 hours will elapse between collection and testing, the specimen should be stored frozen.

Reagents, Supplies, and Equipment

A systemic lupus erythematosus test kit is available from ICL Scientific, Fountain Valley, CA.

The test kit contains:

1. Serascan SLE reagent with dropper cap assembly. Contains deoxyribonucleoprotein extracted from calf thymus and coated on stabilized animal erythrocytes. Store at 2° to 8°C and do not use if the reagent becomes contaminated. Do not use if evidence of freezing is apparent.
2. Capillary pipettes
3. Applicator sticks
4. Glass slide. It is essential that the glass slide be clean. Before use, wash it thoroughly with mild detergent, rinse several times with distilled water, and dry
5. Positive control (human)
6. Negative control (human)

Note: The latex reagent and the controls contain sodium azide as a preservative. The usual warnings, therefore, apply to the disposal of these reagents (see Method 1).

Additional equipment required:

Timer (or stopwatch)

Procedure

Note: All reagents, controls, and test sera must be at room temperature prior to testing.

1. Ensure that the slide to be used is clean.
2. Fill a capillary pipette (provided with the kit). Hold the pipette perpendicular to the slide above the appropriate square, and deliver 1 free-falling drop onto the slide.
3. Repeat step 2, using both the positive and the negative control sera.
4. Resuspend the latex reagent by gentle mixing. Replace the screw-top cap with the dropper assembly. Subsequent resuspension of the reagent should be performed by dispelling the reagent from the dropper and gently inverting the vial until the suspension is homogenous.
5. Add 1 drop of the SLE reagent to each of the divisions containing a serum specimen and the positive and negative controls.
6. Using separate applicator sticks, mix each specimen and control serum with the SLE reagent in a circular manner over the entire area within the division of the slide.
7. Slowly tilt the slide back and forth for 1 minute. Place the slide on a flat surface and allow it to stand undisturbed for 1 minute. (Note: These times are important.)
8. Observe for agglutination.
9. Wash the glass slide thoroughly with mild detergent and rinse several times with distilled water.

Interpretation

Assuming that the controls give the expected results, agglutination indicates a positive result, and lack of agglutination indicates a negative result.

Discussion

False results can result from failure to observe the test mixture at the appropriate times. Note that the serum from patients with SLE has been shown to contain several antinuclear antibodies. A specific diagnosis, therefore, must depend on a correlation of laboratory results and clinical findings. There is no single test that has been shown to be completely reliable for the diagnosis of SLE.

METHOD 4: QUANTITATIVE DETERMINATION OF IgG AND IgM ANTIBODIES TO DEOXYRIBONUCLEOPROTEIN (DNP) IN HUMAN SERUM

Principle

This procedure is an indirect enzyme-labeled immunoassay for determination of IgG and IgM antibodies to deoxyribonucleoprotein (DNP) using antigen-coated microwells as a solid phase. Calf thymus-derived DNP antigen is coated onto the wells of the microplate. Diluted test samples are added to the coated wells and incubated. During incubation, antibodies to DNP present in the sample bind to the antigen-coated well. After washing to remove unbound material, antibodies to human IgG and IgM labeled with alkaline phosphatase (conjugate) are added. The conjugate binds to any antibodies bound to DNP. The well is washed to remove unbound conjugate and incubated with *p*-nitrophenyl phosphate. The *p*-nitrophenyl phosphate is hydrolyzed by alkaline phosphatase to form *p*-nitrophenol, a yellow-colored end product with an absorbance at 405 nm. The intensity of the absorbance at 405 nm is proportional to the amount of antibody to DNP present in the specimen.

Specimen Collection and Handling

No special preparation of the patient is required prior to specimen collection. A minimum of 2 ml of clotted blood is required. The specimen should be centrifuged promptly and an aliquot of serum removed.

Serum specimens should be stored at 2° to 6°C or frozen at −20°C if kept for more than 7 days. Specimens containing visible particulate matter should be clarified by centrifugation prior to testing. Serum samples should *not* be heat inactivated, as this may cause false-positive results.

Reagents, Supplies, and Equipment

Reagents and controls for this test are available in a kit supplied by Sigma Chemical Company, St. Louis, MO. All reagents should be stored at 2° to 6°C.

The kit contains:

1. Antigen wells. Microplate wells coated with calf thymus DNP antigen. The antigen should be stored with desiccant in the reusable plastic bag. Reseal the bag after opening.
2. Holder for wells.
3. Sample diluent. This buffered protein solution contains surfactant and blue dye, pH 7.5. It also contains absorbent (heat-aggregated human IgG) and 0.1 per cent sodium azide as a preservative.
4. Calibrator. This is a human serum containing antibodies to DNP. The content (IU/ml) is indicated on the label. It contains 0.1 per cent sodium azide as a preservative.
5. Conjugate. This solution contains goat antibodies to human IgG and IgM labeled with calf alkaline phosphatase. It contains a pink dye and 0.02 per cent sodium azide as a preservative.
6. Substrate. This solution contains *p*-nitrophenyl phosphate, disodium hexahydrate 1 mg/ml, pH 9.6. The substrate may develop a slight yellow color upon storage. Do not use if absorbance of the undiluted substrate is greater than 0.4 at 405 nm when measured against water using a microplate reader or a spectrophotometer with a 1-cm lightpath.
7. Wash concentrate. This is a buffer solution concentrate with surfactant. It contains 0.1 per cent sodium azide as a preservative. The wash solution is prepared by adding the contents of the wash concentrate bottle to 1 liter of deionized water. Mix well.
8. Stop solution. Alkaline solution pH 12.0. Store at room temperature. *Note: This stop solution causes irritation to eyes and skin. Avoid contact with eyes, skin, and clothing. Avoid breathing the vapor. Wash thoroughly after handling.*
9. Positive control. Human serum containing antibodies to DNP.
10. Negative control. Human serum containing no detectable antibodies to DNP.

Note: With the exception of the wash solution, do not interchange reagents from different lots.

Additional equipment and supplies required:

1. Spectrophotometer that accommodates a 1-ml volume, or microplate reader capable of accurately measuring absorbance at 405 nm
2. Pipetting device for the accurate delivery of 5 μl, 100 μl, and 200 μl
3. Timer
4. 1 liter measuring cylinder
5. Squeeze bottle for dispensing wash solution
6. Dilution plates or tubes
7. Test tubes or cuvettes, 1.0 ml

Procedure

1. Dilute calibrator, positive and negative controls, and test samples by combining 5 μl of each with 200 μl sample diluent in labeled tubes or dilution plates.
2. Place the desired number of antigen wells in the holder.
3. Using a pipette tip, mix the samples and diluent by drawing up and expelling 2 or 3 times. Transfer 100 μl of each diluted specimen to the appropriate antigen well.
4. Include 1 well that contains only 100 μl sample diluent. This serves as the reagent blank and is used to zero the photometer.
5. Allow the plate to stand at room temperature (18° to 26°C for 30 ± 2 minutes).
6. Shake out or aspirate contents of wells. Wash the wells by filling them with wash solution from a squeeze bottle and shaking out or aspirating. Wash 3 times. Drain the wells on a paper towel to remove excess fluid. Note: Thorough washing is necessary to achieve accurate results. Avoid bubbles.
7. Place 2 drops (or 100 μl) conjugate into each well, including the reagent blank well.
8. Allow to stand at room temperature for 30 minutes (± 2 minutes).
9. Wash wells by repeating step 6.
10. Place 2 drops (or 100 μl) of substrate into each well, including the reagent blank well.
11. Repeat step 8.
12. Place 2 drops (or 100 μl) of stop solution into each well.
13. Read and record absorbance of each test at 405 nm within 2 hours after the reaction has been stopped.

Microplate reader: Set absorbance at 405 nm to zero with water as a reference. Read and record absorbance of reagent blank (A blank). Then set absorbance to zero with the reagent blank as reference. Read and record absorbance of samples (A sample) and calibrator (A calibrator).

Spectrophotometer: Completely remove contents of each well and transfer to cuvette or test tube. Add 800 μl of deionized water to each sample and mix. Set absorbance at 405 nm to zero with water as a reference. Read and record the absorbance of each sample including the reagent blank. Subtract the absorbance of the reagent blank for the absorbance of each sample.

Calculation

Concentration of IgG and IgM antibodies to DNP in samples is calculated as follows:

$$\text{Antibody concentration (IU/ml) in sample} = \frac{\text{A sample}}{\text{A calibrator}} \times \text{IU/ml of calibrator}$$

Interpretation

Results are reported in International Units (IU) per ml standardized to the World Health Organization antinuclear factor serum (homogeneous), human, First Reference Preparation, 1970.

Positive: equal to or greater than 40 IU/ml.
Negative: less than 40 IU/ml.

Discussion

The absorbance values will vary with the temperature of the room and the incubation time. Absorbance value or reagent blank when read against water at 405 nm should be less than 0.4 using a microplate reader, or less than 0.09 using a spectrophotometer with a 1-cm lightpath. The absorbance value of the calibrator should be greater than or equal to 0.5 using a microplate reader when the assay is performed at 22°C. The assay value of the positive control should be within the range printed on the label. The negative control should be less than 40 IU/ml. If these requirements are not satisfied, the test results may be inaccurate and the tests should be repeated.

Specimens giving absorbance values above that

of the calibrator should be diluted appropriately and reassayed. The value obtained should be multiplied by the dilution factor.

Biological false-positives can be obtained because antinuclear antibodies occur at low titers in other disorders (e.g., chronic hepatitis, periarteritis nodosa, dermatomyositis, scleroderma, and drug sensitivities).

Antibodies to nuclear components occur in many connective tissue disorders. Idiopathic SLE is characterized by the presence of antibodies to double-stranded DNA and to DNP. Patients with drug-induced SLE, however, usually lack antibodies to double-stranded DNA, although they do have antibodies to DNA and histones.

This procedure should therefore be taken as an aid to diagnosis. Laboratory findings should be correlated with clinical findings before diagnosis is considered definite.

Rheumatoid Arthritis

Characteristics of the Disease

Rheumatoid arthritis (RA) is a chronic inflammatory disease, primarily affecting the joints and periarticular tissues. Although certain areas of the body show a particular susceptibility to inflammation, it appears likely that no body system or tissue is entirely exempt. Apart from the joints, the most commonly affected areas are other synovium-lined spaces such as tendon sheaths, the subcutaneous tissues at sites of pressure or friction, the heart and blood vessels, and the lungs. The highest incidence of the disease is in women between the ages of 30 to 50 years.

The pathologic changes during the disease process include a proliferation of a synovial membrane with the formation of granulation tissue that extends as a vascular "pannus" layer from the margin toward the center of the affected joint. The articular cartilage, too, gradually becomes replaced by fibroid granulation tissue, and focal collections of macrophages and lymphocytes are found in the synovial membrane, the joint capsule, and the periarticular tissues, or in the form of subcutaneous nodules, which occur in approximately 20 per cent of patients and have a characteristic structure.

Other clinical manifestations of the disease include the following:

1. Hypochromic anemia, often providing clear evidence of a hemolytic process without demonstrable erythrocyte abnormality.
2. Characteristic changes in the serum protein pattern.
3. Toxemia, demonstrated primarily by a considerably increased sedimentation rate of blood erythrocytes.
4. Generalized lymphadenopathy. Enlargement of the spleen and lymph nodes is occasionally seen, although in most cases of RA, the lymph node enlargement is accompanied by other evidence of hypersplenism, and lymph node enlargement may be generalized. (A similar state may occur in childhood in Still's disease, in which the spleen and lymph nodes are invariably enlarged. This disease, however, differs in so many of its clinical features from RA that it possibly represents a distinct entity.)

The general clinical manifestations of RA include nonspecific findings of fatigue, weight loss, weakness, mild fever, and anorexia. All patients experience morning stiffness and joint pain that improves through the day. The inflammatory joint changes, which most often affect the small joints, may result in loss of function or permanent deformity. In patients with high titers of rheumatoid factor (RF) (see below), vasculitis, rheumatoid nodules (round or oval firm masses located in the subcutaneous tissue near joints), and Sjögren's syndrome may be manifest.

Despite continued study of the disease throughout the world, the cause of RA remains unknown. It is generally accepted that the immunologic reactions (discussion follows) plays an important, probably essential part in the pathogenesis of the disease, although the antigen(s) involved remain elusive.

Characteristics of Rheumatoid Factors

The clinical and histologic features of RA provide no more than suggestive evidence of immunologic involvement in the disease. A variety of immunologically oriented investigations, however, have provided more compelling evidence.

For more than 25 years, evidence has accumulated suggesting that several abnormal proteins circulate in the blood of patients with RA. These proteins, because of their obvious correlation with the disease, became collectively known as *rheumatoid factor* (RF). They are now generally accepted as a group of immunoglobulins that interact specifically with the Fc portion of IgG molecules (i.e., *anti-antibodies*). Immune complexes are formed, either IgG aggregates or IgM-IgG complexes, and the classical pathway of complement is activated and amplified by the alternative pathway of complement. The inflammatory response proceeds via the bioactive complement fragments (and with the aid of T cells), and inflammatory cells enter the synovial space and release intracellular products that damage the synovium. The pannus production (mentioned above) is a consequence of the inflammatory response. This abnormal growth of synovial cells follows enzymatic destruction of the cartilage.

Rheumatoid factors can occur in nonrheumatoid individuals with chronic infective conditions (e.g., LE, infectious hepatitis, chronic hepatic disease, syphilis); likewise, animal homologues of these factors can be induced by repeated infection (Abruzzo and Christian, 1961). On the basis of these facts, the probable stimulus is the presence of IgG configurationally changed by combination with antigen. The stimulus in cases of RA is presumably the same. It is interesting to note, however, that RF in chronic infective states virtually disappears when the infection is overcome by appropriate therapy, whereas in cases of RA, the RF persists indefinitely, providing evidence of a persistent infective agent, or, alternatively, the persistence of another antigen whose combination with IgG constitutes an adequate stimulus.

The correlation between RF and RA remains an intriguing yet unsolved problem. Even if one accepts the autoantibody nature of RF, it does not obviously follow that any of the disease manifestations result from autoimmune processes. It is indeed possible that RF could be the *consequence* of infection with an *unrecognized agent* and without any pathologic significance. Moreover, patients with various conditions, such as sarcoidosis, that are associated with hypergammaglobulinemia, may show high titers. Finally, RA may occur in patients with hypogammaglobulinemia; these patients lack detectable RF in their serum, as well

as having very low levels of ordinary 7S gamma globulin.

Serologic Tests

Tests for RA are designed to detect certain macroglobulins in the patient's serum that react with normal human IgG or normal animal IgG (i.e., rheumatoid factors). The majority of tests use particular carriers (e.g., erythrocytes, latex, and bentonite particles) that transform the reaction between RF and IgG into visible aggregation. In essence, all the tests are designed to detect antibody to immunoglobulin, but they are not identical, because sometimes human and sometimes animal immunoglobulin is used as the coating for the particles. In some circumstances, the different tests give different results; therefore, one can postulate that a number of rheumatoid factors with different specificities are involved.

Included among the various serologic tests for the detection of RF are the latex fixation test (Singer and Plotz, 1956), the sheep cell agglutination test (Rose *et al.*, 1948), the sensitized alligator erythrocyte test (Cohen *et al.*, 1958), the bentonite flocculation test (Bloch and Bunim, 1959), and the concanavalin A and complement fixation test for the detection of IgG RA factor (Tanimoto *et al.*, 1976).

Of these tests (with the exception of the last, which is specific for IgG RF), the latex fixation and the sheep cell agglutination tests are the most popular. A number of preparations for use in rapid slide tests are also available.

METHOD 1: RHEUMATOID ARTHRITIS TEST

The following procedure is modified from the Rheuma-Fac Rheumatoid Arthritis Test (Latex) product insert, ICL Scientific, Fountain Valley, CA.

Principle

This test is based on the reaction between patient antibodies in the serum (rheumatoid factor) and an antigen derived from gamma globulin. Latex reagent (the antigen) consists of a stabilized latex suspension coated with albumin and chemically bonded with denatured human gamma globulin. If rheumatoid factors are present in the serum, macroscopic agglutination will be visible when the latex reagent and the serum are mixed. It should be noted that positive tests may be observed in disorders such as lupus erythematosus, Sjögren's syndrome, syphilis, and hepatitis.

Specimen Collection and Preparation

No special preparation of the patient is required prior to specimen collection. A minimum of 2 ml of clotted blood is required. The specimen should be centrifuged promptly and an aliquot of serum removed.

The specimen may be refrigerated at 2° to 8°C for no longer than 72 hours. If a delay greater than this occurs before testing, the specimen should be frozen at −18°C or below. Frozen serum should be rapidly thawed at 37°C.

Reagents, Supplies, and Equipment

The kit contains:

1. Latex reagent with dropper assembly. This is a suspension of stabilized polystyrene latex particles coated with human albumin and chemically bonded with denatured human gamma globulin. Do not freeze. Store at 2° to 8°C.
2. Glycine-saline buffer (pH 8.2 ± 0.1). Store at 2° to 8°C.
3. Capillary pipettes
4. Applicator sticks
5. Glass slide
6. Positive control serum (human)—prediluted. The value of the control in IU/ml is printed on the vial label and is established by comparison with a reference preparation that was calibrated using the World Health Organization (WHO) International Reference Preparation of Rheumatoid Arthritis Serum. The positive control should not be used as a standard for titration because the predilution varies from lot to lot. Store at 2° to 8°C.
7. Negative control serum (human)—prediluted. Store at 2° to 8°C.

Additional equipment required:

1. Stopwatch (or timer)
2. 10 × 75 mm test tubes
3. Serologic pipettes (1 ml graduated) and safety pipettor
4. Light source

Procedure (Qualitative Slide Test)

Note: All reagents and specimens must be at room temperature prior to testing.

1. Prepare a 1:20 dilution of patient serum in glycine-saline buffer, i.e., 0.1 ml of serum and 1.0 ml of diluent, and thoroughly mix the tube contents.
2. Using one of the capillary pipettes provided, fill approximately two thirds of the pipette with diluted serum. Deliver 1 free-falling drop of the diluted serum from the pipette (held perpendicularly) to the center of 1 of the oval divisions of the slide.
3. Add 1 drop of positive control and 1 drop of negative control to the appropriately labeled divisions of the slide.
4. Mix the latex reagent and add 1 drop of reagent to the patient specimen and to each of the controls.
5. Mix each specimen with a separate applicator stick. All the contents of the mixtures are to spread evenly over the entire area of their respective divisions on the slide.
6. Tilt the slide back and forth, slowly and evenly, for 2 minutes.
7. Place the slide on a flat surface and observe immediately for macroscopic agglutination, using a direct light source.

Interpretation of Results

Agglutination of the latex suspension is a positive result that indicates the presence of rheumatoid factor (RF) in the specimen.

The absence of visible agglutination and the presence of opaque fluid constitutes a negative reaction.

The strength of a positive reaction may be graded as follows:

1+   Very small clumping with an opaque fluid background.
2+   Small clumping with a slightly opaque fluid in the background.

3+ Moderate clumping with fairly clear fluid in the background.

4+ Large clumping with a clear fluid background.

Procedure (Quantitative Tube Test)

Note: The quantitative test should be performed on all positive samples.

1. Label 10 12 × 75 mm test tubes (1 to 10) for the reference preparation. (Note: This reference preparation is used to establish a unit value in International Units (IU) per ml for quantitative determinations of serum specimens. The value assigned to RA Reference Preparations is derived from the World Health Organization International Reference Preparation of Rheumatoid Arthritis Serum.

2. Label 10 12 × 75 mm test tubes (1 to 10) for the patient's serum.

3. Pipette 1.9 ml of glycine-saline buffer diluent into the first tube of each set of tubes.

4. Pipette 1.0 ml of glycine-saline buffer diluent into each of the remaining tubes in each set.

5. Pipette 0.1 ml of the reference preparation to the first tube of the reference set of tubes. Mix and transfer 1.0 ml from tube 1 to tube 2 and continue this procedure through tube 9. Mix and discard 1.0 ml of the dilution from tube 9. Tube 10 is a reagent negative control.

6. Pipette 0.1 ml of the patient's serum to the first tube of the reference set of tubes. Mix and transfer 1.0 ml from tube 1 to tube 2 and continue this procedure through tube 10. Mix and discard 1.0 ml of the dilution from tube 10.

7. To each tube of both sets of tubes, add 1 drop of well-mixed latex reagent.

8. Mix the contents of each tube thoroughly and incubate at 37°C for 15 minutes.

9. Following incubation, centrifuge all tubes at 600 to 900 rcf (relative centrifical force) for 2 minutes, or for 5 to 10 minutes at a lower rcf. The rcf can be calculated by using the following formula:

$$rcf = 28.38 \ (R) \left(\frac{N}{1000} \right)^2$$

R = radius of rotor in inches

N = revolutions per minute

10. Gently shake each tube to resuspend the precipitate until an even suspension is achieved. Examine each tube for the presence of macroscopic agglutination by observing against a dark or black background under an oblique light.

In reporting results as a titer, use the same lot of latex reagent to establish titer range. Any change in the reagent lot will necessitate reestablishment of the titer in order to ensure reproducible results. It is necessary to run the RA reference preparation only once with each series of specimens.

Calculations

To calculate the results of the quantitative method in International Units (IU) per ml based on the value of the reference preparation, use the following formula:

$$\frac{\text{IU/ml of RA reference} \times \text{titer of patient's serum}}{\text{Titer of RA reference}}$$

Interpretation

Titers less than 1:20 are considered to be negative for rheumatoid factors. Positive reactions have been shown to be present in RA patients with titers ranging from 1:20 to 1:40,950.

Notes on the Procedure

False-positive results may occur if specimens are lipemic, hemolysed, or heavily contaminated with bacteria. The appearance of a positive result may also be produced if the reaction time is longer than 2 minutes, due to a drying effect.

False-negative results may be caused by high levels of CRP (antigen excess) when undiluted specimens are used. A 1:5 dilution of serum is also tested for this reason.

Biologic false-positive results can be manifested by disorders such as lupus erythematosus, Sjögren's syndrome, syphilis, and hepatitis. A small number of positive reactions have been noted in abnormalities such as periarteritis nodosa, rheumatic fever, osteoarthritis, tuberculosis, arthritis type undetermined, myositis, and polymyalgia rheumatica.

It should also be noted that parallel titrations

must be performed under similar conditions, since variations in any one set of titrations may affect the values obtained.

Slide and tube dilution methods may give different results because tube methods are more sensitive. Use of the RA reference preparation will compensate for this difference by standardizing the test results through the assignment of IU/ml to each specimen.

METHOD 2: QUANTITATIVE DETERMINATION OF IgM RHEUMATOID FACTOR IN HUMAN SERUM

Principle

This is an indirect enzyme-labeled immunoassay using microwells as a solid phase. Human immunoglobulin G (IgG) is coated onto wells of microplates. Diluted test samples are added to the coated wells and incubated. During incubation, rheumatoid factor present in the sample will bind to the IgG-coated well. After washing to remove unbound material, antibodies to human IgM labeled with alkaline phosphatase (conjugate) are added. The conjugate binds to the rheumatoid factor bound to IgG. The well is washed to remove unbound conjugate and incubated with p-nitrophenyl phosphate. The p-nitrophenyl phosphatase is hydrolyzed by alkaline phosphatase to form p-nitrophenol, a yellow-colored end product with absorbance maximum at 405 nm. The intensity of absorbance at 405 nm is proportional to the amount of IgM rheumatoid factor present in the specimen. Results are reported in international units (IU) per ml standard to the World Health Organization (WHO).

Establishing the presence of rheumatoid factor is useful in supporting the differential diagnosis of rheumatoid arthritis from other chronic inflammatory arthritides. The frequency of IgM rheumatoid factor is 70 to 80 per cent in patients with clinical features of rheumatoid arthritis. Determination of rheumatoid factor is also important in the prognosis and therapeutic management of this disease. Rheumatoid factor, however, has been associated with some bacterial and viral infections, such as hepatitis and infectious mononucleosis, and some chronic infections such as tuberculosis, parasitic disease, subacute bacterial endocarditis, and cancer. Ele-

vated values may also be observed in the normal elderly population.

Specimen Requirements

A minimum of 2 ml of clotted blood is required. The specimen should be centrifuged promptly and an aliquot of serum recovered. If the test cannot be performed immediately, the specimen may be stored at 2° to 8°C for no longer than 72 hours. If additional delay occurs, the serum should be frozen at −20°C or below. Frozen serum should be thawed rapidly at 37°C. Specimens containing visible particulate matter should be clarified by centrifugation prior to testing. The serum sample should not be heat-activated prior to testing.

Reagents, Supplies, and Equipment

SIA Rheumatoid Factor Kit Reagents are available commercially from Sigma Chemical Co., St. Louis, MO.

Note: Store reagents at 2° to 6°C.

1. Antigen wells. Microplate wells coated with human IgG. Store antigen wells with desiccant in the reusable plastic bag. Reseal the bag after opening.
2. Holder for wells
3. Sample diluent. Buffered protein solution containing surfactant and blue dye, pH 7.5. Contains 0.1 per cent sodium azide as a preservative.
4. Calibrator. Human serum containing IgM rheumatoid factor. Content (IU/ml) indicated on the label. This constituent contains 0.1 per cent sodium azide as a preservative.
5. Conjugate. Goat antibodies to human IgM labeled with calf alkaline phosphatase. This solution contains a pink dye and 0.02 per cent sodium azide as a preservative.
6. Substrate. Contains p-nitrophenyl phosphate, disodium hexahydrate 1 mg/ml, pH 9.6. The substrate may develop a slight yellow color upon storage. Do not use if absorbance of the undiluted substrate is greater than 0.4 at 405 nm when measured against water using a microplate reader or a spectrophotometer with a 1 cm lightpath.
7. Wash concentrate. Buffer solution concentrate

with surfactant. This solution contains 0.1 per cent sodium azide as a preservative. The wash solution is prepared by adding the contents of wash concentrate bottle to 1 liter of deionized water. Mix well.

8. Stop solution. This is an alkaline solution, pH 12.0. Store at room temperature. It should be noted that this stop solution causes irritation to eyes and skin. Avoid contact with eyes, skin, and clothing. Avoid breathing the vapors. Wash thoroughly after handling.

9. Positive control. Human serum containing IgM rheumatoid factor. Content (IU/ml) indicated on the label. The serum contains 0.1 per cent sodium azide.

10. Negative control. Human serum containing no detectable IgM rheumatoid factor. The serum contains 0.1 per cent sodium azide.

Note: Do not interchange reagents from different lots.

Procedure

1. Dilute calibrator, positive and negative controls, and test samples by combining 2 μl of each with 200 μl sample diluent in labeled tubes or dilution plates.

2. Place the desired number of antigen wells in holder.

3. Using a pipette tip, mix the samples and diluent by drawing up and expelling 2 or 3 times. Transfer 100 μl of each diluted sample to the appropriate antigen well.

4. Include one well that contains only 100 μl sample diluent. This serves as the reagent blank and is used to zero the photometer.

5. Allow the plate to stand at room temperature (18° to 26°C) for 20 ± 2 minutes.

6. Shake out or aspirate contents of wells. Wash wells by filling them with wash solution from a squeeze bottle and shaking out or aspirating. Wash 3 times. Drain wells on paper towel to remove excess fluid. (Note: Thorough washing is essential to achieve accurate results. Avoid bubbles.)

7. Place 2 drops (or 100 μl) conjugate into each well, including the reagent blank well.

8. Allow to stand at room temperature for 20 minutes (± 2 minutes).

9. Wash wells by repeating step 6.

10. Place 2 drops (or 100 μl substrate) into each well, including the reagent blank well.

11. Repeat step 8.

12. Place 2 drops (or 100 μl) stop solution into each well.

13. Read and record absorbance of each test at 405 nm within 2 hours after reaction has been stopped.

Microplate reader: Set absorbance at 405 nm to zero with water as a reference. Read and record absorbance of reagent blank (A blank). Then set absorbance to zero with a reagent blank as a reference. Read and record absorbance of samples (A sample) and calibrator (A calibrator).

Spectrophotometer: Completely remove contents of each well and transfer to cuvette or test tube. Add 800 μl of deionized water to each sample and mix. Set absorbance at 405 nm to zero with water as a reference. Read and record the absorbance of each sample including the reagent blank. Subtract the absorbance of the reagent blank for absorbance of each sample.

Calculations

IgM rheumatoid factor concentration:

$$\text{(IU/ml) in specimen} = \frac{\text{A sample}}{\text{A calibrator}} \times \text{IU/ml of calibrator}$$

Interpretation

Reference ranges should be established by each laboratory to reflect the characteristics of the population of the area in which it is located.

If the IgM rheumatoid factor value (IU/ml) is less than 20, report as negative for IgM rheumatoid factor.

If this value is greater than 20, report as positive for IgM rheumatoid factor.

A value greater than 60 is indicative of rheumatoid arthritis.

Procedure Notes

Specimens giving absorbance values above that of the calibrator should be diluted appropriately with sample diluent and reassayed. The value obtained should then be multiplied by the dilution factor.

The absorbance values will vary with room temperature and incubation time. The absorbance value of the reagent blank when read against water at 405 nm should be less than 0.4 using a microplate reader, or less than 0.09 using a spectrophotometer with a 1-cm lightpath. The absorbance value of the calibrator should be greater than or equal to 0.5 using a microplate reader when the assay is performed at 22°C. The assay value (IU/ml) on the positive control should be within the range shown on the label. The negative control should be less than 15 IU/ml. If these requirements are not satisfied, test results may be inaccurate, and the assay should be repeated.

Biologic false-positive results may be obtained in a variety of disorders, such as systemic lupus erythematosus (SLE).

METHOD 3: THE LATEX-FIXATION TEST FOR RHEUMATOID FACTORS

Latex suspension, RA plasma fraction, and RA buffer are available from Difco Laboratories, Detroit, MI.

Materials

1. Test serum. The test serum need not be inactivated, although inactivated serum may be used.
2. Latex suspension. This is a standardized suspension of particles 0.81 μ in diameter.
3. RA plasma fraction II. This is purified human IgG.
4. RA buffer. This is an isotonic buffer with a pH of 8.2 when rehydrated.
5. 10 × 75 mm test tubes (round bottomed)

Preparation of Antigen

1. To determine the milliliters of buffer required, multiply the number of serum samples to be tested by 3 and add 3 (e.g., if 10 samples are to be tested, [10 × 3] + 3 = 33 ml of buffer).
2. Divide the number of milliliters of buffer required (e.g., 33) by 20 (1.65). This is the amount of RA plasma fraction II required.
3. Divide the number of milliliters of buffer required

(e.g., 33) by 100 (0.33). This is the amount of latex suspension required.
4. In the example given above (i.e., with 10 samples), mix 33 ml of RA buffer with 1.65 ml of RA plasma fraction II and add 0.33 ml of latex suspension. This will be the "antigen" to use in the test.

Method

1. Set up 3 test tubes in a test tube rack for *each* test serum.
2. Add 1.9 ml of test serum to tube 1, mix and transfer 1.0 ml to tube 2, mix and transfer 1.0 ml to tube 3, and discard 1.0 ml from this tube.
3. Add 1.0 ml of the "antigen" (as previously prepared) to each tube.
4. Shake and incubate the tubes at 56°C for 2 hours.
5. Centrifuge at 2,300 rpm for 4 minutes.
6. Read macroscopically for agglutination.

Interpretation

Any agglutination in tubes 2 and 3 is considered positive. The report will state "positive" or "negative"; no titer is reported.

Controls

1. Antigen control: 1.0 ml of RA buffer and 1.0 ml of antigen. This should give no agglutination.
2. Positive serum control. Using positive control serum (commercial), set up as with test serum. This should give agglutination in tubes 2 and 3.
3. Negative serum control. Using negative control serum (commercial), set up as with test serum. This should give no agglutination.

METHOD 4: THE SHEEP CELL AGGLUTINATION TEST FOR RHEUMATOID FACTORS

Materials

1. Test tubes—12 × 100 mm
2. Rabbit anti-sheep erythrocyte hemolysin (50 per cent glycerinated)
3. 2 per cent sheep erythrocytes

4. 0.85 per cent saline
5. Patient's serum—inactivated

Estimation of the Minimal Hemagglutinating Dose (MHD)

1. Prepare the sheep erythrocytes by washing the cells 3 times with 0.85 per cent saline. After the third washing, centrifuge the cells for 10 minutes at 2,500 rpm. Prepare a 2 per cent suspension.
2. Set up 6 test tubes. Place 0.5 ml of 0.85 per cent saline into tubes 2 through 6. Prepare a 1:100 dilution of anti-sheep erythrocyte hemolysin by adding 0.2 ml of 50 per cent glycerinated hemolysin to 9.8 ml of 0.85 per cent saline. Mix well and place 0.5 ml into tubes 1 and 2.
3. Mix the contents of tube 2 and transfer 0.5 ml to tube 3. Mix the contents of tube 3 and transfer 0.5 ml to tube 4. Continue mixing and transferring, and discard 0.5 ml from tube 6. The dilutions are 1:100 to 1:3,200.
4. To each tube add 0.5 ml of 2 per cent sheep erythrocytes and 1.0 ml of 0.85 per cent saline.
5. Mix the tubes and place in a 37°C water bath for 1 hour, followed by overnight incubation in the refrigerator at 2° to 4°C.
6. Observe for agglutination. The last tube in which agglutination is observed is the endpoint. The dilution of hemolysin in this tube corresponds to the agglutinating titer of the hemolytic serum (i.e., the MHD).

The Sensitization of Sheep Erythrocytes

1. Add one half MHD to an equal volume of 2 per cent sheep erythrocytes (e.g., if the MHD is 1:200, prepare a 1:400 dilution of anti-sheep erythrocyte hemolysin).
2. To a volume of 2 per cent sheep erythrocytes, add an equal volume of diluted hemolysin while constantly stirring. (The volume of sheep erythrocytes to be prepared will depend upon the number of tests to be performed.)
3. Incubate the suspension at room temperature for 45 to 60 minutes (for 10 minutes at 37°C followed by 30 minutes at room temperature). This now represents a 1 per cent suspension of sensitized erythrocytes.

Method

1. Collect a fasting blood specimen, allow to clot, and separate the serum.
2. Set up 2 sets of 10 test tubes (i.e., 20 tubes). Mark one set "sensitized" and the other set "unsensitized."
3. Place 0.9 ml of saline into the first tube of each set and 0.5 ml of saline into each of the remaining 9 tubes of each set.
4. For each set, place 0.1 ml of the patient's serum into tube 1. Mix well and transfer 0.5 ml to tube 2. Continue mixing and transferring, and discard 0.5 ml from tube 9 of each set. The dilutions are 1:10 to 1:2,560.
5. Place 0.5 ml of the 1 per cent suspension of sensitized sheep erythrocytes into each tube of the "sensitized" set. (The 1 per cent suspension is prepared by diluting the 2 per cent suspension 1:2 in saline.)
6. Mix all tubes and incubate in a 37°C water bath for 1 hour, followed by overnight incubation in the refrigerator at 2° to 4°C.
7. Read for agglutination. The endpoint is the highest dilution of the serum giving at least a 1+ reaction. The results are expressed in terms of the geometric difference between serum titers with the "sensitized" and "unsensitized" erythrocytes. This "differential agglutination titer" (DAT) is calculated as follows:

$$DAT = \frac{\text{Serum titer with sensitized erythrocytes}}{\text{Serum titer with unsensitized erythrocytes}}$$

Interpretation

The DAT is reported in Rose units. A titer higher than 16 units is regarded as characteristic of sera from patients with RA.

METHOD 5: THE 1-MINUTE LATEX AGGLUTINATION TEST FOR THE QUALITATIVE AND QUANTITATIVE DETERMINATION OF RHEUMATOID FACTOR IN SERUM (RHEUMATEX)

Two test kits are in common use as rapid screening techniques for RA. These kits are provided by Wampole Laboratories, Cranbury, NJ, and are known as "Rheumatex" and "Rheumaton."

Specimen Collection and Preparation

Blood for this test should be collected aseptically by venipuncture into a clean tube without anticoagulant. The blood should be permitted to clot for at least 10 minutes at room temperature (20° to 25°C) before use. Rim the clot, and centrifuge at 1,000 × g for 10 minutes or until the supernatant fluid is free of cells. No special preparation of the serum is required; however, specimens that are grossly hemolyzed or that show gross lipemia or turbidity must not be used. (Note: Plasma must not be used for this test.)

If the specimen testing is delayed, the specimen should be stored refrigerated (2° to 8°C) for no longer than 24 hours. If the delay between specimen collection and testing is longer than 24 hours, store the specimen frozen at −20°C. If the specimens are to be mailed, add sodium azide to a concentration of 0.1 per cent as a preservative. As with most biologic materials, repeated freezing and thawing should be avoided. If turbidity is apparent upon thawing, the specimen should be clarified by centrifugation prior to use.

Materials

The following materials are provided:

Note: All materials must be stored in the refrigerator (2° to 8°C) when not in use. Do not freeze.

1. Rheumatex latex reagent (latex particles sensitized with human IgG)—contains buffer and preservative, 0.1 per cent sodium azide. Shake well before using.
2. Concentrated diluent 20 × (glycine-saline buffer)—contains preservative, 0.1 per cent sodium azide. Dilute 1:20 with distilled water prior to use as required for assay.
3. Positive control (RA factor–positive serum, human)—contains buffer, stabilizer, and preservative, 0.1 per cent sodium azide.
4. Negative control (RA factor–negative serum, human)—contains buffer, stabilizer, and preservative, 0.1 per cent sodium azide.

The following materials are required but are not provided:

1. Stirrers
2. Conventional test tubes
3. Distilled water
4. Serologic pipettes
5. Glass slides

Method

Note: The following precautions should be taken:

1. All reagents and specimens should be at room temperature prior to use.
2. Care should be taken to avoid contamination of reagents with each other or with the test specimens.
3. The latex reagent should be gently and well shaken prior to use. Expel the contents of the dropper, and refill.
4. The positive control and negative control should be run in parallel with the unknown specimen. Do not dilute the controls before testing.
5. Because traces of detergent or previous specimens may adversely affect the results, use only a thoroughly clean glass slide. Use only distilled water to clean the slide, and do not use detergent.
6. The results must be read at 1 minute; failure to do so may cause erroneous results.

Qualitative Slide Procedure

1. Prepare a 1:20 working solution of the concentrated diluent with distilled water, as required.
2. Dilute specimen 1:20 with the prepared diluent. Place 1 drop (approximately 50 μl) of the diluted specimen on a section of the slide.
3. Place 1 drop of positive control on a section of the slide. On another section of the slide, place 1 drop of negative control.
4. Add 1 drop of well-shaken latex reagent to each section.
5. Mix each section separately. Use a new stirrer for each section.
6. Rock the slide back and forth gently and evenly for 1 minute at a rate of 8 to 10 times per minute.
7. Observe for agglutination *immediately* at 1 minute, using an indirect oblique light source.
   Interpretation follows.

Quantitative Slide Procedure

1. Serum to be titrated should be serially diluted (1:20, 1:40, etc.) with prepared diluent. At least 6 more dilutions should be prepared.

TABLE 14–4. Prepared Dilutions in the Quantitative Tube Procedure for the Detection of Rheumatoid Factor in Serum

Tube No.	Dilution	Tube No.	Dilution
1	1:20	7	1:1,280
2	1:40	8	1:2,560
3	1:80	9	1:5,120
4	1:160	10	Positive control
5	1:320	11	Negative control
6	1:640		

2. Place 1 drop of each specimen dilution onto successive sections of the slide. Test each specimen dilution as described in the section entitled Qualitative Procedure, steps 4 through 7.

Interpretation

Positive sera show readily visible agglutination. A weakly positive serum may show very fine granulation or partial clumping. Negative sera appear uniformly turbid.

In the quantitative procedure, the last dilution to show positive agglutination on the slide is taken as the RA factor titer. For example, if the 1:80 dilution of the specimen is positive while higher dilutions are negative, the titer is 1:80. (Reference: Rheumatex package insert. Wampole Laboratories, Cranbury, NJ.)

Quantitative Tube Procedure

The qualitative test procedure described above can also be performed using test tubes as follows:

Materials

The following materials are required but are not provided:

1. Test tubes—12 × 75 mm
2. 37°C water bath
3. Centrifuge capable of 1,000 × g

Method

1. Prepare a 1:20 working dilution of the concentrated diluent with distilled water as required.

2. Label 11 test tubes 1 through 11, and place them in a test tube rack.
3. Pipette 1.9 ml of prepared diluent into tube 1, 1.0 ml of prepared diluent into tubes 2 through 9, and 0.8 ml of prepared diluent into tubes 10 and 11.
4. Add 0.1 ml of specimen to tube 1. Mix and transfer 1.0 ml of this mixture to tube 2. Mix and transfer 1.0 ml of this mixture to tube 3. Continue serially diluting in this manner through tube 9. Discard 1.0 ml from tube 9. Pipette 0.2 ml of the positive control into tube 10 and 0.2 ml of the negative control into tube 11. The prepared dilutions are as shown in Table 14–4.
5. Add 1 drop of well-shaken latex reagent to each tube.
6. Shake each tube, and incubate it for 15 minutes in a 37°C water bath.
7. Centrifuge the tubes at 1000 × g for 2 minutes.
8. Gently shake each tube until the sediment is dislodged from the bottom. Once the sediment is suspended, carefully tilt each tube back and forth until an even suspension is obtained. Do not use automatic mixing devices.
9. Examine all tubes for macroscopic agglutination against a dark background using an oblique light.

Interpretation

The highest dilution at which agglutination can still be observed is considered the titer. If a secondary standard of the International Reference Preparation of Rheumatoid Arthritis Serum, such as Wampole's Rheumatoid Factor Reference Preparation, is used, the results can be expressed in IU per ml, using the following equation:

$$\text{IU RA factor/ml of specimen} = \frac{\text{IU/ml standard} \times \text{titer of specimen}}{\text{Titer of standard}}$$

When using RF latex tests, a titer of 80 or greater is generally considered a positive reaction, a titer of 20 or 40 is considered a weakly positive reaction, and, if there is no agglutination at 1:20, the specimen should be considered negative for rheumatoid factor, even if subsequent dilution shows agglutination.

Note: The tube dilution procedure is more sensitive than the slide procedure. Consequently, differences in the raw titer will be seen between the tube titration and slide procedures.

METHOD 6: THE 2-MINUTE HEMAGGLUTINATION SLIDE TEST FOR THE QUALITATIVE AND QUANTITATIVE DETERMINATION OF RHEUMATOID FACTOR IN SERUM OR SYNOVIAL FLUID (RHEUMATON)

Specimen Collection and Preparation

Fresh serum should be used. If serum cannot be tested within 24 hours after collection, it should be stored frozen. If the sample to be tested is to be mailed, a preservative such as sodium azide, 0.1 per cent, or thimerosal, 1:10,000, should be used. In the frozen state, serum may be kept for extended periods of time. Specimens must be clear and free from particulate material. Sera must be examined, and if not clear, they should be centrifuged before use.

This test can also be performed using synovial fluid, comparable results have been reported with the sera of the same patients. Satisfactory results have been obtained using hyaluronidase to reduce the viscosity of the test material and without the use of enzyme pretreatment. In addition, the use of heparin in synovial fluid to prevent clots has been found not to interfere with the test.

Materials

The following materials are provided:

1. Rheumaton reagent (stabilized sheep erythrocytes sensitized with rabbit gamma globulin, 3 per cent)—contains buffer and 0.1 per cent sodium azide as preservative. Shake well before use.
2. Positive control (RA factor–positive serum, human)—contains saline and 0.1 per cent sodium azide as preservative.
3. Negative control (RA factor-negative serum, human)—contains saline and 0.1 per cent sodium azide as preservative.
4. Calibrated capillary tubes with rubber bulbs
5. Glass slides

The following materials are required, but are not provided:

1. Disposable stirrers
2. Distilled water or isotonic saline (0.85 per cent sodium chloride)

Qualitative Procedure

1. Fill the capillary to the mark with the patient's serum, and expel it into the center of a section of the slide.
2. Add 1 drop of Rheumaton reagent to the sample.
3. Mix with disposable stirrer, spreading over the entire section. Use a clean disposable stirrer for each mixture.
4. Rock the slide gently with a rotary motion for 2 minutes, and observe immediately for agglutination.
5. If agglutination is evident, dilute the serum specimen 1 volume to 10 volumes using either distilled water or isotonic saline (0.85 per cent sodium chloride in distilled water), and repeat the test.

Quantitative Procedure

Dilute the serum sample with isotonic saline (0.85 per cent sodium chloride), starting with a 1:10 dilution and making progressive twofold serial dilutions up to 1:1,280, as follows:

1. Place 8 small test tubes (12 × 75 mm) in a test tube rack and label them 1 through 8.
2. To tube 1 add 1.8 ml of saline. To tubes 2 through 8, add 1.0 ml of saline.
3. Add 0.2 ml of serum to be tested to tube 1, mix, and transfer 1.0 ml of this serum-saline mixture to tube 2. Mix the contents of tube 2, and transfer 1.0 ml of this mixture to tube 3. Continue mixing and transferring in this manner through tube 8. Discard 1.0 ml from tube 8.
4. Test each dilution (1:10 through 1:1,280) as described under Qualitative Procedure above.

Interpretation

In the qualitative procedure, serum samples that contain serologically detectable RF will agglutinate with the Rheumaton reagent.

In the quantitative procedure, the last dilution to

show positive agglutination on the slide is taken as the titer.

Note: Absence of agglutination with the diluted serum in the quantitative procedure (i.e., 1:10) following a positive test with the undiluted serum indicates a very low RF titer such as may exist in a variety of other diseases, namely LE, endocarditis, tuberculosis, syphilis, sarcoidosis cancer, viral infections, and diseases affecting the liver, lung, or kidney. RF has been detected in approximately 75 per cent of clinically diagnosed RA cases.

When testing undiluted serum, both RF as well as high-titer sheep agglutinins (as encountered in infectious mononucleosis and serum sickness) may also agglutinate in this test using Rheumaton reagent, by virtue of their reaction with cell antigens rather than with the rabbit gamma globulin coating the erythrocytes. In doubtful cases, tests for infectious mononucleosis should be carried out (see discussion in Chapter 12).

Ankylosing Spondylitis

Ankylosing spondylitis (AS) is a systemic rheumatic disorder that affects 10 times more men than women and begins most often between the ages of 20 and 40 years. It is characterized by inflammation of the synovial and spinal apophyseal (synovial) joints, causing back pain. In some instances, however, the disease begins in peripheral joints and (although rarely) with acute iridocyclitis.

Evidence of an unusually high frequency of the inherited antigen HLA-B27 in patients with AS (96 per cent of patients, 50 per cent of first-degree relatives) has provided overwhelming confirmation of a genetic linkage in this disorder, as has long been suspected yet never proved.

The pathogenesis of AS is not fully understood, but it is suspected that variable inciting factors (e.g., ulcerative colitis, regional enteritis, Reiter's syndrome, psoriasis), which have shown frequent, although hitherto unexplained associations with the disorder, might cause spondylitis in an individual possessing the HLA-B27 antigen. The disease may then result in a self-destructive attack of the immune response against "altered self."

Diagnosis of AS is based on the presence of the clinical and radiologic signs of the disease.

Necrotizing Angiitis (Vasculitis)

Necrotizing angiitis encompasses a group of disorders characterized by segmental inflammation of arteries, namely polyarteritis nodosa (PN), hypersensitivity angiitis, Henoch-Schönlein purpura, Wegener's granulomatosis, Takayasu's disease, and giant cell arteritis. Of these, PN and hypersensitivity angiitis are difficult to distinguish, although PN is seen more often in males and involves both medium and small arteries, whereas hypersensitivity angiitis involves only the small arteries. Marked cutaneous involvement usually suggests hypersensitivity angiitis, which is often caused by drugs (notably penicillin and sulfonamides).

Henoch-Schönlein purpura affects the small arteries of the skin, joints, and gastrointestinal tract and is frequently accompanied by purpura, gastrointestinal bleeding, and focal glomerulonephritis. Deposits of IgA, C_3, and fibrin-fibrinogen in capillaries and connective tissue of the dermis have recently been reported and may prove useful in diagnosis. Of the other disorders mentioned, Wegener's granulomatosis is characterized by vasculitis in the upper respiratory tract, lung, and kidney; in Takayasu's disease, the vasculitis occurs in the aorta and its major branches; and in giant cell arteritis, it occurs in the temporal and other cranial arteries.

In PN, 30 to 40 per cent of patients reveal the presence of immune complexes of HBsAg (hepatitis B surface antigen) in affected tissues. Otherwise, the etiology of these conditions is unknown. At present, biopsy obtained from the affected area is the only means of confirming the diagnosis.

The laboratory diagnosis is aided by findings of elevated erythrocyte sedimentation rates (the most consistent finding in all types of vasculitis), anemia, moderate leukocytosis, and (possibly) reduced complement levels. When associated with other diseases (e.g., SLE), findings consistent with that disease are sought.

Polymyositis and Dermatomyositis

Polymyositis is a condition that is characterized by degeneration and inflammation of skeletal muscle, the disease being manifested by weakness of the muscles of the shoulders, hips, and neck, usually associated with muscle pain and tenderness.

Common associated findings include dysphagia, Raynaud's phenomenon, and arthritis. The disease primarily affects females, its peak incidence occurring in the young and in those of late middle age. It is characterized histologically by myofiber necrosis, the phagocytosis of degenerating muscle cells, and infiltration by chronic inflammatory cells. An associated connective tissue disease (e.g., SLE, RA) is found in some individuals. Laboratory findings include elevated serum muscle enzymes (creatine kinase), abnormal electromyographic tracings, polyclonal hypergammaglobulinemia, rheumatoid factor, antinuclear antibody, myoglobulinemia, increased erythrocyte sedimentation rate (ESR), and increased urine creatine (Fye and Sack, 1987). Diagnosis is aided by a finding of elevated creatine kinase levels and erythrocyte sedimentation rate, and by muscle biopsy. Specific ANA are PM-1, associated with polymyositis-progressive systemic sclerosis overlap syndrome, and Jo-1, which is the serum antibody most often detected in patients with polymyositis (Nakamura *et al.*, 1985).

Dermatomyositis is a form of polymyositis with involvement of the skin. In this condition, the symmetric weakening and atrophy of the muscles of the shoulders, hips, neck, and trunk are accompanied by a maculopapular or eczema-like skin rash. The etiology of the disease is unknown, although some cases are associated with malignant neoplasms or connective tissue disease. Dysphagia and symptoms typical of systemic sclerosis (discussion follows) may be produced by involvement of the esophagus.

Progressive Systemic Sclerosis (Scleroderma)

Progressive systemic sclerosis (PSS) (also called *scleroderma*) is a chronic disease of the connective tissue, characterized by diffuse fibrosis involving the skin and several internal organs (lungs, heart, kidney, and gastrointestinal tract), inflammatory and degenerative changes of the skin and viscera, and vascular abnormalities. PSS may be associated with Sjögren's syndrome and thyroiditis. The disease usually occurs in adults (20 to 60 years) and affects females two to three times more frequently than males. Raynaud's phenomenon (pain in the extremities when exposed to cold temperatures) is the most common symptom (affecting more than

90 per cent of patients). The disease may occur in a benign or rapidly progressive form, the latter form resulting in death within a few years, the major cause being irreversible renal disease.

CREST syndrome is a milder form of scleroderma manifested by *c*alcinosis, *R*aynaud's phenomenon, *e*sophageal dysmotility, *s*clerodactyly, and *t*elangiectases.

Laboratory findings include polyclonal hypergammaglobulinemia and ANA, with speckled or nucleolar pattern. Scl-70 antibody is a marker ANA detected in 15 to 20 per cent of patients, whereas centromere antibody is a marker antibody for the CREST variety with a frequency of 70 to 90 per cent. Hematologic studies show anemia; urinalysis is usually normal (except in the presence of renal disease). Although the etiology is unknown, evidence for an antigen-mediated pathogenesis is suggested by increased levels of immunoglobulin (IgG) and ANA (40 to 70 per cent). Between 25 and 33 per cent of affected individuals have positive tests for syphilis; positive LE cell reactions also occur. Pulmonary function tests may show increased residual volume and decreased maximal breathing capacity. Esophageal hypomotility and diverticuli are often revealed by X-ray examination.

Mixed Connective Tissue Disease

Mixed connective tissue disease (MCTD) is a syndrome that has the combined clinical features of RA, SLE, PSS, and polymyositis. Typically, patients have positive ANA of the speckled pattern and high titers of antibody to extractable ribonucleoprotein (anti-RNP antibodies). In addition, RF, elevated ESR, and hypergammaglobulinemia are usually present, whereas anti-DNA and anti-Sm are usually absent.

Sjögren's Syndrome

Sjögren's syndrome (SS) most often occurs secondary to RA, scleroderma, polymyositis, or SLE. In its primary form, SS manifests itself in the form of dry eyes (keratoconjunctivitis sicca) and dry mouth (xerostomia).

Sjögren's syndrome is characteristically revealed through remarkable immunologic reactivity detected in the serum. LE cells, ANA (usually a speckled or diffuse pattern), RA factor, and hypergammaglobulinemia are frequently present, and, in addition, antibodies against RNA, salivary duct, lacrimal gland, smooth muscle, mitochondria, and thyroid gland may be found. There is an increased frequency of renal tubular acidosis, and lymphoma may also develop, particularly in patients with the primary form of SS.

An association between the antigen HLA-Dw3 and primary SS has been found. Diagnosis is confirmed by salivary technetium pertechnetate scintiscanning, which is more sensitive that sialography and labial biopsy.

Specific ANA include SS-B (in primary Sjögren's syndrome), SS-A (associated with SLE), and rheumatoid arthritis nuclear antigen (associated with rheumatoid arthritis) (Nakamura *et al.*, 1985; Rodnan and Schumacher, 1983).

ORGAN-SPECIFIC AUTOIMMUNE DISEASES

Organ-specific autoimmune diseases are those diseases in which the major effect involves a single organ (Table 14–5). The diagnosis of these diseases is aided by serologic tests, which are used to detect the presence of antibodies to tissue-specific antigens.

Autoimmune Diseases of the Blood

Autoimmune Hemolytic Anemias

All the formed elements of the blood may be involved in autoimmune reactions. The autoimmune hemolytic anemias (AHA) are a group of anemias characterized by a hemolytic process involving red cell–specific antibodies in the serum.

The study of the AHA takes place primarily in the immunohematology laboratory. The brief description given here is included for the sake of completeness; readers are referred to the list of general references at the end of this chapter for more detailed coverage.

Autoimmune Hemolytic Anemia (Warm Type). This is the most common of the AHA, consisting of idiopathic and secondary types. The disease affects both sexes and people of all ages. The anemia is caused by antibodies primarily of the IgG class, which show limited complement-fixing ability and react (in the vast majority of cases) with Rh or

TABLE 14–5. Autoimmune Diseases That Are Organ Specific

Organ	Disease
Blood	Autoimmune hemolytic anemias Autoimmune thrombocytopenic purpura Neutropenia Lymphopenia Autoimmune aplastic anemia
Kidneys	Goodpasture's syndrome Systemic lupus erythematosus Acute streptococcal nephritis Berger's disease Membranoproliferative glomerulonephritis
Endocrine (thyroid)	Autoimmune thyroiditis (Hashimoto's disease) Primary myxedema Thyrotoxicosis (Graves' disease) Addison's disease Parathyroid disease Early-onset diabetes
Pancreas	Diabetes mellitus
Adrenals	Addison's disease
Parathyroids	Idiopathic hypoparathyroidism
Ovary and testis	Allergic orchitis
Nervous system	Disseminated encephalomyelitis Idiopathic polyneuritis Landry's paralysis Multiple sclerosis
Stomach and intestines	Pernicious anemia Gastric atrophy Regional ileitis (Crohn's disease) Ulcerative colitis Gluten-sensitive enteropathy Sjögren's syndrome
Liver	Chronic aggressive hepatitis Drug-induced liver diseases Primary biliary cirrhosis Portal cirrhosis
Muscle	Myasthenia gravis Polymyositis Multiple sclerosis
Eye	Phacogenic uveitis Sympathetic ophthalmia Sjögren's syndrome
Skin (dermis)	Pemphigus vulgaris Bullous pemphigoid Cicatricial pemphigoid Dermatitis herpetiformis Systemic lupus erythematosus
Heart	Post-cardiotomy syndrome Post-myocardial infarction syndrome (Dressler's syndrome)

extractable nuclear antigens. The idiopathic form accounts for more than half of the cases of AHA, and although the etiology remains obscure, on long-term follow-up, some of these patients are found to have lymphoma. In the secondary type, anemia occurs in association with one of many diseases or after the use of drugs. In 30 to 40 per cent of cases, the patient's red cells are coated (sensitized) with IgG only; in 50 per cent of cases, the red cells are coated with IgG and complement; and in 10 to 20 per cent of cases, the red cells appear to be coated only with complement. In each case, IgG and complement are readily detected by the indirect antiglobulin (Coombs') test with broad spectrum anti-human globulin.

Autoimmune Hemolytic Anemia (Cold Type). In the cold agglutinin group, antibodies are primarily IgM, reacting best at 0° to 4°C, with lesser activity at higher temperatures, becoming dissociated at 37°C. These antibodies have the ability to fix complement and are usually directed against the I antigen, the i antigen, and (rarely) the Sp_1 antigen. These antibodies, particularly anti-I, are found in such diseases as primary atypical pneumonia (*Mycoplasma pneumoniae*), infectious mononucleosis, and cold agglutinin disease. The clinical lesions include anemia, the severity of which is dependent upon the thermal activity of the antibody. Renal failure from hemolysis is rare. The disease is associated with cirrhosis, malignant diseases, infectious mononucleosis, mycoplasma infections, and sarcoidosis. On long-term follow-up, some patients are found to have overt lymphoma.

Paroxysmal Cold Hemoglobinuria. The cold autohemolysins (Donath-Landsteiner-type) found in this group of AHA were first described in patients with tertiary syphilis. The antibodies are cold agglutinins of the IgG class, which fix complement and are directed against the P antigen. Because complement fixation is avid, most cells are lysed before they reach phagocytic cells, and the result is rapid intravascular hemolysis when the body or part of the body is cooled below the critical temperature (15° to 20°C). Hemolysis may occur, with hemoglobinuria, fever, chills, hypotension, and abdominal and back pain.

Drug-Induced Hemolysis. There are four basic mechanisms that can cause drug-induced coating of red cells with accompanying hemolysis.

Drug Absorption. In this mechanism, the drug binds strongly to any protein, including red cell membrane proteins, which produces a drug–red cell–hapten complex that can stimulate the production of antibodies. The formed antibody is specific for the complex, and no reaction will take place unless the drug is absorbed onto the erythrocytes.

Penicillin is one of the drugs that displays drug absorption, although massive doses of the drug, injected intravenously, are needed to coat the erythrocytes sufficiently for antibody attachment to occur.

A positive direct antiglobulin test is seen in about 3 per cent of affected patients, and less than 5 per cent of patients will develop hemolytic anemia as a result. Red cell hemolysis is extravascular and slow, and the condition, which will abate when the drug is discontinued, is not life threatening. (Note: there is no connection between this type of antibody production and allergic penicillin sensitivity caused by the production of IgE.)

Other drugs that display drug absorption are cephalothin (Keflin), and quinidine.

Immune Complex. A variety of drugs display immune complexing. The drug and antibody form a complex, which then attaches nonspecifically to red cells. Complement is activated, which results in intravascular hemolysis. The immune complex may dissociate from the red cell membrane after complement activation and attach to another red cell, thus allowing a small amount of drug to produce a severe anemia. The hemolytic process disappears when the offending drug is discontinued.

Membrane Modification. In this mechanism, the drug alters the membrane so that there is nonspecific absorption of globulins, including IgG, IgM, and IgA, and complement. Hemolysis is not a frequent complication. Drugs of the cephalosporin type are implicated in this mechanism.

Autoantibody Formation. A formed autoantibody recognizes a part of the red cell and therefore reacts with most normal red cells in this mechanism. Some of these autoantibodies have specificity (e.g., Rh type) although most do not. The implicated drugs are methyldopa (Aldomet), levodopa, and mefanamic acid (Ponstel). Antibody production stops when the drug is discontinued.

Etiology and Laboratory Diagnosis of AHA. The etiology of AHA is unknown. It has been postulated, however, that drugs and viruses may in some way alter the antigenic structure of the red cell membrane, rendering the erythrocyte susceptible to hemolysis. Genetically determined susceptibility to develop autoantibodies has also been postulated; this may be associated with certain immunologic abnormalities.

The major diagnostic criteria used in the laboratory to distinguish AHA from other forms of anemia are the presence of spherocytes in the peripheral blood smear and a positive direct antiglobulin (Coombs') test (for method, see Bryant, 1982). The type of AHA is determined by the temperature of the agglutination reactions.

Autoimmune Thombocytopenic Purpura (AITP)

Patients with thrombocytopenia associated with normal, or possibly increased, numbers of megakaryocytes in the bone marrow were termed as having *idiopathic thrombocytopenic purpura (ITP)*. In view of the evidence that the condition is due to the formation of autoantibodies, the term *autoimmune thombocytopenic purpura* has now become more common, using the abbreviation AITP rather than ATP to avoid confusion with the abbreviation for adenosine triphosphate.

Harrington *et al.* (1951) were the first to demonstrate the presence of anti-platelet factor in the plasma of patients with AITP. These investigators found that plasma from an AITP patient, when transfused to an affected individual, resulted in a profound fall in the recipient's platelet count.

The serologic tests for AITP include:

The Antiglobulin Consumption Test. This test (Dixon *et al.*, 1975) gives a very high percentage of positive results; however, it is also positive in various disease states not necessarily associated with an increased rate of platelet destruction (e.g., SLE). Certain modifications of the antiglobulin consumption test have been found to give varying, though encouraging, results in cases of AITP. These include modifications suggested by Rosse *et al.* (1980) and by Nel and Stevens (1980), which used an enzyme-linked antibody.

Hymes *et al.* (1979) described an antiglobulin consumption test method in which platelets were frozen, thawed, and sonicated. The IgG was then extracted and applied to wells of microtiter plates, to which it stuck. Rabbit anti-human IgG was then added to the plates, followed by ^{125}I-labeled staphylococcal protein. The wells were then removed

and counted. This method was found to be very sensitive and has the advantage of being able to use platelets stored at $-20°C$ before testing. A similar type of method found to be almost equal in sensitivity but using enzyme-linked antiglobulin serum was described by Hedge *et al.* (1981). In this technique, IgG was extracted from platelets and bound to anti-human IgG, previously coated onto polystyrene. The amount of platelet-associated IgG was then estimated by adding the enzyme reagent (anti-human IgG coupled with alkaline phosphatase) together with a suitable substrate.

The Platelet Immunofluorescence Test. The original platelet immunofluorescence test was plagued with the problem of nonspecific immunofluorescence. A modification of the technique was described by von dem Borne *et al.* (1978), which overcame this difficulty through the pretreatment of platelets with paraformaldehyde. In the latter method, paraformaldehyde-treated platelets are incubated with serum, then washed and incubated with antiglobulin serum labeled with fluorescein-isothiocyanate. After incubation, the cells are washed again, then examined under a fluorescence microscope. The test appears to be more sensitive than the antiglobulin consumption test, yet it also does not give positive results in all cases of AITP.

The Radioactive Antiglobulin Test. Soulier *et al.* (1975) and Mueller-Eckhardt *et al.* (1978) described the use of a ^{125}I-labeled antiglobulin test for the detection of platelet antibodies. The use of this test in cases of AITP revealed that only about 80 per cent of patients with the disease had a raised platelet-associated IgG (PAIgG) level, whereas an increased level of PAIgG was not confined to AITP but was also found in chronic liver disease, leukemia, myeloma, and other diseases (Mueller-Eckhardt *et al.*, 1980). Like the platelet immunofluorescence test, this test appears to be more sensitive than antiglobulin consumption, yet it does not give positive results in all cases of AITP.

Helmerhorst *et al.* (1980) performed a comparison test on a small number of patients using the three procedures just discussed and concluded that the platelet immunofluorescence test was the most sensitive of the three and that the higher percentage of positive results observed with the antiglobulin consumption test indicated the nonspecificity of that test in the detection of red cell–bound antibody. These investigators therefore recommend that a positive result with the immunofluorescence test (or the radioactive antiglobulin test) provides strong support for a diagnosis of AITP (although the diagnosis is not ruled out by a negative test), whereas a positive antiglobulin consumption test alone does not establish a diagnosis of AITP.

Neutropenia

This is a disease in which there is a decrease in the number of neutrophilic leukocytes in the blood below the lower reference limit of 2,000 per mm³ for caucasians and 1,300 per mm³ for blacks. The disease is therefore characterized by susceptibility to infection. The surface antigens of the neutrophil are probably causative, although it is possible that the disease is produced by several mechanisms, including decreased or ineffective neutrophil production in the bone marrow, increased loss of neutrophils from the peripheral blood, and "pseudo" neutropenia in which there is a shift from the circulating granulocyte pool to the marginal granulocyte pool.

Neutropenia can result from the administration of drugs (particularly by cancer chemotherapy, but also as an idiosyncratic response to many other drugs). It can also be caused by exposure to radiation. The disease is associated with acute leukemias, many infections, RA, congestive splenomegaly, and vitamin B_{12} deficiency. There are also several forms of congenital neutropenia, which, in young children, have a guarded prognosis. However, resistance to infection improves if children survive infancy, which is presumed to reflect compensatory development of antibody and cell-mediated responses, both of which are functionally intact in most of these patients.

The primary neutropenias can be diagnosed on the basis of age of onset, history of exposure to toxic substances or drugs, family history, and blood or bone marrow analysis. Immunologically mediated neutropenia is better established by determining the presence of serum leukoagglutinins or specific anti-neutrophil antibody.

Lymphocytopenia

This is a disease in which there is a decrease in the proportion of lymphocytes in the blood, characterized by secondary immunodeficiency. The T lymphocytes are preferentially depleted from the circulation to a greater extent than are the B lymphocytes. In addition, there is a selective depletion of certain T cell subpopulations, as determined by phenotypic markers as well as by functional capabilities. The probable antigens are lymphocyte-specific surface antigens; the antibody is much like heterologous anti-lymphocyte globulin.

Autoimmune Aplastic Anemia

This disease occurs in about one third of all patients with aplastic anemia (a type of anemia in which there is complete absence of reticulocytes in the blood and of all types of erythroblasts in the bone marrow). It is probable that the stem cell–specific antigens are involved. The immunity seems to be T cell mediated.

Autoimmune Diseases of the Kidney

An inflammatory reaction within the kidney can result in any one of four types of immunologically mediated renal disease:

Type I (Anaphylactic). Although no specific renal disease has been definitely ascribed to Type I hypersensitivity, it has been preliminarily implicated in mediating a form of renal disease associated with Henoch-Schönlein purpura, because IgE deposition in the glomeruli of patients with this disease has been noted. The acceptance of IgE as a pathogenic factor requires more extensive confirmation, however. It is likely that Type I hypersensitivity plays at least a contributing role in certain forms of reversible renal transplant rejection and in interstitial nephritis of methicillin-induced nephritis.

Type II (Cytotoxic). Injury to the kidney results from tissue antigen-antibody combination that activates complement and other systems of inflammation. Anti-GBM (glomerular basement membrane) disease is a good example in which antibody to GBM is produced and antibody and complement are deposited in linear fashion along the GBM. If the anti-GBM reacts with the other basement membranes (e.g., the lung) as well, injury to the pulmonary capillary bed occurs. The syndrome of anti-GBM–mediated immune renal failure and pulmonary hemorrhage is known as *Goodpasture's syndrome.* The deposition of antibody and complement in linear fashion along the GBM can be shown by direct immunofluorescence (Fig. 14–2).

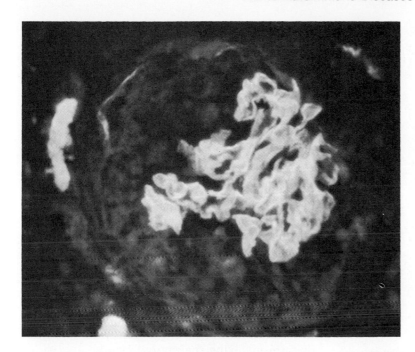

Figure 14–2. A photomicrograph of the kidney of a patient with Goodpasture's syndrome demonstrated by direct fluorescence microscopy. (From Bellanti, J. A.: Immunology III. Philadelphia, W. B. Saunders Company, 1985, p. 432.)

Tubulointerstitial renal disease occurs when the anti basement membrane is directed against the tubular basement membrane (TBM). Anti-TBM antibodies are associated with such disorders, as anti-GBM disease, SLE, and renal transplant rejection.

Hyperacute renal allograft rejection is a form of Type II-mediated renal disease that affects the entire kidney. It is associated with high levels of pre-existing HLA antibodies of the transplant. It is likely that the injury to the kidney results from a Type II attack by anti-HLA against HLA antigens of the renal transplant, which are widely distributed.

Type III (Immune Complex). Deposition of immune complexes formed in the glomeruli of kidneys is the basis of the majority of immunologically mediated renal diseases, even though the immunologic specificity is not directed toward the antigens of the kidney itself. The antigen-antibody complexes deposit in the glomerular capillary wall (immune-complex glomerular renal disease) or in the tubulointerstitium (immune complex tubulointerstitial renal disease).

A classic example of immune complex disease of the kidney is SLE, in which the antigen-antibody-complement complexes form in the blood, deposit in the glomeruli in granular distribution, and activate complement, thus inducing inflammation and activating the clotting system.

Acute post-streptococcal glomerulonephritis is another form of immune-complex disease. In this, the antigen resides in the wall of the streptococcus (usually group A beta-hemolytic streptococci, particularly types 12 and 49). Infection induces the production of antibody that combines with the streptococcal antigens, and these complexes deposit in the glomerular capillary wall. An acute glomerular inflammatory response ensues, with activation of complement, release of lysozymes from polymorphonuclear cells, and subsequent tissue injury.

Both exogenous antigens (i.e., bacterial, viral, parasitic, foreign serum, and drugs) and endogenous antigens (i.e., nuclear antigens and tumor antigens) may induce immune-complex glomerulonephritis (Table 14–6).

Type IV (Cell Mediated). Cell-mediated immune renal injury is best exemplified by renal allograft rejection, in which sensitized lymphoid cells attack the graft, with immune renal injury resulting. The reaction occurs throughout the kidney, and soluble substances are released by lymphoid cells. These soluble substances (called *lymphokines*) may cause an inflammatory response, thus reducing tissue injury.

It is also possible that chronic glomerulonephritis may fall into the category of Type IV hypersensitivity. It has been hypothesized that the release of

TABLE 14–6. Exogenous and Endogenous Antigens Associated with Type III Immune Renal Injury

Antigen	Examples
Exogenous	
Bacterial	Post-streptococcal GN
	Staphylococcal
Viral	Chickenpox
	Hepatitis B
Parasitic	Malaria
	Toxoplasmosis
Foreign serum	Serum sickness
Drugs	Heroin nephropathy (?)
Endogenous	
Nuclear antigens	Systemic lupus erythematosus
Tumor antigens	Carcinoembryonic antigen

Slightly modified from Bellanti, J. A.: Immunology III. Philadelphia, W. B. Saunders Company, 1985, p. 434.

renal tissue antigens after acute glomerulonephritis may result in cell-mediated hypersensitivity to those antigens. This hypothesis is supported by studies showing that, on exposure to renal tissue antigens by lymphoid cells from patients with chronic glomerulonephritis, migration inhibitory factor (MIF) is released.

Other Forms of Immune Renal Disease

A number of renal diseases have been described that do have apparent immunologic bases, yet do not fit into any of the categories, just described. Two of them are IgG-IgA nephropathy (Berger's disease) and membranoproliferative or mesangio-capillary glomerulonephritis.

In IgG-IgA nephropathy (Berger's disease), renal biopsy shows IgG and IgA deposits in mesangial areas of the glomerulus, with subsequent mesangial cell hyperplasia. The cause of deposition in this disease is not known. It has been suggested from studies in rabbits that the mesangium may be capable of clearing small amounts of immune complexes during early antigen-antibody production when the level of complexes is small, but that after saturation of other mononuclear phagocytic systems (e.g., the liver and spleen), complexes may begin to accumulate in the capillary wall and extraglomerular sites.

Membranoproliferative glomerulonephritis ap-

pears to result from the deposition of activated complement components within the kidney, the complement possibly activated through the alternative pathway (see Chapter 3). The direct activation of C3 is likely to be related to a heat-stable gamma globulin in the serum known as *nephritic factor*, which is capable of cleaving C3 to C3b directly. In this form of renal disease, C3 is deposited densely within the capillary wall of the glomerulus. The disease does not in all instances proceed to kidney failure, but patients who do develop renal failure and receive transplants are at risk of the disease recurring in the transplant.

Autoimmune Diseases of the Endocrine Organs

Autoimmune disease has been associated with all the endocrine organs, although the most extensively studied and most frequently occurring are diseases involving the thyroid gland.

Autoimmune Diseases of the Thyroid

The diseases of the thyroid gland in which autoimmune factors are involved are *lymphocytic thyroiditis (Hashimoto's thyroiditis)* and *thyrotoxicosis (Graves' disease)*.

Autoimmune Thyroiditis (Hashimoto's Thyroiditis). This is the most common form of thyroiditis occurring at any age, although it usually occurs in patients between the ages of 35 and 55 years. It is 5 to 10 times more frequent in females than in males.

Initially, the symptom is enlargement of the thyroid gland, which is usually painless and may develop gradually over a number of years. If the enlargement is great, dysphagia, choking, and dyspnea may result. The enlargement is generally diffuse, although it may be nodular; in some cases, the lesion may occur as a solitary nodule.

The disease is characterized histologically by an intense infiltration of the thyroid stroma and follicles by lymphocytes and plasma cells, and by degeneration and regeneration of the thyroid parenchyma. Immunologically, circulating antibodies as well as lymphoproliferative responses to various constituents of thyroid are commonly seen. In addition to these circulating antibodies (which may represent autoimmune phenomena), antibodies have been described in this disease (and in Graves' disease, discussion follows) that appear to regulate cellular activity and may in fact contribute to the hyperthyroidism. These include:

1. Long-acting thyroid stimulator (LATS). This has an *in vivo* ability to enhance the release of thyroid hormone. It is an IgG immunoglobulin that is detected by means of bioassay. The antibody is formed against a thyroid protein and mimics most actions of thyrotropin. Not all patients with Hashimoto's thyroiditis have detectable levels of LATS; none is detected in normal individuals.
2. LATS protector activity (LPA). This has the ability to prevent the neutralization of LATS by an inactivator normally present in human thyroid extract.
3. Thyroid-stimulating immunoglobulins (TSI). These appear to represent autoantibodies directed against thyrotropin receptors, which are capable of binding to the receptor and stimulating the production of cyclic AMP and the excessive production of thyroid hormone. TSI has been detected in 15 per cent of patients with Hashimoto's thyroiditis.

Whether or not these activities represent three distinct antibodies (or whether they may be different manifestations of the same antibody specificity, differing only in the methods required for their detection) remains unclear.

There are many immunologic tests that are useful in the detection of thyroid antibodies. Antithyroglobulin antibodies can be detected by precipitation, latex agglutination, the tanned red cell (TRC) test, and radioimmunoassay. Microsomal antibodies can be detected using complement fixation, cytotoxicity tests, immunofluorescence of unfixed thyroid epithelial cells, radioimmunoassay, and hemagglutination tests. The second antibody of acinar colloid, a protein that is distinct from thyroglobulin, is also detected by immunofluorescence. This antibody is not specific for Hashimoto's thyroiditis and is seen in patients with thyrotoxicosis and cancer of the thyroid. Immunofluorescence on living suspensions of human thyroid cells has revealed thyroid-specific cell surface antibodies; the significance of these antibodies is unknown.

Tests of thyroid function, including T_3 (triiodothyronine) and T_4 (thyroxine) levels, T_3-resin uptake, and ^{131}I uptake are usually in the range of low to normal in this disorder; in such cases, the most sensitive test for hypothyroidism is the measurement of thyroid-stimulating hormone (TSH) levels.

A useful test for the detection of anti-thyroid antibody (ATA) in the sera of patients with chronic thyroiditis (including Hashimoto's thyroiditis and Graves' disease) is the CSI ATA Immunopath Fluoro-Kit (Clinical Sciences Inc., Whippany, NJ), which uses an indirect fluorescent antibody method and is designed as a screening test for all three ATA. This test should be run on every patient with a goiter, because 10 to 20 per cent of adult patients with chronic thyroid disease may have negative results when tested with the hemagglutination technique, and the latter test is only reactive with the thyroglobin antigen, whereas the CSI ATA Immunopath test is capable of detecting all three organ-specific antibodies simultaneously.

Myxedema. This is a condition associated with hypothyroidism and characterized by the collection of hydrated mucopolysaccharides in the dermis and in other tissues of the body. The diagnosis of this disease is based on the clinical signs and measurement of the serum levels of triiodothyronine (T_3) and thyroxine (T_4). Frequently, there is also hypercholesterolemia and increased serum levels of TSH.

Thyrotoxicosis (Graves' Disease). An association between Hashimoto's thyroiditis and Graves' disease is becoming more and more frequently recognized, because the two conditions frequently exist together in the same patient and may represent different manifestations of a common spectrum. Graves' disease is now considered to be a multisystem disorder consisting of three components:

1. Hyperthyroidism due to diffuse goiter
2. Infiltrative ophthalmopathy (exophthalmos)
3. Infiltrative dermopathy (localized pretibial myxedema)

These components may present in combination with each other or, in some cases, individually. Infiltrative ophthalmopathy and infiltrative dermopathy occur most frequently in adult patients in whom a higher incidence of antibodies is found.

The three ATA previously described (see Hashimoto's thyroiditis) are also present in Graves' disease. LATS is detected in about 50 per cent of patients with Graves' disease, and TSI is detected in about 90 per cent of these patients.

The CSI ATA Immunopath Fluoro-Kit described above for autoimmune thyroiditis (Hashimoto's thyroiditis) is also used for the detection of ATA in Graves' disease.

Autoimmune Diseases of the Pancreas

Diabetes Mellitus

There is increasing evidence that autoimmune mechanisms play a role in insulin-dependent diabetes mellitus (IDDM) early in the disease (Boitard et al., 1986; Eisenbarth, 1986). An immunoglobulin has been found in the serum of these patients that (when IgG, IgA, or IgM) appears to inhibit binding of insulin to its receptor, and, when IgG, appears to contribute to insulin allergy.

Radioimmunoassay of insulin concentrations is a useful test, facilitated through the production of insulin antibodies in animals.

Thyroid and gastric autoantibodies have also been found in the sera of diabetic patients without clinical thyroid disease or pernicious anemia. These antibodies are primarily found in juvenile-onset diabetes and are usually insulin-dependent and often insulin-resistant. They are more frequently detected in females.

Approximately 60 to 85 per cent of patients with IDDM have cytoplasmic staining of the beta cells of the pancreas.

Autoimmune Disease of the Adrenals

Autoantibodies to adrenal tissues, detectable by immunofluorescence or complement fixation, have been reported in patients with Addison's disease. The significance of these findings is not known.

Autoimmune Disease of the Parathyroids

Antibodies to thyroid, adrenal, and gastric tissues have been detected in a disorder known as *idiopathic hypoparathyroidism*, which occurs more frequently in children than in adults and is more common in females than in males. Hypoparathyroidism may be accompanied by certain associated disorders, including idiopathic Addison's disease,

pernicious anemia, alopecia totalis, and moniliasis. When clusters of two or more of these associated diseases are present, it appears that an autosomal recessive mode of transmission of an underlying defect may be involved. Hypoparathyroidism is also associated with development failure of the thymus-dependent immune system in DiGeorge's syndrome.

Autoimmune Disease of the Ovary and Testis

Alper and Garner (1985) and Miyaka et al. (1987) have reported evidence of autoimmunity in 30 to 50 per cent of patients with premature ovarian failure. Assays for anti-ovarian antibodies are limited to research laboratories.

Anti-sperm antibodies have been found in the sera of some infertile couples (Mathur, 1985; Meinertz and Hjort, 1986). They have also been detected in the serum and semen of individuals after vasectomy (Meinertz and Hjort, 1986) but only occasionally in those with primary testicular agenesis. The mechanisms by which such antibodies lead to infertility are still unclear.

Autoimmune Diseases of the Nervous System

The best-studied autoimmune disease of the central nervous system is acute disseminated encephalomyelitis. Other autoimmune conditions of the nervous system include idiopathic polyneuritis (Guillain-Barré syndrome), Landry's paralysis, and multiple sclerosis (MS).

Disseminated Encephalomyelitis. This is a disease characterized by fever, photophobia, blindness, muscle weakness, decreased consciousness, seizures, paresis, loss of appetite, and sphincter disturbance. Increased protein and lymphocytosis are seen in the cerebrospinal fluid. The condition may develop subsequent to infection by either bacterial or viral agents, but viral infections (e.g., measles, mumps, and rubella) are much more common as predisposing causes. Following infection, there is a latent period of 5 to 30 days before the onset of disease. Various immunizations (notably smallpox or rabies) may precipitate the disease.

Circulating antibody to encephalitogenic factors has been demonstrated by a number of techniques, but now there is rather clear evidence that the *major* pathologic change in experimental allergic encephalomyelitis (EAE) is mediated by sensitized lymphocytes.

Idiopathic Polyneuritis. Also known as Guillain-Barré syndrome, idiopathic polyneuritis is another form of neurologic disease that has immunologic features. The disease, which is of unknown etiology, is characterized by peripheral nerve involvement. The disease may follow a variety of infectious diseases, or it may occur subsequent to immunization (e.g., swine influenza immunization).

Landry's Paralysis. This is another form of polyneuritis that produces a weakness and sensory loss in the limbs as a result of inflammation in the peripheral nerves.

Multiple Sclerosis. This is a slowly progressive disease of the central nervous system of unknown cause, usually beginning in early adult life, which is characterized by disseminated, patchy demyelination of the brain and spinal cord. The disease results in a number of neurologic symptoms and signs, and it may relapse and remit over long periods of time. A number of infectious disease pathogens have been implicated in MS, but the precise cause remains unclear. An immunologic mechanism, however, is suggested by the presence of lymphocytes in early lesions and plasma cells, and macrophages in older lesions. The finding of an elevated spinal fluid gamma globulin in 80 per cent of patients is a distinguishing feature of the disease. About 90 per cent of patients with MS have oligoclonal banding, although this is not specific for MS, since it can also be demonstrated in viral meningitis, neurosyphilis, SLE with central nervous system involvement, and other immunologic diseases of the central nervous system (Mehl and Penn, 1986).

No specific treatment of MS is available, and death is usually due to some intercurrent disease.

Autoimmune Diseases of the Stomach and Intestines

Diseases of the stomach and intestines that are triggered by an immunologic response include pernicious anemia, gastric atrophy, regional ileitis, ulcerative colitis, and gluten-sensitive enteropathy (celiac disease).

Pernicious Anemia. This is a disorder characterized by inflammation of the gastric mucosa with inability to secrete hydrochloric acid, intrinsic factor, and pepsin, followed by the development of macrocytic anemia. The disease is characteristically associated with the presence of parietal cell antibody or intrinsic factor antibody or both in patients with atrophic gastritis. Antibody has recently been found in the gastric juice, and lymphoid cells have been found in infiltrate gastric mucosa. An antibody that, when mixed with intrinsic factor, interferes with the absorption of vitamin B_{12} has been found in the sera of patients with pernicious anemia (PA). Whether these antibodies are the cause or the result of the disease is not known. The clear link, however, between the presence of these antibodies and the clinical disease and the fact that pernicious anemia will respond to steroid therapy lend evidence for the autoimmune nature of the disease.

Serologic tests in cases of PA include complement fixation or immunofluorescence (for the detection of antibodies directed against the microsomal fraction of gastric mucosal cells), and blocking and binding antibody tests (to detect the antibodies that bind with preformed intrinsic factor B_{12} complex, binding antibody, or those that block the combination of intrinsic factor with antibody, blocking antibody). The tests for these antibodies are important in differentiating PA from other causes of megaloblastic anemia.

Gastric Atrophy. Atrophic gastritis affects about 20 to 30 per cent of the adult population, apparently progressing from a lesion of superficial gastritis. The incidence of the disorder increases with age, as do the gastric autoantibodies. Parietal cell antibodies and intrinsic factor antibody occurring in this case would cause PA. Their presence is particularly associated with other diseases of autoimmunity (e.g., Graves' disease, myxedema, insulin-dependent diabetes, Addison's disease), and they occur with increased frequency in the families of patients with PA, thyroid diseases, and other autoimmune disorders.

Regional Ileitis (Crohn's Disease). Although suspected, an autoimmune basis has not been substantiated in this disease, which is characterized by granulomatous inflammatory changes of the ileum that sometimes also involve other parts of the gastrointestinal tract. Antibodies to heterologous colon have been demonstrated in regional ileitis.

Ulcerative Colitis. The pathogenesis of ulcerative colitis is unknown, but it is thought to be auto-immune on the basis of circulating antibody to colonic tissue, probably triggered by enteric infection. The fact that females are more affected than males suggests a genetic predisposition in this disorder. The disease primarily affects the large bowel and is characterized by bloody diarrhea, abdominal pain, weight loss, and anemia.

An IgM hemagglutinin, a precipitating antibody, and an immunofluorescent antibody are the three kinds of antibodies that have been demonstrated against colonic tissue, although their significance in the pathogenesis of ulcerative colitis is not clear. The lymphocytes from affected patients cause cytotoxicity to cells in culture (although antibody-containing serum does not); this suggests that cell-mediated immune mechanisms may be more important than humoral antibody in the pathogenesis of this disease.

Gluten-Sensitive Enteropathy (Celiac Disease). This disorder is characterized by malabsorption of fats and carbohydrates. The ingestion of the gliadin fraction of gluten (a protein found in grains) appears to cause diarrhea in these patients, although it is not known how this effect is mediated. A hypersensitivity reaction may also occur to the gliadin fraction itself. High-titer antibodies to gliadin (IgA and IgM) have been detected in affected patients. In addition, the finding that IgA deficiency occurs more frequently in celiac patients than in the general population is probably related to common factors underlying the two conditions. An association between gluten-sensitive enteropathy (GSE) and HLA-Dw3 and B8 has been reported.

Autoimmune Diseases of the Liver

Liver diseases with immunologic features include viral hepatitis (acute and chronic), drug-induced liver diseases, biliary cirrhosis, and portal cirrhosis. Of these, the most important are infectious hepatitis (type A) and serum hepatitis (type B) (see Chapter 7).

Hepatitis. See Chapter 7.

Drug-Induced Liver Diseases. The use of a number of different drugs can induce liver disease in hypersensitive individuals. Two forms of drug-induced liver disease are seen: (1) a toxic form and (2) a true hypersensitivity reaction. Antibodies have been detected in the toxic form, although not in the hypersensitivity form. The disease can only be treated through the discontinuation of the offending drugs.

Primary Biliary Cirrhosis. The term *cirrhosis* refers to liver disease characterized pathologically by loss of the normal microscopic lobular architecture with fibrosis and nodular regeneration. The term is sometimes used to refer to chronic interstitial inflammation of any organ. Primary biliary cirrhosis is a rare form of biliary cirrhosis of unknown etiology, occurring without obstruction or infection of the major bile ducts, sometimes occurring after the administration of certain drugs (e.g., chlorpromazine, arsenicals). The disease primarily affects middle-aged women and is characterized by chronic cholestasis with pruritus, jaundice, and hypercholesterolemia, with xanthomas and malabsorption.

Portal Cirrhosis. Also known as Laennec's cirrhosis, this is the form of liver disease that is closely associated with chronic excessive alcohol ingestion.

Autoimmune Diseases of the Muscle

Polymyositis (dermatomyositis) has been discussed with the systemic autoimmune conditions; the other muscular disorder considered to be autoimmune in nature is myasthenia gravis, which is associated with thymic abnormalities and affects the voluntary muscles, causing muscle weakness and fatigability. The disease can occur in a transitory neonatal form and has been described in infants born of myasthenic mothers. It commonly affects young females, with a peak incidence in those between 10 and 20 years; the peak incidence in males is between the ages of 60 and 70 years. Juvenile and adult cases are chronic, although signs and symptoms are variable. Thymic abnormalities consisting of hyperplasia and plasma cell infiltration occur in 80 per cent of patients. Evidence indicates that there is a thymic polypeptide factor that acts to inhibit neuromuscular transmission at the myoneural junction. Antibodies to neuromuscular receptors have also been described.

Serum antibodies directed against muscle may be detected by a variety of tests, including direct and indirect immunofluorescence, complement fixation, precipitation, and tanned-cell hemagglutination.

MS can also be classified as an autoimmune disease affecting the muscles (see earlier discussion in this chapter under autoimmune diseases of the nervous system).

Autoimmune Diseases of the Eye

Autoimmune phenomena have been implicated in three diseases of the eye: (1) phacogenic uveitis, which affects the lens; (2) sympathetic ophthalmia, which affects the uvea; and (3) autoimmune reaction involving the lacrimal gland (Sjögren's syndrome).

The eye is isolated anatomically and contains a variety of antigens that normally are not in contact with the circulation (so-called sequestered antigens). The release of lens protein into the circulation as a result of trauma or surgery may result in both inflammatory and immunologic events leading to the destruction of the lens. Inflammatory cells are found within the lesions, and anti-lens antibody is found within the circulation and aqueous humor of the affected individual.

Sympathetic ophthalmia typically follows penetrating injuries of the globe. The injured eye subsequently may develop an endophthalmitis characterized by diffuse lymphocytic infiltration of the uvea. The unaffected eye (sympathetic eye) may spontaneously develop a similar lesion several days or weeks later. Anti-uveal antibody has been demonstrated in some patients.

Autoimmune Diseases of the Skin

The typical immunologic fluorescent staining patterns seen in those diseases of the skin that have an autoimmunologic basis are shown in Table 14–7.

Pemphigus Vulgaris. In this disease, the loss of intracellular bridges in the epidermis is associated with autoantibodies directed against antigens located in the intercellular zones between adjacent epidermal cells.

Bullous Pemphigoid. This is another skin disease in which blisters arise subepidermally, but the autoantibodies react with constituents in the zona pellucida of the basement membrane in the epidermis rather than the intercellular cement.

Dermatitis Herpetiformis. This disease is characterized by grouped vesicles surmounted on an erythematous base involving predominantly the exterior surfaces of the back and arms. The HLA-B8 antigen has been found in approximately 75 to 80 per cent of patients with this disease. The examination of the perilesional skin of patients with the disease has shown a granular deposition of IgA (in 95 per cent of patients) as well as C3, C5, properdin, and properdin factor B. IgG and early components of complement are infrequently noted. These findings suggest that the major activation of complement in the disease may be via the alternative pathway.

Systemic Lupus Erythematosus. The skin manifestations of SLE are seen in both the systemic and the chronic discoid forms of the disease. In chronic discoid lupus, the skin lesions consist of a sharply circumscribed scaling erythematous dermatitis in which follicular plugging, telangiectasia, and atrophy are commonly seen. In both SLE and discoid lupus, immunoglobulins and complement are found in granular deposition at the dermal-epidermal junction. In chronic discoid lupus, this deposition is confined to the involved areas of skin,

TABLE 14–7. Immunofluorescent Staining Pattern in Autoimmune Diseases of the Skin Illustrating Demonstration of Immunoglobulins (Ig) and Complement (C)

	Direct					Indirect		
	Intercellular		Basement Membrane					Basement
Disease	IgG	C	IgG	IgA	IgM	C	Intercellular	Membrane
Dermatitis herpetiformis	−	−	+	++++	0	+	0	0
SLE (involved and uninvolved skin)	−	−	++++	+	+	+	0	0
Discoid lupus (uninvolved skin only)	−	−	++++	+	+	+	0	0
Bullous pemphigoid	−	−	++++	+	+	+	0	+
Pemphigus vulgaris	++++	+	−	−	−	−	+	0

From Bellanti, J. A.: Immunology III. Philadelphia, W. B. Saunders Company, 1985, p. 439.

whereas in SLE, the deposition is seen both in involved and uninvolved areas.

Autoimmune Diseases Affecting the Heart

Injury to the myocardium appears to result in subsequent autoimmune disease of the heart. When this follows surgery it is known as *postcardiotomy syndrome,* and when it follows coronary occlusion it is known as *postmyocardial infarction syndrome (Dressler's syndrome).* In both conditions, there is an association with autoantibodies against heart muscle.

CONCLUSION

The autoimmune diseases are in effect a collection of disorders that have in common the activation of autoimmune phenomena. The relationship of these autoimmune phenomena to the diseases is not well understood. It is possible that these diseases are under genetic control, as evidenced by the abnormal sex ratios that several of them show, and that they represent disorders of suppression or regulation of the lymphoid system.

JUST THE FACTS

Introduction

1. Normal individuals generally do not produce destructive responses to their own tissues.
2. When an immunologic reaction occurs in the host to his own tissues, the disorder is known as an *autoimmune disease.*
3. An autoantibody is directed against a "self" antigen.
4. An autoimmune response often does not result in disease and frequently occurs in otherwise healthy individuals.
5. It is thought that autoimmune diseases result from tissue injury caused by autoimmune responses.
6. It is common to see autoimmune phenomena in association with infectious diseases, yet there is no evidence that this response results in a self-perpetuating protracted autoimmune disease.

7. Some autoimmunity is necessary and beneficial to the host.
8. An MHC molecule must accompany an antigen to initiate an immune response.
9. Regulation of an immune response occurs by idiotype–anti-idiotype interaction.

Possible Mechanisms in the Initiation of Autoimmune Diseases

1. The *forbidden clone theory* postulates that a clone of changed or altered lymphocytes arises through cell mutation. These cells lack foreign surface antigen and therefore are not destroyed by normal lymphocytes.
2. The *altered antigen theory* postulates that altered surface antigen can be treated by chemical, physical, or biologic means as well as by mutation, which would result in an autoimmune response when a portion of the immune response is directed against the altered antigen.
3. The *sequestered antigen theory* postulates that certain antigens are "hidden" in the circulation. Exposure to these antigens in later life through trauma or infection results in autoimmune disease.
4. The *immunologic deficiency theory* is based on the loss or deficiency of immunoregulation. Normal individuals who develop autoimmune disease therefore have an underlying immune deficiency that renders them susceptible to autoimmune states (this can be compared with loss of "tolerance").
5. The *cross-reactive antigen theory* postulates that, because of the size of antigenic determinants, complex foreign structures could possess structural parents that are similar or identical to self structures. This cross-reactivity may be sufficient to initiate autoimmune disease.

Criteria for Autoimmune Diseases

1. Autoimmune diseases can involve more than one organ (systemic) or a single organ (organ-specific).
2. Criteria for autoimmune diseases are:
   a. The autoimmune response must be regularly associated with the disease.
   b. It must be possible to induce a replica of the disease in laboratory animals.
   c. The immunopathologic changes observed in

the natural and experimental diseases should parallel each other.

   d. It should be possible to transfer the autoimmune illness from the diseased individual to a normal recipient through the transfer of serum or lymphoid cells.

3. In some cases it is only possible to state that autoantibodies are often "associated" with the disease.

Genetic Control of Autoimmune Diseases

1. Certain immune disorders are characterized by predominance in females and in families.
2. Whether an autoimmune disease is a genetic trait can be determined by family studies and population studies.
3. A link between the disease and HLA is found when family members with a presumed autoimmune disease are found to share common HLA haplotypes.
4. The autoimmune disease with the highest relative risk (the criteria for HLA-disease relationship) is ankylosing spondylitis.

Systemic Autoimmune Diseases
Systemic Lupus Erythematosus (SLE)

1. SLE occurs primarily in women and has a strong hereditary tendency.

Characteristics of SLE

1. SLE is a generalized disorder of unknown cause that expresses itself as a vasculitis.
2. Diagnosis has been made in patients of all ages, but the disease usually affects adults between the ages of 20 and 40 and affects females four times more frequently than males.
3. There is a higher incidence of SLE in blacks than in whites.
4. SLE is an immune complex disease.
5. The immune complexes are believed to be the result of depressed suppressor T-cell function, allowing for the overproduction or inappropriate production of autoantibodies.
6. The most important immune complexes are DNA–anti-DNA.
7. The autoimmune reaction seen in SLE is believed to come under genetic influence.

8. There is no common clinical pattern for SLE.
9. Usual clinical manifestations include fever, weight loss, malaise, and weakness.
10. Arthritis is common. Joint involvement is symmetrical and rarely deforming and can involve almost any joint.
11. Skin lesions are also common, usually a red rash across the nose and upper cheeks.
12. More serious internal lesions involve the kidneys, blood vessels, blood cells, and heart.
13. Joint pain may affect several joints bilaterally.
14. At least 50 per cent of patients have central nervous system involvement.
15. Renal involvement occurs in the majority of cases. Resultant kidney disease is the primary cause of death.
16. Five classes of glomerulonephritis are associated with SLE.
17. There is no cure for SLE. Steroids and immunosuppressive drugs often help in controlling its course.

Laboratory Observations in SLE

1. The most striking laboratory observation is the presence of antinuclear antibodies (ANA).
2. ANA are usually IgG but may be IgM or IgA.
3. Because of ANA, patients may have a false-positive serologic test for syphilis, hemolytic anemia with a positive antiglobulin test, leukopenia, and thrombocytopenia.
4. The most relevant laboratory observation is the LE cell phenomenon.
5. LE cells are polymorphonuclear leukocytes found in the bone marrow and peripheral blood.
6. The LE factor is a 7S IgG antibody, which reacts with anti-DNA and complement.
7. The LE factor is found in more than 95 per cent of SLE patients.
8. The LE factor is not specific as an indicator of SLE. It is also present in the serum of patients suffering from certain other autoimmune diseases.
9. Several different specificities of ANA have been found in SLE patients: antibodies to DNA, DNA-histone, RNA, and ENA.
10. Certain ENAs have a high degree of specificity for SLE (notably Sm and MA antigens)
11. 25 per cent of patients with SLE have Sm antibodies.

12. Many other antibodies are found in SLE patients (e.g., antibodies reacting with nPNP, PCNS, Sjögren's syndrome antigens, histone antigens, and others).

Etiology of SLE

1. SLE arises spontaneously. It may be genetic or induced by certain drugs.
2. It is believed that estrogens may play a potentially harmful role in disease development and progression.
3. Environmental factors, bacterial infections, and viral infections are capable of inducing or exacerbating the signs and symptoms of SLE.
4. An association with HLA-B8, HLA-DRw2, and HLA-DRw3 has been reported.
5. In individuals who are genetically predisposed to the disease, viral infections are thought to be an important etiologic factor.
6. SLE occurs primarily in women and has a strong hereditary tendency.

Serologic Tests for SLE

1. In the laboratory, the tests for SLE involve the demonstration of the LE cell (no longer widely used) and the detection of ANA.
2. The detection of ANA is not diagnostic of SLE, but ANA absence may be used as a means of ruling out the disease.
3. The methods applied to the diagnosis of SLE include methods of detecting antibodies to DNA and nucleoprotein (radioimmunoassay and hemagglutination assays).

Rheumatoid Arthritis (RA)

Characteristics of RA

1. RA is a chronic inflammatory disease primarily affecting the joints and periarticular tissues.
2. Certain body areas show particular susceptibility to inflammation, but it appears that no body system or tissue is entirely exempt.
3. Besides the joints, the most commonly affected areas are other synovium-lined spaces.
4. The highest incidence of the disease is in women between the ages of 30 and 50.
5. Clinical manifestations include the formation of a vascular "pannus."
6. Other clinical manifestations include hypochromic anemia, characteristic changes in the serum protein pattern, toxemia (increased sedimentation rate), and generalized lymphadenopathy.
7. General clinical manifestations include fatigue, weight loss, weakness, mild fever, and anorexia.
8. Joints may lose function or be permanently deformed.
9. In patients with high titers of RF, vasculitis, rheumatoid nodules, and Sjögren's syndrome may be manifest.
10. The cause of RA is unknown, as are the involved antigens.

Characteristics of Rheumatoid Factors

1. Several proteins circulate in the blood of patients with RA, known collectively as rheumatoid factor (RF).
2. RA interact specifically with the Fc portion of IgG molecules.
3. Immune complexes are formed (IgG aggregates or IgM-IgG complexes) and the classical pathway of complement is activated and amplified by the alternative pathway of complement.
4. The inflammatory response proceeds via the bioactive complement fragments (with the aid of T cells), and inflammatory cells enter the synovial space and release intracellular products that damage the synovium.
5. Rheumatoid factors can occur in nonrheumatoid individuals with chronic infective conditions.
6. The correlation between RF and the disease RA remains unsolved.

Serologic Tests for RA

1. Rheumatoid arthritis test, based on the reaction between patient antibodies (rheumatoid factor) and an antigen derived from gamma globulin.
2. Quantitative determination of IgM rheumatoid factor in human serum.
3. The latex-fixation test for rheumatoid factors.
4. The sheep cell agglutination test for rheumatoid factors.
5. The 1-minute latex agglutination test for the qualitative and quantitative determination of rheumatoid factor in serum (Rheumatex).
6. The 2-minute hemagglutination slide test for the qualitative and quantitative determination of

rheumatoid factor in serum or synovial fluid (Rheumaton).

Ankylosing Spondylitis (AS)

1. This is a systemic rheumatic disorder characterized by inflammation of the synovial and spinal apophyseal joints, causing back pain.
2. AS affects 10 times more men than women and begins most often between the ages of 20 and 40 years.
3. There is evidence of a genetic linkage between AS and HLA-B27.
4. Diagnosis of AS is based on the presence of the clinical and radiologic signs of the disease.

Necrotizing Angiitis (Vasculitis)

1. Necrotizing angiitis encompasses a group of disorders characterized by segmental inflammation of arteries, namely polyarteritis nodosa (PN), hypersensitivity angiitis, Henoch-Schönlein purpura, Wegener's granulomatosis, Takayasu's disease, and giant cell arteritis.
2. PN and hypersensitivity angiitis are difficult to distinguish.
3. PN is seen more often in males and involves both medium and small arteries. Hypersensitivity angiitis involves small arteries only.
4. Hypersensitivity angiitis is often caused by drugs (penicillin and sulfonamides). From 30 to 40 per cent of patients reveal the presence of immune complexes of HBsAg in affected tissues.
5. Henoch-Schönlein purpura affects the small arteries of the skin, joints, and gastrointestinal tract.
6. Wegener's granulomatosis is characterized by vasculitis in the upper respiratory tract, lung, and kidney.
7. Takayasu's disease involves vasculitis in the aorta and its major branches.
8. Giant cell arteritis involves vasculitis in the temporal and other cranial arteries.
9. Elevated sedimentation rates are an aid to diagnosis.

Polymyositis and Dermatomyositis

1. Polymyositis is a condition characterized by degeneration and inflammation of skeletal muscle.
2. It is commonly associated with dysphagia, Raynaud's phenomenon, and arthritis.
3. Its peak incidence occurs in the young and in those of late middle age.
4. Laboratory findings include elevated serum muscle enzymes, abnormal electromyographic tracings, polyclonal hypergammaglobulinemia, rheumatoid factor, antinuclear antibody, myoglobulinemia, increased erythrocyte sedimentation rate, and increased urine creatine.
5. Specific ANA include PM-1, associated with polymyositis-progressive systemic sclerosis overlap syndrome.
6. Jo-1 is the serum antibody most often detected.
7. Dermatomyositis involves the skin.
8. Symmetric weakening and atrophy of the muscles of the shoulders, hips, neck, and trunk are accompanied by maculopapular or eczema-like skin rash. The etiology is unknown.

Progressive Systemic Sclerosis (Scleroderma)

1. PSS is a chronic disease of the connective tissue, characterized by diffuse fibrosis involving the skin and several internal organs, inflammatory and degenerative changes of the skin and viscera, and vascular abnormalities.
2. The disease usually occurs in adults between the ages of 20 and 60 years.
3. Females are affected two to three times more frequently than males.
4. Raynaud's phenomenon is the most common symptom.
5. CREST syndrome is a milder form of scleroderma.
6. Laboratory findings include polyclonal hypergammaglobulinemia and ANA with speckled or nucleolar pattern.
7. Sc1-70 antibody is a marker ANA detected in 15 to 20 per cent of patients.
8. Centromere antibody is a marker for the CREST variety in 70 to 90 per cent of patients.
9. An antigen-mediated pathogenesis is suggested by increased levels of IgG and ANA.
10. From 25 to 30 per cent of affected individuals have a positive test for syphilis.
11. Positive LE cell reactions also occur.

Mixed Connective Tissue Disease

1. MCTD is a syndrome that has the combined clinical features of RA, SLE, PSS, and polymyositis.
2. Patients have positive ANA and high titers of anti-RNP antibodies.
3. RF, elevated ESR, and hypergammaglobulinemia are usually present.
4. Anti-DNA and anti-Sm are usually absent.

Sjögren's Syndrome

1. SS often occurs secondary to RA, scleroderma, polymyositis, or SLE.
2. In its primary form, it manifests itself in the form of dry eyes and dry mouth.
3. There is remarkable immunologic reactivity in the serum.
4. An association between HLA-Dw3 and primary SS has been found.
5. Specific ANA include SS-B in primary disease, SS-A associated with SLE, and rheumatoid nuclear antigen associated with rheumatoid arthritis.

Organ-Specific Autoimmune Diseases
Autoimmune Diseases of the Blood

Autoimmune Hemolytic Anemias

1. The autoimmune hemolytic anemias are a group of anemias characterized by a hemolytic process involving red-cell specific antibodies in the serum.
2. AHA may occur as "warm" type (the most common) where antibodies (IgG [40 per cent of cases], IgG and complement [50 per cent of cases], or complement only [10 per cent of cases]) react best at warm temperatures, and the "cold" type, where antibodies (primarily IgM) react best at 0° to 4°C.
3. Paroxysmal cold hemoglobinuria involves cold IgG antibodies that fix complement and lyse cells before they reach phagocytic cells, resulting in rapid intravascular hemolysis when the body or part of the body is cooled below the critical temperature (15° to 20°C).
4. Drug-induced hemolysis may occur as a result of:
   a. Drug absorption (drug binds strongly to any protein producing a drug–red cell–hapten complex that can stimulate antibody production).
   b. Immune complex (drug and antibody form a complex, which then attaches nonspecifically to red cells and activates complement, resulting in intravascular hemolysis).
   c. Membrane modification (drug alters the membrane so that there is nonspecific absorption of globulins).
   d. Autoantibody formation (formed autoantibody recognizes a part of the red cell and reacts with most normal red cells).

Autoimmune Thrombocytopenic Purpura (AITP)

1. AITP is manifest through the presence of anti-platelet factor that results in a fall of the patient's platelet count.
2. Serologic tests include the antibody consumption test, the platelet immunofluorescence test, and the radioactive antiglobulin test.

Neutropenia

1. This disease is characterized by a decrease in the number of neutrophilic leukocytes in the blood, resulting in susceptibility to infection.
2. The surface antigens of the neutrophil are probably causative, although it is possible that the disease is produced by several mechanisms.
3. Drugs can cause neutropenia.
4. The disease can also be caused by exposure to radiation.
5. Immunologically mediated neutropenia is established by determining the presence of serum leukoagglutinins or specific antineutrophil antibody.

Lymphocytopenia

1. This disease is characterized by a decrease in the proportion of lymphocytes in the blood, characterized by secondary immunodeficiency.
2. T lymphocytes are preferentially depleted.
3. The probable antigens are lymphocyte-specific surface antigens; the antibody is much like heterologous anti-lymphocyte globulin.

Autoimmune Aplastic Anemia

1. This occurs in about one third of all patients with aplastic anemia, characterized by complete absence of reticulocytes and of all types of erythroblasts in the bone marrow.
2. Stem cell–specific antigens are probably involved. The immunity seems to be T-cell mediated.

Autoimmune Diseases of the Kidney

1. The four types of immunologically mediated renal disease are anaphylactic (type 1), cytotoxic (type II), immune complex (type III), and cell mediated (type IV).

Other Forms of Immune Renal Disease

1. Two diseases that have apparent immunologic bases yet do not fit into the above categories are Berger's disease (IgG-IgA nephropathy) and membranoproliferative or mesangiocapillary glomerulonephritis.

Autoimmune Diseases of the Endocrine Organs

1. The most frequently occurring of these are diseases involving the thyroid gland.

Autoimmune Diseases of the Thyroid

1. These include lymphocytic thyroiditis (Hashimoto's thyroiditis) and thyrotoxicosis (Graves' disease).
2. Hashimoto's thyroiditis is the most common form, involving enlargement of the thyroid gland.
3. It usually occurs in patients 35 to 55 years of age.
4. It is 5 to 10 times more frequent in females than in males.
5. Circulating antibodies as well as lymphoproliferative responses to various constituents of thyroid are commonly seen.
6. In addition, anti-thyroid antibodies (ATA) have been described that appear to regulate cellular activity and may contribute to hyperthyroidism, including:
   a. Long-acting thyroid stimulator (LATS) (IgG).
   b. LATS protector activity.
   c. Thyroid-stimulating immunoglobulins (autoantibodies).
7. Anti-thyroglobulin antibodies can be detected by precipitation, latex agglutination, the tanned red cell test, and radioimmunoassay.
8. Microsomal antibodies can be detected using complement fixation, cytotoxicity tests, immunofluorescence of unfixed thyroid epithelial cells, radioimmunoassay, and hemagglutination.
9. Tests of thyroid function are usually in the range of low to normal in this disorder.
10. Myxedema is associated with hypothyroidism and characterized by a collection of hydrated mucopolysaccharides in the dermis and other tissues of the body.
11. Graves' disease frequently exists with Hashimoto's thyroiditis in the same patient.
12. Graves' disease is now considered to be a multisystem disorder consisting of hyperthyroidism due to diffuse goiter, infiltrative ophthalmopathy, and infiltrative dermopathy.
13. The three ATA previously described (point 6) are also present in Graves' disease.

Autoimmune Diseases of the Pancreas

Diabetes Mellitus

1. Antibodies to insulin have been found in the sera of diabetic patients, which may contribute to insulin allergy (if IgE) or insulin resistance (if IgG, IgA, or IgM).
2. Thyroid and gastric autoantibodies have also been found in the sera of diabetic patients without clinical thyroid disease or pernicious anemia.

Autoimmune Disease of the Adrenals

1. Autoantibodies to adrenal tissues, detectable by immunofluorescence or complement fixation, have been reported in patients with Addison's disease.

Autoimmune Disease of the Parathyroids

1. Antibodies to thyroid, adrenal, and gastric tissues have been detected in idiopathic hypoparathyroidism.

2. This disorder occurs more frequently in children than in adults and is more common in females than in males.
3. The disorder may be accompanied by certain associated disorders (idiopathic Addison's disease, pernicious anemia, alopecia totalis, and moniliasis).

Autoimmune Disease of the Ovary and Testis

1. Autoimmunity has been found in 30 to 50 per cent of patients with premature ovarian failure.
2. Anti-sperm antibodies have been found in the sera of some infertile couples and in the serum and semen of individuals after vasectomy.

Autoimmune Diseases of the Nervous System

1. Disseminated encephalomyelitis
   a. Characterized by fever, photophobia, blindness, muscle weakness, decreased consciousness, seizures, paresis, loss of appetite, and sphincter disturbance.
   b. May develop subsequent to infection by either bacterial or viral agents.
   c. Viral infections (measles, mumps, and rubella) are more common predisposing causes.
   d. The incubation period is 5 to 30 days.
   e. Immunizations (notably smallpox or rabies) may precipitate the disease.
   f. Circulating antibody to encephalitogenic factors has been demonstrated.
   g. The major pathologic change in experimental allergic encephalomyelitis is mediated by sensitized lymphocytes.
2. Idiopathic Polyneuritis
   a. Also known as Guillain-Barré syndrome.
   b. Of unknown etiology, characterized by peripheral nerve involvement.
   c. May follow a variety of infectious diseases, or may occur subsequent to immunization (e.g., swine influenza immunization).
3. Landry's Paralysis
   a. Another form of polyneuritis.
   b. Produces weakness and sensory loss in the limbs as a result of inflammation in the peripheral nerves.
4. Multiple Sclerosis

   a. Slowly progressive disease of the central nervous system and muscles.
   b. Cause unknown, usually begins in early adult life.
   c. Characterized by disseminated, patchy demyelination of the brain and spinal cord.
   d. The precise cause remains unclear.
   e. Elevated spinal fluid gamma globulin is found in 80 per cent of patients.
   f. 90 per cent of patients have oligoclonal banding, but this is not specific for MS.
   g. No specific treatment is available. Death usually results from some intercurrent disease.

Autoimmune Diseases of the Stomach and Intestines

1. Pernicious Anemia
   a. Characterized by inflammation of the gastric mucosa with inability to secrete hydrochloric acid, intrinsic factor, and pepsin, followed by the development of macrocytic anemia
   b. Antibody in gastric juice and lymphoid cells, when mixed with intrinsic factor, interferes with the absorption of vitamin B_{12}.
   c. It is not known if this antibody is the cause or the result of the disease.
   d. Pernicious anemia will respond to steroid therapy.
   e. Serologic tests include complement fixation or immunofluorescence and blocking and binding antibody tests.
2. Gastric atrophy.
3. Regional ileitis (Crohn's disease).
4. Ulcerative colitis.
5. Gluten-sensitive enteropathy (celiac disease).

Autoimmune Diseases of the Liver

1. Liver diseases with immunologic features include viral hepatitis (acute and chronic), drug-induced liver disease, biliary cirrhosis, and portal cirrhosis.
2. Portal cirrhosis is closely associated with chronic excessive alcohol intake.

Autoimmune Diseases of the Muscle

1. These include polymyositis (dermatomyositis) (discussed above), myasthenia gravis (which is

associated with thymic abnormalities and affects the voluntary muscles, causing weakness and fatigability), and multiple sclerosis (discussed above).
2. Myasthenia gravis commonly affects young females, with a peak incidence in those between 10 and 20 years; the peak incidence in males is between the ages of 60 and 70 years. Serum antibodies against muscle may be detected by direct and indirect immunofluorescence, complement fixation, precipitation, and tanned-cell hemagglutination.

Autoimmune Diseases of the Eye

1. Phacogenic uveitis (which affects the lens).
2. Sympathetic ophthalmia (which affects the uvea).
3. Autoimmune reaction involving the lacrimal gland (Sjögren's syndrome).

Autoimmune Diseases of the Skin

1. Pemphigus vulgaris (loss of intracellular bridges).
2. Bullous pemphigoid (subepidermal blisters).
3. Cicatrical pemphigoid (variant of bullous pemphigoid).
4. Dermatitis herpetiformis (grouped vesicles surmounted on an erythematous base involving predominantly the exterior surfaces of the back and arms).
5. Systemic lupus erythematosus (skin manifestations are seen in both the systemic and the chronic discoid forms of the disease).

Autoimmune Diseases Affecting the Heart

1. Injury to the myocardium appears to result in subsequent autoimmune disease.
2. When this follows surgery, it is known as postcardiotomy syndrome.
3. When it follows coronary occlusion, it is known as postmyocardial infarction syndrome (Dressler's syndrome).
4. In both conditions, there is an association with autoantibodies against heart muscle.

Conclusion

1. Autoimmune diseases have in common the activation of autoimmune phenomena.
2. The relationship of these autoimmune phenomena to the diseases is not well understood.
3. It is possible that these diseases are under genetic control, evidenced by the abnormal sex ratios that several of them show, and that they represent disorders of suppression or regulation of the lymphoid system.

Review Questions

Multiple Choice

Choose the phrase, sentence, or symbol that completes the statement or answers the question. More than one answer may be correct in each case. Answers are given at the end of this book.

1. The theories that have been proposed to explain the mechanisms that initiate autoimmune diseases include:
   (a) the forbidden clone theory
   (b) the altered antigen theory
   (c) the altered antibody theory
   (d) the immunologic deficiency theory
   (Possible Mechanisms in the Initiation of Autoimmune Diseases)

2. Which of the following represent Koch's postulates:
   (a) All autoimmune diseases are either systemic or organ specific
   (b) The autoimmune response must be regularly associated with the disease
   (c) It must be possible to induce a replica of the disease in laboratory animals
   (d) The autoantibodies in autoimmune disease must play a central role in the cause
   (Criteria for Autoimmune Diseases)

3. The immune response gene is closely linked to the:
   (a) Rh locus on chromosome 1

(b) MHC locus on chromosome 4
(c) MHC locus on chromosome 6
(d) ABO locus on chromosome 9
(Genetic Control of Autoimmune Diseases)

4. Systemic lupus erythematosus:
   (a) is a disease of the connective tissue
   (b) occurs primarily in women
   (c) has a strong hereditary tendency
   (d) occurs primarily in adults between the ages of 20 and 40
   (Systemic Lupus Erythematosus)

5. The LE cell:
   (a) is a polymorphonuclear leukocyte
   (b) is found in the bone marrow and peripheral blood of patients with systemic lupus erythematosus
   (c) is always engulfed by the phagocyte and fills its cytoplasm
   (d) when free in stained blood, is often surrounded by viable neutrophils, producing a rosette formation
   (Systemic Lupus Erythematosus: Laboratory Observations)

6. The LE factor:
   (a) is a 7S IgG antibody
   (b) reacts with DNA
   (c) is found in 4 per cent of SLE patients
   (d) is found in 60 per cent of normal individuals
   (Systemic Lupus Erythematosus: Laboratory Observations)

7. Rheumatoid factor:
   (a) represents proteins found in the blood of patients with rheumatoid arthritis
   (b) shows no particular correlation with rheumatoid arthritis
   (c) is generally accepted to be a group of immunoglobulins that react with the Fc portion of IgG molecules
   (d) can occur in non-rheumatoid individuals
   (Characteristics of Rheumatoid Factors)

8. The tests for rheumatoid arthritis:
   (a) are designed to detect rheumatoid factor
   (b) usually use particulate carriers that transform the reaction between RF and IgG into visible aggregation
   (c) are designed to detect antibody to immunoglobulin
   (d) always give identical results
   (Rheumatoid Arthritis: Serologic Tests)

9. Which of the following would be classified as a systemic autoimmune disease?
   (a) autoimmune aplastic anemia
   (b) ankylosing spondylitis
   (c) vasculitis
   (d) mixed connective tissue disease
   (Other Systemic Autoimmune Diseases)

10. Autoimmune hemolytic anemia of the warm type:
    (a) is the most common form of AHA
    (b) affects both sexes and all ages
    (c) is more prevalent in males than in females
    (d) is caused by antibodies primarily of the IgM class
    (Autoimmune Diseases of the Blood)

11. The serologic tests for autoimmune thrombocytopenic purpura include:
    (a) the antiglobulin (Coombs') test
    (b) the antiglobulin consumption test
    (c) the platelet immunofluorescence test
    (d) the radioactive antiglobulin test
    (Autoimmune Thrombocytopenic Purpura)

12. Neutropenia:
    (a) is an autoimmune disease of the blood
    (b) is characterized by susceptibility to infection
    (c) is probably caused by surface antigens on the neutrophil
    (d) may be caused by decreased neutrophil production in the bone marrow
    (Neutropenia)

13. The four types of immunologically mediated renal diseases are:
    (a) anaphylactic
    (b) cytotoxic
    (c) genetic
    (d) systemic
    (Autoimmune Diseases of the Kidney)

14. Long-acting thyroid stimulator (LATS):
    (a) is an IgG immunoglobulin
    (b) can be detected by means of bioassay
    (c) is found in 30 per cent of normal individuals
    (d) is found in detectable levels in all patients with Hashimoto's thyroiditis
    (Autoimmune Diseases of the Thyroid)

15. LATS is detected in:
    (a) about 50 per cent of patients with Graves' disease
    (b) all patients with Hashimoto's thyroiditis
    (c) about 20 per cent of patients with Graves' disease
    (d) all patients with Graves' disease
    (Thyrotoxicosis [Graves' Disease])

16. Which of the following diseases affects the nervous system?
    (a) pernicious anemia
    (b) Landry's paralysis
    (c) multiple sclerosis
    (d) gastric atrophy
    (Autoimmune Diseases of the Nervous System)

17. Autoimmune diseases of the skin include:
    (a) pemphigus vulgaris
    (b) bullous pemphigoid
    (c) dermatitis herpetiformis
    (d) systemic lupus erythematosus
    (Autoimmune Diseases of the Skin)

Answer "True" or "False"

1. In systemic autoimmune diseases, the major effect involves a single organ.
   (Criteria for Autoimmune Diseases)

2. There is a relationship between the presence of the HLA-B27 antigen in an individual and the occurrence of the disease ankylosing spondylitis.
   (Genetic Control of Autoimmune Diseases)

3. Systemic lupus erythematosus and rheumatoid arthritis are two distinct diseases showing completely different clinical signs and symptoms.
   (Systemic Lupus Erythematosus)

4. About 75 per cent of patients with systemic lupus erythematosus develop hypocomplementemia.
   (Systemic Lupus Erythematosus: Laboratory Observations)

5. Rheumatoid factors can occur in non-rheumatoid individuals with chronic infective conditions.
   (Rheumatoid Arthritis: Characteristics of Rheumatoid Factors)

6. Necrotizing angiitis is a systemic autoimmune disease that affects the arteries.
   (Necrotizing Angiitis [Vasculitis])

7. Portal cirrhosis is closely associated with chronic excessive alcohol ingestion.
   (Autoimmune Diseases of the Liver)

8. Autoimmune diseases affecting the heart are not associated with autoantibodies against heart muscle.
   (Autoimmune Diseases Affecting the Heart)

GENERAL REFERENCES

Abbas, A.K., Lichtman, A.H., and Prober, J.S.: Cellular and Molecular Immunology. Philadelphia, W. B. Saunders Company, 1991.

Baron, E.J., and Finegold, S.M.: Bailey and Scott's Diagnostic Microbiology, 8th ed. St. Louis, C. V. Mosby Company, 1990.

Bennington, J.L.: Saunders Dictionary and Encyclopedia of Laboratory Medicine and Technology. Philadelphia, W. B. Saunders Company, 1984.

Dorland's Illustrated Medical Dictionary, 27th ed. Philadelphia, W. B. Saunders Company, 1988.

Henry, J.B.: Clinical Diagnosis and Management by Laboratory Methods. Philadelphia, W. B. Saunders Company, 1991.

Sheehan, C.: Clinical Immunology: Principles and Laboratory Diagnosis. Philadelphia, J. B. Lippincott Company, 1990.

Turgeon, M.L.: Immunology and Serology in Laboratory Medicine. St. Louis, C. V. Mosby Company, 1990.

15

Fungal Antibody Tests, Febrile Antibody Tests, and Viral Antibody Tests

OBJECTIVES

The student shall know, understand, and be prepared to explain:
1. The fungal antibody tests for:
    a. Histoplasmosis
    b. Aspergillosis
    c. Coccidioidomycosis
    d. North American blastomycosis
    e. Candidiasis
    f. Sporotrichosis
2. The febrile antibody tests
3. The viral antibody tests, specifically
    a. Complement fixation
    b. Latex fixation
    c. Precipitation
    d. Neutralization
    e. Immunofluorescence
    f. Hemagglutination
    g. A brief description of the virus antigens and antibodies detected with other tests, to include direct and immune electron microscopy, enzyme immunoassay, inhibition, radioimmunoassay, hemadsorption immunosorbent technique, and cDNA probes.

FUNGAL ANTIBODY TESTS

Fungal serologic tests often play an important role in the diagnosis of mycotic infections, in spite of the fact that the evidence of infection they provide is often only tentative.

In performing such tests, the issue of false-negative results and false-positive results must be kept in mind. False-negative results can occur when blood is drawn at an inappropriate time or if blood is obtained from a patient who is immunosuppressed by chemotherapy or underlying diseases and whose antibody production is therefore diminished. False-positive results may occur because many of the antigens used for testing are crude extracts of the fungi that contain many common components that cross-react with other fungi (e.g., the antigens for *Histoplasma capsulatum* are similar to those of *Blastomyces dermatitidis* and *Coccidioides immitis*). A patient with histoplasmosis will sometimes present positive results with *all* antigens. As a safeguard against these false reactions, it is advisable to repeat serologic testing at 2 to 3 week intervals. This way, a rise in antibody titer to the antigen of the fungal agent under suspicion can be confirmed. (Note: Generally the antibody titer is greater to the antigen from the organism that is the actual cause of infection, even in cases where all antigens give positive results.)

The proper collection and transportation of specimens (if these are being referred to reference laboratories) is important. Serum that is aseptically collected from at least 10 ml of blood is adequate for most serologic testing. The sample should be as fresh as possible: if storage is required, the sample can be satisfactorily stored at 4°C for short periods of time or at −20°C or colder when longer storage is necessary. When transported, serum and cerebrospinal fluid samples should be packed in dry or wet ice to prevent bacterial contamination (alternatively, a preservative [e.g., thimerosal] should be added).

Several species of fungi are associated with respiratory diseases in humans that are acquired by inhaling spores from exogenous reservoirs, including dust, bird droppings, and soil. A selected number are briefly described here, focusing on those for which serologic tests can be performed.

Histoplasmosis

This disease is a granulomatous infection caused by *Histoplasma capsulatum*. The species name is a misnomer, because the organism does not possess true capsule.

The source of human infection is believed to be from the soil, especially when it is laden with excreta from chickens, birds, or bats ("cave fever"). Most commonly, human infection results from inhalation of spore-laden dust.

The disease is often difficult to diagnose, because it presents as a broad spectrum, ranging from asymptomatic (the acute phase characterized by nonproductive cough and shortness of breath), to a chronic pulmonary disease of long duration (characterized by chronic cavitary lesions in some adults, chronic cough, low-grade fever, and occasionally hemoptysis), to a disseminated form in which pulmonary symptoms may be minimal, but hepatosplenomegaly and diffuse lymphadenopathy are usually present in varying degrees of severity, due to propensity of fungus to invade the cells of the mononuclear phagocyte system. The disseminated disease is also characterized by fever, anemia, leukopenia, weight loss, and lassitude (Paya, 1987). The initial indication of the disease may be solitary or multiple ulcerations of the mucous membranes. Any of the viscera may be involved. If the disease affects the adrenal glands, this can lead to Addison's disease and, if undiagnosed, may have a fatal outcome. Patients with AIDS may experience rapid and fatal dissemination. Fulminant pulmonary disease can mimic *Pneumocystis carinii* infections. Atypical cutaneous lesions such as papules, pustules, folliculitis, and perirectal ulcers may herald the disease. Fungemia is common, and in some patients intracellular organisms may be seen within circulating monocytes when examining peripheral blood smears.

A definite diagnosis requires the isolation in culture and microscopic identification of the fungus, as well as serologic evidence.

Kauffmann (1966) described the use of immunodiffusion for the detection of histoplasmin. In this test, H and M bands appearing together are indicative of active infection, with the M band on its own indicating early infection or chronic infection (the M band may also appear after a recent skin test). The H band appears later than the M band and disappears earlier, and its disappearance may indicate regression of the infection. This test is useful for screening purposes.

Carlisle and Saslaw (1958) described a latex agglutination test for histoplasmosis that also detects histoplasmin, but the test is unreliable due to a high number of false-positive and false-negative reactions.

A complement fixation test for histoplasmosis was described by Hazen *et al.* (1970). It is generally considered that a diagnosis made with a combination of history, physical examination, and delayed hypersensitivity skin testing is confirmed by a rise in complement-fixing antibodies to *Histoplasma* antigens. Titers of 8 and 16 (dilution 1:8, 1:16) are highly suspicious of infection, but a titer of 32 or greater is usually indicative of active infection. Rising titers indicate progressive infection, and decreasing titers indicate regression. Some disseminated infections are nonreactive in the complement-fixation test. Recent skin tests in individuals who have had prior exposure to *H. capsulatum* will cause a rise in the complement-fixation titer in 17 to 20 per cent of persons. Cross-reactions in the complement fixation test occur in patients having aspergillosis, blastomycosis, and coccidioidomycosis, but titers are usually lower. For this reason, several follow-up serum samples should be tested at 2 to 3 week intervals.

For a review of histoplasmosis, see Wheat (1988).

Aspergillosis

This refers to any disease of humans and animals that is caused by a species of the genus *Aspergillus*, the etiologic agents being *Aspergillus fumigatus*, *Aspergillus niger*, *Aspergillus flavus*, *Aspergillus terreus*, and other species. Of these many species, only seven or eight are pathogenic for humans and, of these, *Aspergillus fumigatus* is the most important (Fig. 15–1), being responsible for about 90 per cent of infections.

The clinical disease manifestations include pulmonary aspergillosis (the major symptom being hemoptysis), allergic bronchopulmonary aspergillosis (which most commonly develops in persons who develop hypersensitivity to aspergilli antigens after repeated exposures), fungus ball (in which congenital bronchial cysts or cavitary lesions caused by tuberculosis, bronchiectasis, or carcinoma may become colonized with one of the aspergilli, notably *A. fumigatus*), and external otomycosis (in which an aspergillus, notably *A. niger,* may become colonized within a cerumen plug in the external auditory canal).

The disease caused by *Aspergillus fumigatus* is an acute or chronic inflammatory granulomatous infection of the sinuses, bronchi, lungs, and occasionally other parts of the body. It has been recognized as an occupational disease among those who handle and feed squabs and among those who handle furs and hair.

In culture, *Aspergillus* grows rapidly at 37°C on common mycologic laboratory media; however, it is sensitive to cyclohexamine. Species identification of *Aspergillus* is made microscopically. In the presence of suspicious symptoms, the same species of *Aspergillus* must be recovered from multiple samples of respiratory secretions before the diagnosis can be established.

Serologically, skin reactions and immunodiffusion are useful tools for identification, especially if the culture is negative. Precipitin formation by immunodiffusion is useful in patients with pulmonary eosinophilia, severe allergic aspergillosis, and aspergillomas. One or more precipitin bands are suggestive of active infection. The precipitin bands have been shown to correlate with complement-fixation titers—the greater the number of bands, the higher the titer. Precipitins can be found in 95 per cent of fungus ball cases and 50 per cent of the allergic bronchopulmonary cases. When aspergillomas are surgically removed, the precipitin bands disappear. In invasive aspergillosis, the patient is usually immune-deficient; therefore, antibody detection is complicated. The sensitivity of immunodiffusion can be increased by using a battery of antigens from several species of *Aspergillus*, as well as serum concentration. The ELISA procedure is currently being used to detect IgE and IgG anti-

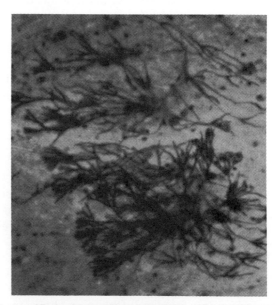

Figure 15–1. *Aspergillus fumigatus.* (From Freeman, B.: Burrows Textbook of Microbiology. Philadelphia, W. B. Saunders Company, 1985.)

bodies in patients' sera (see further discussion in Chapter 5).

Coccidioidomycosis

This disease is also known as desert fever, San Joaquin fever, and valley fever. It occurs in primary pulmonary, primary cutaneous, and disseminated forms. It is generally contracted from the inhalation of soil or dust containing the arthrospores of the causative agent, *Coccidioides immitis.*

In culture, *C. immitis* grows on Sabouraud's glucose agar from arthrospores or spherules. After 2 or 4 days of incubation, a cottony white, moist colony with aerial mycelia develops and gradually turns brown with age.

Several serologic tests are available: the tube precipitin test, complement fixation test, latex agglutination test, and immunodiffusion. Of these, the tube precipitin test is positive in more than 90 per cent of the primary symptomatic cases.

The complement fixation test becomes positive later than the tube precipitin test and is more effective in determining disseminated disease. Titers as low as 2 and 4 (dilutions 1:2 and 1:4) have been seen in active infection—titers of 16 or greater are indicative of active infection. When low titers are encountered, the tests should be repeated at 2 to 3 week intervals. Cross-reactions occur in patients having histoplasmosis, and false-negative results occur in patients with solitary pulmonary lesions. The titer parallels the severity of infection.

Immunodiffusion tests give results that usually correlate with those observed with the complement fixation test. They can be used as screening tests and should be confirmed by performing complement fixation.

The latex agglutination test is highly sensitive and rapid but is not as specific as the tube precipitin test. The precipitins, which occur during the first 3 weeks of infection, are diagnostic but not prognostic. This is a useful screening test for precipitins in early infection. False-positive results are frequently seen when diluted serum or cerebrospinal fluid specimens are used.

North American Blastomycosis

This chronic fungal disease is usually secondary to pulmonary involvement. The causative agent is *Blastomyces dermatitidis.* It is marked by suppurating tumors in the skin or by lesions in the lungs, bones, subcutaneous tissues, liver, spleen, and kidneys.

On incubation at room temperature in Sabouraud's glucose medium or in blood agar without cyclohexamine at 37°C, a white, filamentous colony forms, with white mycelia. Growth of *B. dermatitidis* is slow and may range from a few days to 1 month. Serologic diagnosis is problematic due to high cross-reactivity, with antigenic components of the organisms causing histoplasmosis and coccidioidomycosis. Two tests, immunodiffusion and complement fixation, have been used in serodiagnosis. Immunodiffusion, in this regard, is claimed to yield better results than complement fixation (Busey and Hinton, 1967); however, the complement fixation test may provide prognostic value. Titers of 8 and 16 are highly suggestive of active infection; titers of 32 and greater are indicative. Cross-reactions occur in patients having coccidioidomycosis or histoplasmosis, although titers are usually lower. A decreasing titer is indicative of regression. Most patients (75 per cent) having blastomycosis have negative tests. There is a good fluorescent antibody test specific for the yeast phase of *B. dermatitidis.*

Candidiasis

The genus *Candida* contains many species, including *C. albicans, C. tropicalis, C. krusei, C. parakrusei, C. stellatoidea,* and *C. guilliermondi.* It is a genus of yeastlike fungi characterized by production of mycelia but not ascospores. The term *candidiasis* refers to any fungal infection involving the genus *Candida.* Of the many species, only *C. albicans* is considered to be pathogenic for humans, but other species are encountered in pathologic conditions. The fungus is found in the lesions of thrush.

Infections with *Candida* species are endogenous. Various species of *Candida* colonize the skin, gastrointestinal tract, and mucous membranes. Clinical disease may arise in conditions in which there is a modification of host defenses or suppression of the normal bacterial flora. Some of the conditions predisposing to candidiasis are pregnancy, diabetes mellitus, indwelling venous catheters, chronic debilitating diseases, and prolonged therapy with broad-spectrum antibiotics. In addition, virtually 100 per cent of AIDS patients have oral candidiasis.

The clinical disease manifestations are cutaneous candidiasis (involving the skin), mucous membrane candidiasis (involving the vaginal and oral mucous membranes), pulmonary candidiasis (involving the bronchial mucosa), endocarditis, and fungemia.

Candida grows on most laboratory media at room temperature. *C. albicans* produces a germ tube after incubation in serum at 37°C for 2 hours. On cornmeal agar, *C. albicans* produces chlamydospores.

Chew and Theus (1967) described a precipitation test for the detection of antibodies to *Candida*, but the test appears to be of little practical value because of the high incidence of *Candida* antibodies in apparently healthy individuals.

Precipitating antibodies prepared from protoplasts are more specific as indicators of *Candida* antibody than are antigens prepared from whole cells (Venezia and Robertson, 1974). Agglutination tests using suspensions of *C. albicans* are of little value because of the incidence of antibodies in normal individuals. Moreover, an inhibitor of agglutination has been found in some individuals with candidiasis (Louria *et al.*, 1972); therefore, even negative agglutination tests are of dubious value. Immunodiffusion and counterimmunoelectrophoresis tests are difficult to interpret (again, because of the high percentage of precipitins in the normal population).

In spite of these difficulties, however, the serologic diagnosis of candidiasis is evolving as a tool for laboratory diagnosis, mainly because high titers of antibodies to intracellular antigens of *Candida* are indicative of systemic disease.

Sporotrichosis

This chronic progressive, subcutaneous lymphatic (rarely respiratory) mycosis is caused by the fungus *Sporothrix schenckii*. The disease takes three forms: lymphatic, disseminated, and respiratory—the lymphatic form being the most common. It is characterized by a "sporotrichotic chancre" at the site of inoculation followed by the development and formation of subcutaneous nodules along the lymphatics draining the primary lesions. The infection is associated with injuries caused by thorns or splinters. Handlers of peat moss are susceptible to the disease, especially when working in rose gardens. The fungus also grows saprophytically on mine timbers as well as on other pieces of wood.

In culture, *S. schenckii* grows readily in Sabouraud's glucose agar at room temperature or in blood agar at 37°C. At 37°C the organism exists as a cigar-shaped yeast, whereas at room temperature it is mold. *S. schenckii* is resistant to cyclohexamine.

Serologically, a fluorescent antibody staining technique is available for the identification of *S. schenckii*. Two of the most sensitive identification tests are the yeast cell and the latex particle agglutination tests (Welsh and Dolan, 1973), which utilize lyophilized whole yeast cells in a buffer suspension and several dilutions of patient serum with agglutination checked after 1 hour. In this test, titers of 80 or greater usually indicate active infection. Some cutaneous infections present negative tests, whereas extracutaneous infections present positive tests. There is also a skin test available that uses a derivative of *S. schenckii* called *sporotrichin*, which produces a tuberculin-type reaction.

FEBRILE ANTIBODY TESTS

Several diseases are detected by the so-called Weil-Felix test (Table 15–1). These diseases as well as several others are collectively known as the *febrile diseases*.

One of the earliest tests of diagnostic value, known as the Widal test, was developed by Widal and Sicard in 1896. This test is still widely used for the detection of antibodies in typhoid fever, brucellosis, and tularemia (Corbel and Cullen, 1970; Damp *et al.*, 1973).

The Weil-Felix test, developed by Weil and Felix (1916), is based on the fact that certain strains of *Proteus vulgaris* most probably share antigens with several of the *Rickettsia* species that produce febrile diseases, such as typhus. Three strains of *Proteus vulgaris* have been found to be useful in diagnosing rickettsial diseases; these have been labeled OX-2, OX-19, and OX-K. By testing suspensions of all three strains, it is possible to detect antibodies against a number of rickettsial diseases (see Table 15–1).

As will be noted in Table 15–1, the Weil-Felix test does not distinguish between antibodies to *Rickettsia prowazekii*, *R. mooseri*, and *R. rickettsii*.

TABLE 15–1. Weil-Felix Reactions in Rickettsial Disease

Organism	Disease	*Proteus* Strain Used and Degree of Reaction		
		OX-2	OX-19	OX-K
R. prowazekii	Epidemic typhus, Brill's disease	+	++++	0
R. mooseri (R. typhi)	Murine typhus	+	++++	0
R. rickettsii	Rocky Mountain spotted fever	+	++++	0
R. akari	Rickettsialpox	0	0	0
R. tsutsugamushi	Tsutsugamushi disease (scrub typhus)	0	0	++++
R. quintana	Trench fever	0	0	0
R. burnetii (Coxiella burnetii)	Q fever	0	0	0

Clinical symptoms must therefore be studied in conjunction with serologic results.

Q fever agglutinins may be detected by a capillary agglutination test described by Luoto (1953). This test uses embryo-cultured *Coxiella burnetii*, which is suspended in saline, inactivated with formalin, and finally stained with hematoxylin and standardized. Similar test antigens have been developed for psittacosis or ornithosis, but they are not widely available. Laboratory diagnosis of Q fever, however, is preferably made using the complement fixation test.

VIRAL ANTIBODY TESTS

Many diseases of humans now recognized as caused by viruses, such as smallpox and yellow fever, have been known for centuries. Several additional major illnesses of humans (and other animals) are viral in nature, including influenza, measles, mumps, poliomyelitis, and so forth (Table 15-2).

Serologic tests used for the detection of viral antibodies include complement fixation, latex fixation, precipitation, neutralization, immunofluorescence, and hemagglutination. Tests vary greatly in their diagnostic usefulness. The reader is also referred to various sections of this book in which tests for viruses are discussed in detail.

Complement Fixation

The interaction of viral protein and antibody often fixes complement, and because sensitive methods for the titration of complement are available, this provides a convenient and accurate method of measuring the amount of either viral antigen or antibody to such antigens. Complement fixation is useful too in the detection of viral antibodies, because it is less complex, less time consuming, and less costly than other techniques.

In the modern serology laboratory, complement fixation can be used to detect the antibody to the antigens of adenovirus, the antibody to types 3 and 5 of arbovirus, the antibody to coxsackie A and B types, the antibody to echovirus, the antibody to herpes simplex virus types 1 and 2, the antibodies to types A, B, and C influenza, the antibody to Japanese encephalitis virus, the antibody to measles (rubella) virus, the antibody to mumps virus (soluble antigen), the antibody to reovirus, the antibody to respiratory syncytial virus, and the antibody to varicella-zoster virus (see Table 15–2).

In addition, the antibody to poliovirus types 1, 2, and 3 can be detected with the complement fixation inhibition (neutralization) test.

Latex Fixation Tests

Aubert *et al.* (1962) reported studies of viral antibody titrations using latex suspensions. These tests have not gained wide acceptance, however, except in the detection of HBsAg, in which latex fixation is often used as a screening test for blood donors.

Precipitation

Because of the difficulty in preparing purified antigens, few satisfactory precipitation tests have

TABLE 15–2. Tests for Viral Antigens and Antibodies

Test	Organism
Complement fixation	Adenovirus
	Arboviruses
	Coxsackie virus
	Echoviruses
	Herpes simplex viruses (1 and 2)
	Influenza A, B, C
	Japanese encephalitis virus
	Lymphocytic choriomeningitis virus
	Rubella virus
	Mumps virus
	Reovirus
	Respiratory syncytial virus
	Varicella-zoster virus
Complement fixation inhibition	Poliovirus types 1, 2, 3
Latex fixation	Hepatitis virus
Precipitation	Not generally used
Neutralization	Echovirus
	Herpes simplex viruses (1 and 2)
	Visna virus
Inhibition	Polyomaviruses
Indirect fluorescent antibody	Arboviruses
	Coronaviruses
	Herpes simplex viruses (1 and 2)
	Lymphocytic choriomeningitis virus
Direct fluorescent antibody	Respiratory syncytial virus
Hemagglutination	Echoviruses
Hemagglutination inhibition	Echoviruses
	Rubella virus
	Polyomaviruses
	Reovirus
	Influenza viruses A, B, C
	Mumps virus
	Vaccina virus
	Smallpox virus
	Newcastle disease virus
Latex particle agglutination	Rubella virus
	Rotavirus
	Cytomegalovirus
Direct electron microscopy	Adenovirus
	Rotavirus
Immune electron microscopy	Norwalk virus
Enzyme immunoassay	Arboviruses
	Herpes simplex viruses (1 and 2)
	Influenza A, B, C
	Japanese encephalitis virus
	Rubella virus
	Mumps virus
	Norwalk virus
	Polyomaviruses
	Respiratory syncytial virus
	Rotavirus
	Varicella-zoster virus
	Cytomegalovirus
Radioimmunoassay	Norwalk virus
	Parvoviruses
cDNA probe	Papillomaviruses
Hemadsorption immunosorbent technique	Parainfluenza

For tests for hepatitis viruses, see Chapter 7.

been developed. Chew and Theus (1967) described a double-diffusion test for adenoviral antibody, and Mata (1963) described an agar cell culture precipitation test, which is an adaptation of the Elek diffusion test using Eagle's medium. Although these methods have merit, they have never been widely used.

Neutralization

A number of distinctly different neutralization techniques have been developed in the field of virology. Lennette and Schmidt (1969) have described these procedures in some detail. Another method, essentially the same as the *in vivo* tests, uses embryonated eggs instead of animals for the inoculation of virus and of antibody mixtures. This *in ovo* method is now mainly of historic value. Some viruses produce distinct "pocks" on some of the membranes of embryonated eggs; this fact has been used in the development of so-called pock reduction tests. In this technique, the allantoic membrane is dropped to allow the outer surface to be inoculated. Inocula of certain virus suspensions may be titrated to produce a determinable number of pocks during a specific time period and then mixed with test sera just prior to inoculation. When the test serum contains antibodies to the pock-producing virus, a reduction in the number of pocks produced is an indicator of the quantity of antibody present.

The tissue-culture neutralization test is useful in virology and has been adapted to a microtitration method (Rosenbaum *et al.*, 1963). Sterile microplates are available for this test from Baltimore Biological Laboratories, Baltimore, MD, and Cooke Engineering, Alexandria, VA. The test, while economically practical, is highly sophisticated and requires extensive experience to perform. (Note: This tissue culture neutralization test has been adapted for use in the determination of diphtheria antibodies [Quevillon and Chagnon, 1973].)

Dulbecco (1952) used plaque reduction tests with some success in viral antibody determination. In this technique, monolayers of cell cultures are inoculated with virus suspensions and immediately overlaid with an agar-gel medium, which prevents the virus particles released from infected cells from moving via the medium to cells other than the immediately adjacent ones. Patches of infected cells (plaques) therefore develop underneath the agar surface. Each live virus particle will, in theory, produce one plaque, and the plaques may be counted to determine the number of viable viruses. To determine the number of antibodies in the test serum, viral suspensions are mixed with dilutions of test serum prior to inoculation onto the cell culture; this results in a reduced number of plaques. The reduction is proportional to the number of antibodies in the test serum. Kenyon and McManus (1974) have shown that the number of plaques produced by *Rickettsia*, unaffected by some antisera, can be reduced in the presence of antiglobulins to the antiserum.

A metabolic inhibition test was proposed by Salk *et al.* (1954). It has some distinct advantages over the conventional tissue culture neutralization test, but it also has serious shortcomings that greatly limit its practical usefulness. The test is based on the fact that certain viruses inhibit the metabolic processes of living cells that are suspended in a culture medium, resulting in a readily observable pH change of the cell culture medium. When viruses are mixed with antisera, no pH change occurs. The test is easy to read and appears to be more sensitive than other tissue culture neutralization tests; only a few viruses bring about the pH change, however, and in some instances pH changes may occur in the absence of virus.

In the modern serology laboratory, neutralization can be used to detect the antibody to echovirus, herpes simplex viruses 1 and 2, and the antibody to the visna virus (see Table 15–2).

Immunofluorescence

Immunofluorescence has been widely used in the detection of rubella-specific IgM (Iwakata *et al.*,

1972), cytomegalic inclusion virus in smears from urinary sediments (Hanshaw, 1969), herpes simplex in clinical specimens (Nahmias *et al.*, 1971), and IgM specific for Epstein-Barr virus (Banatvala *et al.*, 1972). These tests are highly useful and have become important tools in viral diagnostic testing. Practical limitations include the difficulty in maintenance and standardization of virus-infected cells, the stability of these cells, and the problem of nonspecific reactions.

The indirect fluorescent antibody test is used to detect the antibodies to arboviruses (IgG and IgM), antibodies to strain OC-43 229E of coronaviruses, herpes simplex viruses 1 and 2 (IgM), and IgM and IgG antibodies of lymphocytic choriomeningitis virus in serum (IgM only in cerebrospinal fluid).

The direct fluorescent antibody test is used to detect the respiratory syncytial virus (antigen).

Hemagglutination

Hirst's report (1942) of the phenomenon of viral hemagglutination quickly led to the development of the hemagglutination-inhibition (HI) test for the detection and titration of viral antibodies in patient's sera and for the identification of specific viruses. This test has in recent years become the most practical for determining the immune status of an individual against rubella and in the serologic diagnosis of rubella viral infections. The HI test can be used in any situation involving viruses that agglutinate (e.g., influenza, mumps, vaccina, smallpox, Newcastle disease, rubella). It is also useful in the detection of antibody to echovirus, polyomaviruses, and reovirus. In principle, the test involves the attachment of antibody molecules to the viral particles, subsequently hindering the absorption of viral particles to erythrocytes. Failure of hemagglutination to occur constitutes a positive test. HI is also useful in the identification of virus isolates by mixing known antiserum dilutions with fixed quantities of unknown hemagglutinating viral suspensions (see Table 15–2).

Others

Other tests that can be used in the detection of virus antigens or antibodies include direct electron microscopy to detect adenovirus and rotavirus; immune electron microscopy to detect Norwalk virus; enzyme immunoassay to detect the antibodies to arboviruses (IgG and IgM in serum and cerebrospinal fluid), herpes simplex virus (IgG), influenza (IgM, IgG, and IgA antibody to types A, B, and C), Japanese encephalitis (IgM and IgG), rubella virus (IgM and IgG), mumps virus (IgM and IgG), Norwalk virus (IgM and IgG), polyomaviruses (BK virus), respiratory syncytial virus (IgM and IgG), rotavirus (IgM and IgG), varicella-zoster virus (IgM and IgG), and cytomegalovirus; inhibition to detect the antibody to polyomaviruses; radioimmunoassay to detect the antigen to Norwalk virus and the antibody to parvoviruses; hemadsorption immunosorbent technique to detect the IgM antibody to parainfluenza; and cDNA probes to detect the human papillomaviruses. A summary of the tests used to detect viral antigens and antibodies is given in Table 15–2.

JUST THE FACTS

Fungal Antibody Tests

1. The evidence of mycotic infection that serologic tests may provide is often only tentative, although they often play an important role in diagnosis.
2. False-negative results can occur when blood is drawn at an inappropriate time or if blood is obtained from a patient who is immunosuppressed by chemotherapy or underlying diseases.
3. False-positive results may occur because of cross-reaction.
4. As a safeguard against false reactions, serologic testing should be repeated at 2 to 3 week intervals.
5. Proper collection and transportation of specimens is important.
6. Serum that is collected from at least 10 ml of blood is adequate for most testing.
7. Serum can be stored at 4°C for short periods and at −20°C or colder for longer periods.
8. When transported, serum and cerebrospinal fluid should be packed in dry or wet ice (or a preservative should be added) to prevent bacterial contamination.

Histoplasmosis

1. This is a granulomatous infection caused by *Histoplasma capsulatum.*
2. The source of human infection is believed to be from soil, especially when it is laden with excreta from chickens, birds, or bats. Human infection most commonly results from inhalation of spore-laden dust.
3. The disease presents as a broad spectrum ranging from an acute, asymptomatic form to a chronic pulmonary form, to a disseminated form.
4. The disseminated form is the most serious.
5. AIDS patients may experience rapid and fatal dissemination.
6. The disease can mimic *Pneumocystis carinii* infections.
7. A definite diagnosis requires isolation in culture and microscopic identification of the fungus, as well as serologic testing.
8. Serologic testing includes immunodiffusion, latex agglutination, and complement fixation.

Aspergillosis

1. The etiologic agents are *Aspergillus fumigatus* (the most important), *A. niger, A. flavus, A terrus,* and other species.
2. *Aspergillus fumigatus* is responsible for about 90 per cent of infections.
3. The clinical disease manifestations include pulmonary aspergillosis, allergic bronchopulmonary aspergillosis, fungus ball, and external otomycosis.
4. In the diagnosis of suspicious symptoms, the same species of *Aspergillus* must be recovered from multiple samples of respiratory secretions.
5. Serologically, skin reactions and immunodiffusion are useful. The ELISA procedure is currently being used to detect both IgE and IgG antibodies in patients' sera.

Coccidioidomycosis

1. This disease is also known as desert fever, San Joaquin fever, and valley fever.
2. It occurs in primary pulmonary, primary cutaneous, and disseminated forms.

3. It is generally contracted from the inhalation of soil or dust containing the arthrospores of the causative agent *Coccidioides immitis.*
4. The available serologic tests are the tube precipitin test (positive in 90 per cent of cases), complement fixation (which becomes positive later), latex agglutination (which is highly sensitive and rapid but not as specific as tube precipitation), and immunodiffusion (which gives results that usually correlate with those observed with complement fixation).

North American Blastomycosis

1. This disease is usually secondary to pulmonary involvement.
2. The causative agent is *Blastomyces dermatitidis.*
3. Serologic diagnosis is complicated by a high degree of cross-reactivity, with antigenic components of the organisms causing histoplasmosis and coccidioidomycosis.
4. Serologic tests include immunodiffusion (claimed to yield better results than complement fixation) and complement fixation (which may provide prognostic value). Most patients, however, have negative tests.
5. There is a good fluorescent antibody test specific for the yeast phase of *B. dermatitidis.*

Candidiasis

1. The term candidiasis refers to any fungal infection involving the genus *Candida,* of which there are many species.
2. Only *C. albicans* is considered to be pathogenic for humans, but other species are encountered in pathologic conditions.
3. Infections are endogenous.
4. Some of the conditions predisposing to candidiasis are pregnancy, diabetes mellitus, indwelling venous catheters, chronic debilitating diseases, and prolonged therapy with broad-spectrum antibiotics.
5. Virtually 100 per cent of AIDS patients have oral candidiasis.
6. The clinical disease manifestations are cutaneous candidiasis, mucous membrane candidiasis, pulmonary candidiasis, endocarditis, and fungemia.
7. Serologic tests include precipitation (for the detection of antibodies). The test is of little value because of the high incidence of antibodies in apparently healthy individuals.
8. Other serologic tests include agglutination, immunodiffusion, and counterimmunoelectrophoresis. All of these tests are of dubious value.
9. Serologic testing is evolving as a tool for diagnosis because high titers of antibodies to intracellular antigens of *Candida* are indicative of systemic disease.

Sporotrichosis

1. This chronic, progressive, subcutaneous lymphatic (rarely respiratory) mycosis is caused by *Sporothrix schenckii.*
2. The disease can be lymphatic (most common), disseminated, and respiratory.
3. Infection is associated with injuries caused by thorns or splinters. Handlers of peat moss, especially when working in rose gardens, are susceptible.
4. The fungus grows on mine timbers and on other pieces of wood.
5. Serologically, a fluorescent antibody staining technique is available for the identification of *S. schenckii.*
6. Two of the most sensitive identification tests are the yeast cell and the latex particle agglutination tests.
7. A skin test is also available that uses a derivative of *S. schenckii* called *sporotrichin* and produces a tuberculin-type reaction.

Febrile Antibody Tests

1. Several diseases detected by the Weil-Felix test (as well as several others) are known as febrile diseases.
2. The Widal test is used for the detection of antibodies in typhoid fever, brucellosis, and tularemia.
3. The use of the Weil-Felix test in rickettsial diseases is summarized in Table 15–1.
4. Q fever agglutinins may be detected by a capillary agglutination test that uses embryo-cultured *Coxiella burnetii.*
5. The laboratory diagnosis of Q fever, however, is preferably made using the complement fixation test.

Viral Antibody Tests

1. Serologic tests used for the detection of viral antibodies include:
   a. *Complement fixation.* This is a convenient and accurate method of measuring the amount of either viral antigen or antibody to such antigens.
   b. *Latex fixation tests.* These are not widely accepted but are used as a screening test for the detection of HBsAg in blood donors.
   c. *Precipitation.* Few precipitation tests have been developed because of the difficulty in preparing purified antigens. Tests that have been described are not widely used.
   d. *Neutralization.* A number of techniques have been developed, including pock reduction tests, a tissue-culture neutralization test (which has been adapted to a microtitration method), plaque reduction tests, and a metabolic inhibition test (which is of limited practical value because it relies on a pH change, and only a few viruses bring about this change when suspended in culture medium. In addition, pH changes may occur in the absence of virus).
   e. *Immunofluorescence.* This test has been widely used in the detection of rubella-specific IgM, cytomegalic inclusion virus in smears from urinary sediments, herpes simplex in clinical specimens, and IgM specific for Epstein-Barr virus. The tests are highly useful and are important tools in viral diagnostic testing, although there are some practical limitations (difficulty in maintenance and standardization of virus-infected cells, the stability of these cells, and the problem of nonspecific reactions).
   f. *Hemagglutination.* The hemagglutination-inhibition test is most practical for determining the immune status of an individual against rubella and the serodiagnosis of rubella viral infections. It has also been used in any situation involving viruses that agglutinate (influenza, mumps, vaccina, smallpox, Newcastle disease, rubella).
   g. *Others.* Other tests include direct and immune electron microscopy, enzyme immunoassay, inhibition, radioimmunoassay, hemadsorption immunosorbent technique, and cDNA probes (see Table 15–2).

Review Questions

Multiple Choice

Choose the phrase, sentence, or symbol that completes the statement or answers the question. More than one answer may be correct in each case. Answers are given at the end of this book.

1. The detection of histoplasmin antibodies can be achieved using:
   (a) the immunodiffusion test
   (b) hemagglutination tests
   (c) neutralization tests
   (d) none of the above)
   (Histoplasmosis)

2. The serologic tests that are considered useful in the serologic diagnosis of aspergillosis include:
   (a) skin tests
   (b) immunodiffusion
   (c) precipitation
   (d) ELISA
   (Aspergillosis)

3. The causative agent of coccidioidomycosis is known as:
   (a) *Coccidioides immitis*
   (b) *Coccidioides amitis*
   (c) *Coccidioides dermatitidis*
   (d) *Coccidioides guilliermondi*
   (Coccidioidomycosis)

4. Which of the following members of the genus *Candida* is considered to be pathologic for humans?
   (a) *C. tropicalis*
   (b) *C. parakrusei*
   (c) *C. albicans*
   (d) *C. guilliermondi*
   (Candidiasis)

5. Which of the following fungal diseases is caused by *S. schenckii?*
   (a) coccidioidomycosis
   (b) sporotrichosis

(c) blastomycosis
(d) none of the above
(General)

6. The Widal test is used for the detection of:
   (a) Q fever agglutinins
   (b) strains of *Proteus vulgaris*
   (c) antibodies in typhus fever
   (d) antibodies in typhoid fever
   (Febrile Antibody Tests)

7. In which of the following fungal diseases is the fungus encountered in the lesions of thrush?
   (a) North American blastomycosis
   (b) candidiasis
   (c) aspergillosis
   (d) histoplasmosis
   (Fungal Antibody Tests)

8. Which of the following is not a strain of *Proteus vulgaris* useful in diagnosing rickettsial disease?
   (a) OX-2
   (b) OX-19
   (c) OX-K
   (d) OX-4
   (Febrile Antibody Tests)

9. The pack reduction test is:
   (a) a neutralization technique
   (b) a complement fixation technique
   (c) an immunofluorescent technique
   (d) a precipitation technique
   (Viral Antibody Tests)

10. Oral candidiasis is seen in 100 per cent of patients with:
    (a) diabetes mellitus
    (b) indwelling venous catheters
    (c) prolonged therapy with broad-spectrum antibiotics
    (d) AIDS
    (Candidiasis)

Answer "True" or "False"

1. Histoplasmosis is caused by *Histoplasma capsulatum.*
   (Fungal Antibody Tests)

2. Aspergillus is sensitive to cyclohexamine.
   (Fungal Antibody Tests)

3. Complement fixation cannot be used as a test for coccidioidomycosis.
   (Fungal Antibody Tests)

4. Growth of *B. dermatitidis* on blood agar or in Sabouraud's glucose medium may take as long as 1 month.
   (Fungal Antibody Tests)

5. The genus *Candida* contains only one species, *C. albicans.*
   (Fungal Antibody Tests)

6. Immunofluorescence has been widely used in the detection of rubella-specific IgM.
   (Viral Antibody Tests)

GENERAL REFERENCES

Baron, E.J., and Finegold, S.M.: Bailey and Scott's Diagnostic Microbiology, 8th ed. St Louis, C. V. Mosby Company, 1990.

Bennington, J.L.: Saunders Dictionary and Encyclopedia of Laboratory Medicine and Technology. Philadelphia, W. B. Saunders Company, 1984.

Dorland's Illustrated Medical Dictionary, 27th ed. Philadelphia, W. B. Saunders Company, 1988.

Henry, J.B.: Clinical Diagnosis and Management by Laboratory Methods. Philadelphia, W. B. Saunders Company, 1991.

Turgeon, M.L.: Immunology and Serology in Laboratory Medicine. St. Louis, C. V. Mosby Company, 1990.

16

Lyme Disease

OBJECTIVES

The student shall know, understand, and be prepared to explain:
1. A brief history of Lyme disease
2. The etiology of Lyme disease
3. The incidence of Lyme disease
4. The mode of transmission of Lyme disease
5. The characteristics of Lyme disease
6. Treatment and prevention of Lyme disease
7. Antibody development in Lyme disease
8. The laboratory diagnosis of Lyme disease

A BRIEF HISTORY OF LYME DISEASE

Lyme disease was first reported in 1977. It is so called because of an outbreak of "pseudojuvenile rheumatoid arthritis" in four young boys living in Lyme, Connecticut. At first this outbreak was considered to represent a "new" condition, yet it appears in retrospect that the first symptom of Lyme disease, the rash known as *erythema chronicum migrans* (ECM), was recognized in Sweden in 1908. This same rash was noted in other parts of Europe, as were other symptoms that frequently followed ECM's eruption.

In 1969 this "European" rash was reported in a Wisconsin physician who was bitten by a tick while hunting. This rash had been seen in Americans who had traveled in Europe but otherwise the condition was virtually unknown in the United States.

In 1975 physicians at the U.S. Navy base in Groton, Connecticut, reported seeing four patients with a rash similar to ECM, and at around the same time the four children from Lyme were reported

to the Connecticut State Department of Health and to a rheumatologist at Yale University.

Since 1975 Lyme disease has become the most prevalent tick-borne disease in the United States (see Disease Characteristics, below).

ETIOLOGY

In 1983 Burgdorfer isolated a previously unrecognized spirochete, now known as *Borrelia burgdorferi,* which is transmitted by the bite of certain ixodes ticks that are part of the *Ixodes ricinus* complex. This agent was identified as the etiologic agent of Lyme disease. Several genera of ticks act as vectors in the United States, including *Ixodes pacificus* in California and other western states and *I. dammini* in the northeastern and midwestern states. Endemic areas of disease have, in fact, been identified in 14 states, as well as in Europe (where the etiologic agent is *I. ricinus*), Asia (where the etiologic agent is *I. persulcatus*), and Australia (Burgdorfer, 1986). The spirochete has been recovered from the blood, cerebrospinal fluid, and skin lesions of patients, and (rarely) from joint fluid (Steere *et al.*, 1984).

The preferred hosts of the ixodes ticks are the white-tailed deer and the white-footed mouse, although they have been found on at least 30 types of wild animals and 49 species of birds. It is not known if illness develops in wild animals, but clinical Lyme disease does occur in domestic animals (e.g., dogs, horses, and cattle).

INCIDENCE

Between 1977 and 1988 a three- to eightfold increase in the incidence of Lyme disease was reported in Connecticut residents, the number growing to 22 per 100,000 population. From 1987 to 1988 the average annual incidence of reported Lyme disease in the United States was 1.4 per 100,000, with New York reporting 57 per cent of these cases. Ninety-two per cent of cases in the United States, in fact, were reported from just eight states (New York, New Jersey, Pennsylvania, Connecticut, Massachusetts, Rhode Island, Wisconsin, and Minnesota). Seven states, all located west of the 100th meridian, had not reported any cases of Lyme disease. The total number of cases reported to the Centers for Disease Control from 1987 to 1988 (from 43 states) was 6,876. Of these, 4,507 cases were reported in 1988, which represented twice the number reported in 1987 and nine times the number reported in 1982 (when a systematic system of national surveillance was established).

In 1990 the number of cases in the United States had swelled to 7,997, an increase of 1,121 over the number reported in 1988, which represented 3.2 per 100,000 population. (Figures for 1991 were not available at the time of this writing.) Forty-six states were then reporting incidence. By 1991, all states had reported an incidence of the disease (Centers for Disease Control, Colorado; personal communication, 1991).

MODE OF TRANSMISSION

As mentioned (see Etiology, above), *Borrelia burgdorferi* is transmitted by the bite of a tick. All stages of tick can harbor the spirochete and transmit disease. The disease is usually contracted during the summer, when the nymphal form of the tick, which is most likely to transmit disease, is active and people are in the woods and dressed in light clothing. During this stage, the tick is very tiny, about the size of a pinhead, and is therefore easily overlooked. The tick needs to be attached for a minimum of 24 hours before disease transmission is possible.

DISEASE CHARACTERISTICS

Lyme disease is a multisystem illness that involves the skin, nervous system, heart, and joints. It is characterized by three stages, not all of which occur in any given patient (Duray and Steere, 1988).

Stage 1: Cutaneous Involvement. The characteristic red, annular skin lesion (erythema chronicum migrans, or ECM) appearing at the site of the tick bite (and sometimes at distant sites as well) is the most common finding in the first stage of the disease. It is most commonly located on the thigh, groin, or axilla, or may be located on the face, particularly in children. Subsequently, about 50 per cent of untreated patients develop secondary skin lesions (disseminated lesions and lymphocytoma) within days to weeks after the onset of ECM, and some may progress to late skin lesions (acrodermatitis chronica atrophicans, or ACA), although these are more commonly seen in Europe than in the United States.

Another early manifestation of Lyme disease is a borrelia lymphocytoma, which is a tumor-like violaceous swelling or nodule at the base of the earlobe or the nipple, caused by a dense lymphocytic infiltrate of the dermis. In conjunction with other symptoms, this lesion, which occurs at the site of the tick bite, may be confused with lymphoma.

Patients may experience headache, fever, muscle and joint pain, and malaise during this stage.

Stage 2: Neurologic and Cardiac Involvement. This stage begins within weeks to months after infection. It may include arthritis, but the most important features are neurologic disorders and carditis. Neurologic disorders, which may include aseptic meningitis, cranial nerve palsies, peripheral radiculoneuritis, and peripheral neuropathy, occur in about 15 per cent of untreated patients, occurring within 2 to 8 weeks after the onset of disease. Lyme carditis occurs in about 8 per cent of untreated patients. The abnormalities, which occur within 2 to 6 weeks following initial infection and may in some cases be the initial manifestation of the disease, are usually short-lived (days to weeks) and generally do not require permanent cardiac pacing. Arrhythmia can occur, although this is less common, which may cause the condition to be mistaken for acute rheumatic fever.

Stage 3: Joint Involvement. The final stage of the disease is usually characterized by chronic arthritis, which may persist for years. During this stage, there may be involvement of the joints with intermittent oligoarthritis, peripheral neuritis, myositis, and a variety of chronic skin lesions.

Notes. There is considerable overlap between the stages of Lyme disease—a patient may have one or all of the manifestations and the disease may not become symptomatic until the second or third stage. The majority of affected patients have ECM, and about 25 per cent have arthritis, whereas neurologic and cardiac involvement is infrequent.

In some cases of Lyme disease there may be ocular involvement, which may manifest as cranial nerve palsies, optic neuritis, panophthalmitis with loss of vision, and choroiditis with retinal detachment.

The Centers for Disease Control definition for Lyme disease contracted in endemic areas is the presence of ECM and a positive serologic test for antibody to *Borrelia burgdorferi*. The serologic results of neurologic, cardiac, or arthritic manifestations are not taken into account.

There is no uniform pattern of congenital malformations in the maternal-fetal transmission of the disease.

TREATMENT AND PREVENTION

The first-choice drugs for therapy in cases of Lyme disease are phenoxymethyl penicillin or erythromycin. If initial treatment fails, broad-spectrum cephalosporins, particularly ceftriaxone and chloramphenicol, have been successful (Barbour, 1988).

It should be noted that treatment may result in lack of antibody response in the patient, which allows for reinfection. In some cases, treatment has been reported to fail completely, especially in patients with chronic disease.

The best preventive strategies include the use of insect repellent and careful inspection for ticks on a daily basis during outdoor activity in high-risk areas.

ANTIBODY DEVELOPMENT

Antibodies against *B. burgdorferi* are usually not detected in a patient's serum until 2 to 4 weeks after the appearance of symptoms. At this time there is a slow rise in titer of IgM and a concomitant rise in IgG. These antibodies both last for several years. Anti-*B. burgdorferi* antibodies (IgG) should be present in the serum of patients with Lyme arthritis. These same patients have negative tests for serum antinuclear antibodies, rheumatoid factor, and syphilis (using the VDRL test).

LABORATORY DIAGNOSIS

The diagnosis of Lyme disease is usually established clinically with serologic confirmation. Numerous laboratory techniques are available. In the early stages of the disease laboratory findings are nonspecific (an elevated sedimentation rate, elevated serum IgM levels, and mildly elevated hepatic transaminase levels).

Culture of the spirochete may be attempted, but the yield is low, and therefore this method is unreliable for diagnosis. If culture is attempted, the periphery of the annular lesion of erythema chronicum migrans, blood, and cerebrospinal fluid provide the best specimens. The resuspended plasma, cerebrospinal fluid, or macerated tissue biopsy is inoculated into a tube of modified Kelly's medium (BSK II) and incubated tightly capped for one month at 33°C. Blind subcultures are performed weekly from the lower portion of the broth to fresh media, and the cultures are examined by darkfield microscopy for the presence of spirochetes. The organism may also be visualized in tissue sections stained with Warthin-Starry silver stain and in blood and cerebrospinal fluid stained with acridine orange, specific fluorescent stain, or Giemsa (Barbour, 1988).

The most practical serologic tests for the detection of antibodies to *B. burgdorferi* include latex agglutination (available commercially as a test kit), indirect fluorescent antibody staining methods (IFA), and enzyme-linked immunosorbent assays (ELISA) for total immunoglobulins or IgM and IgG antibodies. To characterize immune response and for diagnosis, immunoblotting techniques can be used in conjunction with ELISA. Western blot analysis can verify reactivity of antibody to major surface or flagellar proteins of *B. burgdorferi*.

There are several disadvantages to the current techniques, however. These include low sensitivity (e.g., IFA and ELISA during the first 3 weeks of infection) and lengthy processing times. In addition, antigenic similarity causes the antibody produced by patients with Lyme disease to cross-react with other spirochetal antigens, leading to false-positive and false-negative results (Magnarelli *et al.*, 1987). Finally, it has been found that 15 per cent of patients with Lyme disease fail to produce antibodies and therefore would give negative results in serologic tests (Dattwyler *et al.*, 1988; Grodzicki and Steere, 1988).

JUST THE FACTS

A Brief History of Lyme Disease

1. Lyme disease is so called because of an outbreak of the disease in four young boys living in Lyme, Connecticut.
2. In retrospect, the first symptom of Lyme disease was recognized in Sweden in 1908.
3. The first symptom is a rash known as *erythema chronicum migrans* (ECM).
4. In 1969 this "European" rash was reported in Wisconsin.
5. The rash (prior to this) had been seen only in Americans who had traveled in Europe.
6. In 1975 physicians at the U.S. Navy base in Groton, Connecticut, reported seeing four patients with a rash similar to ECM.
7. At the same time, the four boys from Lyme were reported.
8. Since 1975 Lyme disease has become the most prevalent tick-borne disease in the United States.

Etiology

1. *Borrelia burgdorferi* is the etiologic agent of Lyme disease.
2. The agent is a spirochete, transmitted by the bite of certain ixodes ticks that are part of the *I. ricinus* complex.
3. Several genera of ticks act as vectors.
4. Endemic areas have been identified in 14 states as well as in Europe, Asia, and Australia.
5. The spirochete has been recovered from the blood, cerebrospinal fluid, skin lesions, and (rarely) joint fluid of patients.
6. The preferred host of the ixodes ticks are the white-tailed deer and the white-footed mouse, although they have been found in at least 30 types of wild animals and 49 species of birds.
7. Clinical Lyme disease occurs in domestic animals (dogs, horses, cattle).

Incidence

1. From 1987 to 1988 the average annual incidence of reported Lyme disease in the United States was 1.4 per 100,000. The total number of cases (from 43 states) was 6,876. Seven states (all located west of the 100th meridian) reported no incidence of the disease.
2. In 1990 there were 7,997 cases of the disease, representing 3.2 per 100,000 population.
3. Forty-six states were reporting incidence in 1990.
4. By 1991 all states had reported an incidence of the disease.

Mode of Transmission

1. All stages of tick can harbor *Borrelia burgdorferi* and transmit disease.
2. The disease is usually contracted during the summer, when the nymphal form of the tick (most likely to transmit disease) is active and people are in the woods and dressed in light clothing.
3. During this stage, the tick is tiny and easily overlooked.
4. The tick needs to be attached for a minimum of 24 hours before disease transmission is possible.

Disease Characteristics

1. Lyme disease is a multisystem illness.
2. It involves the skin, nervous system, heart, and joints.
3. It is characterized by three stages.
4. Not all stages occur in any given patient.
5. Stage 1 is characterized by a red, annular skin lesion (erythema chronicum migrans, or ECM) appearing at the site of the tick bite (and sometimes in distant sites as well).
6. ECM is commonly located on the thigh, groin, or axilla. It may be located on the face, particularly in young children.
7. About 50 per cent of untreated patients develop secondary skin lesions (disseminated lesions and lymphocytoma) within days to weeks after the onset of ECM, and some may progress to late skin lesions (acrodermatitis chronica atrophicans) although these are more common in Europe than in the United States.
8. Another early manifestation is a borrelia lymphocytoma. This lesion may be confused with lymphoma.
9. Patients may experience headache, fever, muscle and joint pain, and malaise during Stage 1.
10. Stage 2 begins weeks to months after infection.
11. It may include arthritis, but the most important features are neurologic disorders (including aseptic meningitis, cranial nerve palsies, peripheral radiculoneuritis, and peripheral neuropathy) and carditis (usually short lived).
12. Neurologic disorders occur in about 15 per cent of untreated patients, occurring within 2 to 8 weeks after the onset of disease.
13. Lyme carditis occurs in about 8 per cent of untreated patients. It may include arrhythmia, in which case the condition may be mistaken for acute rheumatic fever.
14. Stage 3 involves the joints.
15. It is usually characterized by chronic arthritis, which may persist for years.
16. There is considerable overlap between the stages of Lyme disease.
17. The disease may not be symptomatic until the second or third stage.
18. The majority of patients have ECM.
19. About 25 per cent have arthritis.
20. Neurologic and cardiac involvement is infrequent.
21. There may be ocular involvement in Lyme disease.
22. Lyme disease is defined by the CDC (in endemic areas) as the presence of ECM and a positive serologic test for antibody to *B. burgdorferi*.
23. There is no uniform pattern of congenital malformations in the maternal-fetal transmission of the disease.

Antibody Development

1. Antibodies against *B. burgdorferi* are not usually detected in a patient's serum until 2 to 4 weeks after the appearance of symptoms.
2. At this time IgM rises in titer slowly with a concomitant rise in IgG.
3. These antibodies last for several years.
4. The IgG antibody should be present in patients with Lyme arthritis.
5. These same patients have negative tests for serum antinuclear antibodies, rheumatoid factor, and syphilis (by VDRL test).

Laboratory Diagnosis

1. In the early stages of the disease laboratory findings are nonspecific (elevated ESR, serum IgM levels, and hepatic transaminase levels).
2. Culture is not usually successful.
3. Serologic tests include latex agglutination, indirect fluorescent antibody staining methods, and enzyme-linked immunosorbent assays (ELISA).
4. Immunoblotting techniques can be used to characterize immune response and for diagnosis (used in conjunction with ELISA).
5. Western blot analysis can verify reactivity of antibody to major surface or flagellar proteins of *B. burgdorferi*.
6. Disadvantages of the current techniques include:
   a. Low sensitivity (e.g., IFA and ELISA during the first 3 weeks of infection).
   b. Lengthy processing times.
   c. Cross-reaction, leading to false-positive and false-negative results.
   d. 15 per cent of patients fail to produce antibodies and therefore would give negative results in serologic tests.

Review Questions

Multiple Choice

Choose the phrase, sentence, or symbol that completes the statement or answers the question. More than one answer may be correct in each case. Answers are given at the end of this book.

1. Lyme disease:
   (a) is so called because of an outbreak of the condition in Lyme, Connecticut
   (b) was prevalent in the United States in 1908
   (c) is a condition found only in the United States
   (d) has become the most prevalent tick-borne disease in the United States
   (A Brief History of Lyme Disease)

2. The etiologic agent of Lyme disease is:
   (a) *Borrelia dammini*
   (b) *Borrelia burgdorferi*
   (c) *Borrelia ricinus*
   (d) None of the above
   (Etiology)

3. In 1991 in the United States, Lyme disease had been reported in:
   (a) 43 states
   (b) 46 states
   (c) 7 states
   (d) all states
   (Incidence)

4. Lyme disease is transmitted:
   (a) by the nymphal form of tick
   (b) usually during the summer months
   (c) usually during the winter months
   (d) by direct person-to-person contact
   (Mode of Transmission)

5. The majority of patients with Lyme disease have:
   (a) erythema chronicum migrans
   (b) arthritis
   (c) neurologic disorders
   (d) cardiac disorders
   (Disease Characteristics)

6. Antibodies against *B. burgdorferi*:
   (a) are usually not detected until 2 to 4 weeks after the appearance of symptoms
   (b) are IgM only
   (c) are IgG only
   (d) are IgM and IgG
   (Antibody Development)

7. The most practical tests for Lyme disease include:
   (a) culture of the spirochete
   (b) latex agglutination
   (c) enzyme-linked immunosorbent assays
   (d) indirect fluorescent antibody staining methods
   (Laboratory Diagnosis)

Answer "True" or "False"

1. The first symptom of Lyme disease was recognized in Sweden in 1908.
   (A Brief History of Lyme Disease)

2. The etiologic agent of Lyme disease in Europe is *I. dammini*.
   (Etiology)

3. In 1990 46 U.S. states were reporting cases of Lyme disease.
   (Incidence)

4. The tick needs to be attached for a minimum of 2 hours before Lyme disease transmission can occur.
   (Mode of Transmission)

5. There is no overlap between the stages of Lyme disease—patients exhibit only one manifestation of the disease at a time.
   (Disease Characteristics)

6. Phenoxymethyl penicillin or erythromycin are the first choice drugs for therapy in cases of Lyme disease.
   (Treatment and Prevention)

7. IgM and IgG antibodies against *B. burgdorferi* last in the patient's circulation for several years.
   (Antibody Development)

8. Western blot analysis can verify the reactivity of antibody to major surface or flagellar proteins of *B. burgdorferi*.
   (Laboratory Diagnosis)

GENERAL REFERENCES

Baron, E.J., and Finegold, S.M.: Bailey and Scott's Diagnostic Microbiology, 8th ed. St. Louis, C. V. Mosby Company, 1990.

Benach, J.L., and Bosler, E.M. (Eds.): Lyme Disease and Related Disorders. Ann. NY Acad. Sci., *539*:1–513, 1988.

Dorland's Illustrated Medical Dictionary, 27th ed. Philadelphia, W. B. Saunders Company, 1988.

Henry, J.B.: Clinical Diagnosis and Management by Laboratory Methods. Philadelphia, W. B. Saunders Company, 1991.

Steere, A.C.: Lyme Disease. N. Engl. J. Med., *321*:9, 1989.

Turgeon, M. L.: Immunology and Serology in Laboratory Medicine. St. Louis, C. V. Mosby Company, 1990.

17

Miscellaneous Serology

OBJECTIVES

The student shall know, understand, and be prepared to explain:

1. Opsonocytophagic tests
2. Bacteriolysin
3. The characteristics of rubella
4. The available serologic tests for rubella
5. Skin tests, specifically:
    a. General characteristics
    b. The performance of skin tests
    c. The *Trichinella spiralis* skin test
    d. The tuberculin skin test
    e. The brucellergin skin test
    f. The coccidioidin skin test
    g. The Frei test
    h. The histoplasmin skin test
    i. The Schick test
    j. The toxoplasmin skin test
    k. The *Trichinella* skin test
    l. Vollmer's patch test
    m. Delayed hypersensitivity skin tests
6. The classification of streptococci
7. Elek's diffusion test
8. The detection and identification of immunoglobulin and other serum proteins
9. Toxoplasmosis
10. Tests for the detection of antibody to *Toxoplasma gondii*
11. Pregnancy testing
12. Laboratory tests for pertussis (whooping cough)
13. Serologic tests for leptospira
14. General laboratory techniques, including:
    a. Complement fixation
    b. Complement fixation inhibition
    c. Hemagglutination inhibition
15. The collection and preservation of sheep blood
16. The preparation of sheep red cell hemolysin
17. The preparation and preservation of complement
18. The preparation of red cell concentrations

Introduction

Many diseases, disorders, and serologic procedures exist that are of interest to the student of serology. The purpose of this chapter is to acquaint the student with these and to offer a list of references that might prove useful if any subsection demands further study within a course outline.

OPSONOCYTOPHAGIC TESTS

The presence in a patient's serum of opsonins against certain bacteria is demonstrated by mixing the patient's fresh, citrated blood with a saline suspension of the bacteria. The mixture is incubated at 37°C for 20 minutes, and a drop of sedimented cells is then smeared on a glass slide, allowed to dry, and stained with any good stain. Subsequently, the number of bacteria present within a certain number of segmented neutrophil leukocytes (phagocytes) is counted in order to determine the opsonic power of the patient's blood. One to 20 phagocytized bacteria indicate slight phagocytosis; 41 or more indicate marked phagocytosis.

The "opsonic index" is an expression of the opsonic power of the patient's blood in relation to the opsonic power of normal blood. Opsonocytophagic tests are occasionally used in cases of brucellosis (in conjunction with the agglutination test or the skin test), but they are of doubtful diagnostic value in this disease.

BACTERIOLYSIN

A bacteriolysin is an antibody that causes the dissolution of bacteria. These bacteriolysins are found in the blood serum of animals that are naturally immune to a particular antigen as well as in those that have been artificially immunized against an antigen by injection. Unlike antitoxin, which neutralizes soluble toxin, bacteriolysin destroys the bacterial cell itself. In order for the bacteriolytic reaction to take place, complement is necessary (unlike toxin-antitoxin neutralization).

In 1894 Pfeiffer demonstrated that when cholera vibrio organisms are intraperitoneally injected into a guinea pig previously immunized against cholera, the organisms gradually lose their motility, become swollen, and disintegrate (known as Pfeiffer's phenomenon). Metchnikoff later showed that the same phenomenon can be detected *in vitro* by mixing cholera vibrios in a test tube with peritoneal fluid (or serum) from an immunized guinea pig.

Lysins have been produced for a variety of cells other than bacterial and are highly specific. If red blood cells of an animal or human are injected into an animal of a different species, hemolysins are developed that are specific for those cells. This test is useful in court trials where it is necessary to determine whether blood stains are of human or animal origin.

RUBELLA

Characteristics of Rubella

Acquired rubella (also known as German measles or 3-day measles) is caused by an enveloped, single-stranded RNA virus of the togavirus family, originally isolated in 1962. The disease is highly contagious and is transmitted through respiratory secretions.

Widespread rubella immunization has decreased the incidence of rubella, although elimination of the disease is hampered by the number of people who are not vaccinated and by vaccination failures.

The signs and symptoms of rubella vary greatly from one individual to another, and therefore diagnosis is based on clinical manifestation *and* serologic testing. The acquired infection has an incubation period of 10 to 21 days, and victims are contagious for 12 to 15 days, beginning 5 to 7 days before the appearance of a rash. The acute form usually lasts from 3 to 5 days and requires minimal treatment, with permanent effects being extremely rare. The manifestations of the disease are usually mild. There is a prodromal period of catarrhal symptoms, followed by involvement of the retroauricular, posterior cervical, and postoccipital lymph nodes, followed by the characteristic maculopapular rash on the face and then on the neck and trunk. A low fever (less than 101°F) is usually present. When the disease occurs in older children and in adults, self-limiting arthralgia and arthritis are common.

Rubella infection in pregnant women, particularly in the first trimester, can have devastating effects on the fetus. Infection *in utero* can cause fetal death or manifestation of rubella syndrome, which presents a spectrum of congenital defects. Ten to 20 per cent of newborns infected *in utero* fail to survive past the first 18 months of life. Fetal abnormalities include encephalitis, hepatomegaly, bone defects, mental retardation, cataracts, thrombocytopenic purpura, cardiovascular defects, splenomegaly, and microcephaly. Multiple defects may be seen in different organs. Most have low birth weight and fail to thrive.

Although some infants manifest nearly all of the defects, others exhibit few or none. Almost all affected children develop immunity, although about one third lose antibody and become susceptible in later childhood to acquired infection. If this occurs, however, it follows the typical benign course. Vaccination, therefore, may still be necessary.

Both IgM and IgG antibodies appear as the result of primary rubella infection. The IgM antibody becomes clinically undetectable within 4 to 5 weeks, whereas the IgG antibody remains present and protective indefinitely.

Serologic Tests for Rubella

The most widely used technique for the detection of antibodies to rubella is the hemagglutination inhibition test. This test is marketed as "Rubindex" by Ortho Diagnostics, Raritan, NJ. Other tests include the passive latex agglutination test (marketed as "Rubrascan" by Becton Dickinson Microbiology Systems, Cockeysville, MD) and the semiquantitative immunoassay (an indirect enzyme-labeled immunosorbent assay using microwells as a solid phase) for determination of IgG antibodies to rubella virus (marketed by Sigma Chemical Company, St. Louis, MO). Latex procedures provide a more rapid and convenient alternative to hemagglutination inhibition. Enzyme immunoassay (which can be used to measure total antibody, IgG or IgM) and fluorescent immunoassay (which gives quantitative results) appear to be as reliable as hemagglutination inhibition. Passive hemagglutination methods are not licensed for serodiagnosis of recent rubella infection, although they are faster and less complex than hemagglutination inhibition. The complement fixation test is unsuitable in rubella testing, because the CR antibody disappears after infection.

Hemagglutination inhibition (HI) antibodies rise rapidly, often reaching a peak level within 5 to 7 days of the onset of rash and remaining at a high level for a long period of time. The hemagglutination inhibition test is based on the ability of the rubella virus to agglutinate the erythrocytes of certain species. Antibodies to the rubella virus inhibit this agglutination and can be quantitated by exposing serially diluted test sera to rubella virus antigen and recording those dilutions in which agglutination does not take place.

Complete inhibition of agglutination represents a positive test and is indicated by the formation of a red cell button at the bottom of the well. The highest dilution at which hemagglutination is still completely inhibited represents the antibody titer. A titer of 8 (dilution 1:8) or greater indicates a positive reaction. A fourfold or greater increase in titer between two specimens collected at least 1 or 2 weeks apart indicates a recent rubella infection. No increase in titer between two specimens usually indicates a previous rubella infection.

The absence or low levels of rubella HI antibody indicate susceptibility to rubella virus. If rubella antibodies appear within 7 days following exposure to infection, prior infection with rubella virus can be presumed. If rubella antibodies are absent in a sample at the time of exposure, yet are found to be present in a second sample taken 3 to 4 weeks later, a rubella infection that has resulted from exposure can be presumed. A negative result in this second sample indicates that the infection has not occurred.

Congenital rubella infections can be confirmed serologically through the observation of persisting antibody, above and beyond that passively transferred from mother to infant during fetal life, especially if this antibody is present in the infant's blood during the first months after birth.

SKIN TESTS

Skin tests are still in common use, yet *in vitro* allergen tests are now available against a wide variety of allergens using radioimmunoassay techniques. These tests (RAST tests) should be used whenever possible in place of intradermal testing.

Skin tests are usually carried out in allergic or

immunologic conditions (e.g., diphtheria, scarlet fever, and so forth).

The Performance of Skin Tests

Three types of skin tests can be used, namely:

1. *Intradermal.* These tests are commonly used for tuberculin, histoplasmin, coccidioidin in adults, and so on.
2. *Scratch.* These tests are commonly used in testing for pollen or food allergens.
3. *Patch.* These tests are sometimes used for tuberculin tests in children, but are not as reliable as the intradermal tests. The success of the patch tests depends upon the ability of the diagnostic material to diffuse into the skin.

For obvious reasons, only sterile instruments and materials should be used in skin testing. The skin should be cleansed using 70 per cent alcohol. Skin tests are usually carried out on the flexor surface of the forearm, but other areas of the skin are just as reliable.

Skin tests are available for the following conditions: trichinosis, hydatid cyst, schistosomiasis, filariasis, leishmaniasis, mumps, influenza, lymphogranuloma venereum (Frei test), coccidioidomycosis, sporotrichosis, histoplasmosis, certain skin infections by the fungi, primary allergies, serum sickness, tuberculosis (Pirquet's, Vollmer's, Mendel's, Mantoux tests), undulant fever, tularemia, diphtheria (Schick test), scarlet fever (Dick test), glanders (mallein test), brucellosis, chancroid, North American blastomycosis, and others.

Commonly Used Skin Tests

Trichinella Spiralis (Pork Trichina) Skin Test

In a typical case of *Trichinella spiralis*, in which uncomplicated trichinosis has run a course of 2 weeks or more, sensitivity to *Trichinella* substance develops and can be detected by injection of *Trichinella* extract. The antigen used for the test is a 1:10,000 dilution of a saline extract of larvae of *Trichinella spiralis* freed from the tissues of the host in which the parasites were developed in the laboratory.

METHOD 1: *TRICHINELLA SPIRALIS* SKIN TEST

Method

1. A small volume of the antigen (0.1 ml or less) is injected intramuscularly on the forearm some distance from the elbow.
2. As a control, a similar injection is made with the saline solution used for extracting the larvae.

Interpretation

A positive skin reaction (indicating infection with *trichinellae* at some time, usually within the past 5 years or so) is of the immediate type. It is characterized by the development, within 20 minutes, of an elevated wheal, or edematous blanched area, from 8 to 15 mm in diameter, from which pseudopods may or may not radiate into the surrounding area of pronounced erythema. The contrast between the reaction to the antigen and the control solution constitutes the criterion for reading the results of the test.

The Tuberculin Skin Test

Purified protein derivative (PPD) in first, second, and intermediate strengths is available commercially.

One tenth of a milliliter of PPD is injected intradermally, forming a wheal. The test is read at 48 hours. A positive reaction is characterized by an area of definite palpable induration or edema. Redness can be disregarded. A positive test indicates the presence of a tuberculous focus in the body but does not distinguish between an active and an inactive lesion. A negative test practically rules out the existence of tuberculous infection at any age.

Brucellergin Skin Test

One tenth of a milliliter of antigen is injected intradermally and read at 48 hours. Readings are similar to the tuberculin skin test (previously described). A positive reaction occurs as a tender edematous plaque 1 to 6 cm in diameter. Positive tests denote the occurrence of infection without indication as to its activity.

Note: If agglutination tests are to be performed later, the skin test should *not* be performed, because it will stimulate the production of specific agglutinins.

Coccidioidin Skin Test

One tenth of a milliliter of a 1:100 solution is used. The solution is injected intradermally and read at 48 hours. The reading is similar to the tuberculin skin test (previously described).

Note: Previous pulmonary infection must be ruled out if the test is used to diagnose the cutaneous form of the disease because sensitization persists for a long period of time.

Frei Test (Lymphogranuloma Venereum)

One tenth of a milliliter each of antigen and control are injected intradermally and read after 48 hours. A positive test is characterized by an infiltrated inflammatory area with a small, well-defined papule not smaller than 7 mm in diameter.

Note: This test is not *specific* for lymphogranuloma venereum because of antigenic similarity to other viruses in this group.

Note: The patient should be asked about allergy to eggs, because the source of the injected material is infected chick embryo.

Histoplasmin Skin Test

For this test, undiluted filtrate is used. One tenth of a milliliter is injected intradermally and read at 48 hours. Readings are similar to the tuberculin test previously described. A high incidence of positive histoplasmin skin tests has been observed in certain areas of the United States, especially the midwest.

Schick Test

This test is used to indicate blood levels of diphtheria antitoxin. It involves the intradermal injection of a quantity of diphtheria toxin equal to one fiftieth of the guinea pig minimal lethal dose in one arm (the test site) and of an equal quantity of heat-inactivated diphtheria toxin in the other arm (the control site). A positive reaction appears as an area of redness that appears in 24 to 36 hours at the test site only and persists for 4 to 5 days, leaving an area of brownish pigmentation. This indicates a lack of immunity to diphtheria. A pseudoreaction involving an area of redness appearing at both sites and usually disappearing within 48 hours without residual pigmentation or a negative reaction indicates immunity.

Toxoplasmin Skin Test

One tenth of a milliliter each of antigen and control are injected in the flexor part of the arm and read at 48 hours. A positive test reveals induration of 100 mm or more with the control site negative.

Note: Material for the skin test cannot be obtained commercially.

Trichinella *Skin Test*

One tenth of a milliliter of allergen is injected intradermally. The test reveals an immediate reaction within 20 minutes, characterized by a wheal with an areola of hyperemia. A control should be run in parallel with the test, which must be negative for the result to be considered valid. This test is positive in almost 100 per cent of cases. It becomes positive approximately 2 weeks after contact and remains positive for several years. The positive reactions, however, cannot be considered *conclusive*, particularly if other parasites are present.

Vollmer's Patch Test

This test for tuberculous infection is used mainly for children because it is painless. The test is made by applying a specifically prepared tape, which has three small squares, the middle one being the control and other two being infiltrated with sensitivity agent. The tape is applied to either the flexor part of the arm or on the sternum and is left in place for 48 hours without wetting, after which time it is removed and read. A positive reaction consists of a red area with tiny vesicles. A negative reaction cannot be regarded as *excluding* tuberculous infection. The test has a further disadvantage in that the redness of a positive reaction can be confused with a simple reaction to the adhesive tape itself.

Delayed Hypersensitivity Skin Tests

Delayed hypersensitivity skin tests are an excellent measure of T-cell function because they measure the ability to recognize and present antigen, mobilize the T cells, and generate an inflammatory response. The major disadvantage is that the test is unreliable in infants (who have not had sufficient exposure to respond to antigens) and therefore is of no use at a time when T-cell functional assessment is very important. The test also has many technical shortcomings, although the use of multiple, antigen-coated, plastic puncture rings has obviated many of these (Kniker *et al.*, 1985).

CLASSIFICATION OF STREPTOCOCCI

Lancefield (1933) developed a method of serologic differentiation of human and other groups of hemolytic streptococci by means of precipitin reactions between solutions of the carbohydrate extracted from streptococcal cells and antisera prepared by immunizing rabbits with heat-killed suspensions of streptococci. The separation of hemolytic streptococci into distinct categories by this technique resulted in a classification related to the most characteristic source of the organisms. Thus group A is composed of strains usually pathogenic for humans, group B is composed of strains from bovine mastitis, group C is composed of strains commonly found in streptococcal diseases of lower animals, and so on. Groups A through O have been established.

Two other schemes of classification have been devised. Unfortunately, these schemes overlap and are therefore potentially confusing. One scheme divides the streptococci into physiologic divisions—pyogenic, viridans, lactic, and enterococcal. In the second scheme they are classified according to their hemolytic reactions—those that completely hemolyze the red cells about their colonies are called β-hemolytic, those that partially hemolyze the red cells are α-hemolytic, and those that do not hemolyze the red cells at all are γ-hemolytic.

In comparing these two latter schemes, the *pyogenic* group includes the β-hemolytic human and animal pyogenes, the *viridans* group includes the α-hemolytic, potentially pathogenic organisms occurring as normal flora in the human upper respiratory tract, the *lactic* group includes saprophytic forms associated with the souring of milk, and the *enterococcus* group includes organisms with variable hemolysis that are normal flora of the intestinal tract.

Both clinically and in the laboratory, these three classification schemes serve a useful purpose, and therefore it is generally not possible to eliminate any one of them completely.

ELEK'S DIFFUSION TEST

Elek (1948) devised a special modification of the double-diffusion method in two dimensions for demonstrating the toxigenicity of a given strain of *Corynebacterium diphtheriae*. In this method, diffusion is achieved in agar, with a special culture medium known as Elek's medium (preparation of Elek's medium follows). A strip of filter paper is soaked in diphtheria antitoxin and embedded in the agar in a Petri plate. The culture or cultures under study are then planted perpendicularly to the strips (Fig. 17–1).

At A-B (see Fig. 17–1), there is streaked a known toxigenic strain of *C. diphtheriae*. At X-Y is streaked the strain of *C. diphtheriae* under test. With the group of toxin-producing organisms, the toxin diffuses outward from the culture and at right angles to the line of diffusion of the antitoxin from the filter paper. A line of precipitation will form at the sites of cross-diffusion where antigen and antibody are in equal proportions. This precipitation line, which arises when a positive toxigenic organism is placed in the streak X-Y, will give an identical reaction and will so join with the similar line that arises from the reaction between the antitoxin and the known toxigenic strain in the streak A-B.

A simplification of this technique was described by Maniar and Fox (1968). This simplification of the Elek's method is given below.

METHOD 2: ELEK'S DOUBLE-DIFFUSION TEST

Materials

1. Test culture—a viable *C. diphtheriae* culture
2. Antitoxin—diphtheria antitoxin containing 4,000 IU per ml

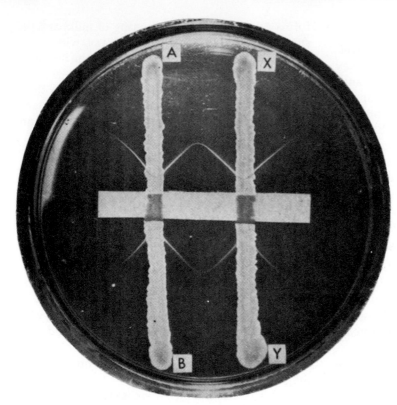

Figure 17–1. Elek's method for demonstrating toxigenicity of an unknown strain of *Corynebacterium diphtheriae*. (From Humphrey, J. H., and White, R. G.: Immunology of Students of Medicine, 3rd ed. Oxford, Blackwell Scientific Publications, 1970.)

3. Control culture—a toxin-producing strain of *C. diphtheriae*
4. Elek's medium (preparation method follows)
5. Sterile distilled water
6. Sterile filter-paper strips (0 × 1.0 cm Whatman filter paper No. 1)
7. Sterile Petri dishes

Preparation of Elek's Medium

Preparation A

Proteose peptone—4 gm
Maltose—0.6 gm
Lactic acid—0.14 ml
Distilled water—100 ml
Dissolve and adjust pH to 7.8.

Preparation B

Agar—3 gm
Sodium chloride—1 gm
Distilled water—100 ml
Dissolve by heat, filter, and adjust pH to 7.8.

Preparation C

Cisamino acid—1 gm
Tween 80—1 ml
Glycerol—1 ml
Distilled water—100 ml
Shake gently, heat to 50°C, dispense in 3.0 ml vials, and autoclave at 115°C for 15 minutes. Store at 4°C.

Mix equal parts of preparation A and preparation B, distribute 20 ml portions in screw-capped tubes, and sterilize by flowing steam for 30 minutes on 3 successive days. Store indefinitely at 4°C. For use, melt 1 tube, cool to below 55°C, and add 3.0 ml of preparation C. Pour plates.

Procedure

1. Aseptically mix 1.9 ml of sterile distilled water and 0.1 ml of antitoxin in a Petri dish.
2. Aseptically dip a filter-paper strip into the mixture until it is completely wet, and transfer it to an empty Petri dish for 30 minutes.
3. Apply a relatively dry strip to the center of a plate of solidified Elek's medium.

4. Inoculate the test culture in streaks perpendicular to the paper strip (see Fig. 17–1).
5. Inoculate at least 1 similar streak using the control culture.
6. Incubate at 35°C for up to 72 hours.
7. Read every 24 hours. The control culture should demonstrate lines of precipitation. Similar lines of precipitation by test cultures are indicative of toxin production by those cultures.

THE DETECTION AND IDENTIFICATION OF IMMUNOGLOBULIN AND OTHER SERUM PROTEINS

Specific immunoglobulins, as well as a wide range of other serum proteins, may be detected and identified by immunoelectrophoresis and single radial immunodiffusion tests.

The principle of immunoelectrophoresis has been described earlier in this text in Chapter 5. Figure 17–2 shows the use of the test in immunoglobulin class differentiation and detection.

Single radial immunodiffusion offers a much more accurate procedure for the identification and measurement of immunoglobulin (Mancini *et al.*, 1965). The test is based on the fact that when antigen diffuses from a well into agar containing suitable antiserum, the concentration of antigen continuously falls until the point is reached at which the reactants are in optimal proportions, and a ring of precipitation is formed. The higher the concentration of antigen, the greater the diameter of the ring (Fig. 17–3).

By incorporating standards of known antigen concentration in the plate, a calibration curve can be obtained and used to determine the amount of antigen in the unknown sample.

Absolute values can be determined with the use of plates from commercial companies. These plates can also be used, in most instances, for the detection of several other plasma or serum proteins.

In addition to the immunoglobulins, several proteins (e.g., albumin, haptoglobin, ceruloplasmin, α-2-macroglobulin, β-lipoprotein, transferrin, α-1-antitrypsin) can be detected and identified with the use of immunoelectrophoresis and radial immunodiffusion tests. Techniques are essentially the same with the substitution of suitable antibody in each case.

METHOD 3: IMMUNOGLOBULIN QUANTITATION BY IMMUNODIFFUSION

Materials

1. Radial immunodiffusion plates (RID) (available commercially)
2. Reference sera (available commercially)
3. 5-μl pipettes
4. Two-cycle semilog graph paper
5. Measuring device (available commercially)

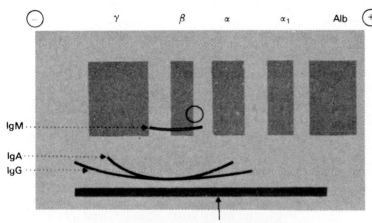

Figure 17–2. Demonstration of major immunoglobulin classes by immunoelectrophoretic analysis. (From Roitt, I.: Essential Immunology, 2nd ed. Oxford, Blackwell Scientific Publications, 1974.)

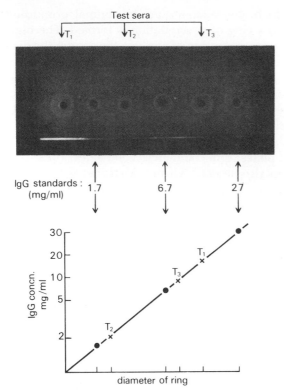

Figure 17–3. Single radial immunodiffusion. Relation of antigen concentration to size of precipitation ring formed. (From Roitt, I.: Essential Immunology, 2nd ed. Oxford, Blackwell Scientific Publications, 1974.)

Method

1. Allow the RID plates and reference sera to reach room temperature.
2. Dispense 5 μl of each of the 3 reference sera into wells, and repeat by adding 5 μl of test serum into a well.
3. Cover the plate. Place in a ziplock bag, and incubate at room temperature on a level surface for 18 hours (± 1/2 hour).
4. Measure the precipitin ring diameter to the nearest 0.1 mm.
5. Plot the reference sera concentrations against the zone diameter, and determine the concentration of the test sample from a graph.

TOXOPLASMOSIS

The causative organism of toxoplasmosis, *Toxoplasma gondii*, is one of the most common infectious agents of humans in the world. Since its isolation in 1908 in a North African rodent, the gondii, many species of birds, reptiles, and mammals have been found to harbor it.

Humans are infected with *Toxoplasma gondii* from the following sources:

Human

1. Mother to fetus.
2. Immunosuppression (induced or developmental)—organ transplantation or activation of quiescent infections.
3. Transfusion.

Animal

1. Ingestion of infected meat, especially mutton or pork.
2. Soil contamination by oocysts from domestic and feral cat feces.

Unknown

1. Acquisition by vegetarians?
2. Age, sex, and geographic differences.
3. Other—undefined.

Congenital toxoplasmosis is a disease with a very wide range of manifestations—so much so, in fact, that it must be considered in the differential diagnosis of almost all types of obscure illness occurring during early infancy. The symptoms are sometimes nonspecific (including anemia, splenomegaly, jaundice, fever, hepatomegaly, adenopathy, and vomiting), and because of this, toxoplasmosis is easily misdiagnosed on clinical grounds, even in sick infants who have the generalized form of the disease.

Tests for the Detection of Antibody to *Toxoplasma Gondii*

Toxoplasma gondii is difficult to culture and therefore diagnosis must be supported by serologic tests. Serologically, the demonstration of elevations of toxoplasma antibodies indicates infection. Antibodies can be demonstrated within the first 2 weeks after infection. These antibodies fall slightly but persist for many months, only declining to low levels after many years. Both IgG and IgM antibodies can be detected serologically. The presence of

IgM to *T. gondii* indicates active infection. In newborns, the presence of IgM antibodies also suggests active infection since IgM is not capable of crossing the placenta and therefore the antibodies are fetal in origin.

Note: Both clinical and laboratory findings in this disease resemble infectious mononucleosis.

Laboratory procedures for the *T. gondii* antibody include indirect fluorescent antibody (IFA), indirect hemagglutination (IHA), enzyme-linked immunoassay (EIA), complement fixation, and the Sabin-Feldman dye test. Of these, EIA is considered by many to be the method of choice. IFA is also commonly used, although the IFA titers have usually fallen in the second to fourth month, whereas EIA titers are usually elevated for 4 to 8 months. Also, IgM measured by EIA for toxoplasma-specific antibodies is positive in about 75 per cent of infants with proven congenital infection, compared with only 25 per cent positivity with IgM evaluation by the IFA method. Complement fixation is particularly useful when early sera are not available for specific IgM tests, since it commonly shows a fourfold rise in titer with sera taken during each of the first 3 months following the onset of symptoms. The Sabin-Feldman dye test is useful because it is sensitive and specific and has been diagnostic in problem cases, and because the titer peaks very early (usually in less than 4 weeks) and is persistent. The hemagglutination technique is least useful because an increase in titer usually takes 4 to 10 weeks.

A test kit for the quantitative determination of IgM antibodies to *Toxoplasma gondii* is available from Sigma Diagnostics, Sigma Chemical Company, St. Louis, MO. The test kit contains all of the chemicals required for performance of the test, but the laboratory should also have a spectrophotometer that accommodates a 1 ml volume or a microplate reader capable of accurately measuring absorbance at 405 nm, a pipetting device for the accurate delivery of 5 µl, 100 µl, and 200 µl volumes, a timer, a 1-liter measuring cylinder, squeeze bottle for dispensing wash solution, dilution plates or tubes, and 1 ml test tubes or cuvettes.

PREGNANCY TESTING

A number of serologic tests have been used in pregnancy testing, each designed to detect minute amounts of human chorionic gonadotropin (HCG) when it appears in the urine during the first few weeks of pregnancy.

The methods most commonly used now are based on the agglutination inhibition test developed by Noto and Miale (1964). This test consists of incubation of the patient's urine with anti-HCG, followed by the addition of latex particles coated with HCG. If HCG is present in the urine it neutralizes the antibody so that no agglutination of the latex particles is seen. If no HCG is present in the urine, agglutination occurs between the anti-HCG and HCG-coated latex particles.

The test gives reliable results about 42 days after the onset of the last normal menstrual period but is not reliable after the first trimester of pregnancy. The first morning urine specimen is required, and it should have a specific gravity of at least 1.015. It should be not more than 12 hours old from the time of collection; fresh urine may be frozen and tested later. Chorioepithelioma, hydatidiform mole, or excessive ingestion of aspirin may give false-positive results.

A number of test kits are available (Warner/Chilcott Laboratories, Morris Plains, NJ; Ortho Diagnostics, Raritan, NJ; and Organon Inc., West Orange, NJ) that give equally satisfactory results.

Home pregnancy kits utilize some of the discussed immunoassays. Manufacturers claim that these kits give 90 per cent accuracy (Hicks and Iosefsohn, 1989), although it is probably still true that laypersons experience more difficulty in performing and interpreting these tests than would qualified technologists.

LABORATORY TESTS FOR PERTUSSIS (WHOOPING COUGH)

The etiologic agent of pertussis, *Bordetella pertussis* (formerly known as *Haemophilus pertussis*), was isolated by Bordet and Gengou in 1906. It is a small, nonmotile, gram-negative rod. The detection of pertussis agglutinins can be made with suspensions of 10^9 organisms per milliliter of freshly isolated cultures of *B. pertussis* serotype 1,3 in saline, added in 0.4-ml volumes to equal volumes of serum dilutions. After incubation for 18 hours in a 37°C water bath, tests are read with a magnifying glass. The titer is expressed as the highest dilution yielding complete agglutination.

Complement fixation tests are more sensitive for pertussis antibody testing, although they are more complicated. (See Diagnosis of whooping cough: comparison of serologic tests with isolation of *Bordetella pertussis*. A combined Scottish study. Br. Med. J., 4:637, 1970.) In addition, a direct fluorescent antibody stain is available for the detection of *B. pertussis* in smears made from pharyngeal material. This reagent has proven very efficient for early diagnosis of cases of whooping cough (Young *et al.,* 1987; Welsh *et al.,* 1986).

An enzyme immunoassay for detection of antibody to *B. pertussis* has been shown to be valuable in diagnosing culture-negative patients (Steketee *et al.,* 1988). Commercial variations of this test are available from Labsystems-USA, Chicago, IL.

SEROLOGIC TESTS FOR LEPTOSPIRA

The leptospiroses are a group of diseases produced by a large number of antigenically distinct members of the genus *Leptospira*. At least 80 different serotypes and subserotypes of the genus have been identified. Several species of *Leptospira* are associated with human infection (Table 17–1). In addition to these pathogenic species, the genus also contains saprophytes, which are collectively designated as *Leptospira biflexa*.

Human leptospirosis can be definitely established either by isolating the disease agent from typical clinical specimens (e.g., blood and cerebrospinal fluid) or by demonstrating a significant rise in leptospiral antibody titer by serologic tests. Tests include the leptospiral agglutination test (Cole, 1973) and the hemagglutination test (Sulzer and Jones, 1973). The agglutination test requires microdilution plates available commercially. The hemagglutination test uses a soluble antigen coupled to sheep erythrocytes that are then fixed with glutaraldehyde. The sensitized cells are claimed to be stable for at least 1 year. (See Sulzer and Jones [1973] for the test procedure.) An enzyme-linked immunosorbent assay (ELISA) test for IgM antibody is available commercially.

TABLE 17–1. Leptospira Species Capable of Causing Human Infection

Species	Disease
L. australis	Canefield fever Field fever Mud fever Pomona fever
L. autumnalis	Akiyami Autumnal fever Fort Bragg fever Seven-day fever
L. bataviae	Ricefield fever Swineherd's disease Weil's disease
L. hebdomadis	Akiyami B Feld-fieber (field fever) B Seven-day fever
L. icterohaemorrhagiae	Infectious or leptospiral jaundice Weil's disease
L. canicola	Canicola fever
L. pyrogenes	Canefield fever Leptospirosis febrilis

GENERAL LABORATORY TECHNIQUES

Complement Fixation

Methods of complement fixation include manual techniques, test tube techniques, and automated micro methods (slow fixation and rapid fixation). The standard micro method that uses 0.025 ml of all reagents will be described here. The volumes and procedure can easily be adapted from this procedure to suit any specific requirements.

METHOD 4: COMPLEMENT FIXATION

Materials

1. Hemolysin—This is a serum that contains antibodies to sheep erythrocytes (see preparation of sheep red cell hemolysin, later).
2. Sheep erythrocytes (see collection and preservation of sheep blood, later).
3. Alsever's solution—This is prepared with 1,000 ml distilled water, 0.55 gm citric acid, 8.0

gm sodium citrate, 4.2 gm sodium chloride, and 20.5 gm dextrose.

4. Citrate solution—This is prepared with 2.08 gm sodium citrate and 2.5 gm dextrose in 100 ml distilled water.
5. Diluent—Veronal-buffered saline is most commonly used. This is prepared with 85.0 gm sodium chloride, 5.75 gm diethybarbituric acid, and 3.75 gm sodium barbital in 2,000 ml distilled water.
6. Microtiter plates (available commercially).
7. Complement—Usually from guinea pig serum (see preparation and preservation of complement, later).
8. Antigens—A variety are used, available commercially.
9. Antigen medium (normal antigen)—This is necessary when testing for viral antibodies and is prepared in the same way as viral antigen except that normal cells (rather than virus-infected cells) are used. The medium serves as a control to test each serum for cellular antibodies, which lead to false-positive results.
10. Test serum—Patient's serum, inactivated at 56°C for 30 minutes. Stored sera (i.e., for more than 1 day) should be inactivated before use (10 minutes at 60°C). Because antibody titers will decrease on storage and cause the sera to become anticomplementary, they should not be stored for long periods of time (see preparation and preservation of complement, later).

Preliminary Tests

Preliminary tests to determine the efficiency of the many reagents used in the complement fixation test should be carried out on each new batch of reagent.

Hemolysin

A titration of hemolysin should be performed whenever a new batch of cells of a new hemolysin is used.

1. Dilute the hemolysin 1:1,000.
2. Set up 1 row of 8 test tubes in a test tube rack.
3. Make the following dilutions of hemolysin in buffered saline:

Tube No.	Hemolysin	Buffered Saline	Dilution
1	1.0	0	1,000
2	0.66	0.34	1,500
3	0.5	0.5	2,000
4	0.33	0.67	3,000
5	0.25	0.75	4,000
6	0.166	0.834	6,000
7	0.125	0.875	8,000
8	0	1.0	0

4. Using separate pipettes for each tube, add 1.0 ml of a 2 per cent suspension of sheep erythrocytes to each tube. Mix.
5. Allow to stand (sensitize) at room temperature.
6. Dilute complement 1:10.

TABLE 17–2. Complement Dilutions in Complement Fixation

Dilutions of Hemolysin	Dilutions of Complement								
	1:10	1:15	1:20	1:30	1:40	1:60	1:80	1:120	0
0	4	4	4	4	4	4	4	4	4
1:8,000	2	3	4	4	4	4	4	4	4
1:6,000	1	1	1	2	2	3	3	3	4
1:4,000	tr	0	0	0	1	2	3	3	4
1:3,000	0	0	0	1	2	3	3	3	4
1:2,000	0	0	0	0	0	tr	2	3	4
1:1,500	0	0	0	0	0	0	1	3	4
1:1,000	0	0	0	0	0	tr	1	3	4

Interpretation
0=Complete hemolysis   2=50% cells
tr=10% cells   3=75% cells
1=25% cells   4=100% cells (no hemolysis)

7. Set up 1 row of 8 test tubes in a test tube rack.
8. Make the same dilutions of complement as made for hemolysin (step 3).
9. Deliver 0.025 ml of complement dilutions into the wells of a microplate, as shown in Table 17–2.
10. Add 0.05 ml of saline to each well as a substitute for the serum and antigen in the actual tests.
11. Allow plates to stand at 37°C for 90 minutes.
12. After incubation, deliver 0.025 ml of the sensitized cells (step 5) in a checkerboard fashion (as in step 9).
13. Shake gently but firmly. Incubate at 37°C for 30 minutes. Shake again at 15 minutes and on removal from the incubator.
14. Read. (Note: Plates need not be read immediately but may be left for several hours at room temperature if desired.)

Complement

Each new batch of complement should be titrated as follows:
1. Set up 10 test tubes in a test tube rack.
2. Dilute complement 1:10.
3. Make the following dilutions of complement in saline:

Tube No.	Complement	Saline	Dilution
1	1.0	0	1:10
2	0.66	0.34	1:15
3	0.5	0.5	1:20
4	0.33	0.67	1:30
5	0.25	0.75	1:40
6	0.16	0.84	1:60
7	0.12	0.88	1:80
8	0.08	0.92	1:120
9	0.06	0.94	1:160
10	0	1.0	0

4. Mix and deliver 0.025 ml of each dilution into separate wells in a row of wells on a microplate.
5. Incubate plate at 37°C for 90 minutes.
6. After incubation, deliver 0.025 ml of sensitized cells in a checkerboard fashion (see step 12 under titration of hemolysin).
7. Shake gently but firmly and incubate at 37°C for 30 minutes. Shake at 15 minutes and again on removal from the incubator.

8. Read. The HD_{50} (hemolytic dose, 50 per cent) is taken as the dilution that gives 2+ hemolysis (50 per cent). In the actual test, 2.5 HD_{50} is used. This is derived by dividing the dilution showing 50 per cent hemolysis by 2.5.

Antigen

Each batch of new antigen should be subject to all three of the following titrations:

Anticomplementary Titration

1. Add 0.025 ml of diluent to wells 2 through 9 of a microplate.
2. Add 0.025 ml of antigen to wells 1 and 2. Mix and serially dilute to well 9. Discard 0.025 ml of the final dilution in well 9.
3. Add 0.025 ml of diluent to all wells.
4. Add 0.025 ml of complement (2.5 HD_{50}) to each well and shake gently.
5. Incubate. (Some systems require overnight incubation at 4°C; others require 2 hours at room temperature. Such requirements are usually indicated in the instruction inserts with commercial antigens. As a general rule, bacterial, influenzal, and chlamydial antigens require 2 hours at room temperature; all others give better results if incubated overnight at 4°C.)
6. Add 0.25 ml of sensitized sheep erythrocytes to all wells.
7. Shake gently and place in a 37°C water bath for 30 minutes.
8. Read. No fixation should occur in any well. If, however, a slight degree of fixation is noted in the first or second well, the antigen may still be used if the maximal reactivity titer is high.

Hemolytic Titration

1. Repeat steps 1 and 2 under anticomplementary titration.
2. Add 0.05 ml of diluent to each well.
3. Add 0.025 ml of sensitized sheep erythrocytes to all wells.
4. Place immediately in a 37°C water bath for 30 minutes.
5. Read. No hemolysis should occur in any well. If a small degree of hemolysis occurs in a very low titer, however, the antigen may still be used if the maximal specific reactivity is to a higher titer.

Reactivity Titration

1. Set up a block titration by serially diluting a positive serum and the antigen in test tubes and then distributing 0.025 ml of each into the wells of a microplate in a checkerboard fashion.
2. Add 0.025 ml of complement (2.5 HD_{50}) to all wells.
3. Set up controls as described under test controls (later).
4. Incubate as for long or short fixation (see step 5 under anticomplementary titration).
5. Add 0.025 ml of sensitized sheep erythrocytes to all wells.
6. Shake and place in a 37°C water bath for 30 minutes.
7. Read. A calculation is made to determine two antigenic units per 0.025 ml. The *antigenic unit* is read as the highest dilution of the hyperimmune serum that gives a 4+ reaction in the presence of the highest dilution of antigen.

Procedure

1. Deliver 0.75 ml of diluent to well 1 and 0.025 ml to wells 2 through 7 of 1 row of wells in a microplate.
2. Add 0.025 ml of test serum to well 1. Mix and transfer 0.025 ml of the mixture to well 2 through to well 6. Wells 7 and 8 serve as serum controls. Discard 0.025 ml of the final 1:128 dilution in well 6.
3. Add 0.025 ml of antigen (2 units) to each of wells 1 through 6. Add 0.025 ml of antigen medium to well 8, if necessary (see antigen medium under materials).
4. Add 0.025 ml of complement (2.5 HD_{50}) to each well.
5. Incubate as required (see step 5 under anticomplementary titration).
6. Add 0.025 ml of sensitized sheep erythrocytes to each well.
7. Shake and place in a 37°C water bath for 30 minutes.
8. Read. The titer is expressed as the highest serum dilution that will allow fixation of enough complement to prevent 50 per cent of cell lysis, provided that all controls give the appropriate results (see test controls, following).

Test Controls

1. Antigen hemolytic control—0.025 ml of antigen, 0.05 ml of diluent, no complement, 0.025 ml of sensitized erythrocytes. Correct reading, 4+ (no hemolysis).
2. Antigen anticomplementary control—0.025 ml of antigen, 0.025 ml of diluent, 0.025 ml of complement, 0.025 ml of sensitized erythrocytes. Correct reading, 0 (complete hemolysis).
3. Complement controls:
   a. 0.05 ml of diluent, 0.025 ml of complement, 0.025 ml of sensitized erythrocytes. Correct reading, 0 (complete hemolysis).
   b. 0.065 ml of diluent, 0.01 ml of complement, 0.025 ml of sensitized erythrocytes. Correct reading, 2+ (50 per cent hemolysis).
4. Cell control (also diluent control)—0.075 ml of diluent, 0.025 ml of sensitized erythrocytes. Correct reading, 4+ (no hemolysis).
5. Known positive and negative serum controls—Correct reading positive serum, 4+ (no hemolysis) up to its titer. Correct reading negative serum, 0 (complete hemolysis).
6. Test serum—antigen medium control: well 7 of the actual test. Correct reading, 0 (complete hemolysis).
7. Test serum—anticomplementary control: well 8 of the actual test. Correct reading, 0 (complete hemolysis).

METHOD 5: COMPLEMENT FIXATION INHIBITION

Materials

As for complement fixation. In addition, an indicator antibody is used.
1. Indicator antibody—Serum that will fix complement in the presence of the test antigen.
2. Test sera—Usually avian samples that fail to fix complement in the presence of the test antigen.

Preliminary Tests

The same preliminary tests are required as described under complement fixation. In addition, the indicator antibody needs to be titrated prior to use, as follows:

1. Prepare serial twofold dilutions of the indicator serum in 0.025 ml volumes in a row of wells in a microplate.
2. Add to each well 0.025 ml volumes of antigen containing two CF units each.
3. Add 0.025 ml of 2.5 HD_{50} complement to each well.
4. Incubate as required (see step 5 under anticomplementary titration).
5. Add 0.025 ml of sensitized erythrocytes to each well.
6. Shake gently and reincubate at 37°C for 30 minutes.
7. Read. The highest serum dilution that will fix 100 per cent of the complement (no hemolysis) is taken as 1 unit of indicator antibody.

Procedure

1. Proceed with steps 1, 2, and 3 as described under the procedure for complement fixation.
2. Add 0.025 ml of the indicator antibody serum as determined by titration, to each of wells 1 through 6. Add 0.01 ml of antigen medium to well 7, if necessary.
3. Add 0.025 ml of complement (2.5 HD_{50}) to each well.
4. Incubate as required.
5. Add 0.025 ml of sensitized erythrocytes to each well.
6. Shake gently.
7. Place in a 37°C water bath for 30 minutes.
8. Read. The titer is read as the highest dilution of test serum that will completely inhibit complement fixation. This will be the last well in which complete lysis is demonstrated.

Test Controls

In addition to the controls discussed under complement fixation, the following must also be incorporated in each test run:

1. Test serum—Antigen control: 0.025 ml of test serum, 0.025 ml of antigen, 0.025 ml of diluent, 0.025 ml of complement, and 0.025 ml of sensitized erythrocytes. Correct reading, 0 (complete hemolysis).
2. Test serum—Indicator antibody control: 0.025

ml of each of the following: diluent, indicator antibody, complement, and sensitized erythrocytes. Correct reading, 0 (complete hemolysis).
3. Antigen—Indicator antibody control: 0.025 ml of each of the following: diluent, antigen, indicator antibody, complement, and sensitized erythrocytes. Correct reading, 4+ (no hemolysis).
4. Antigen medium—Indicator antibody control (if necessary): 0.025 ml of each of the following: diluent, antigen medium, indicator antibody, complement, and sensitized erythrocytes. Correct reading, 0 (complete hemolysis).

METHOD 6: HEMAGGLUTINATION INHIBITION

Materials

1. Test serum—Nonspecific agglutinins present in normal serum must be removed before use (method to follow).
2. Antigen—Commercially available. Antigens must be titrated before used (method to follow).
3. Red cells—See Table 17–3 for species recommended with the particular antigen. Make up 50 per cent and 0.05 per cent suspension in appropriate dilution.
4. Diluent—0.85 per cent saline or HEPES-saline-albumin-gelatin (HSAG) diluent (preparation of HSAG diluent given later).
5. Test tubes or microplates—10 × 75 round bottomed test tubes or V-bottomed microplates (available commercially).
6. Diluting loops—For microplate technique.
7. Positive and negative control sera.

Preliminary Procedures

The procedure described here uses 0.1-ml volumes of all reagents. Volumes will differ depending upon whether tubes or microplates are used but can be adjusted according to the technique chosen. Temperature and incubation times will also differ depending upon the virus used, as will the erythrocytes used. General instructions given in this procedure can be adjusted to suit the virus under test by the technologist engaged in the testing (see Table 17–3).

TABLE 17–3. Cells, Incubation Times, and Temperatures for Various Hemagglutination-Inhibition Systems

Virus	Erythrocytes	Time for Ab-Ag Reaction	Time for Agglutination	Temperature of Incubation (°C)
Influenza Parainfluenza Mumps Sendai Reovirus	Human—Group O	15 min	60	20
Enterovirus	Human—Group O	15 min	60	4
Measles (Rubeola)	Rhesus or vervet monkey	15 min	90	37
Rubella	Baby chick at 4°C	60 min	90	4
Adenovirus	Rhesus monkey	15 min	90	37
Vaccinia Smallpox	Chicken	30 min	90	20

Preparation of Erythrocytes

See preparation of red cell concentrations later in this chapter.

Preparation of HSAG Diluent (If Required)

Solution A

1. HEPES (N-2-hydroxyethyl-piperazine-N-2-ethanesulfonic acid)—29.8 gm
2. Sodium chloride—40.95 gm
3. Calcium chloride ($CaCl_2 \cdot 2H_2O$)—0.74 gm
4. Distilled water—1,000 ml

Dissolve the chemicals in 900 ml of distilled water. Adjust the pH with approximately 12 ml of 1 N sodium hydroxide to 6.5. Add more distilled water to bring to 1,000 ml. Sterilize by filtration and store at 4°C.

Solution B

1. Bovine albumin powder—25 mg
2. Distilled water—1,000 ml

Dissolve the albumin in 900 ml of water and adjust the volume to 1,000 ml. Sterilize by filtration and store at 4°C.

Solution C

1. Gelatin—25 mg
2. Distilled water—1,000 ml

Dissolve the gelatin. Sterilize in an autoclave at 120°C for 15 minutes and store at 4°C.

HSAG diluent is prepared by mixing 200 ml of solution A, 500 ml of solution B, and 100 ml of solution C in 200 ml of sterile distilled water. Adjust the pH to 6.2 with 1 N sodium hydroxide or hydrochloric acid if necessary. Store at 4°C for up to 2 months.

Titration of Antigen

1. Set out 10 tubes in a test tube rack.
2. Add 0.1 ml of diluent to each tube.
3. Deliver 0.1 ml of antigen to tube 1, mix, transfer 0.1 ml to tube 2, and so on. Discard 0.1 ml of the final dilution in tube 9.
4. Add 0.1 ml of diluent to each tube.
5. Add 0.1 ml of 0.5 per cent erythrocytes to each tube. (The same erythrocyte suspension should be used in this preliminary test and in the actual test.)
6. Shake (microplates must be shaken on a mechanical vibrator for 1 minute).
7. Incubate.
8. Read. The cell control (tube 10) should show no hemagglutination. The antigen titer (1 unit) is the

reciprocal of the highest dilution yielding complete hemagglutination. In the actual test, 4 units of antigen must be used. These are obtained simply by dividing the true titer by 4.

Removal of Nonspecific Agglutinins

1. To 1.0 ml of test serum add one drop (0.03 ml) of 50 per cent erythrocytes. (These should be of the same species required for the test antigen; refer to Table 17–3.)
2. Shake and leave at room temperature for 15 minutes.
3. Centrifuge at 1,500 rpm for 10 minutes.
4. Aspirate the supernatant fluid.

Removal of Nonspecific Inhibitors

Absorption with Kaolin

1. Mix 1.0 ml of test serum (the supernatant fluid collected in the removal of nonspecific agglutinations) with 1.0 ml of a 50 per cent suspension of acid-washed kaolin in saline.
2. Leave for 30 minutes at room temperature, shaking periodically.
3. Centrifuge at 1,500 rpm for 15 minutes.
4. Collect the clear supernatant fluid.

This method removes all nonspecific inhibitors. It does not, however, lend itself well to the absorption of sera to be tested against some viral antigens, such as rubella.

Absorption with Heparin-Manganese Chloride

1. Prepare a mixture of equal volumes of 5,000 units (USP) per milliliter of sodium heparin and a filtration-sterilized solution of 19.8 per cent manganese chloride ($MnCl_2 \cdot 4H_2O$). This solution may be stored at 4°C for up to 2 weeks.
2. Mix 0.2 ml of test serum (the supernatant fluid removed in the removal of nonspecific agglutinins) with 0.4 ml of HSAG diluent.
3. Add 0.2 ml of the heparin-manganese chloride solution.
4. Shake and incubate at 4°C for 15 minutes.

5. Centrifuge at 4°C for 15 minutes at 1,500 rpm.
6. Aspirate the supernatant fluid.

Note: When making dilutions in the actual test, the first method given will dilute the test serum 1:2, and the second method 1:4.

Procedure

1. Set up 10 test tubes in a test tube rack. (A microplate may also be used.)
2. Deliver 0.1 ml of treated test serum to tubes 1, 2, and 10 and 0.1 ml of diluent to tubes 2 through 10.
3. Mix the contents of tube 2, transfer 0.1 ml to tube 3, mix and transfer 0.1 ml to tube 4, and so on up to tube 9. Discard 0.1 ml of the final dilution in tube 9. Tube 10 will serve as the serum-erythrocyte control. Serum treated with kaolin will yield dilutions of 1:2 to 1:512; serum treated with heparin-MnCl₂ will yield dilutions of 1:4 to 1:1,024.
4. Add 0.1 ml of antigen (containing 4 units) to tubes 1 through 9.
5. Shake and incubate as required (see Table 17–3).
6. Add 0.1 ml of 0.5 per cent erythrocytes to all tubes.
7. Shake and incubate as required (see Table 17–3).
8. Read. The antibody titer is the reciprocal of the highest serum dilution in which 50 per cent or more of the hemagglutination is inhibited.

Test Controls

1. Test serum-erythrocyte control—Tube 10 of each series of test serum dilutions should show no hemagglutination.
2. Antigen control—0.1 ml of diluent, antigen, and erythrocytes. Final result, complete hemagglutination.
3. Red cell control—0.2 ml of diluent and 0.1 ml of erythrocytes. Final result, no agglutination.
4. Positive and negative serum controls—Set up in the same manner as the test sera. These should read their exact, known titers.

COLLECTION AND PRESERVATION OF SHEEP BLOOD

Blood is collected from the jugular vein of the animal, defibrinated, and stored at 4°C. The sheep red cells may be stored for 1 week provided that no hemolysis becomes visible. If sheep red cells are difficult to obtain, they may be collected in Alsever's solution or citrate in larger volumes and stored at 4°C for approximately 1 month. Cells should not be used until after stabilization, which takes 2 to 3 days of storage at 4°C.

Before use, the cells must be filtered through two layers of cotton gauze and washed three times in buffered saline, with centrifugation of the cells at 2,000 rpm each time. After each washing, the buffy coat of white cells should be removed with a pipette. Any red cells that stick to the side of the tube should be removed with a wooden applicator stick. After the final washing the supernatant fluid must be perfectly clear. This final suspension is centrifuged for 15 to 20 minutes to pack the cells.

To sensitize the cells, a 2 per cent suspension of cells is made up in diluent. An equal volume of hemolysin dilution is prepared, and these two are mixed by pouring the *cells* into the *hemolysin* and then pouring back and forth from one bottle to the other about 10 times. The mixture is then left to sensitize for 30 minutes at 37°C.

PREPARATION OF SHEEP RED CELL HEMOLYSIN

The method of preparing sheep red cell hemolysin is to inject whole sheep blood intracutaneously into rabbits and then to inoculate washed sheep cells intravenously. Sheep red cell hemolysin is readily available commercially, however, and is usually supplied as a 50 per cent glycerinated suspension. A dilution of 1:100 is made by adding 2.0 ml of glycerinated hemolysin to 94.0 ml of buffered saline and then adding 4.0 ml of 5 per cent phenol solution as a preservative. The dilution constitutes the stock solution and is stable for about 3 months at 4°C.

PREPARATION AND PRESERVATION OF COMPLEMENT

Complement, usually from guinea pig serum, is available from many commercial houses. It must be stored in a cold room at 4°C or in an ice bath while tests are being carried out. In a dried state, it can be stored indefinitely in a cold room at 4°C. Dissolved in distilled water, it should be stored at −20°C. When preparing dilutions of complement, care should be taken to avoid excess shaking or vigorous pipetting because this can cause inactivation.

PREPARATION OF RED CELL CONCENTRATIONS

Blood collected in anticoagulant from a human, sheep, or other source is washed in three volumes of diluent (saline) by mixing, centrifuging at 1,500 rpm for 15 minutes, and aspirating until the supernatant is completely clear. The cells are resuspended to a 50 per cent suspension in diluent and can be stored at 4°C for up to 2 weeks. For more tests, the required suspensions may be made directly from the 50 per cent suspension in diluent. If more exact suspensions are required, a standardization procedure should be performed as follows:

METHOD 7: PREPARATION OF RED CELL CONCENTRATIONS

1. Prepare solutions of cyanmethemoglobin (CMG) in CMG diluent reagent containing 80, 60, 40, 20, and 0 mg CMG per 100 ml.
2. Read each solution in a spectrophotometer at the 540-nm wavelength. Plot the readings on regular graph paper against milligrams per 100 ml of the standard CMG. This should produce a straight line.
3. Calculate the factor to be used for determining the target optical density (OD). The factor will be the sum of the concentrations of the standards (80+60+40+20+0) divided by the sum of the OD readings obtained.
4. Calculate the target OD. The target OD is the target number of milligrams of CMG per 100 ml divided by the factor obtained in step 3. Once

the targets and factors for a given cell suspension have been established, they can be used for all subsequent standardizations, provided that the spectrophotometer is not moved or jarred.

JUST THE FACTS

Opsonocytophagic Tests

1. Opsonocytophagic tests detect the presence in a patient's serum of opsonins against certain bacteria.
2. The opsonic power of a patient's blood in relation to the opsonic power of normal blood is known as the "opsonic index."
3. Opsonocytophagic tests are occasionally used in cases of brucellosis, although they are of doubtful diagnostic value in the disease.

Bacteriolysin

1. A bacteriolysin is an antibody that causes the dissolution of bacteria.
2. Bacteriolysins are found in the blood serum of animals who are naturally immune to a particular antigen, as well as in those who have been artificially immunized against an antigen by injection.
3. Bacteriolysins destroy the bacterial cell itself.
4. Complement is necessary for the reaction to take place.
5. Lysins have been produced for a variety of cells other than bacterial and are highly specific.

Rubella

1. Acquired rubella (German measles or 3-day measles) is caused by an enveloped, single-stranded RNA virus of the togavirus family.
2. The disease is highly contagious and is transmitted through respiratory secretions.
3. Vaccination has decreased the incidence of rubella.
4. Signs and symptoms vary greatly from one individual to another.
5. The incubation period in acquired rubella is 10 to 21 days.
6. Patients are contagious for 12 to 15 days, beginning 5 to 7 days after the appearance of a rash.

7. The acute form usually lasts from 3 to 5 days.
8. The disease requires minimal treatment, and permanent effects are rare.
9. Symptoms include enlarged lymph nodes, rash, and low fever.
10. When the disease occurs in older children and adults, self-limiting arthralgia and arthritis are common.
11. Rubella infection in pregnant women can have devastating effects on the fetus.
12. Both IgM and IgG antibodies appear as the result of primary rubella infection. The IgM antibody becomes clinically undetectable within 4 to 5 weeks, while the IgG antibody remains present and protective indefinitely.

Serologic Tests for Rubella

1. Hemagglutination inhibition is the most widely used test.
2. Other tests include passive latex agglutination, the semiquantitative immunoassay (an indirect enzyme-labeled immunosorbent assay using microwells as a solid phase), fluorescent immunoassay (which gives quantitative results), and passive hemagglutination.
3. Complement fixation is unsuitable in rubella testing, because the CR antibody disappears after infection.

Skin Tests

1. Skin tests are usually carried out in allergic or immunologic conditions.
2. There are three types of skin tests: intradermal, scratch tests, and patch tests.
3. The commonly used skin tests are the *Trichinella spiralis* (pork trichina) skin test, the tuberculin skin test, the brucellergin skin test (which should not be performed if agglutination tests are to be performed later because it will stimulate the production of specific agglutinins), the coccidioidin skin test, the Frei test for lymphogranuloma venereum, the histoplasmin skin test, the Schick test (used to indicate blood levels of diphtheria antitoxin), the toxoplasmin skin test, the trichinella skin test, Vollmer's patch test (for tuberculosis infection and used mainly for children because it is painless), and delayed hypersensitivity skin tests (which measure T-cell function).

Classification of Streptococci

1. Three schemes have been developed to classify streptococci:
   a. Lancefield grouping separates hemolytic streptococci into distinct categories by means of precipitin reactions between solutions of the carbohydrate extracted from streptococcal cells and antisera prepared by immunizing rabbits with heat-killed suspensions of streptococci. The scheme differentiates between human and other groups of hemolytic streptococci.
   b. The second scheme divides streptococci into physiologic divisions (pyogenic, viridans, lactic, and enterococcal).
   c. The third scheme classifies streptococci according to their hemolytic reactions—those that completely hemolyze red cells about their colonies are called β-hemolytic, those that partially hemolyze are α-hemolytic, and those that do not hemolyze at all are γ-hemolytic.
2. All three schemes are useful, and it is generally not possible to eliminate any one of them completely.

Elek's Diffusion Test

1. This is a modification of the double-diffusion method in two dimensions for demonstrating the toxigenicity of a given strain of *Corynebacterium diphtheriae*.

The Detection and Identification of Immunoglobulin and Other Serum Proteins

1. Specific immunoglobulins, as well as a wide range of other serum proteins, may be detected and identified by immunoelectrophoresis and single radial immunodiffusion tests.

Toxoplasmosis

1. The causative organism of toxoplasmosis is *Toxoplasma gondii.*
2. It is found in a North African rodent, many species of birds, reptiles, and mammals.
3. Sources of infection are human (mother to fetus, immunosuppression, transfusion), animal (ingestion of infected meat—especially mutton or pork, and soil contamination by oocysts from domestic and feral cat feces), and others.
4. Congenital toxoplasmosis has a very wide range of manifestations and because of this it is easily misdiagnosed, even in sick infants who have the generalized form of the disease.

Tests for the Detection of Antibody to Toxoplasma Gondii

1. Both IgG and IgM antibodies to *Toxoplasma gondii* can be detected serologically.
2. The presence of IgM to *T. gondii* indicates active infection.
3. Laboratory procedures include indirect fluorescent antibody (IFA), indirect hemagglutination (IHA), enzyme-linked immunoassay (EIA), complement fixation (CF), and the Sabin-Feldman dye test.
4. Of these, enzyme-linked immunoassay is considered by many to be the method of choice, because titers are elevated for 4 to 8 months, and because IgM measured by this technique for *Toxoplasma*-specific antibodies is positive in about 75 per cent of infants with proven congenital infection, compared to only 25 per cent positivity with IgM evaluation by the IFA method.
5. IFA titers have usually fallen in the second to fourth month.
6. Complement fixation is useful when early sera are not available for specific IgM tests, since it commonly shows a fourfold rise in titer with sera taken during the first 3 months following the onset of symptoms.
7. The Sabin-Feldman dye test is useful because the titer peaks very early and is persistent. It is also sensitive and specific and has been diagnostic in problem cases.
8. The hemagglutination technique is least useful because an increase in titer usually takes 4 to 10 weeks.

Pregnancy Testing

1. Serologic tests are used to detect minute amounts of human chorionic gonadotropin (HCG) when it appears in the urine during the first few weeks of pregnancy.

2. The methods used are based on the agglutination inhibition test.
3. The test gives reliable results about 42 days after the onset of the last normal menstrual period but is not reliable after the first trimester of pregnancy.
3. A number of test kits are available.
4. Home pregnancy kits are claimed to give 90 per cent accuracy.

Laboratory Tests for Pertussis (Whooping Cough)

1. *Bordetella pertussis* is the etiologic agent for pertussis.
2. Tests include the detection of pertussis agglutinins, complement fixation, a direct fluorescent antibody stain for the detection of *B. pertussis* in smears made from pharyngeal material, and enzyme immunoassay, which is valuable in diagnosing culture-negative patients.

Serologic Tests for *Leptospira*

1. The leptospiroses are a group of diseases produced by a large number of antigenically distinct members of the genus *Leptospira*.
2. Several species are associated with human infection (see Table 17–1).
3. Human leptospirosis can be definitely established by isolating the disease agent from typical clinical specimens (blood or cerebrospinal fluid).
4. Serologic tests, which demonstrate a significant rise in leptospiral antibody titer, include the leptospiral agglutination test, the hemagglutination test, and an enzyme-linked immunosorbent assay test for IgM antibody.

Review Questions

Multiple Choice

Choose the phrase, sentence, or symbol that completes the statement or answers the question. More than one answer may be correct in each case. Answers are given at the end of this book.

1. The expression of the opsonic power of a patient's blood in relation to the opsonic power of "normal" blood is known as:
   (a) the opsonic factor
   (b) the opsonic expression
   (c) the opsonic index
   (d) none of the above
   (Opsonocytophagic Tests)

2. Bacteriolysins:
   (a) are antibodies that cause the dissolution of bacteria
   (b) are found in the blood stream of animals who are naturally immune to a particular antigen
   (c) are found in the blood stream of animals who have been artificially immunized against an antigen by injection
   (d) destroy the bacterial cell itself in the presence of complement
   (Bacteriolysin)

3. Acquired rubella has an incubation period of:
   (a) 2 to 3 days
   (b) 10 to 21 days
   (c) 40 to 50 days
   (d) 10 to 21 hours
   (Characteristics of Rubella)

4. The most widely used technique for the detection of antibodies to rubella is:
   (a) the complement fixation test
   (b) passive hemagglutination
   (c) hemagglutination inhibition
   (d) none of the above
   (Serologic Tests for Rubella)

5. Intradermal skin tests are commonly used for:
   (a) tuberculin
   (b) histoplasmin
   (c) coccidioidin
   (d) all of the above
   (The Performance of Skin Tests)

6. Delayed hypersensitivity skin tests:
   (a) are an excellent measure of B-cell function
   (b) are an excellent measure of T-cell function
   (c) are unreliable in infants
   (d) measure the ability of T cells to recognize and present antigen
   (Delayed Hypersensitivity Skin Tests)

7. In the classification of streptococci, the pyogenic group includes:
(a) the β-hemolytic human and animal pyogens
(b) the α-hemolytic, potentially pathogenic organisms occurring in normal flora in the human upper respiratory tract
(c) saprophytic forms associated with the souring of milk
(d) organisms with variable hemolysis that are normal flora of the intestinal tract
(Classification of Streptococci)

8. Human infection by *Toxoplasma gondii* can occur:
(a) from mother to fetus
(b) in immunosuppression
(c) through the ingestion of infected pork
(d) through transfusion
(Toxoplasmosis)

9. Antibodies developed in response to *T. gondii* infection are:
(a) IgG only
(b) IgM only
(c) IgG and IgM
(d) IgE
(Tests for the Detection of Antibody to Toxoplasma Gondii*)*

Answer "True" or "False"

1. Rubella infection in pregnant women can have devastating effects on the fetus.
(Characteristics of Rubella)

2. The complement fixation test is useful for rubella testing *after* infection.
(Serologic Tests for Rubella)

3. The Schick test is used to indicate blood levels of diphtheria antitoxin.
(Schick Test)

4. The Elek's diffusion test method demonstrates the toxigenicity of a given strain of *Corynebacterium diphtheriae*.
(Elek's Diffusion Test)

5. The presence of IgM to *Toxoplasma gondii* indicates active infection.
(Tests for Detection of Antibody to Toxoplasma Gondii*)*

6. Human chorionic gonadotropin appears in the urine after the first trimester of pregnancy.
(Pregnancy Testing)

7. The etiologic agent of pertussis is *Bordetella pertussis*.
(Laboratory Tests for Pertussis [Whooping Cough])

8. Leptospira is not associated with human infection.
(Serologic Tests for Leptospira)

GENERAL REFERENCES

Baron, E.J., and Finegold, S.M.: Bailey and Scott's Diagnostic Microbiology, 8th ed. St. Louis, C.V. Mosby Company, 1990.
Dorland's Illustrated Medical Dictionary, 27th ed. Philadelphia, W. B. Saunders Company, 1988.
Freeman, B.A.: Burrows Textbook of Microbiology, 27th ed. Philadelphia, W. B. Saunders Company, 1985.
Henry, J.B.: Clinical Diagnosis and Management by Laboratory Methods. Philadelphia, W. B. Saunders Company, 1991.
Sheehan, C.: Clinical Immunology: Principles and Laboratory Diagnosis. Philadelphia, J. B. Lippincott Company, 1990.
Turgeon, M. L.: Immunology and Serology in Laboratory Medicine. St. Louis, C. V. Mosby Company, 1990.

Bibliography

Aach, R.D., Grisham, J.W., and Parker, C.W.: Detection of Australia antigen by radioimmunoassay. Proc. Natl. Acad. Sci. U.S.A., *68*:1056, 1971.

Aach, R.D., Hacker, E.J., and Parker, C.W.: Recognition of hepatitis B antigen determinants by a double-label radioimmunoassay: A sensitive means of subtyping hepatitis B antigen. J. Immunol., *III*:381, 1973.

Aach, R.D., Szmuness, W., Mosley, J.W. *et al.*: Serum alanine aminotranferase of donors in relation to the risk of non-A, non-B hepatitis in recipients: The transfusion-transmitted viruses study. N. Engl. J. Med., *304*:989, 1981.

Abernathy, R.S., and Heiner, D.C.: Precipitation reactions in agar gel in North American blastomycosis. J. Lab. Clin. Med., *57*:177, 1966.

Abernethy, T.J., and Francis, T., Jr.: Studies on the somatic C-polysaccharide of pneumococcus. I. Cutaneous and serologic reactions in pneumonia. J. Exp. Med., *69*:69, 1937.

Abruzzo, J.C.L., and Christian, C.L.: The induction of a rheumatoid factor-like substance in rabbits. J. Exp. Med., *114*:791, 1961.

Aiya, S.K., and Gallo, R.C.: Three novel genes of human T-lymphotropic virus type III: Immune reactivity of their products with sera from acquired immune deficiency syndrome patients. Proc. Natl. Acad. Sci. USA, *83*:1553, 1986.

Albert, E.D.: The HLA system: Serologically defined antigens. Clin. Immunobiol., *3*:237, 1977.

Allison, A.S.: Self-tolerance and autoimmunity in the thyroid. N. Engl. J. Med., *295*:821, 1976.

Almeida, J.D., Rubenstain, D., and Scott, E.J.: New antigen-antibody system in Australia-antigen-positive hepatitis. Lancet, *2*:1225, 1971.

Alper, C.A., Abrahamson, N., Johnston, R.B., Jandl, J.H., and Rosen, F.S.: Studies *in vitro* and *in vivo* on the abnormality in the metabolism of C3 in a patient with increased susceptibility to infection. J. Clin. Invest., *49*:1975, 1970.

Alper, C.A., Bloch, K.J., and Rosen, F.S.: Increased susceptibility to infection in a patient with type II essential hypercatabolism of C3. N. Engl. J. Med., *288*:601, 1973.

Alper, C.A., and Rosen, F.S.: Complement and clinical medicine. *In* Vyas, G.N., Stites, D.P., and Brecher, G. (Eds.): Laboratory Diagnosis of Immunologic Disorders. New York, Grune & Stratton, 1975.

Alper, M.M., and Garner, P.R.: Premature ovarian failure: Its relationship to autoimmune disease. Obstet. Gynecol., *66*:27, 1985.

Alter, H.J., Holland, P.V., and Purcell, R.H.: Counterelectrophoresis for detection of hepatitis-associated antigen: Methodology and comparison with gel diffusion and complement fixation. J. Lab. Clin. Med., *77*:1000, 1971.

Alter, H.J., Purcell, R.H., Feinstone, S.M., Holland, P.V. Morroe, A.G.: Non-A, non-B hepatitis: A review and interim report of an ongoing prospective study. *In* Vyas, G.N., Cohen, S.N., and Schmid, R. (Eds.): Viral Hepatitis: A Contemporary Assesment of Etiology, Epidemiology, Pathogenesis and Prevention. Philadelphia, Franklin Institute Press, 1978, pp. 359,689.

Alter, H.J.: The dominant role of non-A, non-B in the pathogenesis of post-transfusion hepatitis: A clinical assessment. Clin. Gastroenterol., *9*:155, 1980.

Anderson, H.C., and McCarthy, M.: Determination of the C-reactive protein in the blood as a measure of the activity of disease process in acute rheumatic fever. Am J. Med., *8*:445, 1950.

Andujar, J.J., and Mazurek, E.E.: The Plasmacrit (PCT) test on capillary blood. Am. J. Clin. Pathol., *31*:197–204, 1959.

Asano, T., *et al.*: Viremia and neutralizing antibody response in infants with exanthem subitum. J. Pediatr., *114*:535, 1989.

Asher, T.M., and Shigekawa, J.M.: Technical evaluation of CR-test. Scientific Report No. 2. Costa Mesa, Hyland Laboratories.

Aubert, E., Pavilanis, V., and Starkey, O.H.: Virus antibody titrations using latex suspensions. Can. J. Public Health, *53*:206, 1962.

Bach, F.H., and Good, R.A.: Inflammation. *In* Bach, F.H. (Ed.): Clinical Immunobiology. New York, Academic Press, 1980, p. 139.

Bach, F.H., and Van Rood, J.J.: The major histocompatibility complex—genetics and biology. N. Engl. J. Med., *295*:806, 872,927, 1976.

Banacerraf, B.: Role of major histocompatibility complex in genetic regulation of immunologic responsiveness. Transplant. Proc., *9*:825, 1977.

Banatvala, J.E., Best, J.M., and Walker, D.K.: Epstein-Barr virus-specific IgM in infectious mononucleosis, Burkitt's lymphoma, and nasopharyngeal carcinoma. Lancet, *1*:1205, 1972.

Barbour, A.G.: Laboratory aspects of Lyme borreliosis. Clin. Microbiol. Rev., *1*:399, 1988.

Barker, L.F., Peterson, M.R., and Murray, R.: Application of the microtiter complement fixation technique to studies of hepatitis-associated antigen in human hepatitis. Vox Sang., *19*:211, 1970.

Barré-Sinoussi F., Chermann, J.C., Rey, F. et al.: Isolation of a T-lymphotropic retrovirus from a patient at risk for acquired immunodeficiency syndrome (AIDS). Science, *220*:868, 1983.

Barrett, J.T.: Textbook of Immunology, 4th ed. St. Louis, C.V. Mosby, 1991.

Barrett, J.T.: Textbook of Immunology, 5th ed. St. Louis, C.V. Mosby, 1988, pp. 29,103,146.

Baseman, J.B.: The biology of *Treponema pallidum* and syphilis. Clin. Microbiol. Newsletter, *5*:517, 1983.

Bennich, H.: Structure of IgE. Prog. Immunol., *2*:49, 1974.

Bergdorfer, W., et al.: Erythema chronicum migrans—a tick-borne spirochetosis. Acta Tropica, *40*:79–83, 1983.

Bernheimer, A.W.: Cytolytic toxins of bacteria. *In* Ajl, S.J., Kadis, S., and Montie, T.C. (Eds.): Microbial Toxins. Vol. 1, Bacterial Protein Toxins. New York, Academic Press, 1970, pp. 183–212.

Bicols, S.W., and Nakamura, R.M.: Agglutination and agglutination inhibition. *In* Rose, N.R., Friedman, H., and Fahey, J.L. (Eds.): Manual of Clinical Laboratory Immunology, 3rd ed. Washington, DC, American Society for Microbiology, 1986, p. 49.

Bier, O.G., Leyton, G., Mayer, M.M., and Heidelberger, M.: A comparison of human and guinea-pig complements and their component fractions. J. Exp. Med., *81*:445, 1945.

Billingham, R.E., Brent, L., and Medawar, P.B.: "Actively acquired tolerance" of foreign cells. Nature, *172*:603, 1953.

Bitter-Suerman, D., Dierich, M., Konig, W., and Hadding, U.: Bypass-activation of the complement system starting with C3. Immunology, *57*:267, 1972.

Bloch, K.J., and Bunim, J.J.: Simple, rapid diagnosic test for rheumatoid arthritis—bentonite flocculation test. J.A.M.A., *169*:207, 1959.

Blount, J.H., and Holmes, K.K.: Epidemiology of syphilis and the non-venereal treponematoses. *In* Johnson, R.C. (Ed.): The Biology of Parasitic Spirochetes. New York, Academic Press, 1975.

Blum, H.E., and Vyas, G.N.: Non-A, non-B hepatitis: A contemporary assessment. Haematologia, *15*:162, 1982.

Blumberg, B.S., Alter, H.J., and Visnich, S.: A new antigen in leukemia sera. J.A.M.A., *191*:541, 1965.

Blumberg, B.S., Sutnick, A.I., and London, W.T.: Hepatitis and leukemia: Their relation to Australia antigen. Bull. N.Y. Acad. Med., *44*:1566, 1968.

Boitard, C., Debray-Sachs, M., and Bach, J.F.: Autoimmune disorders in diabetes. Adv. Nephrol., *15*:281, 1986.

Bonino, F., Smedile, A., and Verme, G.: Hepatitis delta virus infections. Adv. Intern. Med., *32*:345, 1987.

Borsos, T., Circolo, A., and Ejzemberg, R.: Lack of C4 binding by human IgM during activation of the classical pathway. Key Biscayne, Florida, 9th International Complement Workshop, 1981.

Breit, S.N., Wakefield, D., Robinson, J.P., *et al.*: The role of alpha-1-antitrypsin deficiency in the pathogenesis of immune disorders. Clin. Immunol. Immunopathol., *35*:363, 1985.

Brown, D.L., and Cooper, A.G.: The *in vivo* metabolism of radioiodinated cold agglutinins of anti-I specificity. Clin. Sci., *38*:175, 1970.

Bryant, N.J.: An Introduction to Immunohematology, 2nd ed. Philadelphia, W.B. Saunders, 1982.

Burgdorfer, W.: The enlarging spectrum of tick-borne spirochetosis. Rev. Inf. Dis., *8*:932, 1986.

Burnet, F.M., and Fenner, F.: The Production of Antibodies. London, Macmillan, 1941.

Busey, J.F., and Hinton, P.F.: Precipitins in blastomycosis. Am. Rev. Respir. Dis., *95*:112, 1967.

Cabane, J., Thibierge, E., Godeau, P., et al.: AIDS in an apparently risk-free woman. Lancet, *2*:105, 1984.

Cantor, H., and Boyse, E.A.: Regulation of the immune response by T-cell subclasses. Contemp. Top. Immunobiol., *4*:47, 1977.

Chaplin, H. (1980): Personal communication cited by Mollison, P.L.: Blood Transfusion in Clinical Medicine. Oxford, Blackwell Scientific Publications, 1983.

Capra, J.D., Dowling, P.M., Cook, S., and Kunkel, H.G.: An incomplete cold-reactive gamma-G antibody with i specificity in infectious mononucleosis. Vox Sang., *16*:10, 1969.

Caputo, M.J.: Hyland Technical Discussion No. 27. Costa Mesa, Hyland Laboratories, 1975.

Carlisle, H.N., and Saslaw, S.: A histoplasmin latex agglutination test. J. Lab. Clin. Med., *51*:793, 1958.

Carlson, D.A.: AIDS risks and precautions for laboratory personnel. Med. Lab. Observ., Jan. 1988, p. 57.

Carpenter, P.L.: Immunology and Serology, 3rd ed. Philadelphia, W. B. Saunders Company, 1975.

Carrell, R.W.: Alpha-1-antitrypsin: Molecular pathology, leukocytes, and tissue damage. J. Clin. Invest., *78*:1427, 1986.

Cayzer, I., Dane, D.S., Cameron, C.H., and Denning, J.V.: A rapid hemagglutination test for hepatitis B antigen. Lancet, *1*:947, 1974.

Centers for Disease Control Task Force on Kaposi's Sarcoma and Opportunistic Infections: Epidemiologic aspects of the current outbreak of Kaposi's sarcoma and opportunistic infections. N. Engl. J. Med., *306*:248, 1982.

Chambers, L.A., Popovsky, M.A.: Decrease in post-transfusion hepatitis: Contribution of changes in donor screening for ALT and anti-HBc and changes in the general population. Arch. Intern. Med. (in press).

Chaplin, H.: Personal communication cited by Mollison, P.L.: Blood Transfusion in Clinical Medicine. Oxford, Blackwell Scientific Publications, 1983.

Chen, S.: Cells and tissues of the immune system. *In* Sheehan, C. (Ed.): Clinical Immunology: Principles and Laboratory Diagnosis. Philadelphia, J. B. Lippincott Company, 1990, pp. 19–29.

Chen, S.: Hypersensitivity. *In* Sheehan, C. (Ed.): Clinical Immunology: Principles and Laboratory Diagnosis. Philadelphia, J. B. Lippincott Company, 1990, pp. 68–80.

Chew, W.H., and Theus, T.L.: Candida precipitins. J. Immunol., *98*:220, 1967.

Chrystie, I.L., Islam, M.N., Banatvala, J.E., and Cayzer, I.: Clinical evaluation of the turkey-erythrocyte passive-hemagglutination test for hepatitis B surface antigen. Lancet *I*:1193, 1974.

Cinader, B.: Membrane lesions in immune lysis. Surface rings, globule aggregates, and transient openings. J. Cell. Biol., *56*:528, 1973.

Clavel, F., Mansinho, K., Chamaret, S., et al.: Human immunodeficiency virus type 2 infection associated with AIDS in West Africa. N. Engl. J. Med., *316*:1180, 1987.

Cleveland, P.H., and Richmond, D.D.: Enzyme immunofiltration staining assay for immediate diagnosis of herpes simplex virus and varicella-zoster virus directly from clinical specimens. J. Clin. Microbiol., 25:416, 1987.

Cohen, E., Neter, E., Mink, I., et al.: Use of alligator erythrocytes for demonstrating agglutination activating factor in rheumatoid arthritis. Am. J. Clin. Pathol., 20:32–34, 1958.

Cohen, S., and Freeman, T.: Metabolic heterogeneity of human gamma-globulin. Biochem. J., 76:475, 1960.

Cole, J.R., Sulzer, C.R., and Pursell, A.R.: Improved microtechnique for the leptospiral microscopic agglutination test. Appl. Microbiol., 25:976, 1973.

Coons, A.H.: Histochemistry with labeled antibody. Int. Rev. Cytol., 5:1, 1956.

Coons, A.H.: Fluorescent antibody methods. In Danielli, J.F. (Ed.): General Cytochemical Methods, Vol. 1. New York, Academic Press, 1958, pp. 400–422.

Coons, A.H.: The beginnings of immunofluorescence. J. Immunol., 87:499, 1961.

Corbel, M.J., and Cullen, G.A.: Differentiation of the serologic response to Yersinia enterocolitica and Brucella abortus in cattle. J. Hyg. (Cambridge), 68:519, 1970.

Costea, N., Yakulis, V.J., and Heller, P.: Inhibition of cold agglutinins (anti-I) by M. pneumoniae antigens. Proc. Soc. Exp. Biol. (N.Y.), 139:476, 1972.

Crockson, R.A., Payne, C.J., Ratcliff, A.P., and Soothill, J.F.: Time sequence of acute reactive proteins following surgical trauma. Clin. Chim. Acta, 14:435, 1966.

Csonka, G.W.: "Bejel": Childhood treponematosis. Med. Illus. (London), 6:401, 1952.

Dacie, J.V.: The Hemolytic Anemias, 2nd ed. London, J. and A. Churchill Ltd., 1962.

Damp, S.C., Crumrine, M.H., and Lewis, G.E.: Microtiter plate agglutination test for Brucella canis antibodies. Appl. Microbiol., 25:489, 1973.

Daniels, J.C., Larson, D.L. Abston, S., and Ritzmann, S.E.: Serum protein profiles in thermal burns. J. Trauma, 14:153, 1974.

Das, P.C., Hopkins, R., Cash, J.D., and Cumming, R.A.: Rapid identification of hepatitis-associated antigen and antibody by counter-immunoelectro-osmophoresis. Br. J. Haematol., 21:673, 1971.

Dattwyler, R.J., Volkman, D.J., Luft, B.J., et al.: Seronegative Lyme disease: Discussion of specific T- and B-lymphocyte responses to Borrelia burgdorferi. N. Engl. J. Med., 319:1441, 1988.

Davidsohn, I.: Serological diagnosis of infectious mononucleosis. J.A.M.A., 108:289, 1937.

Dawson, S.F.: The significance of the C-reactive protein estimation in streptococcal and allied diseases. Arch. Dis. Child., 32:454, 1957.

Day, N.K., Geiger, H., McLean, R., Michael, A., and Good, R.A.: C2 deficiency: Development of lupus erythematosus. J. Clin. Invest., 52:1601, 1973.

Deinstag, J.L., Feinstone, S.M., Purcell, R.H., Hoofnagle, J.H., Barker, L.E., London, W.T., Popper, H., Peterson, J.M., and Kapikian, A.Z.: Experimental infection of chimpanzees with hepatitis A virus. J. Infect. Dis., 132:532, 1975.

Delaat, A.N.C.: The complement fixation test in virus antibody studies. Can. J. Med. Technol., 26:35, 1964.

DeVita, V.T. Jr., Hellman, S., and Rosenberg, S.A.: AIDS: Etiology, Diagnosis, Treatment and Prevention. Philadelphia, J.B. Lippincott, 1985.

Diaz, L.A., and Provast, T.T.: Dermatologic diseases. In Stite, D.P., Stobo, J.D., and Wells, J.V. (Eds.): Basic and Clinical Immunology, 6th ed. Norwalk, Appleton & Lange, 1987, p. 516.

Dienhardt, F., Holmes, A.W., Capps, R.B., and Popper, H.: Studies on the transmission of human viral hepatitis to marmoset monkeys. J. Exp. Med., 125:673, 1967.

Dixon, R., Rosse, W., and Ebbert, L.: Quantitative determination of antibody in idiopathic thrombocytopenic purpura. N. Engl. J. Med., 292:230, 1975.

Dodd, R.Y.: Reflection of methods for HBsAg, anti-HIV and anti-HBc testing. In Dixon, M.R., and Ellisor, S.S. (Eds.): Selection of Methods and Instruments for Blood Banks. Arlington, American Association of Blood Banks, 91:108, 1987.

Dodd, R.Y.: Screening for hepatitis infectivity among blood donors. A model for blood safety? Arch. Pathol. Lab. Med., 113:227, 1989.

Dodd, R.Y., Popovsky, M.A. et al.: Antibodies to hepatitis B core antigen and the infectivity of the blood supply. Transfusion, 31:443, 1991.

Donaldson, V.H., Rosen, F.S., and Bing, D.H.: Role of the second component of complement (C2) and plasmin in kinin release in hereditary angioneurotic edema (H.A.N.E.) plasma. Trans. Assoc. Am. Physicians. 90:174, 1977.

Drake, M.E., Hampil, B., Pennell, R.B., Spizizen, J., Henle, W., and Stokes, J.: Effect of nitrogen mustard on virus on serum hepatitis in whole blood. Proc. Soc. Exp. Biol. (N.Y.), 80:310, 1952.

Dreesman, G.R., Hollinger, F.B., and Melnick, J.L.: Detection of hepatitis B antigen by counter-immunoelectrophoresis: Enhancing role of homologous serum diluents. Appl. Microbiol., 24:1001, 1972.

Drew, W.L., and Mintz, L.: Rapid diagnosis of varicella-zoster infection by direct immunofluorescence. Am. J. Clin. Pathol., 73:699, 1980.

Dubois, E., Drexler, E., and Arteberry, J.D.: A latex nucleoprotein test for diagnosis of systemic lupus erythematosus. J.A.M.A., 117:141, 1961.

Dulbecco, R.: Production of plaques in monolayer tissue culture by particles of an animal virus. Proc. Natl. Acad. Sci. U.S.A., 38:747, 1952.

Duray, P.H., and Steere, A.C.: Clinical pathologic correlations of Lyme disease by stage. Ann. N.Y. Acad. Sci., 539:65, 1988.

Edelman, G.M.: Antibody structure and molecular immunology. In Kochwa, S., and Kunkel, H.G. (Eds.): Immunoglobulins. Ann. N.Y. Acad. Sci., 190:5, 1971.

Edwards, E.A., and Larson, G.L.: Serologic grouping of hemolytic streptococci by counter-immunoelectrophoresis. Appl. Microbiol., 25:1006, 1973.

Ehrenkranz, N.J., Rubini, J., Gunn R. et al.: Pneumocystis carinii pneumonia among persons with hemophilia A. M.M.W.R., 31:365, 1982.

Eisenbarth, G.S.: Type I diabetes mellitus: A chronic autoimmune disease. N. Engl. J. Med., 314:1360, 1986.

Elek, S.D.: Recognition of toxicogenic bacterial strains in vitro. Br. Med. J., 1:493, 1948.

Ernst, P.B., Underdown, B.J., Beinstock, J.: Immunity in mucosal tissue. In Stites D.P., Stobo, J.D., and Wells, J.V. (Eds.): Basic and Clinical Immunology, 6th ed. Norwalk, Appleton and Lange, 1987, p. 159.

Fahey, J.L., and McKelvy, E.M.: Quantitative determination of serum immunoglobulins in antibody-agar plates. J. Immunol., 94:84, 1965.

Feinstone, S.M., Kapikian, A.Z., and Purcell, R.H.: Hepatitis A. Detection by immune electromicroscopy of a virus-like antigen associated with acute illness. Science, *182*:1026, 1973.

Fiedel, B., and Gewurz, H.: Inhibition of platelet aggregation by C-reactive protein. Fed. Proc. (Abstr.), *34*:854, 1975.

Fike, D.J. Agglutination and agglutination inhibition. *In* Sheehan, C. (Ed.): Clinical Immunology: Principles and Laboratory Diagnosis. Philadelphia, J. B. Lippincott Company, 1990, p. 135.

Fike, D.J.: Major histocompatibility complex. *In* Sheehan, C.: Clinical Immunology, Principles and Laboratory Diagnosis. Philadelphia, J.B. Lippincott, 1990, p. 17.

Fike, D.J.: Antibody structure and function. *In* Sheehan, C. (Ed.): Clinical Immunology: Principles and Laboratory Diagnosis. Philadelphia, J. B. Lippincott Company, 1990, pp. 93–104.

Fike, D.J.: Nature of antigens. *In* Sheehan, C. (Ed.): Clinical Immunology: Principles and Laboratory Diagnosis. Philadelphia, J. B. Lippincott Company, 1990, pp. 105–114.

Fischi, M.A., Richman, D.D., Grieco, M.H., *et al.*: The efficacy of azidothymidine (AZT) in treatment of patients with AIDS and AIDS-related complex. N. Engl. J. Med., *317*:185, 1987.

Fishel, E.E.: Laboratory diagnostic procedures. *In* Cohen, A.S. (Ed.): Rheumatic Diseases. Boston, Little, Brown and Co., 1967, pp. 70–83.

Fisher, A.G., Feinberg, M.B., Josephs, S.F., et al.: The transactivation gene of HTLV-III is essential for virus replication. Nature, *320*:367, 1986.

Fisher, C.L., Gill, C., Forrester, M.G., and Nakamura, R.: Quantitation of acute phase proteins postoperatively. Am. J. Clin. Pathol., *66*:840, 1976.

Foley, J.M.: The nervous system: Degenerative diseases. *In* Robbins, S.L. (Ed.): Pathologic Basis of Disease. Philadelphia, W. B. Saunders Company, 1974, p. 1539.

Forssman, J.: Die Herstellung hochwertiger specifischer Schafhamolysine ohne Verwendung von Schafblut. Ein Beitrag zur Lehre von heterologer Anti-Korperbildung. Biochem. Z., *37*:78, 1911.

Franklin, E.C., and Kinkel, H.G.: Comparative levels of high molecular weight (19S) gamma globulins in maternal and umbilical cord sera. J. Lab. Clin. Med., *52*:724, 1958.

Friedman-Kein, A., Laubenstein, L., Marmor, M., et al.: Kaposi's sarcoma and *Pneumocystis* pneumonia among homosexual men—New York City and California. M.M.W.R., *30*:305, 1981.

Fritz, R.B., and Rivers, S.L.: Hepatitis-associated antigen: Detection by antibody-sensitized latex particles. J. Immunol., *108*:108, 1972.

Fudenberg, H.H., Stites, D.P., Caldwell, J.L., and Wells, J.V.: Basic and Clinical Immunology. Los Altos, Lange Medical Publications, 1976.

Fuller, G.M., and Ritchie, D.G.: A regulatory pathway for fibrinogen biosynthesis involving an indirect feedback loop. *In* Kushner, I., Volanakis, J.E., and Gewurz, H. (Eds.): C-Reactive Protein and the Plasma Protein Response to Tissue Injury. Ann. N.Y. Acad. Sci. *389*:308, 1982.

Fye, K.H., and Sack, K.E.: Rheumatic diseases. *In* Stites, D.P., Stobo, J.D., and Wells, J.V., (Eds.): Basic and Clinical Immunology, 6th ed. East Norwalk, Appleton and Lange, 1987, p. 356.

Gaither, T.A., and Frank, M.M.: Complement. *In* Henry, J.B.: Clinical Diagnosis and Management by Laboratory Methods. Philadelphia, W.B. Saunders, 1991, p. 830.

Gal, K., and Miltenyi, M.: Hemagglutination test for the demonstration of CRP. Acta Microbiol. Acad. Sci. Hung., 3:41, 1955.

Garner, M.F., and Clark, M.E.: The *Treponema pallidum* hemagglutination (TPHA) test. WHO/VDT/RES, 75:332, 1975.

Georg, L.K., Coleman, R.M., and Brown, J.M.: Evaluation of an agar gel precipitin test for the serodiagnosis of actinomycosis. J. Immunol., 100:1288, 1968.

Gershon, R.K.: Immunoregulations by T cells. Miami Winter Symposium, 9:267, 1975.

Glezen, W.P., *et al.*: Acute respiratory disease of university students with special reference to the etiologic role of Herpesvirus hominis. Am. J. Epidemiol., *101*:111, 1975.

Gocke, D.J., and Howe, C.: Rapid detection of Australian antigen by counter-immunoelectrophoresis. J. Immunol., 104:1031, 1970.

Goers, J.W.F., and Porter, R.R.: The assembly of early components of complement on antigen-antibody aggregates and on antibody-coated erythrocytes. Biochem. J., *175*:675, 1978.

Goldberg, L.S., and Barnett, E.V.: Mixed γG-γM cold agglutinin. J. Immunol., 99:803, 1967.

Goldstein, A.L., Thurman, G.B., Cohen, G.H., and Hooper, J.A.: The role of thymosin and the endocrine thymus on the ontogenesis and function of T cells. Miami Winter Symposium, 9:423, 1975.

Goldstein, I.M., Kaplan, H.B., Edelson, H.S. *et al.*: Ceruloplasmin: An acute phase reactant that scavenges oxygen-derived free radicals. *In* Kushner, I., Volanakis, J.E., and Gerwurz, H. (Eds.): C-Reactive Protein and the Plasma Protein Response to Tissue Injury. Ann. N.Y. Acad. Sci. *389*:368, 1982.

Goodman, J.W.: Immunogenicity and antigenic specificity. *In* Stites, D.P., Stobo, J.D., and Wells, J.V. (Eds.): Basic and Clinical Immunology, 6th ed. Norwalk, Appleton and Lange, 1987, p. 20.

Goodman, J.W.: Immunoglobulins I: Structure and function. *In* Stites, D.P., Stobo, J.D., Wells, J.V. (Eds.): Basic and Clinical Immunology, 6th ed. Norwalk, Appleton and Lange, 1987, p. 27.

Gotschlich, E.C., and Edelman, G.M.: C-reactive protein: A molecule composed of subunits. Proc. Natl. Acad. Sci. U.S.A., *54*:558, 1965.

Gotschlich, E.C., and Edelman, G.M.: Binding properties and specificity of C-reactive protein. Proc. Natl. Acad. Sci. U.S.A., *57*:706, 1967.

Gottlieb, M.S., Schroff, R., and Schranker, H.M., et al.: Pneumocystis carinii pneumonia and mucosal candidiasis in previously healthy homosexual men. Evidence of a new acquired cellular immunodeficiency. N. Engl. J. Med, *305*:1425, 1981.

Gottlieb, M.S., Schranker, H.M., Fan, P.T., et al.: *Pneumocystis* pneumonia—Los Angeles. M.M.W.R., *30*:250, 1981.

Govindarjan,S.: Delta hepatitis. What have we learned in the last decade? Lab. Mgt., 26:36, 1988.

Grady, G.F., and Lee, V.A.: Prevention of hepatitis from accidental exposure among the medical workers. N. Engl. J. Med., *293*:1067, 1975.

Gray, D.F.: Immunology. New York, American Elsevier Publishing Co., 1970.

Grodzicki, R.L. and Steere, A.C.: Comparison of immunoblotting and indirect enzyme-linked immunosorbent assay using different antigen preparations for diagnosing early Lyme disease. J. Infect. Dis., *157*:790, 1988.

Groopman, J.E., Chen, F.W., Hope, J.A. *et al.*: Serological characterization of HTLV-III infection in AIDS and related disorders. J. Infect. Dis., *84*:1434, 1986.

Guerrant, R.L., and Dickens, M.D.: Toxigenic bacterial diarrhea: A nursery outbreak involving multiple strains. Fourteenth

Interscience Conference on Antimicrobial Agents and Chemotherapy. Abstr. 130, 1974.

Hanshaw, J.B.: Congenital cytomegalic infection: Laboratory methods of detection. J. Pediatr., 75:1179, 1969.

Harrington, W.J., Minnich, V., Hollingsworth, J.W., and Moore, C.V.: Demonstration of a thrombocytopenic factor in the blood of patients with thrombocytopenic purpura. J. Lab. Clin. Med., 38:1, 1951.

Harris, C., Small, C.B., Klein, R.S., et al.: Immunodeficiency in female sexual partners of men with the acquired immunodeficiency syndrome. N. Engl. J. Med., 308:1181, 1983.

Harrison, R.A., and Lachman, P.L.: The physiologic breakdown of the third component of human complement. Mol. Immunol., 17:9, 1980.

Hayashi, H., and LoGrippo, G.A.: C-reactive protein—potential significance of quantitation in patients with chronic diseases. Henry Ford Hosp. Med. J., 20:91, 1972.

Hazen, E.L., Gordon, M.A., and Reed, F.C.: Laboratory Identification of Pathogenic Fungi Simplified, 2nd ed. Springfield, Charles C Thomas, 1970.

Hedge, U.M., Powell, D.K., Bowes, A., and Gordon-Smith, E.C.: Enzyme-linked immunoassay for the detection of platelet associated IgG. Br. J. Haematol., 48:39, 1981.

Heidelberger, M., and Kendall, F.E.: A quantitative study and a theory of the reaction mechanism. J. Exp. Med., 61:563, 1935.

Heidelberger, M., and Mayer, M.M.: Quantitative studies on complement. Adv. Enzymol., 8:71, 1948.

Helmerhorst, F.M., Bossers, B., Von Dem Borne, A.E.G. Kr., et al.: The detection of platelet antibodies: a comparison of three techniques. Vox Sang. 39:83–92, 1980.

Henry, J.B.: Clinical Diagnosis and Management by Laboratory Methods. Philadelphia, W.B. Saunders, 1991.

Heyward, W.L., and Curran, J.W.: The epidemiology of AIDS in the US. Sci. Am., 259(4):52, 1988.

Hicks, J.M., and Iosefsohn, M.: Reliability of home pregnancy-test kits in the hands of laypersons. N. Engl. J. Med., 320:320, 1989.

Hippert, M., and Bailey, J.W.: The use of immunodiffusion tests in coccidioidomycosis. Tech. Bull. Reg. Med. Technol., 35:155, 1965.

Hirata, A.A., Emerick, A.J., and Boley, W.F.: Hepatitis B virus antigen detection by reverse passive haemagglutination. Proc. Soc. Exp. Biol. Med., 143:761, 1973.

Hirst, G.K.: The quantitative determination of influenza virus and antibodies by means of red cell agglutination. J. Exp. Med., 75:49, 1942.

Holland, P.V., Bancrost, W., and Zimmerman, H.: Post-transfusion viral hepatitis and the TTVS. N. Engl. J. Med., 304:1033, 1981.

Hoofnagle, J.H., Seefe, L.B., and Zimmerman, H.J.: Type B hepatitis after transfusion with blood containing antibody to hepatitis B core antigen. N. Engl. J. Med., 298:1379, 1978.

Hopkins, R., and Das, P.C.: A tanned cell hemagglutination test for the detection of hepatitis-associated-antigen (Au-Ag) and antibody (Anti-Au). Br. J. Haematol., 25:619, 1973.

Hudson, E.H.: Non-Venereal Syphilis. Edinburgh, E. and S. Livingstone, 1958, p. 189.

Hudson, E.H.: Treponematosis and anthropology. Ann. Intern. Med., 58:1037, 1963.

Hughes-Jones, N.C.: Nature of the reaction between antigen and antibody. Br. Med. Bull., 19:171, 1963.

Hugli, T.E. and Muller-Eberhard, H.J.: Anaphylatoxins: C3a and C5a. Adv. Immunol., 26:1, 1978.

Humphrey, J.H., and Dourmashkin, R.R.: Electron microscope studies of immune cell lysis. In Wolstenholme, G.E.W., and Knight, J. (Eds.): Ciba Found. Symp. Complement, London, J. & A. Churchill, 1965.

Humphrey, J.H., and Dourmashkin, R.R.: The lesions in cell membranes caused by complement. Adv. Immunol., 11:75, 1969.

Hunder, G.G., McDuffie, F.C., and Mullen, B.J.: Activation of C3 and factor B in synovial fluids. J. Lab. Clin. Med., 89:160, 1977.

Hunter, E.F., Deacon, W.E., and Meyer, P.C.: An improved test for syphilis—the absorption procedure (FTA-ABS). Public Health Rep., 79:5, 1964.

Hymes, K., Shulman, S., and Karpatkin, S.: A solid-phase radioimmunoassay for bound anti-platelet antibodies. Studies on 45 patients with autoimmune platelet disorders. J. Lab. Clin. Med., 94:639, 1979.

Issitt, P.D.: Antigens defined by antibodies that may lack clinical significance. In Applied Blood Serology, 3rd ed. Miami, Mongomery Scientific Publishing, 1985, p. 422.

Iwakata, S., Rhodes, A.J., and Labzoffsky, N.S.: The significance of specific IgM antibodies in the diagnosis of rubella employing the immunfluorescence technique. Can. Med. Assoc. J., 106:327, 1972.

Jackson, J.B., and Balfour, H.H., Jr.: Practical diagnostic testing for human immunodeficiency virus. Clin. Microbiol. Rev., 1:124, 1988.

Jambazian, A., and Holper, J.C.: Rheophoresis: A sensitive immunodiffusion method for detection of hepatitis associated antigen. Proc. Soc. Exp. Biol. Med., 140:560, 1972.

James K.: Mechanisms of the nonspecific immune response. In Sheehan, C. (Ed.): Clinical Immunology: Principles and Laboratory Diagnosis. Philadelphia, J. B. Lippincott, 1990.

Janda, W.M.: Serologic tests for HTLV-III antibodies: Methods and interpretations. Clin. Microbiol. Newsletter, 7:67, 1985.

Janney, F.A., Lee, L.T., and Howe, C.: Cold hemagglutinin cross-reactivity with Mycoplasma pneumoniae. Infect. Immunol., 22:29, 1978.

Javid, J.: Human haptoglobin. Curr. Top. Hematol., 1:151, 1978.

Jawetz, E., Melnick, J., and Adelberg, E.A.: Review of Medical Microbiology. Los Altos, Lange Medical Publications, 1974.

Jenkins, W.J., Koster, H.G., Marsh, W.L., and Carter, R.L.: Infectious mononucleosis: An unsuspected source of anti-i. Br. J. Haematol., 11:480, 1965.

Jensen, L.P., O'Sullivan, M.K., Gomez-Del-Rio, M., et al.: Acquired immunodeficiency (AIDS) in pregnancy. Am. J. Obstet. Gynecol., 148:1145, 1984.

Jerne, N.K.: Towards a network theory of the immune system. Ann. Immunol. (Paris), 125C:373, 1974.

Jerry, L.M., Kunkel, H.G., and Grey, H.M.: Absence of disulfide bonds linking the heavy and light chains: A property of agenetic variant of γA2 globulin. Proc. Natl. Acad. Sci. U.S.A., 65:557, 1970.

Jodal, U., and Hanson, L.A.: Sequential determination of C-reactive protein in acute childhood pyelonephritis. Acta Pediatr. Scand., 65:319, 1976.

Johannson, B.C., Kindermark, C.O., Triel, E.Y., and Wollheim, F.A.: Sequential changes of plasma proteins after myocardial infarction. Scand. J. Clin. Lab. Invest., 124(Suppl. 29):117, 1972.

Johnson, A.M.: Immunoprecipitation in gels. In Rose, N.R., Friedman, H, Fahey, J.L. (Eds.): Manual of Clinical Immunology, 3rd ed. Washington, DC, American Society for Microbiology, 1986, p. 14.

Johnson, R.C.: Spirochetes. In Howard, B., Klass, J., Rubin, S., et al. (Eds.): Pathogenic Microbiology, 1986, p. 503.

Joklik, W.W., et al. (Eds.): Zinsser Microbiology, 15th ed. Norwalk, Appleton-Century-Crofts, 1972.

Josephs, B.P., et al.: Genomic analysis of the human B-lymphotropic virus (HBLV). Science, 234:601, 1986.

Juji, T., and Yokochi, T.: Hemagglutination technique with erythrocytes coated with specific antibody for detection of Australia antigen. Jpn. J. Exp. Med., 39:615, 1969.

Jushner, I., and Feldmann, G.: Demonstration of C-reactive protein synthesis and secretion by hepatocytes during active inflammation in the rabbit. J. Exp. Med., 148:466, 1978.

Kaplan, M.H., and Volanakis, J.E.: Interaction of C-reactive protein with the complement system. I. Consumption of human complement associated with the reaction of C-reactive protein with pneumococcal C-polysaccharide and with the choline phosphatides, lecithin, and sphingomyelin. J. Immunol., 112:2135, 1974.

Kauffmann, L.: The use of immunodiffusion for the detection of histoplasmin antibodies. Pubic Health Rep., 81:177, 1966.

Kenyon, R.H., and McManus, A.T.: Rickettsial infectious antibody complexes: Detection by antiglobulin plaque reduction technique. Infect. Immun., 9:966, 1974.

Khan, N.C., and Hunter, E.: Detection of human immunodeficiency virus type 1. ACPR, May 1988, p. 20.

Kindermard, C.O.: Stimulating effect of C-reactive protein on phagocytosis of various species of pathogenic bacteria. Clin. Exp. Immunol., 8:941, 1971.

Kline, W.E., Bowman, R.J., McCurdo, K.K.E., et al.: Hepatitis B core antibody (anti-HBc) in blood donors in the United States: Implications for surrogate testing programs. Transfusion, 27:99, 1987.

Kniker, W.T., Lesourd, B.M., McBryde, J.L., and Corriel, R.N.: Cell-mediated immunity assessed by Multitest CMI skin testing in infants and preschool children. Am. J. Dis. Child., 139:840, 1985.

Koneman, E.W., and Roberts, G.D.: Mycotic disease. In Henry, J.B. (Ed.): Clinical Diagnosis and Management by Laboratory Methods, 18th ed. Philadelphia, W. B. Saunders Company, 1991.

Kroof, I.G., and Shackman, N.H.: Levels of C-reactive protein as a measure of acute myocardial infarction. Proc. Soc. Exp. Biol. Med., 86:96, 1954.

Kunkel, H.G., and Prendegast, R.A.: Subgroups of gamma A immune globulins. Proc. Soc. Exp. Biol. Med., 122:910, 1966.

Kushner, I.: The phenomenon of the acute phase response. In Kushner, I, Volanakis, J.E., and Gewurz, H. (Eds.): C-Reactive Protein and the Plasma Protein Response to Tissue Injury. Ann. N.Y. Acad. Sci., 389:39, 1982.

Kushner, I., and Feldman, G.: Demonstration of c-reactive protein synthesis and secretion by hepatocytes during acute inflammation in the rabbit. J. Exp. Med., 148:466, 1978.

Lachmann, P.J., and Pangburn, M.K.: The breakdown of C3bi to C3c and C3e. IXth International Complement Workshop, Key Biscayne, Florida, 1981.

Lakeman, F.D., et al.: Detection of antigen to herpes simplex virus in cerebrospinal fluid from patients with herpes simplex encephalitis. J. Infect. Dis., 155:1172, 1987.

Lancefield, R.C.: A serologic differentiation of human and other groups of hemolytic streptococci. J. Exp. Med., 57:571, 1933.

Lancefield, R.C.: Current knowledge of type-specific M antigens of group A streptococci. J. Immunol., 89:307, 1962.

Landsteiner, K.: Über Beziehungen zwischen dem Blutserum und den Korperzellen. Munch. Med. Wschr., 50:1812, 1903.

Landsteiner, K., and Levine, P.: On the cold agglutinins in human serum. J. Immunol., 12:441, 1926.

Lawton-Smith, J., David, N.J., Indgin, S., et al.: Neuro-ophthalmologic studies of late yaws and pinta. II. The Caracas Project. Br. J. Vener. Dis., 47:226, 1971.

Lazarus, A.H., and Baines, M.G.: Studies on the mechanism of specificity of human natural killer cells for tumor cells: Correlation between target cell transferrin receptor expression and competitive activity. Cell Immunol., 96:255, 1985.

Le, J., and Vilcek, J.: Tumor necrosis factor and interleukin-I: Cytokines with multiple overlapping biological activities. Lab. Invest., 36:234, 1987.

Leach, J.M., and Ruck, B.J.: Detection of hepatitis-associated antigen by the latex agglutination test. Br. Med. J., 4:597, 1971.

LeBouvier, G.L.: The heterogeneity of Australia antigen. J. Infect. Dis., 123:671, 1971.

Lee, C.L., Davidson, I., and Panczyszyn, O.: Horse agglutinins in infectious mononucleosis. Am. J. Clin. Pathol., 49:3, 1968.

Lennette, E.H., and Schmidt, N.J.: Diagnostic Procedures for Viral and Rickettsial Diseases, 4th ed. New York, American Public Health Association, 1969.

Lennette, E.T., Karpatkin, S., and Levy, J.A.: Indirect immunofluorescence assay for antibodies to human immunodeficiency virus. J. Clin. Microbiol., 25:199, 1987.

Levy, J.A., Hoffman, A.D., Kramer, S.M., et al.: Isolation of lymphotropic retroviruses from San Francisco patients with AIDS. Science, 225:840, 1984.

Lofstrom, G.: Comparison between the reactions of acute phase serum with pneumococcus C-polysaccharide and with pneumococcus type 27. Br. J. Exp. Pathol., 25:21, 1944.

Lombardo, J.M.: HIV testing: An overview. ACPR, Nov. 1987, p. 10.

Longbottom, J.L., and Pepys, L.: Pulmonary aspergillosis: Diagnostic and immunologic significance of antigens and C substance in Aspergillus fumigatus. J. Pathol. Bacteriol., 84:141, 1964.

Lopez, C., et al.: Characteristics of human herpesvirus-6. J. Infect. Dis., 157:1271, 1988.

Louria, D.B., Smith, J.K., Brayton, R.G., and Buse, N.: Anticandida factors in serum and their inhibitors. J. Infect. Dis., 125:102, 1972.

Luciw, P.A., Cheng-Mayer, C., and Levy, J.A.: Mutational analysis of the human immunodeficiency virus: The orf-B region down regulates virus replication. Proc. Natl. Acad. Sci. USA, 84:1434, 1987.

Luoto, L.: A capillary agglutination test for bovine Q fever. J. Immunol., 71:222, 1953.

Macdougall, S.L., Shustik, C., and Sullivan, A.K.: Target cell specificity of human natural killer cells. Cell Immunol. 103:352, 1986.

Macleod, C.M., and Avery, O.T.: The occurrence during acute infections of a protein not normally present in the blood. III. Immunologic properties of the C-reactive protein and its differentiation from normal blood proteins. J. Exp. Med., *73*:191, 1941.

Magnarelli, L.A., Anderson, J.F., and Johnson, R.C.: Cross-reactivity in serological tests for Lyme disease and other spirochetal infection. J. Infect. Dis., *156*:183, 1987.

Malin, S.F., and Edwards, J.R.: Detection of hepatitis-associated antigen by latex agglutination. Nature (New Biol.), *235*:182, 1972.

Mancini, G., Carbonara, A.O., and Heremans, J.T.: Immuno-chemical quantitation of antigens by single radial immuno-diffusion. Int. J. Immunochem., *2*:235, 1965.

Mancini, G, Carbonara, A.O. and Heremans, J.F.: Immuno-chemical quantitation of antigens by single radial diffusion. Immunochem., *2*:235, 1965.

Maniar, A.C., and Fox, J.G.: Techniques of an *in vitro* method for determining toxigenicity of *Corynebacterium diphtheriae* strains. Can J. Pub. Health., *59*:297, 1968.

March, R.W., Stiles, G.E., and Forgoine, P.S.: *In* Abstracts of Annual Meeting of American Society for Microbiology, 1974, p. 73.

Marrack, J.R.: The Chemistry of Antigens and Antibodies. London, Medical Research Council, Special Report Series No. 194, 1938.

Marsh, D.G., Meyers, D.A., and Bias, W.B.: Epidemiology and genetics of atopic allergy. N. Engl. J. Med., *305*:1551, 1981.

Martensson, L., and Fudenberg, H.H.: Gm genes and γG-globulin synthesis in the human fetus. J. Immunol., *94*:514, 1965.

Masur, H., Michelis, M.A., Greene, J.B., et al.: An outbreak of community-acquired *Pneumocystis carinii* pneumonia. N. Engl. J. Med., *305*:1431, 1981.

Masur, H., Michelis, M.A., Wormser, G.P., et al.: Opportunistic infection in previously healthy women. Ann. Intern. Med., *97*:533, 1982.

Mata, L.J.: The agar gel culture precipitation test: Its application to the study of vaccinia virus, adenovirus, and herpes simplex virus. J. Immunol., *91*:151, 1963.

Mathur, S.: Immune and immunogenetic mechanisms in infertility. Contrib. Gynecol. Obstet., *14*:138, 1985.

McCarthy, P.L., Frank, A.L., Ablow, R.C., *et al.*: Value of C-reactive protein in the differentiation of bacterial and viral pneumonia. J. Pediatr., *92*:454, 1978.

McGrew, B.E., DuCros, M.J.F., Stout, G.W., and Falcone, V.H.: Automation of a flocculation test for syphilis. Am. J. Clin. Pathol., *50*:52, 1968.

McNamara, A.M.: Viral hepatitis. *In* Sheehan, C. (Ed.): Clinical Immunology: Principles and Laboratory Diagnosis. Philadelphia, J. B. Lippincott Company, 1990.

Mehl, V.S., and Penn, G.M.: Electrophoretic and immuno-chemical characterization of immunoglobulins. *In* Rose, N.R., Friedman, H., and Fahey, J.L. (Eds.): Manual of Clinical Laboratory Immunology, 3rd ed. Washington, DC, American Society for Microbiology, 1986, p. 126.

Meinertz, H., and Hjort, T.: Detection of autoimmunity to sperm. Fertil. Steril., *46*:86, 1986.

Melnick, J.L.: Classification of hepatitis A virus as enterovirus type 72 and of hepatitis B virus as hepadnavirus type 1. Intervirology, *18*:105, 1982.

Meyers, J.D.: Congenital varicella in term infants: Risk reconsidered. J. Infect. Dis., *129*:215, 1974.

Michael, A., and McLean, R.: Evidence for activation of the alternate pathway in glomerulonephritis. Adv. Nephrol., *4*:49, 1974.

Michaelsen, T.E., Frangione, B., and Franklin, E.C.: Primary structure of the "hinge" region of human IgG3. J. Biol. Chem., *252*:883, 1977.

Miller, K.B., and Schwartz, R.S.: Autoimmunity and suppressor T lymphocytes. Adv. Intern. Med., *27*:281, 1982.

Miller, K.B., and Schwartz, R.S.: Familial abnormalities of suppressor-cell function in systemic lupus erythematosus. N. Engl. J. Med., *301*:803, 1979.

Miller, L.H., Mason, S.J. Clyde, D.F., and McGinniss, M.H.: The resistance to *Plasmodium vivax* in blacks. The Duffy blood group genotype FyFy. N. Engl. J. Med., *295*:302, 1976.

Miller, L.H., Mason, S.J., Dvorak, J.A., *et al.*: Erythrocyte reception for (*Plasmodium knowlesi*) malaria: The Duffy blood group determinants. Science, *189*:561, 1975.

Miller, M.E., and Nilsson, U.R.: A familial deficiency of the phagocytosis-enhancing activity of serum related to a dysfunction of the fifth component of complement (C5). N. Engl. J. Med., *282*:354, 1970.

Miller, W.J., *et al.*: Specific immune adherence assay for human hepatitis A antibody. Application to diagnostic and epidemiologic investigations. Proc. Soc. Exp. Biol. Med., *149*:254, 1975.

Miyaka, K.B., Sato, Y., and Takeuchi, S.: Implication of circulating autoantibodies in the genesis of premature ovarian failure. J. Reprod. Immunol., *12*:163, 1987.

Moore, B.P.L., and Maede, D.: Counter-immunoelectrophoresis for detection of hepatitis by antigen and antibody: A technique for large scale use. Can. J. Public Health, *63*:453, 1972.

Morell, A., Skvaril, F., VanLoghem, E., and Kleemola, M.: Human IgG subclasses in maternal and fetal serum. Vox Sang., *2*:481, 1971.

Mortensen, R.F., Osmand, A.P., and Gerwurz.: Effects of C-reactive protein on the lymphoid system. I. Binding to thymus-dependent lymphocytes and alteration of their function. J. Exp. Med., *141*:821, 1975.

Mueller-Eckhardt, C., Kayser, W., Mersh-Baumert, K., *et al.*: The clinical significance of platelet-associated IgG: A study of 298 patients with various disorders. Br. J. Haematol., *46*:123, 1980.

Mueller-Eckhardt, C., Schultz, G., Sauer, K.-H, *et al.*: Studies on the platelet radioactive anti-immunoglobulin test. J. Immunol. Methods, *91*:1, 1978.

Muesing, M.A., Smith, D.H., and Capon, D.J.: Regulation of mRNA accumulation by a human immunodeficiency virus trans-activation protein. Cell, *48*:691, 1987.

Murray, R.: Viral hepatitis. Bull. N.Y. Acad. Med., *31*:341, 1955.

Nagasawa, S., Ichihara, C., and Stroud, R.M.: Cleavage of C4b and C3b inactivator: Production of a nicked form of C4b.C4b' as an intermediate cleavage product of C4b by C3b inactivator. J. Immunol., *125*:578, 1980.

Nahmias, A., Delbuono, I., Pipkin, J., *et al.*: Rapid identification and typing of Herpes simplex virus types 1 and 2 by direct immunofluorescence technique. Appl. Microbiol., *22*:455, 1971.

Nakamura, R.M., Peebles, C.L., Molden, D.P., *et al.*: Autoantibodies to Nuclear Antigens, 2nd ed. Chicago, American Society of Clinical Pathologists Press, 1985.

Nel, J.D., and Stevens, K.: A new method for simultaneous quantitation of platelet-bound immunoglobulin (IgG) and complement (C3)ᵉ employing an enzyme-linked immunosorbent assay (ELISA) procedure. Br. J. Haematol., *44*:281, 1980.

Nelson, R.A.: Factors affecting survival of *Treponema pallidum in vitro*. Am. J. Hyg., *48*:120, 1948.

Nelson, R.A., and Mayer, M.M.: Immobilization of *Treponema pallidum in vitro* by antibody produced in syphilitic infection. J. Exp. Med., *89*:369, 1949.

Nicols, W.S., and Nakamura, R.M.: Agglutination and agglutination inhibition. *In* Rose, N.R., Friedman, H., Fahey, J.L. (Eds.): Manual of Clinical Laboratory Immunology, 3rd ed. Washington, DC, American Society for Microbiology, 1986, p 49.

Niederman, J.C., *et al.*: Clinical and serological features of human herpesvirus-6 infection in three adults. Lancet, 2:817, 1988.

Nisonoff, A., Hopper, J.E., and Spring, S.B.: The Antibody Molecule. New York, Academic Press, 1975.

Noto, T.A., and Miale, J.B.: New immunologic test for pregnancy. Am. J. Clin. Pathol., *41*:273, 1964.

Oppenheim, J.J., Ruscetti, F.W., and Faltynek, C.V.: Interleukin and interferons. *In* Stites, D.P., Stobo, J.D., Wells, J.V. (Eds.): Basic and Clinical Immunology, 6th ed. Norwalk, Appleton and Lange, 1987, p. 82.

Osmond, D.G.: The ontogeny and organization of the lymphoid system. J. Invest. Dermatol. (Suppl.), *85*:2s, 1985.

Oveinnikov, N.M., and Delektorskij, V.V.: Morphology of *Treponema pallidum.* Bull. W.H.O., *35*:223, 1966.

Oveinnikov, N.M., and Delektorskij, V.V.: Further study of ultra-thin sections of *Treponema pallidum* under the electron microscope. Br. J. Vener. Dis., 44:1, 1968.

Overby, L.R., Miller, J.P., Smith, I.D., *et al.*: Radioimmunoassay of hepatitis B virus-associated (Australia) antigen employing ^{125}I-antibody. Vox Sang. (Suppl.), 24.102, 1973.

Owens, R.D.: Immunogenetic consequences of vascular anastomoses between bovine twins. Science, *102*:400, 1945.

Palmer, D.F., and Woods, R.: Qualitation and quantitation of immunoglobulins. Immunology Series No. 3. Atlanta, Centers for Disease Control, U.S. Department of Health, Education and Welfare, 1972.

Paul, J.R., and Bunnell, W.W.: The presence of heterophile antibodies in infectious mononucleosis. Am. J. Med. Sci., *183*:90, 1932.

Paya, C.V., Hermans, P.E., VanScoy, R.E., *et al.*: Repeatedly relapsing disseminated histoplasmosis: Clinical observations during long-term follow-up. J. Infect. Dis., *156*:308, 1987.

Peacock, J.E., Tomar, R.H.: Manual of Laboratory Immunology. Philadelphia, Lea and Febiger, 1980, p. 125.

Pepys, M.B., Drugnet, M., Klass, H.J., *et al.*: Ciba Foundation Symposium 46. Immunology of the Gut. Amsterdam, Elsevier, Excerpta Medica, North Holland, 1977, p. 283.

Perlmann, P.: Cellular immunity: Antibody dependent endotoxicity (K-cell activity). Clin Immunobiol., 3:107, 1976.

Pillemer, L., Blum, L., Lepow, I.H., et al.: The properdin system and immunity. I. Demonstration and isolation of a new system protein, properdin, and its role in immune phenomena. Science, 120:279, 1954.

Pirofsky, B.: Autoimmunization and the Autoimmune Hemolytic Anemias. Baltimore, Williams & Wilkins, 1969.

Platt, W.R.: Maturation of leukocytes and the leukocyte count. *In* Color Atlas and Textbook of Hematology, 2nd ed. Philadelphia, J. B. Lippincott Company, 1979, p. 83.

Polley, M.J., Mollison, P.L., and Soothill, J.F.: The role of 19S gamma globulin blood antibodies in the antiglobulin reaction. Br. J. Haematol., 8:149, 1962.

Popovic, M., Sarngadharan, M.G., Read, E., et al.: Detection, isolation, and continuous production of cytopathic retroviruses (HTLV-III) from patients with AIDS and pre-AIDS. Science, *224*:497, 1984.

Portnoy, J.: Modifications of the rapid plasma reagin (RPR) card test for syphilis for use in large scale testing. Am. J. Clin Pathol., *40*:473, 1963.

Portnoy, J., and Carson, W.: New and improved antigen suspension for rapid reagin test for syphilis. Public Health Rep., *75*:985, 1960.

Portnoy, J., Carson, W., and Smith, C.A.: Rapid plasma reagin test for syphilis. Public Health Rep., *72*:761, 1957.

Portnoy, J., Carson, W., and Smith, C.A.: New and improved antigen suspension for rapid reagin test for syphilis. Public Health Rep., *75*:985, 1960.

Powanda, M.C., and Moyer, E.D.: Plasma proteins and wound healing. Surg. Gynecol. Obstet., *153*:749, 1981.

Prince, A.M.: An antigen detected in blood during the incubation period of serum hepatitis. Proc. Natl. Acad. Sci. U.S.A., *60*:814, 1968.

Provost, P.J., Giesa, P., McAleer, W.J., et al.: Isolation of hepatitis A virus (in vitro) in cell culture directly from human specimens. Proc. Soc. Exp. Biol. Med., *167*:201, 1987.

Purcell, R.H., Holland, P.V., Walsh, J.H., *et al.*: A complement-fixation test for measuring Australia antigen and antibody. J. Infect. Dis., *120*:383, 1969.

Quevillon, M., and Chagnon, A.: Microtissue culture test for the titration of low concentrations of diphtheria antitoxin in minimal amounts of human sera. Appl. Microbiol., *25*.1, 1973.

Rapp, J.H., and Borsos, T.: Molecular Basis of Complement Action. Norwalk, Appleton-Century-Crofts, 1970.

Ratner, L., Haseltine, W., Patarca, R., et al.: Complete nucleotide sequence of the AIDS virus. Nature, *313*:277, 1985.

Rawlinson, K.F., Zubrow, A.B., Harris, M.A., et al.: Disseminated Kaposi's sarcoma in pregnancy: A manifestation of acquired immune deficiency syndrome. Obstet. Gynecol., *63*:25, 1984.

Rawston, J.R., and Farthing, C.P.: A comparison of tests for thyroglobulin antibody. J. Clin. Pathol., *15*:153, 1962.

Redfield, R.R.: The etiology and epidemiology of HTLV-III related disease. Abbott Diagnostics HTLV-III Education Series, 1987.

Reinherz, E.L., and Schlossman, S.: The differentiation and function of human T lymphocytes. Cell *19*:821, 1981.

Ricardo, M.J., and Tomar, R.H.: Humoral immunity: Antibodies and immunoglobulins. *In* Henry, J.B. (Ed.): Clinical Diagnosis and Management by Laboratory Methods, 18th ed. Philadelphia, W. B. Saunders Company, 1991, pp. 809–829.

Riggin, C.H., Beltz, G.A., Hung, C.H., *et al.*: Detection of antibodies to human immunodeficiency virus by latex agglutination with recombinant antigen. J. Clin. Microbiol., *25*:1772, 1987.

Rizzetto, M., Canese, M.G., Arico, S., *et al.*: Immunofluorescence detection of a new antigen-antibody system associated to the hepatitis B virus in the liver and in the serum of HBsAg carriers. Gut, *18*:997, 1987.

Roberts, R.C.: Protease inhibitors of human plasma: Alpha-2-macroglobulin. J. Med., *16*:149, 1985.

Rodnan, G.P., and Schumacher, H.R.: Primer on the Rheumatic Diseases, 8th ed. Atlanta, Arthritis Foundation, 1983.

Roitt, I.: Essential Immunology, 6th ed. Oxford, Blackwell Scientific Publications, 1988.

Roitt, I., Brostoff, J., and Male, D.: Immunology. London, Gower Medical Publishing, 1985.

Rose, H.M., Ragan, C., Pearce, E., et al.: Differential agglutination of normal and sensitized sheep erythrocytes by sera of patients with rheumatoid arthritis. Proc. Soc. Exp. Biol. Med., 68:1, 1948.

Rosenbaum, M.J., Phillips, I.A., Sullivan, E.J. et al.: A simplified method for virus antigen culture procedures in microtitration plates. Proc. Soc. Exp. Biol. Med., 113:224, 1963.

Rosenfield, R.E., Schmidt, P.J., Calvo, R.C., and McGinniss, M.H.: Anti-i, a frequent cold agglutinin in infectious mononucleosis. Vox Sang., 10:631, 1965.

Rosse, W.F., Adams, J.P., and Yount, W.J.: Subclasses of IgG antibodies in immune thrombocytopenic purpura (ITP). Br. J. Haematol., 46:109, 1980.

Rosse, W.F., and Dacie, J.V.: Immune lysis of normal human and paroxysmal nocturnal hemoglobinuria (PNH) red blood cells. II. The role of complement components in the increased sensitivity of PNH red cells to immune lysis. J. Clin. Invest., 45:749, 1966.

Rosse, W.F., Dourmashkin, R., and Humphrey, J.H.: Immune lysis of normal human and paroxysmal nocturnal hemoglobinuria (PNH) red blood cells. III. The membrane defects caused by complement lysis. J. Exp. Med., 123:969, 1966.

Rubinstein, A., Sicklick, M., Gupta, A., et al.: Acquired immunodeficiency with reversed T4/T8 ratios in infants born to promiscuous and drug-addicted mothers. J.A.M.A., 249:2350, 1983.

Salahuddin, S.Z., et al.: Isolation of a new virus, HBLV, in patients with lymphoproliferative disorders. Science, 234:596, 1986.

Salk, J.E., Younger, J.S., and Ward, W.N.: Use of color change of phenol red as the indicator in titrating poliomyelitis virus or its antibody in a tissue culture system. Am. J. Hyg., 60:214, 1954.

Sandoval, O.: Unpublished observations. Cited by Deodhar, S.D., and Valenzuela, R.: C-reactive protein: New findings and specific applications. Lab. Manag., 19(6), 1981.

Sasazuki, T., Kohno, Y., Iwamoto, I., et al.: Association between an HLA haplotype and locus responsive to tetanus toxoid in man. Nature, 272:359, 1978.

Scaletter, R., et al.: A nucleoprotein complement fixation test in the diagnosis of systemic lupus erythematosus. N. Engl. J. Med., 263:226, 1960.

Schmidt, N.J., and Lennette, E.H.: Sensitivity of a 1-day complement fixation test for detection of hepatitis-associated antigen. Health Lab. Sci., 8:238, 1971.

Schuber, J.H., and Hampson, H.C.: An appraisal of serologic tests for coccidioidomycosis. Am J. Hyg., 76:144, 1962.

Schultze, H.E., and Heremans, J.F.: Molecular Biology of Human Proteins with Special Reference to Plasma Proteins, Vol. 1. Amsterdam, Elsevier, 1966.

Schwartz, B.D.: The human major histocompatibility HLA complex. In Stites, D.P., Stobo, J.D., and Wells, J.V. (Eds.): Basic and Clinical Immunology, 6th ed. Norwalk, Appleton and Lange, 1987, p. 50.

Scott, G.B., Buck, B.E., Leterman, J.G., et al.: Acquired immunodeficiency syndrome in infants. N. Engl. J. Med., 310:76, 1984.

Seeff, L.B., et al.: A randomized, double-blind controlled trial of the efficacy of immune serum globulin for the prevention of post-transfusion hepatitis. Gastroenterology, 72:111, 1977.

Sever, J.L.: Application of a micro-technique to viral serologic investigations. J. Immunol., 88:320, 1962.

Shany, S., Bernheimer, A.W., Grushoff, P.S., et al.: Evidence for membrane cholesterol as a common binding site for cereolysin, streptolysin O and saponin. Mol. Cell. Biochem., 3:179, 1974.

Sheehan, C.: Autoimmunity. In Sheehan, C. (Ed.): Clinical Immunology: Principles and Laboratory Diagnosis. Philadelphia, J. B. Lippincott Company, 1990, pp. 318–339.

Shehab, Z.M., and Brunell, P.A.: Enzyme-linked immunosorbent assay for susceptibility to varicella. J. Infect. Dis., 148:472, 1983.

Siegal, F.P., Lopez, C., Hammer, G.S., et al.: Severe acquired immunodeficiency in male homosexuals, manifested by chronic perianal ulcerative herpes simplex lesions. N. Engl. J. Med., 305:1439, 1981.

Siegel, J., Rent, R., and Gewurz, H.: Interactions of C-reactive protein with the complement system. I. Protamine-induced consumption of complement in acute phase sera. J. Exp. Med., 140:631, 1974.

Sim, E., Wood, A.B., Hsiung, L.M., and Sim, R.B.: Pattern of degradation of human complement fragment C3b. FEBS Letters, 132:55, 1981.

Singer, J.M., and Plotz, C.M.: Latex fixation test: Application to serologic diagnosis of rheumatoid arthritis. Am. J. Med., 21:888, 1956.

Smith, S.J., Bos, G., Esseveld, M.R., et al.: Acute phase proteins from the liver and enzymes from myocardial infarction. Clin. Chim. Acta, 81:75, 1977.

Soulier, J.P., Patereau, C., and Drouet, J.: Platelet indirect radioactive Coombs' test. Its utilization of PL^{A1} grouping. Vox Sang., 29:253, 1975.

Stansfield, W.D.: Serology and Immunology: A Clinical Approach. New York, Macmillan, 1981, p. 168.

Steere, A.C., Grodzicki, R.L., Craft, J.E., et al.: Recovery of Lyme disease spirochetes from patients. Yale J. Biol. Med., 57:557, 1984.

Steketee, R.W., Burstyn, D.G., Wassilak, S.G.F., et al.: A comparison of laboratory and clinical methods for diagnosing pertussis in an outbreak in a facility for the developmentally disabled. J. Infect. Dis., 157:441, 1988.

Sternberger, L.A.: In Oslet, A., and Weiss, L. (Eds.): Immunocytochemistry. Englewood Cliffs, Prentice-Hall, 1974.

Sulzer, C.R., and Jones, W.L.: Evaluation of hemagglutination test for human leptospirosis. Appl. Microbiol., 26:655, 1973.

Szmuness, W., Stevens, C.E., Harley, E.J., et al.: Hepatitis B vaccine: Demonstration of efficacy in a controlled clinical trial in a high-risk population in the United States. N. Engl. J. Med., 303:833, 1980.

Tabor, E., et al.: Experimental transmission and passage of human non-A, non-B hepatitis in chimpanzees. In Vyas, G., Cohen, S., and Schmid, R. (Eds.): Viral Hepatitis. Philadelphia, Franklin Institute Press, 1978, p. 419.

Tanimoto, K., Moritoh, T., Azuma, T., et al.: Detection of IgG rheumatoid factor by concanavalin A treatment and complement fixation with IgG rheumatoid factor. Ann. Rheum. Dis., 35:240, 1976.

Tanowitz, H.B., Robbins, N., and Leidich, N.: Hemolytic anemia associated with severe mycoplasma pneumoniae. N.Y. State J. Med., 78:2231, 1978.

Tenveen, J.H., and Feltkamp, T.E.W.: Formalized chicken red cell nuclei as a simple antigen for standardized antinuclear factor determination. Clin. Exp. Immunol., 5:673, 1969.

Test for non-A, non-B hepatitis. ASM News 54:468, 1988.

Theofilopoulos, A.N.: Autoimmunity. *In* Stites, D.P., Stobo, J.D., and Wells, J.V. (Eds.): Basic and Clinical Immunology, 6th ed. East Norwalk, Appleton and Lange, 1987, p. 128.

Tillet, W.S., and Francis, T., Jr.: Serologic reactions in pneumonia with a non-protein somatic fraction of pneumococcus. J. Exp. Med., *52*:561, 1930.

Todd, E.W.: Antigenic streptococcal hemolysin. J. Exp. Med., *55*:267, 1932.

Tomasi, T.B., Jr., Tan, E.M., Solomon, A., and Prendergast, R.A.: Characteristics of an immune system common to certain external secretions. J. Exp. Med., *121*:101, 1965.

Troxel, D.B., Innella, F., and Cohren, R.J.: Infectious mononucleosis complicated by hemolytic anemia due to anti-i. Am. J. Clin. Pathol., *46*:625, 1966.

Tyrell, D.L.J., and Gill, M.J.: Hepatitis. *In* Mandell, L.A., and Ralph, E.D. (Eds.): Essentials of Infectious Diseases. Boston, Blackwell Scientific Publications, 1985, p. 241.

Ueda, K., *et al.*: Exanthem subitum and antibody to human herpesvirus-6. J. Infect. Dis., *159*:750, 1989.

U.S. Department of Health and Human Services: 1985 STD treatment guidelines. Atlanta, Centers for Disease Control, 1985.

Vaerman, J.P., and Heremans, J.F.: Antigenic heterogenicity of human immunoglobulin A proteins. Science, *153*:647, 1966.

Venezia, R.A., and Robertson, R.G.: Efficacy of the Candida precipitin test. Am. J. Clin. Pathol., *61*:849, 1974.

Volankis, J., Clements, W., and Schohenloher, R.: C-reactive protein physical, chemical characterization. J. Immunol. Methods, *23*:285, 1978.

Von Dem Borne, A.E.G. KR.., Verheught, F.W.A., *et al.*: A simple immunofluorescence test for the detection of platelet antibodies. Br. J. Haematol., *39*:195, 1978.

Wain-Hobson, S., Sonigo, P., Danos, O., et al.: Nucleotide sequence of the AIDS virus. L.A.V. Cell, *40*:9, 1985.

Wallace, A.L., and Harris, A.: Reiter treponema. Bull. W.H.O., *36*(Suppl. 2), 1967.

Walsh, L., Davies, P., and McConkey, B.: Relationship between erythrocyte sedimentation rate and serum C-reactive protein in rheumatoid arthritis. Ann. Rheumatol. Dis., *38*:362, 1979.

Wara, D.W., Reiter, E.O., and Doyle, N.E.: Persistent C1q deficiency in a patient with a systemic lupus-like syndrome. J. Pediatr., *86*:743, 1975.

Wassermann, A., Neisser, A., and Bruck, C.: Eine serodiagnostische Reaction bei Syphilis. Dtsch. Med. Wochenschr., *32*:745, 1906.

Weil, W., and Felix, A.: Zur serologischen diagnose des Fleckfiebers. Wien. Klin. Wochenschr., *29*:33, 1916.

Weiner, A.S.: Advances in Blood Grouping, Vol 3. New York, Grune & Stratton, 1970.

Weller, I.A.: Treatment of infections and antiviral agents. Br. Med. J., *295*:200, 1987.

Welsh, R.D., and Dolan, C.T.: Sporothrix whole yeast agglutination test: Low-titer reactions of sera of subjects not known to have sporotrichosis. Am. J. Clin. Pathol., *59*:82, 1973.

Welsh, W.D., Southern, P.M. Jr., and Schneider, N.R.: Five cases of Haemophilus segnis appendicitis. J. Clin. Microbiol., *24*:851, 1986.

West, C.D., Hong, R., and Holland, N.H.: Immunoglobulin levels from the newborn period to adulthood and in immunoglobulin deficiency states. J. Clin. Invest., *41*:2054, 1962.

Wheat, L.J.: Histoplasmosis. Infect. Dis. Clin. North Am., *2* (4):841, 1988.

W.H.O.: Advances in viral hepatitis. Technical Report Series, 602, 1977.

Wilcox, R.R., and Guthe, T.: *Treponema pallidum*. A bibliographic review of the morphology, culture, and survival of *T. pallidum* and associated organisms. Bull. W.H.O., *35*:1, 1966.

Wistreich, G.A., and Lechtman, M.D.: Microbiology and Human Disease. Beverly Hills, Glencoe Press, 1976.

Wollheim, F.A., and Williams, R.C.: Studies on the macroglobulins of human serum. I. Polyclonal Immunoglobulin class M (IgM) increase in infectious mononucleosis. N. Engl. J. Med., *274*:61, 1966.

Wong-Staal, F., Chanda, P., and Ghrayeb, J.: Human immunodeficiency virus: The eighth gene. AIDS Res. Hum. Retrovirol. 3:33, 1987.

Worlledge, S.M., and Dacie, J.V.: Hemolytic and other anaemias in infectious mononucleosis. *In* Carter, R.L., and Penman, H.G. (Eds.): Infectious Mononucleosis. Oxford, Blackwell Scientific Publications, 1969.

Yeager, A.S., *et al.*: Prevention of transfusion-acquired cytomegalovirus infections in newborn infants. J. Pediatr., *98*:281, 1981.

Yoshida, T., Matusi, T., Kobayashi, S., *et al.*: Agglutination test for HIV antibody. J. Clin. Microbiol., *25*:1433, 1987.

Young, S.A., Anderson, G.L., and Mitchell, P.D.: Laboratory observations during an outbreak of pertussis. Clin. Microbiol. Newsletter, *9*:176, 1987.

Zak, S.J., and Good. R.A.: Immunological studies of human serum gamma globulins. J. Clin. Invest., *38*:579, 1959.

Zuck, T.F., Sherwood, W.C., and Bove, J.R.: A review of recent events related to surrogate testing of blood to prevent non-A, non-B posttransfusion hepatitis. Transfusion, *27*:203, 1987.

Zweiman, B., and Lisak, R.P.: Autoantibodies: Autoimmunity and immune complexes. *In* Henry, J.B. (Ed.): Clinical Diagnosis and Management by Laboratory Methods, 18th ed. Philadelphia, W. B. Saunders Company, 1991, pp. 885–911.

Answers

CHAPTER 1: INTRODUCTION: NONSPECIFIC (NATURAL, INNATE) IMMUNITY

MULTIPLE CHOICE

1. c
2. b
3. a,b
4. a,b,d
5. c
6. a,b,c,d
7. a,b,c,d
8. b,c
9. d
10. c,d
11. a,b,c,d
12. d
13. c
14. a,b,c
15. b
16. a,b,c,d
17. a
18. a,b,c

TRUE/FALSE

1. t
2. f
3. t
4. f
5. t
6. f
7. t
8. f
9. t
10. t
11. f
12. t
13. t
14. t
15. f

CHAPTER 2: SPECIFIC IMMUNITY

MULTIPLE CHOICE

1. b
2. a,b,c
3. b
4. a,b,c,d
5. a,b,c
6. d
7. d
8. c
9. a,c
10. a,b,c,d
11. c
12. c
13. a
14. a,b
15. a
16. b,c
17. a,d
18. b

TRUE/FALSE

1. f
2. t
3. t
4. t
5. f
6. f
7. t
8. t
9. f
10. t
11. t
12. t

CHAPTER 3: COMPLEMENT

MULTIPLE CHOICE

1. a,c	6. a	11. c,d
2. c	7. d	12. a,d
3. a,d	8. a,b,c	13. a,c,d
4. c	9. c	14. a,b
5. a	10. a,b	15. c

TRUE/FALSE

1. f	7. t	13. t
2. t	8. t	14. t
3. t	9. f	15. t
4. f	10. t	16. f
5. f	11. t	17. t
6. t	12. f	

CHAPTER 4: THE IMMUNE RESPONSE

MULTIPLE CHOICE

1. a,c	7. a	13. a,b,c,d
2. b,d	8. b,c	14. a,b,c
3. a	9. d	15. c,d
4. a,b	10. c	16. a,b,d
5. c	11. b	17. a,b,c,d
6. d	12. a	

TRUE/FALSE

1. t	7. t	13. t
2. t	8. f	14. t
3. t	9. f	15. f
4. f	10. t	16. t
5. t	11. f	17. f
6. t	12. t	18. f

CHAPTER 5: THE ANTIGEN-ANTIBODY REACTION *IN VITRO*

MULTIPLE CHOICE

1. a,c	7. b	12. d
2. d	8. b,c	13. a,b,c,d
3. b	9. a,c,d	14. b,c
4. a	10. a,b,c,d	15. d
5. a	11. b,c	16. c
6. c		

TRUE/FALSE

1. f	7. f	13. t
2. t	8. t	14. t
3. f	9. f	15. f
4. f	10. t	16. f
5. t	11. f	17. t
6. t	12. t	18. t

CHAPTER 6: SYPHILIS

MULTIPLE CHOICE

1. b	8. a,b,c,d	14. d
2. b,d	9. b	15. d
3. d	10. a,b,c,d	16. a,c
4. a	11. b	17. a,b,c
5. a	12. a	18. a,b,c,d
6. c	13. d	19. a,b,c
7. b,c		

TRUE/FALSE

1. t	6. f	11. t
2. f	7. t	12. t
3. t	8. t	13. f
4. t	9. t	14. f
5. f	10. f	15. f

CHAPTER 7: VIRAL HEPATITIS

MULTIPLE CHOICE

1. a,b,c,d	8. a	15. a,b,c,d
2. a	9. c	16. a,b,c
3. b,c,d	10. b,c	17. a,b,c,d
4. c,d	11. b,c,d	18. a,b,c,d
5. a,b	12. a,b,c,d	19. b,d
6. a,b,d	13. d	20. b
7. a,c	14. a,b,c,d	

TRUE/FALSE

1. t	5. f	8. f
2. t	6. f	9. t
3. f	7. f	10. t
4. t		

CHAPTER 8: C-REACTIVE PROTEIN AND OTHER PLASMA PROTEINS

MULTIPLE CHOICE

1. a,b,d	6. b,d	11. a,b
2. a,b,c,d	7. b,c	12. b
3. b	8. a	13. a,b,c
4. b,c	9. d	14. d
5. a,b,c,d	10. a	15. a,c,d

TRUE/FALSE

1. f	5. t	8. t
2. t	6. f	9. t
3. f	7. t	10. f
4. f		

CHAPTER 9: *STREPTOCOCCUS PYOGENES*

MULTIPLE CHOICE

1. a,b	5. b	9. d
2. a,c	6. a,d	10. c
3. a,c	7. a	11. b,d
4. a,c	8. b	12. b

TRUE/FALSE

1. t	4. t	6. t
2. f	5. f	7. f
3. t		

CHAPTER 10: COLD AGGLUTININS: STREPTOCOCCUS MG

MULTIPLE CHOICE

1. a,d	5. a,c	8. c,d
2. d	6. a,b,c	9. a,c,d
3. a,b	7. b,d	10. a
4. a,c		

TRUE/FALSE

1. t	4. f	7. f
2. t	5. f	8. t
3. f	6. t	

CHAPTER 11: THE HERPES VIRUSES

MULTIPLE CHOICE

1. a,b,c	7. a,b,c	12. c
2. a	8. b,d	13. a,b
3. a,b	9. a,b,c,d	14. c
4. a,b,c,d	10. a,c	15. a,b,c
5. c,d	11. d	16. a
6. d		

TRUE/FALSE

1. t	6. f	11. f
2. f	7. t	12. t
3. f	8. t	13. t
4. t	9. f	14. t
5. t	10. f	

CHAPTER 12: INFECTIOUS MONONUCLEOSIS

MULTIPLE CHOICE

1. d	4. b	7. a,c
2. a,b	5. a,d	8. a,d
3. b	6. a,b	

TRUE/FALSE

1. t   4. t   7. f
2. f   5. f   8. f
3. t   6. t

CHAPTER 13: ACQUIRED IMMUNODEFICIENCY SYNDROME (AIDS)

MULTIPLE CHOICE

1. a,c   6. a,d   11. a,b,c,d
2. a   7. c   12. c
3. b,c   8. a,b,c,d   13. a
4. c   9. b   14. d
5. d   10. c   15. c

TRUE/FALSE

1. t   6. t   11. f
2. f   7. f   12. f
3. t   8. t   13. t
4. t   9. t   14. t
5. t   10. t

CHAPTER 14: AUTOIMMUNE DISEASES

MULTIPLE CHOICE

1. a,b,d   7. a,c,d   13. a,b
2. b,c   8. a,b,c   14. a,b
3. c   9. b,c,d   15. a
4. a,b,c,d   10. a,b   16. a,c
5. a,b,d   11. b,c,d   17. a,b,c,d
6. a,b   12. a,b,c,d

TRUE/FALSE

1. f   4. t   7. t
2. t   5. t   8. f
3. f   6. t

CHAPTER 15: FUNGAL ANTIBODY TESTS, FEBRILE ANTIBODY TESTS, AND VIRAL ANTIBODY TESTS

MULTIPLE CHOICE

1. a   5. b   8. a,b,c
2. a,b,c,d   6. d   9. a
3. a   7. b   10. d
4. c

TRUE/FALSE

1. t   3. f   5. f
2. t   4. t   6. t

CHAPTER 16: LYME DISEASE

MULTIPLE CHOICE

1. a,d	4. a,b	6. a,d
2. b	5. a	7. b,c,d
3. d		

TRUE/FALSE

1. t	4. f	7. t
2. f	5. f	8. t
3. t	6. t	

CHAPTER 17: MISCELLANEOUS SEROLOGY

MULTIPLE CHOICE

1. c	4. c	7. a
2. a,b,c,d	5. d	8. a,b,c,d
3. b	6. b,c,d	9. c

TRUE/FALSE

1. t	4. t	7. t
2. f	5. t	8. f
3. t	6. f	

Glossary

ABO Antigens The antigens of the major blood group system.

Absorption The removal of antibodies from serum by the addition of red cells that possess the corresponding surface antigen.

Accuracy A term used to describe the proximity of the "average" value and the "true" value.

Acquired Incurred because of external factors. Not inherited.

Acquired Agammaglobulinemia Immunodeficiency characterized by a severe decrease or absence of immunoglobulins and occurring in adults with a previously healthy immune system.

Acquired Antigen An antigen that is not genetically determined and is sometimes transient.

Acquired Immunity See *Adaptive Immunity.*

Acquired Immunodeficiency A defect in the normal immune response caused by external factors or as a result of an existing disease or condition (also known as "secondary" immunodeficiency).

Acquired Immunodeficiency Syndrome (AIDS) An immune disorder affecting T4 lymphocytes, caused by the human immunodeficiency virus (HIV).

Activated Macrophage A macrophage from an antigen-sensitized or otherwise stimulated animal.

Active Immunity Immunity that is generated by the actual production of antibody by the host in response to foreign antigen.

Acute A condition of sudden or short duration.

Acute Glomerulonephritis A nonsuppurative sequel to group A streptococcal infection characterized by proteinuria, hematuria, hypertension, and general impaired renal function.

Acute Phase Proteins Plasma proteins whose concentration increases or decreases during inflammation.

Adaptive Immunity Immunity that is developed subsequent to birth. The acquisition of immunity in the form of immunologically competent cells from an immune donor.

Adenocarcinoma A malignant new growth derived from glandular tissue or from recognizable glandular structures.

Adenopathy Swelling or enlargement of the lymph nodes.

Adjuvant A substance that can increase the specific antibody production to, or the degree of sensitization against, an antigen by increasing its size or length of survival in the circulation. A substance (usually injected with an antigen) that improves the immune response, either humoral or cellular, to the antigen.

Adoptive Immunity The transfer of immuno-competent cells from one individual to a second individual to establish immunocompetence in the second individual.

Adsorption The attachment of one substance to the surface of another; in particular, the attachment of antibody to specific receptors on a cell surface.

Afferent Lymphatic Duct The vessel that carries transparent liquid and antigens to the lymph node.

Affinity The tendency for one epitope to unite with one antigen-combining site of an antibody molecule.

Agammaglobulinemia A condition in which all

the immunoglobulins are missing (absent) from a serum.

Agglutination   The aggregation or clumping of cellular or particulate antigens by an antiserum containing antibodies to one or more of the surface antigens.

Agglutinin   An antibody that is capable of causing agglutination with surface antigens.

Agglutinogen   Another term for red cell antigen.

Aggregation   See *Agglutination*.

AIDS   See *Acquired Immunodeficiency Syndrome*.

AIDS-Related Complex (ARC)   The intermediate clinical state following HIV exposure between asymptomatic infection and AIDS.

Alexin   An old term for *Complement*.

Allele   Alternative form(s) of a gene at a particular locus.

Allergen   A substance that causes an allergy (i.e., that stimulates IgE synthesis or causes a delayed hypersensitivity).

Allergy   An altered state of reactivity to an allergen (i.e., usually antigen or hapten). The term is used synonymously with *Hypersensitivity*.

Alloantibody   An antibody that reacts with an antigen from another animal of the *same* species.

Alloantigen   An antigen that is present in other members of one's own species.

Allogenic   Belonging to the same species, yet being of different genetic (and therefore antigenic) type.

Allograft   A tissue graft in which the donor and the recipient are the same individual (or are genetically identical).

Alloimmunization   The immunization of an individual with antigens from within the same species.

Allotype   Genetic variation within a species of the constant region of the heavy or light chain of an immunoglobulin molecule.

Alpha Heavy Chain Disease   The most common heavy chain disease characterized by an infiltration of lymphoid and plasma cells into the small intestines. The disease is common in the Middle East.

Alpha$_1$-Antitrypsin   An acute phase protein that is a serine protease inhibitor.

Alpha$_2$-Macroglobulin   An acute phase protein that is a protease inhibitor.

Alpha-Fetoprotein (AFP)   An oncofetal protein normally produced by fetal liver. In adults, ele-

vated serum levels may indicate hepatoma, testicular teratoblastoma, or other inflammatory disease.

Alternative Complement Pathway   A system for activating complement beginning at C3 and not involving a serologic reaction.

Alveolar   The thin-walled chambers of the lungs that are referred to as pulmonary alveoli.

Amboceptor   Anti-sheep red blood cell antibody that causes hemolysis of sheep red cells in the presence of complement.

Amino Acid   Any one of a class of organic compounds containing the amino (NH_2) group and the carboxyl (COOH) group. Amino acids form the chief structure of proteins.

Amniocentesis   The removal of fluid from the amniotic sac.

Amplification   The generation of C3b in the classical or alternative pathway of complement activation, to provide a feedback loop to increase the activation of C3 through C9 components.

Amyloidosis   A condition of intercellular deposition of an abnormal protein with a waxy, translucent appearance in various tissues.

Anamnestic Response   A rapid rise in immunoglobulin concentration following a second or subsequent exposure to antigen. Also known as a "secondary" or "booster" response.

Anaphylactic Allergy   An allergy that is caused by IgE.

Anaphylactic Shock   A severe allergic reaction.

Anaphylactoid Reaction   A severe reaction to soluble constituents in donor plasma that produces edema.

Anaphylatoxin   Specific peptides from complement fractions 3 and 5 that release histamine from mast cells and basophils. (Note: Originally believed to be a substance that caused histamine release.)

Anaphylatoxin Inhibitor   An enzyme that destroys the biologic activity of C3a and C5a (complement components).

Anaphylaxis   An unexpected, detrimental reaction to a second exposure to antigen in which histamine, serotoxin, etc., are released by reaction of the antigen with IgE on the surface of mast cells.

Anergy   The ability to respond to an antigen (especially in the allergic sense).

Angioedema   Redness and swelling.

Anicteric   Without icterus or lacking a yellow discoloration of the skin and sclera.

Anomalies   Deviations from the normal.

Antenatal   Prior to birth.

Antibody   A globulin formed in response to exposure to an antigen; an immunoglobulin.

Antibody Affinity   See *Affinity.*

Antibody-Dependent Cell-Mediated Cytolysis (ADCC)   An effector mechanism in which cells coated with antibody react with the Fc receptors on lymphocytes to cause target cell damage.

Anti-Core Window   The period of time in which antigen cannot be detected in the circulating blood.

Antigen   A macromolecule that, when introduced into a foreign circulation, will induce the formation of immunoglobulins or sensitized cells that react specifically with that antigen.

Antigen-Antibody Complex   The union of antibody with a homologous antigen.

Antigen Competition   The failure of a mixture of antigens to stimulate as high a titered antiserum to one or more of the antigens, compared with when the antigens are administered independently.

Antigen Determinant Sites   Unique portions of the structure of an antigen that are responsible for its activity.

Antigen-Presenting Cells (APCs)   Accessory cells that present antigen to lymphocytes in conjunction with MHC class II molecules. APCs are required in the initial step of an immune response.

Antigen Valency   The number of antigenic determinants on an antigen.

Antigenic Determinant   The portion of the immunogen molecule that can bind with antibody.

Antigenicity   The ability of a substance to react with immune products.

Antiglobulin Test   A test used to determine the presence of a globulin using an antibody to that globulin.

Anti-Human Globulin   An antibody preparation that contains antibody to a range of globulins (polyspecific) or to a single globulin (monospecific) used to detect sensitized particles.

Antilymphocyte Globulin   A form of immune suppression in which serum contains antibodies directed against lymphocytes.

Antinuclear Antibody (ANA)   An autoimmune antibody directed against a component of the nucleus, commonly found in systemic lupus erythematosus.

Antiserum   A serum containing antibodies.

Antistreptolysin O (ASO)   An antibody produced against streptolysin O, a hemolysin produced by streptococci (particularly group A).

Antitoxin   An antibody (or antiserum) prepared in response to a toxin or toxoid.

Aplastic Anemia   A deficiency of blood cells (e.g., red cells) caused by the lack of cell production in the bone marrow.

APTT   Activated partial thromboplastin time.

ARC   See *AIDS-Related Complex.*

Arteriosclerosis   See *Atherosclerosis.*

Arthralgia   Pain in a joint.

Arthritis   Inflammation of a joint.

Arthropathy   Joint disease.

Arthus Reaction   A necrotic, dermal reaction caused by antigen-antibody precipitation, complement fixation, and neutrophilic inflammation in tissues of an animal inoculated intracutaneously with antigen.

Aseptic   The handling of materials or specimens without the introduction of extraneous microorganisms.

ASO   See *Antistreptolysin O.*

Asthma   A respiratory condition characterized by recurring attacks of difficult or painful breathing and wheezing caused by spasmodic constriction of the larger air passages to or within the lungs (i.e., the bronchi).

Astrocyte   A nerve cell characterized by fibrous or protoplasmic processes. Collectively known as macroglia or astroglia tissue.

Asymptomatic   Without symptoms.

Ataxia   Faulty or irregular muscular action or coordination.

Ataxia Telangiectasis   An autosomal recessive immunodeficiency characterized by variable humoral and cellular immune defects, as well as sinopulmonary infection and ataxia.

Atherosclerosis   A condition of loss of elasticity of the walls of the blood vessels (arteries). Also known as "arteriosclerosis."

Atopic Eczema   Inflammation of the skin, characterized by redness, itching, and weeping. Caused by an allergic reaction.

Atopy   A genetically determined hypersensitivity, usually referring to allergic patients who produce an abnormally large amount of specific IgE when exposed to small concentrations of antigen.

Atrophy   The wasting or lack of growth of tissues or organs.

Attenuation   Weakening the virulence of a pathogenic organism while retaining its viability.

Atypical (Reactive) Lymphocytes   In infectious mononucleosis, suppressor and cytotoxic T lymphocytes capable of recognizing and killing B lymphocytes infected with the Epstein-Barr virus.

Autoantibody   An antibody produced against a "self" antigen.

Autoantigen   A molecule that behaves as a "self" antigen.

Autocoupling Hapten   A hapten that can combine spontaneously with a carrier.

Autofluorescence   The natural fluorescence of a tissue or substrate.

Autograft   Tissue transplanted back to the original donor.

Autoimmune Hemolytic Anemia   A condition in which erythrocytes are destroyed by antibodies to "self" antigens.

Autoimmunity   A condition in which an immune response is stimulated by "self" antigens. The resulting antibodies then react with these self antigens in the same way as they do with foreign antigens, which may result in autoimmune disease.

Autologous   A synonym for "self."

Autonomic Nervous System   The branch of the nervous system that functions without conscious control.

Avascular Necrosis   The death of nonvascular cells or tissues.

Avidity   The tendency for multiple antibodies and multivalent antigens to combine; the cumulative binding strength of all antibody-epitope pairs.

Azathioprine   An immunosuppressive drug that prevents cell division by inhibiting purine metabolism and DNA proliferation.

Azidothymidine   See *AZT.*

AZT (Azidothymidine)   A purine analog that inhibits reverse transcriptase, thus preventing RNA from being converted to DNA. Used to treat HIV infection. Now known as Zidovudine.

B Cell   A lymphocyte from the bursa of Fabricius or that is of the immunoglobulin-forming type.

B Lymphocyte   See *B Cell.*

Bacteremia   An infection of the blood caused by bacterial microorganisms.

Bacteria   Large groups of unicellular microorganisms, existing morphologically as oval or spherical cells (cocci), rods (bacilli), spirals (spirilla), or comma-shaped organisms (vibrios).

Bacteriotropin   An immune opsonin that stimulates phagocytosis of a bacterium, other cell type, or particle.

Basophil   A blood granulocyte whose granules release histamine during anaphylactic reactions.

Becquerel (Bq)   A standardized unit of radioactivity that equals one disintegration per second.

Bence Jones Protein   An immunoglobulin L chain that is found in the urine or blood of patients with a myeloma.

Benign   Nonmalignant.

Beta Particles   Particles emitted from radioisotopes that can be negatively charged electrons (negatrons) or positively charged particles (positrons).

Bilirubin   A breakdown product of erythrocyte catabolism. If high levels of this substance accumulate in the circulation, it will be deposited in lipid-rich tissue (e.g., the brain) and will be manifested by the skin and sclera as jaundice or icterus.

Blast Transformation   The conversion of a B lymphocyte into a plasma cell.

Blastogenic Factor   A lymphokine that stimulates T cell growth.

Blocking Antibody   An antibody that prevents (blocks) the action of another antibody.

Blood Group Antigen   Antigens that are genetically determined and present on the surface of the erythrocytes.

Boivin Antigen   A heat-stable antigen that is extractable from gram-negative bacteria. It can, for the most part, be considered synonymous with "endotoxin."

Bone Marrow   The structure that contains blood-forming (hematopoietic) tissues.

Booster Response   See *Anamnestic Response.*

Bruton's X-Linked Aggammaglobulinemia   A congenital X-linked defect in which B cells fail to mature and secrete immunoglobulin.

Buffer   Any substance(s) in solution that resists changes in pH.

Burkitt's Lymphoma   A undifferentiated malignant neoplasm of B lymphocytes associated with

Epstein-Barr virus infection and found primarily in children in restricted areas of Africa and in New Guinea.

Bursa of Fabricius   A cloacal organ in fowl from which the immunoglobulin-synthesizing B lymphocytes originate.

C-Reactive Protein   An acute-phase protein produced by the liver in early inflammatory response, which is capable of precipitating the C-polysaccharide extract of pneumococcus.

C1 Esterase   An esterase that is formed subsequent to the activation of the C1s component of complement.

Cachectin   A monokine that mediates inflammation (identical to tumor necrosis factor).

CALLA (Common Acute Lymphoblastic Leukemia Antigen)   A 100-kd glycoprotein (CD10) that serves as a useful marker since it is present in 75 per cent of non-T, non-B acute lymphoblastic leukemia and 40 per cent of lymphoblastic lymphoma.

Capping Phenomenon   The movement of antigens on the surface of B lymphocytes to a single position (or locus).

Carcinoembryonic Antigen   A glycoprotein normally synthesized, secreted, and excreted by the gastrointestinal tract. It can be detected in serum in disorders of the gastrointestinal tract.

Carrier   A molecule that, when coupled to a hapten, renders the hapten immunogenic.

Carrier State   The asymptomatic condition of harboring an infectious organism. The term may also refer to a carrier of a recessive gene (i.e., an individual who is heterozygous for a particular gene).

Catecholamines   Biologically active amines (including epinephrine and norepinephrine) that have a marked effect on the nervous and cardiovascular systems, metabolic rate and temperature, and smooth muscle.

CD4   The protein receptor on the surface of a target cell to which the gp120 protein of the HIV viral envelope binds.

Cell-Mediated Immunity   Immunity that is dependent on T lymphocytes and phagocytic cells.

Cellulitis   Inflammation within solid tissues (usually loose tissues beneath the skin) that is manifested by redness, pain, swelling, and interference with function.

Central Lymphoid Tissue   Bone marrow, thymus, and bursa of Fabricius.

Cerebrospinal Fluid (CSF)   The fluid formed by the choroid plexus in the ventricles of the brain and found within the subarachnoid space, the central canal of the spinal cord, and the four ventricles of the brain.

Cerebrovascular Accident   A stroke.

Ceruloplasmin   An acute phase protein that is the principle copper-transporting protein in human plasma.

Chédiak-Higashi Syndrome   A rare inherited autosomal recessive trait characterized by the presence of large granules and inclusion bodies in the cytoplasm of leukocytes.

Chemotaxis   Attraction of leukocytes or other cells by chemicals; with respect to white blood cells, the term can be used synonymously with "leukotaxin."

Cholestasis   The blockage or suppression of the flow of bile.

Chorioretinitis   Inflammation of the choroid and retina of the eye.

Chronic   A condition of long duration.

Circulating Immune Complex   An antigen-antibody complex in the circulation.

Classic Complement Pathway   The major system of complement activation that involves all nine components of complement and is initiated by a serologic reaction.

Coalesce   The fusion of components.

Cold Agglutinin   An agglutinin or hemagglutinin that is active at 4°C but not at 37°C.

Collagen   A protein found in the skin, tendons, bone, and cartilage.

Collagen Disease   Diseases of the skin, tendons, bone, and cartilage (e.g., SLE and RA).

Combining Site   The portion of the Fab fragment that possesses specificity.

Common Immunocyte   Any cell of the lymphoid series that can react with an antigen to produce an antibody or participate in cell-mediated reactions.

Common Thymocyte   Lymphocytes that arise in the thymus and precede mature thymocytes in development.

Competitive Radioimmunosorbent Test   A competitive RIA to detect total IgE.

Complement   A humoral mechanism of nonspecific immune response consisting of at least 14 components that proceed in a cascading sequence of activation, resulting in cell lysis.

Complement Cascade The sequence of activation of plasma proteins that cause lysis of a cell.

Complement Fixation The fixation (or binding) of complement in a reaction with antigen and antibody.

Complementoid An "altered" type of complement (usually partly damaged, e.g., by heating) that is capable of combining with sensitized cells without producing the usual lysis and that is also capable of blocking the normal action of complement.

Con A (Abbr) Concanavalin A.

Concanavalin A A mitogen highly specific for T lymphocytes.

Congenital Rubella Syndrome The passage of rubella virus across the placenta from mother to fetus, possibly resulting in heart disease, cataracts, and neurosensory deafness.

Congenital Syphilis The transfer of *Treponema pallidum* across the placenta, which can result in late abortion, stillbirth, neonatal disease, or latent infection.

Conglutinin A protein that is normally present in bovine serum that reacts with the C3 component of complement.

Conjugate A laboratory substrate prepared by joining two substances together.

Constant Domain The region in an immunoglobulin whose amino acid sequence is identical to the sequence in another region.

Contact Sensitivity Systemic sensitization caused by direct skin contact in which a second encounter with the same antigen results in epidermal inflammation.

Coombs' Test The original term that refers to the antiglobulin test.

Corticosteroid Any of the hormones produced by the outer layer of the adrenal gland, located on top of each kidney.

Counterimmunoelectrophoresis The electrophoresis of antigen and antibody toward one another through a gel medium.

CREST A mild form of scleroderma manifested by calcinosis, Raynaud's phenomenon, esophageal dismotility, sclerodactyly, and telangiectases. The name is formed from the first letters of each of these manifestations.

Cross-Reactive Antigen An antigen so structurally similar to a second antigen that it will react with antibody to the second antigen.

Cryoglobulin Globulin that precipitates from serum at 0° to 4°C.

Curie The traditional unit of radioactivity.

Cutaneous Referring to the skin (epidermis).

Cutaneous Lymphoma A malignant disease characterized by malignant T lymphocytes in the skin.

Cyclosporin An immunosuppressive drug used in transplantation that inhibits Interleukin-2 production and secretion, suppresses helper T-cell activity, and reduces cellular and humoral immunity.

Cytokines Protein molecules secreted by leukocytes that transmit messages to regulate cell growth and differentiation.

Cytomegalovirus A member of the herpes virus family that can cause congenital infections in newborns and a clinical syndrome that resembles infectious mononucleosis.

Cytopenic A severe decrease in hematologic cells.

Cytotoxic T Cells A subpopulation of T lymphocytes that destroy cells by direct cell-to-cell interaction without the presence of antibody.

Cytotoxicity Cell destruction.

Dane Particle A complete hepatitis B virion.

DAT See *Direct Antiglobulin Test*.

Davidsohn Differential Test A hemagglutination test that defines the characteristics of heterophil antibody by guinea pig and beef cell antigens.

Delayed Hypersensitivity Type IV hypersensitivity mediated by lymphokines released from sensitized T lymphocytes.

Delta Agent An RNA virus that causes hepatitis but requires the coexistence of hepatitis B infection.

Dendritic Cells The weakly phagocytic Langerhans cell of the epidermis and similar nonphagocytic cells in the lymphoid follicles of the spleen and lymph nodes, which may be the main agent of T-cell stimulation. The precise region of these cells is unclear.

Density Gradient Centrifugation The most common procedure for the separation of mononuclear cells.

Deoxyribonucleic Acid (DNA) The nuclear acid that forms the main structure of the genes.

Dermatomyositis An inflammatory condition that involves the skin, subcutaneous tissues, and muscles. It is one of the collagen disorders. Necrosis of the muscles is common.

Diapedesis The emigration of cells through a blood vessel well to enter an adjacent tissue.

DIC See *Disseminated Intravascular Coagulation.*

Direct Agglutination An agglutination reaction that occurs through the direct combination of antigen and antibody.

Direct Antiglobulin Test An agglutination procedure that detects *in vivo* sensitization of red cells.

Direct Immunofluorescence An immunofluorescence technique in which an antibody labeled with a fluorochrome reacts with a tissue, cell, or microbial test antigen.

Discoid Lupus The term used to distinguish the benign dermatitis of cutaneous lupus from the cutaneous involvement of SLE.

Disorder An abnormality of body function.

Disseminated Intravascular Coagulation A secondary pathophysiologic state in which coagulation proteins and platelets are consumed in the microcirculation, causing bleeding tendencies. The activated coagulation enzymes also catabolize C3, reducing its serum concentration.

Disulfide Bonds The links between antibody molecule chains.

DNA See *Deoxyribonucleic Acid.*

DNA Amplification An ultrasensitive polymerase chain reaction technique for the detection of HIV-1 that amplifies minute amounts of viral nucleic acid in the DNA of lymphocytes.

Domain A section or region in the peptide chain of an immunoglobulin.

Dysplastic Faulty or abnormal development of body tissue.

Dyspnea Difficulty in breathing.

Dysproteinemia An abnormality of the protein content of the blood.

Early Antigen A "new" antigen expressed by B lymphocytes infected with Epstein-Barr virus in infectious mononucleosis.

Eczema An inflammatory condition of the skin.

Edema Fluid accumulation in the tissues that produces swelling.

Electrophoresis (of serum) The separation of serum proteins according to their rate of travel when an electric current is passed through a buffer solution. The supporting medium can be Whatman paper, starch, or agar gels.

Electrostatic Force The attraction of a positively charged portion of a molecule for a negatively charged portion of a molecule.

Eluate The product of a laboratory separation of an antigen-antibody complex that contains the separated antibody.

Endemic Present at all times.

Endocarditis Inflammation of the inner lining of the heart.

Endodermal Pertaining to the inner layer of a tissue.

Endothelial Cell An epithelial cell that lines body cavities (e.g., the serous cavities, the heart and blood, and lymphatic vessels).

Endotoxemia A condition of having bacterial cell wall heat-stable toxins in the circulation. These toxins are pyrogenic and increase capillary permeability.

Enterocolitis Inflammation of the small intestine and colon.

ENV Gene A gene of a retrovirus that encodes for a polyprotein and contains numerous glycosylation sites.

Enzyme Immunoassay A ligand assay in which the label is an enzyme and the binding reagent is an antibody.

Enzyme-Linked Immunosorbent Assay (ELISA) A serologic test in which one of the reagents is labeled with an enzyme.

Eosinophil A white blood cell that contains cytoplasmic granules with an affinity for acid dyes (also referred to as an "acidophil").

Eosinophilia An increased number of eosinophils in the peripheral blood.

Eosinophilic Chemotactic Factor (ECF) A preformed mediator released from the mast cell during an allergic response that is responsible for attracting eosinophils to the site of activated mast cells.

Epidemiology The study of infectious diseases or conditions in many individuals in the same geographic location at the same time.

Epithelial Cell Skin cell.

Epithelioid Cell Macrophage-derived cell typically found at sites of chronic inflammation.

Epitope An antigenic determinant.

Epstein-Barr Virus A double-stranded enveloped virus belonging to the Herpetoviridae family that is capable of transforming B lymphocytes and then becoming self-perpetuating.

Equivalence Point   The point of dilution in a serologic reaction in which all the antigen and all the antibody are mutually involved in complexes.

Erythema   Redness of the skin caused by inflammation, infection, or injury.

Erythematous   Characterized by erythema.

Erythrocyte   A red cell.

Erythropoiesis   The process of red cell production.

Estrogen   Female sex hormones (estradiol, estriol, and estrone).

Etiology   The study of the causes of a disease.

Extramedullary Hematopoiesis   Erythrocyte production outside of the bone marrow.

Extravascular Destruction   Erythrocyte destruction through phagocytosis and digestion by macrophages of the mononuclear-phagocyte system.

Extrinsic Allergic Alveolitis   See *Hypersensitive Pneumonitis.*

Fab Fragment   The fragment of an antibody molecule that is capable of antigen binding. It consists of a light chain and part of a heavy chain of the molecule.

F(ab')₂   The fragment of an immunoglobulin molecule generated by pepsin cleavage, consisting of two antigen-combining sites joined by disulfide bonds.

Fc Fragment   The fragment of the antibody molecule that, in certain species, can be crystallized. It consists of two pieces of heavy chain.

Fd Fragment   The fragment of the antibody molecule consisting of a light chain and half of a heavy chain.

Febrile Agglutinins   Antibodies produced to bacterial infection in which fever is a prominent feature.

Febrile Disease   A disease characterized by high fever.

Fibroblast   An immature fiber-producing cell of connective tissue.

Fimbriae   Fringed or fingerlike structures.

Flocculation   A specific type of precipitation that occurs over a narrow range of antigen concentration; aggregation of colloidal particles in a serologic reaction (as in syphilis serology).

Flow Cytometry   A method in which a large number of cells pass through an aperture where they are exposed to light or electric current to generate a signal that is measured. The technique is used to detect cell surface markers, cell size, and cell volume.

Fluid Phase Diffusion   A technique in which soluble antigen is layered on top of soluble antibody in a capillary tube and each diffuses toward the other until antibody-antigen complex and precipitate are formed at the interface.

Fluorescence   A form of luminescence in which a molecule absorbs light energy of one wavelength and emits light energy of a lower wavelength in less than 10^{-4} seconds.

Fluorescent Antibody   An antibody (immunoglobulin) that is conjugated to a fluorescent dye for use in ultraviolet microscopy.

Fluorescent Microscope   A modified darkfield microscope that separates excitation wavelengths from emission wavelengths.

Fluorochrome   An organic compound that fluoresces when exposed to short wavelengths of light and that is used to label an antibody so that it can be visualized.

Forbidden Clone Theory   One of the theories used to explain autoimmunity. The theory states that during fetal development those lymphocyte clones that are capable of reacting to self are eliminated.

Forssman Antibody   A heterophil antibody that is stimulated by one antigen and reacts with unrelated surface antigen present on cells from different mammalian species.

Franklin's Disease   Gamma heavy chain disease characterized by the presence of monoclonal protein composed of the heavy chain portion of the antibody molecule.

Fulminant   Occurring very rapidly.

Functional Deletion   A proposed mechanism of immune tolerance in which T-helper cells are absent and therefore cannot help to produce an immune response to T-dependent antigens. This occurs with high concentrations of the antigen.

Gag Gene   A gene of a retrovirus that encodes for the major core structural protein.

GALT   See *Gut-Associated Lymphoid Tissue.*

Gamma Emission   A portion of the electromagnetic radiation spectrum that consists of very short wavelengths originating from an unstable nucleus.

Gamma Heavy Chain Disease   See *Franklin's Disease.*

Gammopathy   An imbalance in immunoglobulin concentration.

Gastroenteritis Inflammation of the lining of the stomach and intestine.

Gestation The period of development and growth of the unborn in viviparous animals.

Giant Cell See *Epithelioid Cell.*

Glial Cell The non-nervous or supportive tissue of the brain and spinal cord.

Globulin A class of proteins to which antibodies belong. They can be separated by electrophoresis into alpha, beta, and gamma fractions.

Glomerulonephritis See *Acute Glomerulonephritis.*

Glomerulus The small structure in the malpighian body of the kidney, composed of a cluster of capillary blood vessels enveloped in a thin wall.

Gm Group An allotypic group based on antigenic changes in H chain antigens of IgG.

Graft-Versus-Host Reaction A reaction resulting from the attack of immunocompetent tissue in a graft against an immunologically compromised host.

Grafting The transfer of cells or organs from one individual to another or from one site to another in the same individual.

Granulocyte A collective term for white blood cells with pronounced cytoplasmic granulation.

Granulocytic Macrophage Colony Stimulating Factor A lymphokine that induces the growth of hematopoietic cells that are committed to become granulocytes or macrophages.

Granuloma A macrophage-derived lesion containing sequestered noxious agents that cannot be eliminated.

Granulomatous Hypersensitivity A cellular reaction that results when microorganisms persist within macrophages.

Granulomatous Lesion A wound composed of granuloma.

Graves' Disease An autoimmune disease of the thyroid in which an antibody to the thyrotropin receptor (thyroid stimulating hormone receptor) stimulates the thyroid.

Guillain-Barré Syndrome A disease of the nerves. Also known as acute idiopathic polyneuritis.

Gummas Lesions commonly seen in tertiary syphilis.

Gut-Associated Lymphoid Tissue Tissue that, with the bone marrow, may play a role in the differentiation of stem cells into B lymphocytes. It functions as the bursal equivalent in humans.

H-2 The major histocompatibility antigen system of mice.

H Antigen The flagella antigens of bacteria.

H Chain (Abbr) The heavy chain of an immunoglobulin. Two such heavy chains exist in the basic four-peptide structure of an immunoglobulin.

H Substance An antigen on human red cells that acts as a precursor for the A and B antigens.

Half-Life The time taken to decrease to half the original value.

Haplotype One half of the histocompatibility genes that are present on one chromosome and are inherited from one parent.

Hapten A nonantigenic material that, when combined with an antigen, conveys a new antigenic specificity on the antigen.

Haptoglobin An acute phase protein that binds irreversibly to free hemoglobin to form a complex that is rapidly cleared from the circulation.

Hashimoto's Thyroiditis An autoimmune thyroid disease characterized by a chronic lymphocytic infiltrate.

HDN (Abbr) See *Hemolytic Disease of the Newborn.*

Heavy Chain See *H Chain.*

Heavy Chain Disease A rare lymphoproliferative disorder characterized by the presence of free heavy chain fragments without light chains.

Helper Cell A subclass of T cells that assists B cells in antibody formation.

Hemagglutination The agglutination (or clumping) of red blood cells, especially by antiserum.

Hemagglutination Inhibition Technique The technique used for the detection of antibodies, which involves the blocking of agglutination of erythrocytes.

Hematopoiesis The production of blood.

Hemolysin An antibody that, in cooperation with serum complement, will cause the hemolysis of erythrocytes.

Hemolysis The lysis of red blood cells by specific antibody and serum complement.

Hemolytic Anemia A disease in circulating erythrocytes caused by the rupture of these cells.

Hemolytic Disease of the Newborn (HDN) A disease of the newborn in which maternal antibodies cross the placenta and contribute to the destruction of fetal red cells.

Hemolyzed Ruptured erythrocytes.

Hemostatic Stoppage of bleeding.

Hepatitis Inflammation of the liver caused by a virus or other agent (e.g., drugs).

Hepatomegaly Enlargement of the liver.

Hepatosplenomegaly Enlarged liver and spleen.

Herpes Virus Any of a group of DNA viruses that cause herpes.

Heterodimer A molecule composed of two unrelated units.

Heterogenous Different. Not originating in the body.

Heteroimmunization The immunization of an individual with antigens from another species.

Heterophil Antibody An antibody produced in response to one antigen that will react with a second, genetically unrelated, antigen. Sometimes spelled "heterophile."

Heterophil Antigen An antigen that is broadly distributed in nature.

Hinge Region The region of the H chain of an immunoglobulin near where the L chain joins it and near the sites of papain and pepsin cleavage. It allows the immunoglobulin to have flexibility.

Histamine A specific chemical compound that is released from mast cells and produces vasodilation, smooth muscle contraction, and edema during anaphylaxis.

Histiocytes Macrophages that are fixed in various tissues and are actively involved in phagocytosis.

Histocompatibility Antigen The antigen on a cell surface that, upon transplantation into a different host, induces a response that leads to graft rejection. Also known as transplant antigen.

Histone A protein found in combination with acidic substances such as nucleic acids.

HIV See *Human Immunodeficiency Virus.*

HLA (Abbr) Human leukocyte antigen. The major histocompatibility antigen system in humans.

Hodgkin's Disease A lymphoma characterized by binucleated Reed-Sternberg cells.

Homogenous The same.

Homology The degree of sameness.

Horror Autotoxicus A term used to describe the inability of an antigen to serve as an autoantigen.

Human Immunodeficiency Virus (HIV) A virus that is causative for AIDS.

Humoral Any fluid or semifluid in the body.

Humoral Immunity Immunity that results from the formation of antibody.

Hutchinsonian Triad The characteristic manifestations of congenital syphilis (notched teeth, interstitial keratitis, and nerve deafness).

Hyaluronidase An enzyme produced by group A β-hemolytic streptococci.

Hybridoma Cell lines created *in vitro* by fusing two different cell types (usually a lymphocyte or plasma cell), one of which is a tumor cell.

Hydrogen Bonding The attraction of two negatively charged atoms for the positively charged hydrogen ion to create a weak bond.

Hydrophilic Water-loving.

Hydrophobic Water-hating.

Hydrophobic Force The attraction between nonpolar groups in an aqueous environment.

Hyperemia An increased flow of blood into the affected area following injury.

Hypergammaglobulinemia Increase in the gamma globulin fraction of plasma protein.

Hypersensitive Pneumonitis A type III hypersensitivity reaction in which inhaled antigens combine with preexisting antibody to initiate inflammation. Also known as extrinsic allergic alveolitis.

Hypersensitivity An unexpected, exaggerated reaction to an antigen. The term is used synonymously with *Allergy.*

Hyperviscosity Increased thickness of substances (e.g., plasma).

Hyperviscosity Syndrome The symptoms resulting from hyperviscosity.

Hypervolemia An increase of total blood volume.

Hypogammaglobulinemia Decreased levels of gamma globulin in plasma.

Hypoplastic Defective or incomplete development of a tissue or organ.

Icteric Pertaining to jaundice.

Idiopathic A disorder or disease of unknown cause.

Idiotopes Antigenic determinants within the variable region of an immunoglobulin molecule.

Idiotype Network The interaction between one product of the immune system (e.g., an antibody) and another product of the immune system (e.g., a second antibody), resulting in the regulation of the production of immune molecules.

IFN (Abbr) See *Interferon.*

Ig Short form for *Immunoglobulin.*

IgA An immunoglobulin that is predominant in secretions and the second most abundant in serum.

IgD An immunoglobulin that is the most abundant on the surface of B lymphocytes and the least abundant in serum.

IgE The homocytotropic antibody that binds to mast cells and is responsible for allergic responses.

IgG The most abundant immunoglobulin in serum; it is predominant in immunity against bacteria and viruses and is the only immunoglobulin to cross the placenta.

IgM An immunoglobulin that is usually produced first in response to antigen challenge. It is the third most abundant in serum.

IL-1 (Abbr) See *Interleukin 1*.

IL-2 (Abbr) See *Interleukin 2*.

Immature B Cell The receptor cell that is finally programmed for insertion of specific IgM molecules into the plasma membrane.

Immediate Hypersensitivity Allergy that is related to IgE or to similar immunoglobulins in lower species (e.g., hay fever, food allergies, certain drug allergies, and other allergies of the intermediate type).

Immune-Associated Antigen An antigen present on B lymphocytes and macrophages and inherited with *Ir Genes* (short form is Ia antigen).

Immune Complex A complex of antigen with antibody (which may involve complement) that can be soluble or can deposit in tissues.

Immune Deficiency Disease A condition in which a defect exists in the ability to detect antigens and/or to produce antibodies against foreign antigens.

Immune Response Any reaction demonstrating specific antibody response to antigenic stimulus.

Immune Response Gene A structural gene in the *Major Histocompatibility Complex* that exerts a regulatory role on the immune response.

Immune Status The measurement of specific antibody to determine if an individual is resistant or susceptible to an infection.

Immune Suppression The suppression of an immunologic response by chemical, physical, or biologic means.

Immune Surveillance Theory The immune response of healthy individuals that eliminates malignant or potentially malignant cells, thereby preventing tumor growth.

Immune System The structures, cells, and soluble constituents that allow the host to recognize and respond to foreign stimulus.

Immune Tolerance The state of being unresponsive to an immunogen.

Immunity The condition of resistance to infection.

Immunization The process by which an antibody is produced in response to antigenic stimulus.

Immunoblast A cell intermediate between the lymphocyte and plasma cell.

Immunocompetence The ability to mount an immune response.

Immunoconglutinin An antibody directed against the antigenic sites of the C3 component of complement that is revealed or created by antigen-antibody fixing of complement.

Immunocyte A cell that is capable of synthesizing immunoglobulin.

Immunodeficiency A dysfunction in blood defense mechanism.

Immunodiffusion A laboratory method for the quantitative study of antibodies.

Immunodominant Region The most potent epitope (antigenic determinant) in an antigen.

Immunofluorescent Assay (IFA) A laboratory method that employs a fluorescent substance in immunologic studies.

Immunogen Antigen.

Immunogenicity The ability of an antigen to produce an immune response.

Immunoglobulin Antibody.

Immunologic Deficiency Theory A theory of autoimmunity that states that a defect in immune regulation is responsible for autoimmunity.

Immunologic Tolerance A failure (or depression) in the immune response on proper exposure to antigen (especially massive doses). Also sometimes known as immune paralysis.

Immunosuppression Reduced activity of T and B lymphocytes and macrophages, including decreased antibody and cytokine production.

Immunosuppressive Agent A drug, chemical, or other mechanism that prevents the immune system from recognizing and responding to foreign stimulus.

Immunotherapy Treatment designed to manipulate the immune system in order to make it more efficient against disease and malignancy.

Impetigo A skin condition caused by streptococci.

Inducer Cell A T-cell subset that causes the maturation of active T-cell subpopulations.

Infarction An area of tissue (e.g., the heart muscle) that undergoes necrosis because of lack of oxygen from the circulating blood. Oxygen deprivation may be caused by narrowing of the blood vessels (stenosis) or a blockage of the blood circulation in the vessel (occlusion).

Infection A pathogenic condition caused by microorganisms.

Infectious Mononucleosis A benign lymphoproliferative disorder.

Inflammation Tissue reaction (redness, tenderness, pain, swelling) to injury by physical or chemical agents, including microorganisms.

Inherited Immunity Immunity resulting from genetic factors (i.e., genetic constitution), not the result of exposure to infectious agents.

Inhibition The prevention of a normal reaction between an antigen and its corresponding antibody, usually because an antigen of the same specificity but from another source is present in the serum.

Innate Immunity Immunity present at birth in all individuals.

Innocent Bystander Cells Cells that may be destroyed through an immune event that is directed against different cells.

In Situ **Hybridization** A laboratory technique for demonstrating the presence of HIV-1 in lymphocytes in primary lymph nodes and peripheral blood from AIDS patients.

Interferon Protein(s) released from a cell that is infected with an intracellular parasite, which protects neighboring cells from invasion by the same or other intracellular parasites.

Interleukin (IL) A monokine that acts on other leukocytes.

Interleukin 1 (IL-1) A monokine that activates T cells and possibly B cells.

Interleukin 2 (IL-2) A monokine that serves as a growth factor for T cells.

Interleukin 3 (IL-3) A lymphokine that stimulates proliferation of cells in the bone marrow.

Interleukin 4 (IL-4) A lymphokine that stimulates proliferation of antigen-activated B cells and induces differentiation of proliferating B cells into antibody-secreting plasma cells. Also known as B-cell growth factor.

Interstitial Pneumonitis An inflammation situated between or in the interspaces of the lung tissue.

Intrarenal Obstruction Obstruction (blockage) in the kidney.

Intrauterine Within the uterus.

Intravascular Coagulation Clot formation within the blood vessels of the circulatory system.

Intravascular Destruction The destruction of red cells within the vessels.

Intravascular Hemolysis The lysis of cells in the vessels of the circulatory system.

Intrinsic Coagulation Mechanism The initial stage of blood coagulation that can be activated by antigen-antibody complexes.

Intrinsic Factor (IF) A substance secreted by the parietal cells of the mucosa in the fundus region of the stomach.

In Vitro Outside the body.

In Vivo Inside the body.

Ir Gene An immune response gene.

Isoantigen An antigen present in another member of one's own species. Also known as *Alloantigen*.

Isoelectric Focusing Separation of molecules on the basis of their charge. Each molecule migrates to the point in a pH gradient where it has no net charge.

Isograft Transplanted tissue between genetically identical individuals.

Isohemagglutinin An antibody of an animal that will agglutinate the red cells of another animal of the same species. Also referred to as isoagglutinin.

Isoimmune Possessing antibodies to antigens of the same system.

Isoimmunization Immunization of an individual with antigens of another individual of the same species.

Isotype A synonym of class (when referring to immunoglobulins).

Isotypic Variant The heavy chain constant region structure associated with the different classes and subclasses of immunoglobulin molecules. Isotypic variants are present in all healthy members of a species.

J Chain A polypeptide chain found attached to a secretory IgA and IgM that may function as a joining chain.

Jaundice The symptom characterized by yellow coloration of the skin and sclera, associated with bilirubinemia, and often seen in hepatitis.

Kahler's Disease Multiple myeloma.

Kaposi's Sarcoma A malignant, metastasizing disorder that primarily affects the skin, frequently observed in AIDS patients.

Kinin A small, biologically active peptide.

Kinin System   A series of serum peptides that are sequentially activated to cause vasodilation and increased vascular permeability.

Kleihauer-Betke Test   A test method used to differentiate between adult and fetal hemoglobin.

Kupffer's Cell   A macrophage of the liver.

L Chain   (Abbr)   The light chain of an immunoglobulin. Two such chains exist in the four-peptide unit of an immunoglobulin.

Lag Period   The period of time between stimulus and reaction.

Laked   Hemolyzed.

Langerhans' Cells   Stellate, dendritic cells found in the stratum spinosum of the skin (epidermis).

Latency   The stage of syphilis characterized by a lack of signs and symptoms, but with positive serologic tests.

Latent   Inactive.

Latent Infection   Persistent infections characterized by periods of reactivation and periods of latency.

Lattice Formation   Crosslinks between sensitized particles.

LC   (Abbr)   See *Langerhans' Cells.*

Lectin   An extract from seeds that possesses the ability to agglutinate red cells (usually directed against a specific antigen).

Leukemia   The malignant proliferation of white blood cells originating in the bone marrow with a peripheral blood phase.

Leukocyte   A white cell.

Leukocytosis   An increase in the total circulating white cell concentration.

Leukopenia   A decrease in the total circulating white blood cell concentration.

Ligand   A molecule that combines with specific complementary configurations of the binding agent (e.g., receptors, proteins, or antibody).

Light Chain   See *L Chain.*

Light Chain Disease (LCD)   A dysproteinemia of the monoclonal gammopathy type in which only kappa or lambda monoclonal light chains or Bence Jones proteins are produced.

Liposome   A particle of fat-like substance held in suspension in tissues.

Localized   Within a specific area.

Locus   The position on a chromosome occupied by a gene.

LPS   (Abbr)   Lipopolysaccharide, the endotoxic portion of the cell wall of most gram-negative bacteria; mitogenic for B lymphocytes.

Lymph Node   An encapsulated collection of lymphocytes and antigen-presenting cells that is a site of antigen interaction, lymphocyte recirculation, and lymphocyte proliferation.

Lymphadenopathy   Enlarged lymph nodes.

Lymphoblast   The most immature stage of a lymphocyte.

Lymphocyte   The agranular leukocyte with sparse cytoplasm and round nucleus derived from the thymus (T type) or bone marrow or bursa (B type) found in lymph, lymph nodes, blood, spleen, etc.

Lymphocyte Recirculation   The process that enables lymphocytes to come in contact with processed foreign antigen and to disseminate antigen-sensitized memory cells throughout the lymphoid system.

Lymphocyte Transformation   The active nucleic acid metabolism and nuclear enlargement of a lymphocyte on contact with antigen.

Lymphocytopenia   A severe decrease in the total number of peripheral blood lymphocytes.

Lymphocytosis   An increase in peripheral blood lymphocytes.

Lymphokine   A soluble protein mediator released by sensitized lymphocytes on contact with an antigen.

Lymphokine-Activated Killer Cell (LAK)   Cells that respond to IL-2, share many cell surface antigens with NK cells, and can lyse target cells.

Lymphoma   A malignant tumor of lymphoid tissue.

Lymphosarcoma   Malignant neoplastic disorders of the lymphoid tissues (excluding Hodgkin's disease).

Lymphotoxins   A family of lymphokines that are cytolytic for target cells.

Lyse   To break apart or dissolve.

Lysis   The irreversible leakage of cell contents following membrane damage.

Lysozyme   An enzyme found in secretions that kills an organism by disrupting the cell wall of bacteria.

Lyt Marker   An antigen marker on T lymphocytes.

M Antigens   Proteins in the cell wall of group A streptococci that determine the serotype and allow the bacterium to adhere to the host cell.

M Component   The serum protein produced in

excessive concentration in cases of myeloma or macroglobulinemia.

Macroglobulin A globulin (protein) with a high molecular weight.

Macrophage A tissue or blood phagocyte, 20 to 80 μm in diameter, containing lysosomes, vacuoles, and partially digested debris in its cytoplasm.

Macrophage Migration Inhibitory Factor (MIF) A lymphocyte product that is chemotactic for monocytes.

Macular Lesion An unraised, discolored spot on the skin.

Maculopapular A lesion that has both macular and papular characteristics.

Major Histocompatibility Complex (MHC) A collection of structural genes associated with transplantation antigens and the immune response.

Malaise A generalized feeling of discomfort.

Malignant Cancerous.

Manifestation The signs and symptoms of a disease or disorder.

Mast Cell A large tissue cell with basophilic granules containing vasoactive amines and heparin. These inflammatory mediations are released when the cell is damaged, which increases vascular permeability and allows complement and phagocytic cells to enter the damaged tissues from the circulating blood.

Mature B Cell A B cell that is concerned with synthesis of circulating antibodies.

Mediator Cell A cell that takes part in immunologic reactions by releasing biochemical substances.

Melanin The pigment that gives hair, eyes, and skin their color.

Melanocyte A cell that produces melanin that can occur abnormally in certain tumors and melanomas.

Memory Cell A cell that responds more quickly to the second exposure to antigen than to the primary exposure and is responsible for the anamnestic response.

Meningovascular Referring to the blood vessels of the covering of the brain and spinal cord.

Mesodermal Referring to the middle layer of a tissue between the ectoderm and the endoderm.

MHC (Abbr) See *Major Histocompatibility Complex.*

MHC Restriction The phenomenon of lympho-cyte activation only in the presence of an antigen and a specific class of MHC molecule.

Microglia The phagocytic cells of the brain.

MIF See *Macrophage Migration Inhibitory Factor.*

Mitogen A substance that stimulates mitosis.

Mitogenic Factor A substance produced by thymic macrophages that includes T-cell development.

Mixed Lymphocyte Culture (MLC) A laboratory technique commonly used to detect MHC class II molecules. It involves the transformation of lymphocytes through exposure to genetically dissimilar lymphocytes.

Monoclonal Antibody The transformation of one clone of B cells to produce one class of immunoglobulin with one specificity.

Monocyte A white blood cell, 12 to 30 μm in diameter, with rounded nucleus. A precursor to macrophages.

Monokine A protein elaborated by a monocyte or macrophage that acts on other host cells.

Mononuclear-Phagocyte System The system of body defenses composed of macrophages and a network of specialized cells of the spleen, thymus, and other lymphoid tissues. Originally known as the reticuloendothelial system (RES).

Monovalent An antigen with only one antigenic determinant.

Morbidity The ratio of sick to healthy persons, or the number of cases of a specific disease in a particular population. Also refers to the condition of being diseased.

Mortality The ratio or rate of death caused by a particular disease.

Multiple Myeloma See *Myeloma.*

Multipotential Stem Cells Precursor cells in the bone marrow that are capable of differentiating into various blood cell types.

Myalgia Pain (tenderness) in the muscle.

Mycoplasma A genus of organisms lacking a cell wall.

Myelitis Inflammation of the spinal cord or bone marrow.

Myeloma A plasma cell neoplasm resulting in excessive production of one or more immunoglobulins.

Myeloma Cell Plasma cell derived from malignant tumor strains.

Myelomatosis Multiple myeloma.

Myeloperoxidase An enzyme in lysosomes that aids intraphagocyte killing.

Myocarditis   An inflammation of the cardiac muscle tissue.

Myosin   One of the two main contractile proteins found in muscles.

Natural Killer Cell (NK Cell)   A population of effector lymphocytes that produces such mediators as interferon and interleukin 2. Formerly called a "null" cell.

Natural Resistance   See *Inherited Immunity.*

Necrosis   The death of cells or a localized group of cells.

Necrotizing Vasculitis   Inflammation of a vessel that results in the destruction of tissue.

Neoantigen   A "new" antigen formed by modification of an "old" antigen by haptenic addition or other means.

Neonate   An infant up to 4 weeks old.

Neoplasm   The growth of new, abnormal tissue (e.g., a tumor).

Neoplastic   Referring to new, abnormal tissue growth.

Nephelometry   A direct measurement of light scattered by particles suspended in solution.

Nephritis   Inflammation of the kidney.

Nephrosis   A condition affecting the kidney (particularly tubular degeneration) that has no accompanying signs or symptoms of inflammation.

Neurologic Sequelae   Morbid nervous system signs and symptoms that follow a disease or are caused by a disease.

Neutropenia   A decrease of neutrophils.

Neutrophil   A leukocyte with granules that are not predominant in their affinity for acid or basic dyes.

NK Cell   See *Natural Killer Cell.*

Nonicteric   See *Anicteric.*

Non-Self   Referring to materials (cells, organs, etc.) that are from a different animal or individual.

Nonsymptomatic   See *Asymptomatic.*

Normal Flora   Microorganisms that normally inhabit areas of the body (e.g., skin, mucous membranes, intestinal tract, etc.).

Nucleocapsid   A virion without a capsule.

Null Cell   See *Natural Killer Cell.*

O Antigen   The surface somatic antigens of bacteria, or one of the antigens of the ABO blood group system.

Oncogenic   Associated with the formation of tumors.

Opportunistic Infection   A microbial disease that infects a debilitated host.

Opsonin   An antibody that attaches to a cellular or particular antigen and that "prepares" it for phagocytosis.

Opsonization   The process of coating an antigen with antibody to provide more effective phagocytosis.

Optimal Proportions   The point of dilution in a serologic reaction that gives a positive reaction.

Osteoclast   A giant, multinucleated cell formed in the bone marrow of growing bones, associated with reabsorption and removal of unwanted tissue.

Osteomyelitis   Inflammation of the bone or bone marrow.

Osteonecrosis   The accelerated destruction of bone tissue.

Otitis Media   Inflammation of the middle ear.

Papule   A small, solid, elevated lesion of the skin.

Paraproteinemia   The presence of protein molecules in plasma that are antigenically similar to, but lack the biologic activity of, normal molecules, especially regarding immunoglobulins.

Passive Hemagglutination   Hemagglutination resulting from antibodies that are directed against antigens adsorbed to their erythrocyte surface.

Passive Immunity   Immunity that results from contribution of protection (e.g., antibody) from one individual to another.

Passive Immunization   The acquisition of immunity through the injection of antibodies or antiserum produced by another animal.

Pathogen   A disease-causing microorganism or agent.

Pathogenesis   The origin of a disease.

Pathogenicity   The ability to cause disease.

Perinatal   Preceding, during, or after birth.

Peripheral Lymphoid Tissue   Lymphoid tissues other than bone marrow, thymus, and bursa.

Petechiae   Small purple hemorrhagic spots on the skin or mucous membranes.

Phagocyte   Any cell that is capable of engulfing or destroying foreign particles such as bacteria.

Phagocytosis   The engulfment of cells or particulate matter by leukocytes, macrophages, or other cells.

Phagosome   A membrane-bound vesicle in a phagocyte containing the phagocytosed material.

Pharynx The throat.

Phlebotomy The removal (withdrawal) of blood from a vein.

Phytohemagglutinin An extract of plants, usually legumes, that will agglutinate red cells.

Plasma The fluid component of blood.

Plasma Cell A cell 10 to 20 μm in diameter that can actively synthesize immunoglobulins and can be distinguished morphologically from similar cells.

Plasmin A proteolytic enzyme that is capable of dissolving formed fibrin clots.

Pluripotent Stem Cell A precursor cell that can differentiate into many different cell types.

PMN (Abbr) See *Polymorphonuclear Neutrophilic Leukocyte.*

Pneumocystis carinii A protozoa that causes interstitial plasma cell pneumonia. Frequently seen as an opportunistic pathogen in cases of AIDS.

Pol Gene A gene of a retrovirus that encodes for reverse transcriptase, endonuclease, and protease activities.

Polyarthritis Inflammation of several joints.

Polyclonal Antibody The increased production of different classes of immunoglobulins due to the transformation of many clones of B cells.

Polymorphism Multiple alleles at a single locus.

Polymorphonuclear Neutrophilic Leukocyte A white blood cell with a granular cytoplasm and a multilobed nucleus that is very active in phagocytosis.

Postnatal After birth.

Postzone The failure of a serologic reaction to occur in extreme dilutions of the antibody.

Precipitation The formation of an insoluble complex of antibody with soluble antigen.

Precursor Substance A substance in a stage of process that precedes a later development.

Prenatal Prior to birth.

Primary Immunodeficiency Dysfunction of an immune organ such as the thymus.

Primary Response The initial response to a foreign antigen.

Primed Immune cells that have been previously exposed to an antigen.

Prognosis A forecast of the probable outcome of a disease, disorder, or condition.

Prophylaxis Prevention or a preventive procedure.

Protein A A protein on the surface of *Staphylococcus aureus* that binds IgG.

Proteinuria Protein (albumin) in the urine.

Proteolytic Enzyme A substance that is able to break apart a protein molecule.

Prozone The failure of a serologic reaction to occur in high concentration of the antibody.

Pseudoagglutination The clumping of cells caused by agents other than antibodies.

Purpura An extensive area of red or dark purple discoloration of the skin.

Pyrogenic Microorganisms that cause the production of pus.

RA (Abbr) Rheumatoid arthritis.

Radioimmunoassay An immunologic test using radiolabeled antigen, antibody, complement, or other reactants.

Radioisotope An atom with an unstable nucleus that spontaneously emits radiation as it decays to a stable nucleus.

Raynaud's Phenomenon Pain in the extremities when exposed to cold temperatures.

Reagin IgE, with specificity for allergens, or syphilitic reagin, with specificity for cardiolipin antigens.

Receptor A cell surface molecule that binds specifically to particular proteins or peptides in the fluid phase.

Regimen A treatment schedule.

Relative Risk The degree of association between a particular HLA antigen and a disease.

Renal Referring to the kidneys.

RES (Abbr) See *Reticuloendothelial System.*

Reticulocyte A type of immature erythrocyte.

Reticuloendothelial Blockade Malfunction of phagocytic cells by prior exposure to phagocytosable particles.

Reticuloendothelial System An old term referring to the mononuclear phagocytic system.

Retinitis Inflammation of the retina of the eye.

Retrovirus An RNA virus that contains *reverse transcriptase*, which enables the virus to make DNA from viral RNA.

Reverse Transcriptase An enzyme found in the single positive-stranded RNA core of a retrovirus.

Rheumatoid Factor (RF) An IgM antibody with specificity towards IgG, which is associated with arthritis.

RIA (Abbr) See *Radioimmunoassay.*

Rubella Syndrome A number of congenital abnormalities (e.g., mental retardation) caused by the rubella virus.

SC (Abbr) See *Secretory Component*.

Secondary Immune Response The cellular and humoral events that occur when an antigen is encountered for a second or subsequent time.

Secondary Immunodeficiency See *Acquired Immunodeficiency*.

Secretory Component A portion of secretory IgA and secretory IgM not present in serum IgA or IgM and not produced in plasma cells. See *Anamnestic Response*.

Secretory Immunoglobulin An immunoglobulin found in colostrum, saliva, mucous secretions, etc., as secretory IgA, or secretory IgM.

Self-Limiting Able to be resolved with time.

Self-Tolerance The ability of the body not to respond to autologous antigens.

Senescence The process of growing old.

Sensitization The induction of an immune response. Also refers to the attachment of antibody to an antigen-coated particle without agglutination.

Sepsis Microbial infection throughout the systemic circulation.

Septicemia The presence of pathogenic microorganisms in the blood.

Sequela A disease caused by a previous disease.

Sequestered Antigen An antigen not found in the circulatory system.

Seroconversion The detection of specific antibody in the serum of an individual in whom the antibody was previously undetectable.

Serum The fluid portion of the blood after the blood clots.

Serum Sickness A reaction caused by the presence of antigen at the time antibody is being formed.

Shared Antigen A cross-reactive antigen (i.e., one that will react with an antibody induced by some other antigen).

Sialic Acid Found on erythrocyte membranes. It produces a negative surrounding charge.

Silent Carrier A disease carrier who has no signs or symptoms of disease.

SLE Systemic lupus erythematosus.

Solid Phase Radioimmunoassay A radioimmunoassay in which one of the reactants is bound to a surface.

Soluble Immune Response Suppressor A lymphokine that suppresses B cells.

Soluble Mediator A lymphokine.

Sor Gene A gene of a retrovirus, the product of which is a protein that induces antibody production in the natural course of infection.

Specificity The special affinity between an antigen and its corresponding antibody.

Spirochete A twisted or spiral bacterium.

Splenomegaly Enlargement of the spleen.

Stasis The complete stopping of blood flow during severe injury.

Streptokinase An enzyme that dissolves clots by converting plasminogen to plasmin.

Subclinical Infection An early or mild form of a disease that has no visible signs.

Substrate A substance upon which another substance (e.g., an enzyme) acts.

Supernatant Fluid above a solid portion.

Suppressor Cell A subclass of T cells that suppresses the capacity of B cells to become immunoglobulin producers.

Surface Immunoglobulin (SIg) The unique surface marker on B cells that is synthesized by the B cell, is expressed on its surface, and serves as the antigen receptor.

Surrogate Testing One test that is performed to indicate indirectly a second infectious or chemical antigen.

Susceptibility Having little resistance.

Symptom An indication of a disorder or disease, or a variation in normal body function.

Symptomatic A departure from normal function or appearance.

Syndrome A collection of symptoms that occur together.

Syngeneic Members of the same species that are genetically identical.

Systemic Throughout the body.

T-Cell-Dependent Antigen An antigen that requires the cooperation of T and B cells to induce specific antibody production.

T-Cell Growth Factor See *Interleukin 2*.

T-Cell-Independent Antigen An antigen that does not require the cooperation of T and B cells to induce specific antibody production.

T Lymphocyte (T Cell) A thymus-derived lymphocyte responsible for cell-mediated hypersensitivity.

Tachycardia An abnormally fast heart rate.

TGGF (Abbr) T-cell growth factor. See *Interleukin 2*.

Th Cell A T-helper cell.

Thrombocytopenia A deficiency of circulating blood platelets.

Thrombosis The formation of a blood clot or thrombus.

Thrombus A clot.

THY 1 Antigen An antigen found on T cells.

Thymosin A hormone-like substance from thymus believed to be the active component of T lymphocytes.

Thymus A gland located near the parathyroid and thyroid whose lymphocytes (T type) regulate cell-mediated hypersensitivity and interact with B cells for immunoglobulin formation.

Titer The greatest dilution of a substance used in a serologic reaction that will produce the desired result.

Tolerance A state of specific nonreactivity to an antigen due to prior exposure to the same antigen under special circumstances. In short, the failure to respond to antigenic stimulus.

Toxoid A toxin treated to preserve its native antigenicity but to eliminate its toxicity.

Trans Prefix meaning across, over, or through.

Ts Cell A T-suppressor cell.

Tumor Swelling; neoplasm.

Turbidimetry The measurement of light transmitted through a suspension of particles.

Ubiquitous Existing everywhere.

Urticaria Hives.

Vaccination The inoculation or ingestion of organisms or antigens to produce immunity to those organisms in the recipient.

Vaccine A suspension of living or dead organisms used as an antigen and injected into individuals as protection against disease.

Van der Waals Force A weak attractive force between the electron cloud of one atom and the nucleus of another atom.

Variable Domain A region in an immunoglobulin whose amino acid sequence is not constant from one molecule species to another.

Varicella Chickenpox.

Vasculitis A group of syndromes that have common clinicopathologic features associated with inflammation in vessel walls.

Venereal Route Disease transmission as a result of sexual activity.

Viral Hemagglutination The agglutination of red blood cells by a virus.

Viremia A systemic (blood) infection caused by a virus.

Virion A virus particle.

Virulence A microorganism's degree of pathogenicity or ability to cause disease.

Waldenström's Macroglobulinemia A myeloma involving IgM or IgM-like molecules.

Warm Agglutinin An antibody (agglutinin) or hemagglutinin that is active at 37° but not at 4°C.

Wassermann Test The first diagnostic test for syphilis. The test is no longer in use.

Witebsky's Postulates A set of conditions that must be met before a disease can be considered to be an autoimmune disease.

Xenoantigen An antigen present in another species.

Xenogeneic Referring to members of different species with different genetic backgrounds.

Xenograft The transplantation of tissue from a donor to a recipient of a different species.

Xenoimmunization The immunization of an individual with antigens from another species (also known as *Heteroimmunization*.

Zidovudine See *AZT.*

Index

Note: Page numbers in *italics* refer to illustrations; page numbers followed by t refer to tables.